EMERGENCY RADIOLOGY
Case Studies

EMERGENCY RADIOLOGY
Case Studies

David T. Schwartz, MD, FACEP

Associate Professor of Clinical Emergency Medicine
New York University School of Medicine
Bellevue Hospital and New York University Medical Center
New York, New York

McGraw-Hill
Medical Publishing Division

New York   Chicago   San Francisco   Lisbon   London   Madrid   Mexico City
Milan   New Delhi   San Juan   Seoul   Singapore   Sydney   Toronto

Emergency Radiology: Case Studies

1 2 3 4 5 6 7 8 9 0 DOCDOC 0 9 8 7

ISBN 978-0-07-140917-9
MHID 0-07-140917-3

This book was set in Times Roman by Aptara, Inc.
The editors were Robert Pancotti, Anne M. Sydor, and Peter J. Boyle.
The production supervisors were Phil Galea and Thomas Kowalczyk.
Production management was provided by Aptara, Inc.
R.R. Donnelley was printer and binder.

This book is printed on acid-free paper.

Cataloging-in-publication data is on file for this title at the Library of Congress.

Dedication

To the NYU/Bellevue Emergency Medicine Residents, past, present, and future. It has been a privilege and pleasure to have worked with the thoughtful and dedicated individuals listed below and to share in their development over the years, their enthusiasm for learning, and their devotion to the care of Emergency Department patients.

Ani Aydin
Nichole Bosson
Whitney Bryant
Louis Cooper
Kelly Doran
Hong Kim
Lauren Kornreich
Michael Madland
Colleen McCarthy
Bryce Meeker
Joshua Mincer
Langley Partridge
Michael Redlener
Teresa Smith
Michael Tocco

Rachel Alt
Brian Baker
Amy Caron
Alfred Cheng
Jimmy Choi
Marie-Laure Geffrard
Jeffrey Glassberg
Aaron Hultgren
Anh Nguyen
Ania Ringwelski
Paulina Sergot
Bradley Shy
Tara Sood-Raviprakash
Michael Van Meter
Chris Wang

Anika Baxter-Tam
Cappi Lay
Anand Swaminathan
Andrew Miner
Rern Lau
Meigra Chin
Taku Taira
Dimitrios Papanagnou
Michael Anana
William Paolo, Jr.
Diana Vo
Rohini Jonnalagadda
Corey Long
Neesha Desai
Kevin Tao
Anwar Al-Awadhi

Dainius Drukteinis
Brian Fletcher
Alice Kwan
Aaron Laskey
Inna Leybell
Greg Lopez
Gigi Madore
Tania Mariani
Jay Mueller
Jesse Rideout
Adam Rosh
Paul Testa
Sara Tuttle
Maria Vasilyadis

Emily Carrier
Turan Catanese-Saul
Nina Chicharoen
Whit Fisher
Jason Kahn
Christina Kirby
Faye Lee
Heather Mahoney
Jeanne Pae
Patricia Rivera
James Rodriguez
Jasper Schmidt
Boris Veysman
Christina Wainwright
Tina Wu

David Beneli
Jennifer Garner
Rajneesh Gulati
Jean Hammel
Edward Jarvis
Mana Kasongo
Stephen Kefalas
John Magnan
Christopher McStay
Benjamin Milligan
Lisa Nocera
Robin Polansky
Patrick Reinfried
Anna S. Shalkham
Silas Smith

Fareed Fareed
Jessica Fleischer-
  Black
Corita Gruzden
James Keating
Erica Kreismann
Felix Leshchinsky
Julie Mayglothling
Maria Raven
Steven Rosonke
Rahul Sharma
Craig Smollin
Michael Stern
Michael Waxman

Lisa Campanella
Amy Chuang
Moira Davenport
Alexis Halpern
Doodnauth Hiraman
Wendy Huang
Barbara Kirrane
Jay Lemery
Mike McGee
Ellie Paras
Rachel Pearl
Seema Rathi
Brian Wexler

Arman Afagh
Nicole Bouchard
Gar Ming Chan
Linda Park
Ian DeSouza
Joanna Garritano
Oren Hirsch
Craig Mochson
Pravene Nath
Linda Regan
Jeffrey Roger
James Sadock
Jessica Stetz
Denise Tyler
Sidney Williamson
Sigrid Wolfram

Rajeev Bais
Sharon Bajwa
Lisa Better
Elizabeth Borock
Antonio Davila
Carol Dersarkissian
Dawn Leighton
Phillip Levy
Nikej Shah
Oronde Smith
Jeremy Sperling

Lars Beattie
William Birdsong
James Burke
Leonico Dilone
Fiona Gallahue
Benjamin Greenblatt
Aaron Hexdall
David Jacobs
Charles Kwon
Lillian Oshva
Salvatore Pardo
Jason Zemmel D'Amore

James Bentler
Ginno Blancaflor
Jose Luis Cervantes
Christopher Cox
William Fernandez
Hossien Joukar
Christopher Lee
Eunhae Park
Stephen C. Pool
Christine Roland
Marc Simmons
Kareen Thompson-Holcomb
Juan Tovar

Nancy Camp
Michael Cetta
Richard Garri
Andrew Garvie
Michael Hockstein
Hanson Hsu
Mona Jaggi
Nancy Kwon
Charles Lawrence
Carol Lee
Olivia Lopez
Seth Manoach
Annabella Salvador
Jeremy Simon

Aaron Barber
Isabel Benavides
G. Richard Bruno
Robert Chang
Steven Heffer
Jason Kearney
Edward Lee
Waiho Lum
Kathryn Parker
Sean Rees
Gabriel Reyes
Susan Stone
Cleo Williams

Gavin Barr
Curt Dill
Jason Hack
Sandra Haynes
Mitchell Heller
Aileen Kennedy
Michael Lee
Karen Portale
Joseph Rella
Manju Rentala

Chris Amrick
Bruce Burstein
Melanie Cerinich
Min Cha
Phil Clement
Oliver Hung
Behdad Jamshahi
Matt Lurin
Eva Prakash
George Southiere

William Costello
Vanessa Price-Davis
Diane Giorgi
Lada Kokan
Ed Kuffner
David Lobel
Jeff Manko
Niall McGarvey
Antonio Mendez
Anthony Shallash

Adrienne Buffalo
Charles Cheng
Lisandro Irizarry
Elizabeth Israel
Mark Kindschuh
Jeff Levine
Rich Levitan
Doug Mailly
Erika Newton
Louisa Oakenell
Dan Sack
Paula Whiteman

CONTENTS

Patient ages are categorized as follows: young adult, 18-40 years;
middle-aged 41-65 years, elderly > 65 years

PREFACE

Working in the Emergency Department is a wonder. There is an extraordinary range of clinical problems to solve and opportunities to attend to patients in need. Diagnostic imaging plays an important role in many clinical situations, although its role must always remain secondary to a carefully performed history and physical examination.

Many different imaging modalities are employed in emergency practice including conventional radiography, CT, ultrasonography and, less often, MRI, nuclear scintigraphy, angiography, and enteric contrast radiography. Nonetheless, conventional radiography remains the most frequently used modality and the one that emergency clinicians are most frequently called upon to interpret. In addition, an understanding of radiographic findings is important to deriving essential information from the radiologist's report and to communicating accurately with medical and surgical colleagues. Conventional radiography is therefore the focus of most of the cases in this book. Noncontrast head CT, which is the chief imaging study for various neurological emergencies, is covered in one section. Other imaging modalities are discussed where they play a role.

This book is based on clinical cases, and is designed to hone the reader's skills in the use and interpretation of radiographs. Easily missed disorders and diagnostic dilemmas are emphasized. Although not exhaustive, the book encompasses many of the major areas in which radiography is helpful in achieving a diagnosis. By limiting the range of topics, these areas can be discussed in greater depth than is possible in an all-inclusive textbook. Such all-inclusive coverage can be found in *Emergency Radiology*, edited by David T. Schwartz and Earl J. Reisdorff (McGraw-Hill, 2000).

The book is divided into seven sections: chest, abdomen, upper and lower extremity, cervical spine, head CT and face. Each section begins with an introductory chapter that discusses the radiographic principles for that region. These include indications for radiography, radiographic views, anatomy, and principles of interpretation.

Each case begins with a description of the patient's clinical presentation and initial radiographic studies. The reader should attempt to interpret the radiographs before proceeding to the discussion. In some instances, a second set of images is provided as the case develops.

A list of suggested reading is provided at the end of each chapter, including both recent and classic articles. These should serve as a starting point for further investigation of the topic. The references are listed alphabetically by author's name and, in many instances, are divided by topic.

Because the cases are initially presented without a final diagnosis, the table of contents identifies only the patient's chief complaint. A second table of contents, located at the end of the front matter on page xiii, lists chapters by diagnosis and should not be consulted until after the cases have been reviewed. This will assist readers in locating the material for later reference. In addition, a comprehensive index is provided in which major topics are indicated by boldface text.

My hope is that the reader will find these cases instructive and engaging, and that they will serve as a stimulus to advance his or her knowledge of diagnostic imaging in emergency medicine practice.

ACKNOWLEDGMENTS

In this multi-year endeavor, there are many individuals to whom I would like to extend my thanks. First and foremost, to my wife Harriet, who offered editorial comments and for whom this longstanding project meant real sacrifice.

To Dr. Lewis R. Goldfrank, who provided continuous support and encouragement and who, despite all his other responsibilities, was able to review and offer suggestions throughout this entire book. To Maureen Gang and Pamela Ryder, who reviewed many chapters and to the EM residents who also read chapters and who, along with EM faculty members, brought many instructive clinical cases to my attention.

I would also like to thank several of the NYU Radiology faculty who were generous with their time and knowledge in the early years of the EM residency—Barry Leitman, Emil J. Balthazar, Cornelia Golimbu, Mahvash Rafii, and Richard Pinto. More recently, the NYU Emergency Radiology faculty, including Alexander Baxter and Mark Bernstein, have been an asset to our residency.

I would also like to thank the ACEP Education Committee and Educational Meetings staff for their assistance in staging Emergency Radiology Workshops at various educational conferences in the past, where many of these cases were first brought together and exhibited.

Finally, I would like to thank the editorial and production staff at McGraw-Hill for their input over many more years than had initially been anticipated. In particular, Andrea Seils was an asset throughout the project, and, more recently, Anne Sydor, Peter Boyle, Robert Pancotti, Sarah Granlund, as well as Denise Showers of Aptara, helped bring this complex project to fruition.

CONTENTS BY DIAGNOSIS

EMERGENCY RADIOLOGY
Case Studies

CHEST RADIOLOGY

Chest radiography is the most commonly ordered imaging test in emergency department patients. It can provide considerable diagnostic information for a wide variety of thoracic disorders. Its diagnostic capabilities are based largely on the contrast between the air-filled lungs and pathological processes that cause fluid accumulation within lung tissue.

Although **chest CT** provides greater anatomical detail of the pulmonary parenchyma and is often used in non-emergency patients with pulmonary disease, the use of chest CT in the ED is limited to certain critical conditions that do not produce distinctive findings on conventional radiography. These include pulmonary embolism and aortic dissection. CT is also used in ED patients with major chest trauma to detect an aortic injury, pneumothorax, hemothorax and pulmonary contusions that may not be evident on the supine portable chest radiographs.

WHEN TO ORDER RADIOGRAPHS

In general, a diagnostic test should be ordered when the disease under consideration produces characteristic findings which help confirm or exclude the suspected disorder. A number of approaches can be used in deciding to order a radiograph.

With a simplistic **"geographic" approach,** radiographs are obtained of the region where the patient is having symptoms, e.g., a chest radiograph in a patient with chest pain. Such an approach is ill-advised because it can lead to diagnostic errors, as well as excessive and unnecessary testing.

Using a **symptom-based approach** to radiograph ordering, the decision to obtain radiographs is based on characteristics of the patient's symptoms, for example whether the chest pain is severe or mild, pleuritic or pressure-like (Rothrock 2002).

However, a more rational **diagnosis-based approach** is to first consider the potential disorders that might be present and then to obtain radiography if the suspected disorder has characteristic radiographic findings, such as pneumonia and pneumothorax. This approach is the most likely to yield clinically useful information and to avoid unnecessary testing. Determining which disorders need investigation in an individual patient

is ultimately based on the clinical judgment, knowledge and experience of the practitioner.

RADIOGRAPHIC VIEWS

Two perpendicular views should be obtained whenever possible. The preferred frontal view is a postero-anterior view **(PA view).** This view is obtained in the radiology suite with the patient standing and the imaging cassette placed against the patient's anterior chest wall. The x-ray beam is directed horizontally and traverses the patient from posterior to anterior. The patient's hands are positioned on the hips, which moves the scapulae laterally and away from the lungs. The patient is instructed to take a full inspiration. The PA view is preferred because the heart and mediastinum are closest to the x-ray imaging cassette and therefore less distorted by magnification.

When the patient is too ill or debilitated to stand for a PA view, an antero-posterior view **(AP view)** is obtained. The patient is in either a lying or sitting position. The sitting position is preferred whenever possible. The x-ray beam is directed downward towards the patient.

The **lateral view** is obtained with the patient standing or sitting. The arms should be raised. The standard lateral view is a *left* lateral view in which the patient's left side is placed against the imaging cassette. In this way, the heart is closer to the cassette and is seen more clearly.

HOW TO READ A RADIOGRAPH

First, examine the radiograph in its entirety looking for obvious and clinically expected findings. Next, a methodical review is performed to obtain complete information from the radiograph.

There are two complementary approaches—systematic and targeted (Table 1). Using a **systematic approach,** each tissue density (air, soft tissue and bone) is examined in all regions of the image. This provides a relatively simple framework for radiograph review that is easily remembered and thorough.

A **targeted approach** is based on the pathological patterns seen on chest radiographs as well as the radiographic manifestations of various thoracic diseases. Using **pattern-recognition,**

TABLE 1

How to Read a Chest Radiograph

A. INITIAL OVERALL REVIEW—Review the image in its entirety
   Look for obvious and expected findings

B. SYSTEMATIC APPROACH
   - Adequacy
      Penetration—Lower thoracic vertebral bodies are faintly visible behind the heart
      Rotation—Medial clavicular heads align with the tips of the spinous processes
      Inspiration—Posterior right 10th or 11th rib is at the *right cardiophrenic sulcus*

   - Bones: Ribs, shoulders, vertebral column
   - Soft tissues: Heart (cardiothoracic ratio), mediastinum, hila, diaphragm
   - Lungs: Use left/right symmetry

   Compare lung markings at each intercostal space with that of the opposite lung

   or

   - Central zone: Heart, mediastinum, trachea, hila, vertebral column
   - Middle zone: Lungs
   - Periphery: Bones and soft tissues of the chest wall and shoulders

C. TARGETED APPROACH

   Pattern recognition—Identify pattern of radiographic abnormality—diffuse airspace filling,
      focal airspace filling, reticular pattern, etc. (see Table 5). A differential diagnosis is then
      derived from the radiographic pattern

   Diagnosis-based—Requires knowledge of the radiographic appearance of the disease clinically
      suspected, e.g., pneumonia, congestive heart failure, pneumothorax (see Table 6)

---

one of several pathological patterns is identified such as airspace filling or a reticular pattern. From the radiographic pattern identified, a differential diagnosis is derived (see Table 5 on p.12) (Reed 2003). Using a **diagnosis-based approach**, disorders suspected based on the clinical examination are specifically sought when reviewing the radiographs (see Table 6 on p.12). This approach depends on knowledge of the radiographic manifestations of thoracic diseases such as pneumonia, pulmonary edema, pneumothorax, and injuries associated with chest trauma.

Both the targeted and systematic approaches are used in radiograph interpretation. A targeted approach is an efficient and effective way to identify both obvious and subtle pathology. A systematic approach provides a complete review of the radiograph, will assure that additional pathology is identified, and provides a step-by-step technique to verify that a radiograph is normal (Loy 2004, Sistrom 2006, Good 1990).

SYSTEMATIC APPROACH TO INTERPRETING A CHEST RADIOGRAPH

A systematic approach provides a step-wise method to review a radiograph. It depends on knowledge of normal radiographic anatomy.

First, the technical **adequacy** of the image is assessed. Then, the **bones, soft tissues** (heart, mediastinum and diaphragm) and, finally, the **lungs** are examined. The bones are examined first so that a skeletal lesion is not overlooked when a more obvious pulmonary abnormality is present. In an alternative scheme, the central region is examined first (heart and mediastinum), then the lungs, and, last, the ribs and chest wall (Table 1).

Adequacy

Three factors are used in assessing the technical adequacy of a chest radiograph: penetration, rotation and level of inspiration (Figure 1).

Penetration   In a properly exposed radiograph, the lower thoracic vertebral bodies should be visible through the superimposed heart. When a radiograph is over-penetrated (too dark), lung pathology may not be visible. When under-penetrated (too light), lung markings appear prominent and could be misinterpreted as abnormal.

Rotation   When the patient is correctly positioned, an anterior midline skeletal structure (center point between the medial

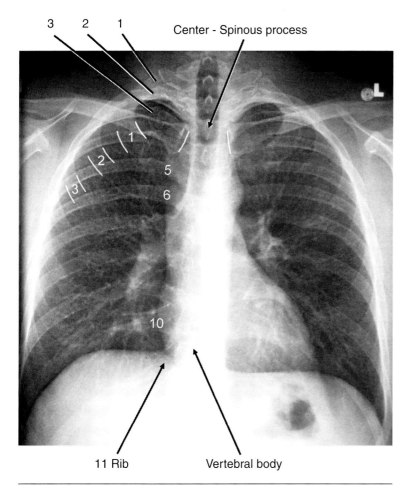

FIGURE 1   Normal PA view in a young adult—Adequacy.

The three factors used to assess adequacy are:

Penetration—The lower vertebral bodies are visible.

Rotation—The spinous processes are centered between the clavicular heads (*white lines*).

Inspiration—The 10th or 11th rib is located at the right cardiophrenic sulcus.

The ribs are counted beginning at the anterior aspects of the first two or three ribs because their posterior aspects overlap and cannot be distinguished. Then, the posterior aspects of ribs 3 to 11 can be counted.

spiration, the posterior aspects of the ribs are counted from the thoracic apex to the diaphragm. Because the posterior aspects of the first, second and occasionally third ribs overlap, the anterior aspects of the first two or three ribs should be located and then the rib contours traced to their posterior aspects. Once the posterior aspects of the first two or three ribs have been identified, the other ribs can be counted (Figure 1).

When the level of inspiration is correct, the lung markings (pulmonary vasculature), heart and mediastinum are clearly depicted. With an incomplete inspiration, the lung markings appear crowded, particularly at the lung bases, and the heart and mediastinum appear widened.

NORMAL RADIOGRAPHIC ANATOMY

Lungs

The right lung has three **lobes**, and the left has two (Figure 2). The **interlobar fissures** separate the lobes—the right lung has the right major (oblique) and minor (horizontal) fissures, and the left lung has the left major (oblique) fissure. Portions of the fissures may be visible on the chest radiograph, appearing as fine white lines on the PA and lateral views (Figure 3).

Each lung is divided into **segments**—nine on the left and ten on the right (Figure 2). These segmental divisions correspond to the branches of the bronchial tree and not divisions within the pulmonary parenchyma. Consequently, although pulmonary parenchymal disorders tend to be localized to one segment, disease processes often spread to adjacent segments. The interlobar fissures, however, are usually not crossed (Hayashi 2001).

clavicular heads) aligns with a posterior midline structure (tips of the spinous processes). When the patient is rotated, the mediastinum appears displaced or widened.

In the absence of rotation or mediastinal shift, the trachea should be in the midline. However, alignment of the trachea over the spinous processes should not be used to assess positioning because the trachea is a mobile structure. For example, if the patient is rotated to the right and the mediastinum is shifted to the left, the trachea overlies the spinous processes and mediastinal shift could be missed.

Inspiration   The posterior aspect of the right tenth or eleventh rib should be at the *right cardiophrenic sulcus* (where the diaphragm intersects the right heart border). To assess in-

Heart

Assessment of **cardiac enlargement** is made using the **cardiothoracic ratio.** The heart at its widest extent should be no greater than half the width of the thorax measured between the inner rib margins at the widest region of the thorax (Figures 3, 4 and 5).

The **heart borders** are formed by particular **cardiac chambers.** On the frontal view, the right heart border represents the *right atrium*, while the left heart border is made up by the *left ventricle* (Figure 3A). A concavity at the superior portion of the left heart border indicates the location of the *left atrial appendage*. When the left atrium is enlarged, a convex bulge appears in this region (Figure 5A). The *right ventricle* is an anterior structure and is therefore only seen on the lateral view,

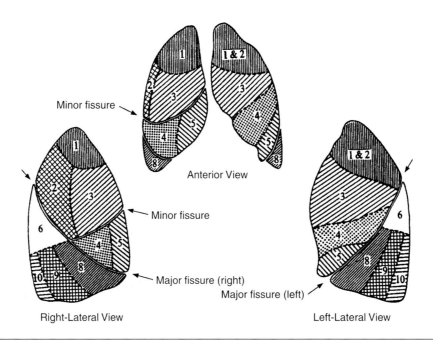

Minor fissure

Anterior View

Minor fissure

Major fissure (right)

Major fissure (left)

Right-Lateral View   Left-Lateral View

FIGURE 2   Lobes, interlobar fissures, and segments of the lungs.

Right upper lobe   1. Apical   2. Anterior   3. Posterior

Right middle lobe   4. Lateral   5. Medial

Right lower lobe   6. Superior   7. Medial basal   8. Anterobasal   9. Lateral basal   10. Posterobasal

Left upper lobe   1 & 2. Apical posterior   3. Anterior   4. Superior lingular   5. Inferior lingular

Left lower lobe   6. Superior   7. Medial basal   8. Anterobasal   9. Lateral basal   10. Posterobasal

[From: Pansky B: *Review of Gross Anatomy*, 6th ed. McGraw Hill, 1996, with permission.]

making up the anterior heart border. The *left atrium* is a posterior structure and is not normally visible on the frontal view (Figure 5B).

When the thorax is abnormally widened as in chronic obstructive pulmonary disease (COPD), the cardiothoracic ratio is not a reliable indicator of cardiac enlargement (Figure 6).

Aorta

The **aortic knob** represents the posterior portion of the aortic arch. In young individuals, the ascending aorta is not normally visible. The left margin of the **descending aorta** is seen inferior to the aortic knob and parallels to the vertebral bodies (Figure 3). Between the inferior margin of the aortic knob and the left pulmonary artery is a small concave fat-containing region known as the **aorticopulmonary window.** This is obliterated or convex when there is mediastinal fluid or adenopathy.

On the **lateral view,** only the aortic arch is normally seen. The descending aorta lies within mediastinal soft tissues and is not visible (Figure 3B).

In **elderly persons,** particularly those with hypertension, the aortic wall is weakened and the aorta becomes dilated (ectatic) and elongated ("uncoiled"). This is known as a **tortuous aorta** (Figure 4). On the PA view, aortic knob is enlarged. The ascending

aorta may be visible as a curved shadow superior to the right heart border and the elongated descending aorta is displaced to the left. On the lateral view, the elongated arc of the descending aorta is seen adjacent to the thoracic vertebrae. The descending aorta is visible because it is adjacent to air-filled lung (visibility of the descending aorta is *not* due to calcification).

Mediastinum

Aside from the heart and aorta, several other **mediastinal structures** are visible on the PA view (Figures 3 and 7).

The **trachea** is a midline air-filled structure that branches at the carina to form the left and right mainstem bronchi. The **left subclavian artery** extends superiorly from the aortic arch. The **descending aorta** extends inferiorly from the aortic knob. The **superior vena cava** forms a faint shadow along the right superior mediastinum.

Mediastinal Pleural Reflection Lines

Several air/fluid interfaces between the lung and mediastinal soft tissue structures are often seen. Distortion or displacement of these contours occurs with accumulation of fluid, lymphadenopathy or masses in the mediastinum (Figure 7).

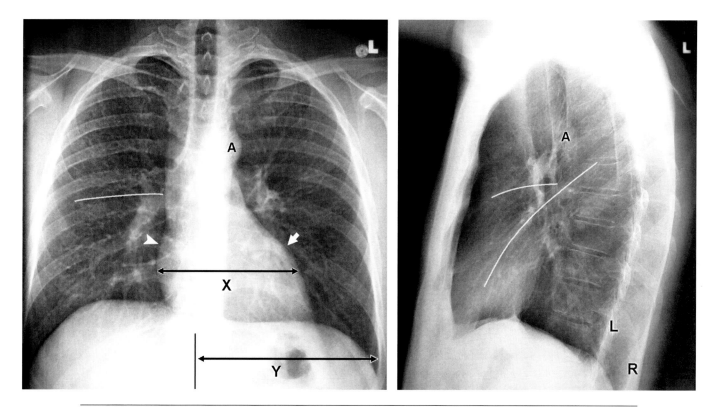

FIGURE 3   Normal PA and lateral radiographs in a young adult.

Heart: The cardiac width (X) is normally less than half the width of the thorax (Y) **(cardiothoracic ratio).** The left heart border is formed by the left ventricle (*arrow*) and the right heart border by the right atrium (*arrowhead*).

Interlobar fissures: On PA view, a white line indicates approximate location of the minor (horizontal) fissure. On the lateral view, the major (oblique) and minor (horizontal) fissures are seen.

Aorta: On the PA view, the aortic knob is small (A). On lateral view, only the aortic arch is visible (A); the descending aorta is not seen because it is within the mediastinal soft tissues.

Ribs: On the lateral view, the **right ribs** (R) are further from the radiograph cassette and therefore magnified and more posterior than the **left ribs** (L).

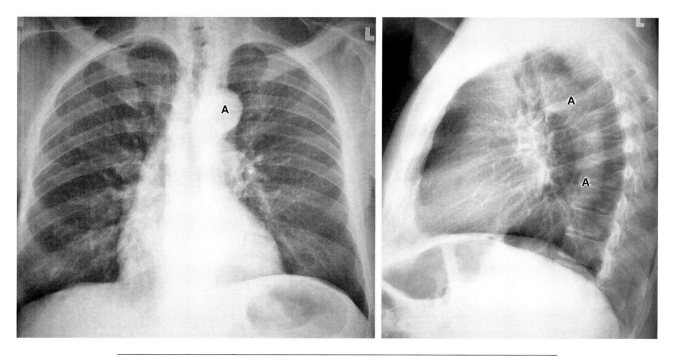

FIGURE 4   Normal PA and lateral radiographs in an elderly adult—Tortuous aorta.
On the PA view, the aortic knob is enlarged (A).
On lateral view, the elongated descending aorta is visible adjacent to thoracic vertebrae (A-A).

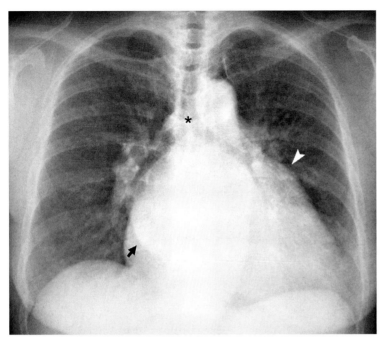 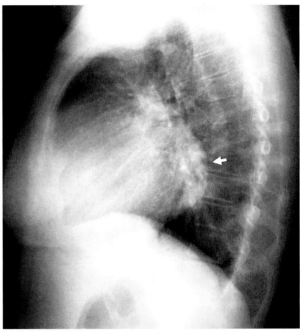

FIGURE 5   **Cardiomegaly in a patient with rheumatic heart disease—Mitral and aortic stenosis.**

Left atrial enlargement causes widening of the angle between the left and right mainstem bronchi at the carina (*asterisk*), convexity at the superior portion of the left heart border due to the enlarged left atrial appendage (*arrowhead*), and a double-density behind the heart at the margin of the left atrium (*arrow*).

On the **lateral view,** the superior portion of the posterior heart border bulges posteriorly due to left atrial enlargement (*arrow*).

Left ventricular enlargement causes an increased cardiothoracic ratio of 60%.

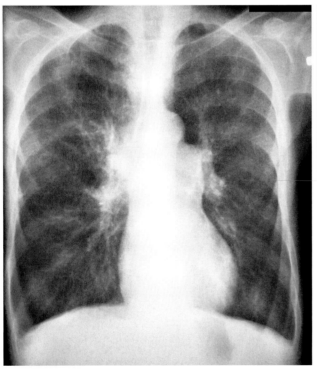 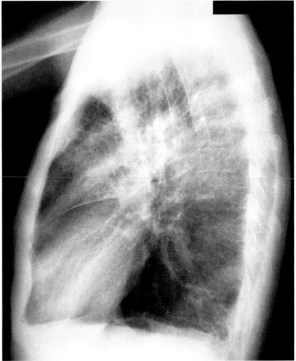

FIGURE 6   **Cardiomegaly without an increased cardiothoracic ratio.**

A 70-year-old man with COPD and cardiomegaly due to **cor pulmonale**. The lungs are hyperexpanded, the thoracic width is increased, and the cardiothoracic ratio is therefore not a reliable indicator of cardiac enlargement.

There are several radiographic signs of **severe COPD.** The diaphragm is flattened on both the PA and lateral views. On the PA view, the tho-

racic height is increased (note the great distance between the aortic knob and the lung apices). On the lateral view, the thoracic anteroposterior diameter is increased.

Pulmonary artery hypertension secondary to COPD causes hilar enlargement due to pulmonary artery distention.

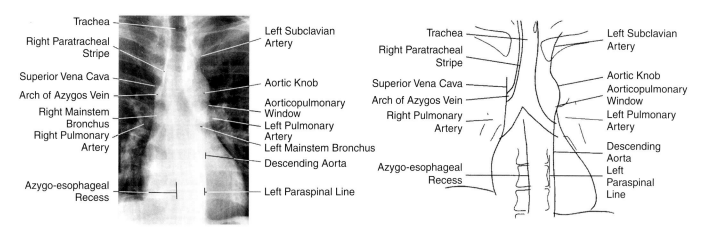

FIGURE 7   Mediastinal anatomy.

Left subclavian artery—A curved shadow that disappears at the superior border of the clavicle.

Right paratracheal stripe—Normally < 5 mm wide; terminates inferiorly at the *arch of the azygos vein.*

Aorticopulmonary window—Space under aortic arch and above superior border of left pulmonary artery.

Left paraspinal line—Up to 15 mm wide; normally disappears above the aortic knob.

Azygo-esophageal recess—Medial surface of the right lung extends into the mediastinum inferior to the arch of the azygos vein and lies against the esophagus (it is not the right side of the descending aorta).

Superior vena cava— Extend superiorly from the right mainstem bronchus.

The **right paratracheal stripe** is a thin layer of connective tissue that lies along the right tracheal wall adjacent to the right lung. It is normally no more than 5 mm thick. The right paratracheal stripe terminates inferiorly at the **arch of the azygos vein** that crosses over the right mainstem bronchus. Widening > 1 cm is a sign of pulmonary venous hypertension (e.g., congestive heart failure).

Inferior to the arch of the azygos vein and carina, the medial surface of the right lung lies against the esophagus forming the **azygo-esophageal recess**. The **left and right paraspinal lines** parallel the margins of the thoracic vertebral bodies. The left paraspinal line normally disappears at the level of the aortic arch.

Hilum

The hila are composed of the *main pulmonary arteries* and the *superior pulmonary veins*, which appear as branching vascular structures (Figures 3 and 7). The lower lobe pulmonary arteries extend for 2 to 4 cm before branching (Figure 8). The *inferior pulmonary veins* enter the left atrium inferior to the hila and do not contribute to hilar density.

Lung Markings

Normal lung markings are pulmonary arteries and veins. These appear as branching vascular structures that become successively finer and disappear within 1 cm of the lung margin (Figure 8). Due to the overlap of blood vessels, normal lung markings can have a reticular or cyst-like appearance. Abnormal lung markings are caused by thickening of the interstitial connective tissues, which are not normally visible.

The **lung markings and hila** are two problematic areas of chest radiology. There is a wide range of normal appearances and abnormalities can be subtle. Identification of abnormalities of the hila or lung markings must therefore be based on an understanding of their normal radiographic anatomy and the changes expected with various pathological processes (discussed in subsequent chapters).

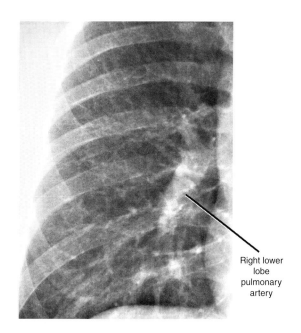

Right lower lobe pulmonary artery

FIGURE 8   Normal hila and lung markings.
Normal lung markings are pulmonary arteries and veins that have a branching vascular appearance. Due to overlap, they can have a reticular or cyst-like appearance. Blood vessels seen on-end appear as small white dots. The lower lobe pulmonary arteries extend 2 to 4 cm from the hilum before branching.

THE LATERAL CHEST RADIOGRAPH

How to Read the Lateral View

A *systematic approach* begins with assessment of the technical **adequacy** of the radiograph. Although there are no clearly defined criteria, penetration, rotation and level of inspiration all affect image quality and interpretation. Next, the **bones** (vertebral bodies, ribs and sternum), **soft tissues** (diaphragm, heart and mediastinum), and **lungs** are examined.

The lateral view is useful to visualize pathology that may not be evident on the PA view (Table 2).

Intrapulmonary opacities (pneumonia or tumors) can sometimes be more easily seen on the lateral view. They also can be localized to a particular segment of the lung.

Normally, the lower vertebral bodies appear more radiolucent (dark) than the superior vertebral bodies because there is more overlying lung and less overlying soft tissue. When the lower vertebral bodies appear more "white," there is a lower lobe infiltrate (postero-basal segment). The retrocardiac and retrosternal regions are also better seen on the lateral than the frontal view (Figure 9).

Mild (interstitial) **pulmonary edema** can be detected on the lateral view buy noting **thickened interlobar fissures.** In addition, **small pleural effusions** may only be seen on the lateral view in the posterior costophrenic sulcus.

Hilar abnormalities, particularly hilar adenopathy, can often be more easily identified on the lateral view. **Cardiomegaly** due to enlargement of the right ventricle and left atrium can be detected on the lateral view.

Radiographic anatomy

The lateral view provides a view of thoracic structures perpendicular to the PA view (Figure 9) (McComb 2002). The left and right **lungs** are superimposed. Portions of the left and right major (oblique) fissures and the minor (horizontal) fissure are often visible (Figure 3B).

The left and right domes of the **diaphragm** are visible and can be differentiated using four criteria. The most reliable method is to identify the right ribs, which are more posteriorly located on the standard left lateral view (Figures 3B, 4B and 5B). The right dome of the diaphragm extends posteriorly to the right ribs at the *posterior costophrenic sulcus.* In addition the left dome of the diaphragm is usually more inferiorly located than the right side, it may be associated with the gastric air bubble, and it tends to disappear anteriorly because it is adjacent to the heart. The right dome of the diaphragm extends to the anterior chest wall.

The **heart** is seen in a different view than on the frontal view (Figure 9). The *right ventricle* forms the anterior heart border. The posterior heart border is formed superiorly by the *left atrium* and, inferiorly, the *left ventricle*. With right ventricular enlargement, the inferior portion of the retrosternal clear space is filled by the heart. With left ventricular enlargement, the heart extends posteriorly into the retrocardiac space to the vertebral bodies. With left atrial enlargement, the superior portion of the posterior cardiac border bulges posteriorly (Figure 5B).

TABLE 2

Useful Findings on the Lateral View

1. Intrapulmonary opacities—pneumonia, tumors

2. Thickened interlobar fissures—interstitial pulmonary edema

3. Small pleural effusion in posterior costophrenic sulcus

4. Hilar abnormalities—adenopathy, masses, increased vascularity

5. Cardiomegaly, heart chamber enlargement, and aortic abnormalities

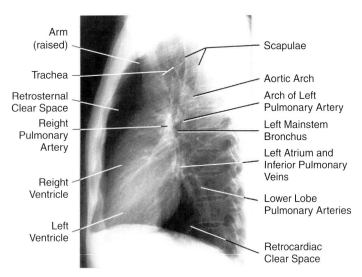

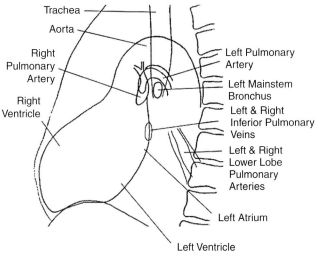

FIGURE 9   The lateral chest radiograph.

The **trachea** and **aortic arch** are visible on the lateral view (Figure 9). In young adults, the **descending aorta** is not seen because it is located within the mediastinal soft tissues (Figure 3B). In an elderly patient with a **tortuous aorta,** the descending aorta is elongated and is visible on the lateral radiograph because it lies next to the vertebrae and adjacent left lung (Figure 4B).

Anterior to the distal trachea and carina, the **right pulmonary artery** forms a radiopaque region (Figure 9). The **left pulmonary artery** arches over the **left mainstem bronchus. The left mainstem bronchus** therefore appears as a radiolucent oval.

Hilar adenopathy can often be readily identified on the lateral view. They are seen as areas of abnormally increased opacity adjacent to the air-filled distal trachea. Normally, the regions posterior and inferior to the distal trachea are radiolucent; when they are radiopaque, there is retrotracheal and subcarinal adenopathy.

The left and right **lower lobe pulmonary arteries** extend inferiorly and posteriorly from the hilum. These can be difficult to distinguish from a lower lobe infiltrate (Figure 9). Inferior to the hilum, along the posterior cardiac border, is a radiopaque area where the **inferior pulmonary veins** are seen on end (Figure 9). These normal vascular structures should not be misinterpreted as pathological lesions.

THE AP PORTABLE CHEST RADIOGRAPH

AP portable chest radiographs are obtained when a patient is unable to stand and cannot be transported to the radiology suite. (Figure 10). Interpretation of an AP chest radiograph uses the same principles as a PA view, although differences in radiographic technique must be taken into account.

Several factors can either obscure or mimic pathological findings on an AP view (Table 3). The AP portable view is frequently technically suboptimal: rotated positioning, poor inspiration, and over-or under-penetrated. These factors can make the heart appear enlarged and the mediastinum appear widened and indistinct. With supine positioning, pleural fluid or a pneumothorax are located, respectively, posterior or anterior to the lung and therefore difficult or impossible to detect. Finally, superimposed extraneous objects can obscure radiographic findings.

Whenever possible, the AP view should be obtained in the *sitting position* because there will be less distortion, the patient is better able to take a full inspiration, and pleural fluid or a (pneumothorax) are more readily identified.

Another shortcoming of portable radiography is that only one view of the thorax is obtained—there is no lateral view to confirm or localize abnormalities seen on the AP view. Subtle radiographic signs of pathology such as the "silhouette sign" are therefore especially important to recognize.

TABLE 3

Distortions on an AP Portable Chest Radiograph

Rotated positioning of the patient—apparent shift of trachea and mediastinum

Poor inspiration—crowded lung markings at the bases

Suboptimal exposure—over or under-penetrated

Cardiac enlargement

Widened and indistinct mediastinum

Pneumothorax and pleural effusion difficult to see on a supine view

Superimposed extrathoracic objects—spine immobilization boards, tubes, monitoring wires, and clips

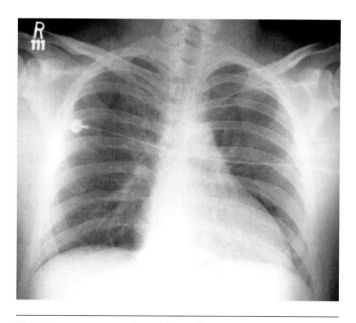

FIGURE 10   A properly performed supine AP portable chest radiograph.

The penetration and level of inspiration are good; the patient is slightly rotated to the left. The cardiac appearance is typical for portable radiogrphy, slightly enlarged and horizontal. The mediastinal structures are not well defined, but do not appear widened. A cardiac monitor lead traverses the chest.

RADIOGRAPHIC PATTERNS OF PULMONARY DISEASE— INCREASED PULMONARY OPACITY

Many pulmonary pathological processes increase or, less commonly, decrease the radiographic opacity of the lungs. Pulmonary disorders that cause fluid accumulation within lung are readily detected on chest radiography. However, diseases such as asthma or pulmonary embolism cause little or no change in pulmonary opacity and radiography generally provides little evidence of their presence.

In evaluating a region of increased opacity, the first step is to determine whether the opacity is within the lung, the pleural space, chest wall, or outside the body. Correlation with the lateral view can help localize an opacity.

There are **three patterns of increased pulmonary opacity**— either the airspaces or interstitial tissues have increased fluid content, or there is diminished aeration of a portion of the lung (known as collapse or atelectasis) (Table 4 and illustrated in subsequent chapters). Airspace-filling can be either localized or diffuse; increased interstitial tissue density has either a reticular or nodular appearance; and with atelectasis, there are signs of lung volume loss.

Infiltrates

An *ill-defined* area of increased pulmonary opacity is often termed an "infiltrate." (*Well-defined* opacities, i.e. those with sharp borders, are referred to as *masses* or *nodules*.) However, "infiltrate" is not a proper radiologic term. It is a histopathological term that refers to infiltration of the lung parenchyma (airspaces or interstitium) with abnormal cellular material (inflammatory or neoplastic cells). Not all ill-defined opacities are infiltrates. For example, airspace pulmonary edema can look radiographically like an infiltrate, but is due to fluid accumulation rather than cellular infiltration of lung tissue. It is therefore preferable to describe the radiographic finding as an "ill-defined opacity" and avoid the term "infiltrate," which has pathological connotations that may or may not be applicable (Patterson 2005, Friedman 1983, Tuddenham 1984).

When there is relatively homogenous opacification of the airspaces of the lung, the radiographic finding can be termed *consolidation*. Unlike the term "infiltrate," consolidation does not have unwarranted pathological implications.

Infiltration of the **interstitial tissues** of the lung with inflammatory or neoplastic cells could be termed an "interstitial infiltrate." However, this usage should be avoided because interstitial pulmonary edema can have a similar radiographic appearance even though it is not truly an infiltrate. It is therefore preferable to describe the lesion's radiographic appearance.

Interstitial lung disorders can have a reticular, nodular or reticulonodular appearance. However, many interstitial lung diseases also involve the airspaces of the lung, resulting in ill-defined opacities of airspace filling. There is thus often a disparity between the histopathology of an interstitial lung disease and its radiographic appearance, e. g.,—patchy multifocal airspace filling rather than an interstitial pattern. High-resolution CT (HRCT) can better characterize a pulmonary pathological process, although it is generally not warranted in the ED (Kazerooni 2001, Gotway 2005).

TABLE 4

Patterns of Increased Pulmonary Opacity

AIRSPACE FILLING

    Localized = segmental
    Diffuse or multifocal

INTERSTITIAL PATTERNS

    Reticular—fine or coarse linear shadows
    Reticulonodular
    Nodular—small (2 to 3 mm), medium, large, or masses (>3 cm)

ATELECTASIS

    Diminished aeration of lung.
    Associated with signs of volume loss

RADIOGRAPHIC FINDINGS AND CLINICAL DIAGNOSIS

Radiography is used in two complementary ways to assist in making a diagnosis. First, by identifying a particular radiographic pattern, a list of potential diagnosis can be generated (Table 5 and Case A) (Reed 2003). Second, based on a patient's clinical presentation, certain disorders will be suspected, and examination of the radiographs is targeted to identifying radiographic signs of the suspected diseases (Table 6). Certain disorders can have subtle radiographic manifestations and the examiner must search carefully for these findings (Case B).

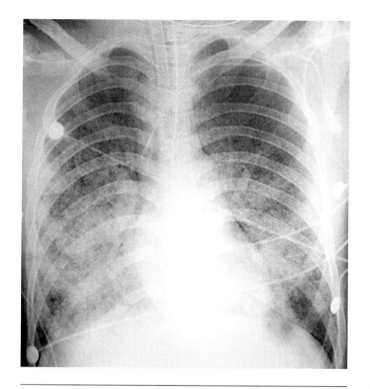

FIGURE 11   Case A

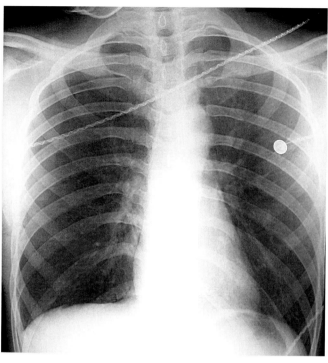

FIGURE 12   Case B

CASE A.
PATTERN RECOGNITION IN RADIOGRAPH INTERPRETATION

A 21-year-old man presented with cough and hemoptysis that had developed over two days. He was previously healthy. He expectorated a teaspoon quantity of blood mixed with clear phlegm. Initially, his respiratory rate was 28, pulse 110, and auscultation of his lungs revealed scattered râles. He was placed in respiratory isolation because of concern about tuberculosis.

While being observed in the ED over the next three hours, he developed increasing respiratory difficulty, hypoxia, and tachypnea that required endotracheal intubation. His temperature rose to 103.6°F.

His chest radiograph is shown (Figure 11).

- What disorders should be suspected based on the clinical presentation and radiographic findings?

CASE B.
TARGETED APPROACH TO RADIOGRAPH INTERPRETATION

A 25-year-old man presented with an abrupt onset of unilateral pleuritic chest pain. He had no prior medical problems. His physical examination was normal, including equal breath sounds bilaterally.

His chest radiograph appears normal (Figure 12).

In this patient, a systematic approach to radiograph interpretation would be time-consuming and could potentially miss the pertinent finding. A targeted review of the radiograph looking for subtle signs of the clinically suspected disorder will lead quickly to the correct diagnosis.

- What is this patient's diagnosis?

TABLE 5

Patterns of Increased Pulmonary Opacity—Differential Diagnosis

A. FOCAL AIRSPACE DISEASE

Pneumonia

Pulmonary embolism: infarction or intrapulmonary hemorrhage

Neoplasm: alveolar cell carcinoma, lymphoma (usually diffuse)

Atelectasis: opacity accompanied by signs of volume loss

B. DIFFUSE or MULTIFOCAL AIRSPACE DISEASE

Pulmonary edema: CHF and non-cardiogenic pulmonary edema

Pneumonia: bacterial, viral, Mycoplasma, Pneumocystis

Hemorrhage: trauma (contusion), immunologic (Goodpasture's), bleeding diathesis, pulm. embolism

Neoplasm: alveolar cell carcinoma, lymphoma

Desquamative interstitial pneumonitis (DIP), alveolar proteinosis

Bat-wing pattern—Central opacification with peripheral clearing—characteristic of pulmonary edema

C. FINE RETICULAR PATTERN

Acute:

Interstitial pulmonary edema

Interstitial pneumonitis: viral, Mycoplasma

(Airspace filling often accompanies interstitial pneumonia and pulmonary edema)

Chronic:

Lymphangitic metastasis, sarcoidosis, eosinophilic granuloma, collagen vascular diseases, inhalation injuries, idiopathic pulmonary fibrosis ("fibrosing alveolitis"), resolving pneumonia

D. COARSE RETICULAR PATTERN—Honeycomb lung—end-stage pulmonary fibrosis

Also seen when pneumonia or pulmonary edema occurs in patients with underlying emphysema

E. RETICULONODULAR PATTERN

A common radiographic pattern that encompasses the same disorders as reticular patterns

F. MILIARY PATTERN—2 to 3 mm well-defined nodules ("micronodular pattern")

Tuberculosis, Fungal, Nocardia, Varicella

Silicosis, Coal Worker's lung, Sarcoidosis, Eosinophilic granuloma

Neoplastic (adenocarcinoma, thyroid)

G. NODULAR PATTERN—Margins of the lesions are generally well-defined. Mass: >3 cm

Neoplasm: metastatic, lymphoma; benign tumors

Fungal or parasitic infection, septic emboli

Rheumatoid nodules, Wegener's granulomatosis

TABLE 6

Radiograph Interpretation Based on Clinical Presentation

SYMPTOM	DISORDERS THAT HAVE CHARACTERISTIC RADIOGRAPHIC FINDINGS
Cough and/or fever	Pneumonia, tuberculosis, cancer
Chest pain	Pneumothorax, aortic dissection, pulmonary embolism, rib fracture, cancer
Dyspnea	Congestive heart failure/pulmonary edema, pulmonary embolism, COPD, pericardial effusion, cancer
Trauma	Aortic injury, pneumothorax, hemothorax, pulmonary contusion, rib fractures

CASE A (CONTINUED).

PATTERN RECOGNITION IN RADIOGRAPH INTERPRETATION: DIFFUSE AIRSPACE FILLING

The radiograph shows diffuse opacification of the airspaces of both lungs (Figure 11). It has a uniform (as opposed to central) distribution. Centrally distributed airspace filling is characteristic of congestive heart failure.

Fluid that fills the airspaces of the lungs may be either an inflammatory exudate (pneumonia), pulmonary edema (cardiogenic or non-cardiogenic), blood or neoplastic cells. Although neoplastic infiltration of the lung usually has an interstitial pattern (nodules or masses), bronchoalveolar cell carcinoma and occasionally lymphoma can fill the airspaces. Miscellaneous causes of airspace filling include desquamative interstitial pneumonitis (DIP) and alveolar proteinosis (Table 5 part B).

In a young man with high fever and diffuse airspace filling, pneumocystis pneumonia related to AIDS is a major concern. However, this patient denied any risk factors for HIV infection.

Among the many causes of **hemoptysis,** pneumonia and bronchitis are most common; tuberculosis and cancer are most feared (although his radiographic findings were not consistent with these disorders); and pulmonary edema usually causes pink, frothy sputum. Other causes of hemoptysis include pulmonary embolism and pulmonary hemorrhagic disorders.

This patient was admitted to the medical intensive care unit and treated with ceftriaxone, azithromycin, trimethoprim/sulfamethoxazole, amikacin, isoniazid, rifampin, pyrazinamide, ethambutol, amphotcricin B, and high-dose corticosteroids. He did not improve. To evaluate microscopic hematuria, a renal consultant ordered the correct diagnostic test—an antiglomerulo-basement membrane antibody. The antibody levels were markedly elevated, which is diagnostic of Goodpasture's syndrome. Emergency plasmapheresis was attempted but the patient did not survive.

Although Goodpasture's syndrome is often considered a disease that primarily causes renal failure, in some cases pulmonary manifestations predominate. Rapid progression of pulmonary hemorrhage is typical.

This case illustrates the use of pattern recognition (diffuse airspace filling) in determining a list of diagnostic possibilities.

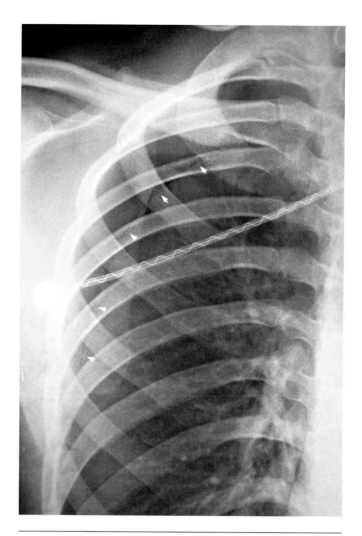

FIGURE 13   Case B (detail)

CASE B (CONTINUED).

TARGETED APPROACH TO RADIOGRAPH INTERPRETATION

In this patient, spontaneous pneumothorax was one of the principal diagnoses suspected. However, there are no obvious radiographic signs of pneumothorax. Examination of the radiograph should therefore be directed to looking for subtle signs of a pneumothorax—a fine line representing the surface of the collapsed lung that parallels the margin of the thorax.

In this patient, a pneumothorax can be seen along the right pleural margin, the side of the patient's chest pain (Figure 13, *arrowheads*).

A targeted approach to radiograph interpretation can provide quick and accurate results. After noting the expected abnormality, the entire radiograph should be reviewed systematically to avoid missing other potentially significant findings.

HARD AND SOFT RADIOGRAPHIC SIGNS

Some radiographic findings have greater diagnostic reliability than others. *Hard signs* clearly show the presence of disease, whereas *soft signs* are less clearly distinguished from normal structures, particularly structures that have a range of normal radiographic appearances such as lung markings and the hila. For example, normal lung markings that are prominent or crowded can have a similar radiographic appearance to pneumonia, an ill-defined pulmonary nodule or mild pulmonary edema.

For an individual patient, the clinician must ultimately decide whether treatment, further testing or follow up is appropriate. Nonetheless, a clear understanding of the radiographic manifestations of various diseases allows subtle but definite pathological findings to be reliably identified.

SUGGESTED READING

Brady WJ, Aufderheide T, Kaplan P: Cardiovascular Imaging, in Schwartz DT, Reisdorff EJ: *Emergency Radiology*, McGraw-Hill, 2000.

Felson B: *Chest Roentgenology*. WB Saunders, 1973.

Fraser RS, Colman N, Muller N, Paré PD: *Synopsis of Diseases of the Chest*, 3rd ed. Saunders, 2005.

Freedman M: *Clinical Imaging: An Introduction to the Role of Imaging in Clinical Practice*. Churchill Livingstone, 1988.

Hansell DM, Armstrong P, Lynch DA, McAdams HP: *Imaging of Diseases of the Chest*, 4th ed. Mosby, 2005.

Harris JH, Harris WH: *The Radiology of Emergency Medicine*, 4th ed. Lippincott Williams & Wilkins, 2000.

Keats TE: *Emergency Radiology*, 2nd ed. Year Book Medical Publishing, 1989.

Muller NL, Colman NC, Paré PD, Fraser RS: *Fraser and Paré's Diagnosis of Diseases of the Chest,* 4th ed. Saunders, 2001.

Novelline RA: *Squire's Fundamentals of Radiology*, 6th ed. Harvard University Press, 2004.

Reed JC: *Chest Radiology: Plain Film Pattern and Differential Diagnosis*, 5th ed. Elsevier, 2003.

Wagner MJ, Wolford R, Hartfelder B, Schwartz DT: Pulmonary Chest Radiology, in Schwartz DT, Reisdorff EJ: *Emergency Radiology*, McGraw-Hill, 2000.

Terminology

Austin J, Morris S, Trapnell D, Fraser RG: The Fleischner society glossary: Critique and revisions. *AJR* 1985;145:1096–1098.

Austin JH, Muller NL, Friedman PJ, et al: Glossary of terms for CT of the lungs: recommendations of the Nomenclature Committee of the Fleischner Society. *Radiology* 1996;200:327–331.

Censullo ML, et al: The "I" word in chest radiography. Why is it such a dirty word? Radiology 2005;237:1121–1124.

Friedman PJ: Radiologic reporting: description of alveolar filling. *AJR* 1983;141:617–618.

Hall FM: Language of the radiology report: Primer for residents and wayward radiologists. *AJR* 2000;175:1239–1242.

Patterson HS, Sponaugle DN: Is infiltrate a useful term in the interpretation of chest radiographs? Physician survey results. *Radiology* 2005;235:5–8.

Tuddenham WJ: Glossary of terms for thoracic radiology: recommendations of the nomenclature committee of the Fleischner Society. *AJR* 1984;143:509–517.

Radiograph Interpretation

Campbell SG, Murray DD, Hawass A, et al: Agreement between emergency physician diagnosis and radiologist reports in patients discharged from an emergency department with community-acquired pneumonia. *Emerg Radiol* 2005;11:242–246.

Good BC, Cooperstein LA, DeMarino GB, et al: Does knowledge of the clinical history affect the accuracy of chest radiograph interpretation? *AJR* 1990;154:709–712.

Loy CT, Irwig L: Accuracy of diagnostic tests read with and without clinical information: A systematic review. *JAMA* 2004;292: 1602–1609.

Sistrom C: Inference and uncertainty in radiology. *Acad Radiol* 2006;13:580–588.

Chest Radiograph Findings

Gibbs JM, Chandrasekhar CA, Ferguson EC, Oldham SAA: Lines and stripes: Where did they go?—From conventional radiography to CT. *Radiographics* 2007;27:33–48.

Hayashi K, Aziz A, Ashizawa K, et al: Radiographic and CT appearances of the major fissures. *RadioGraphics* 2001;21:861–874.

Lupow JB, Sivak SL, Boss D: The accuracy of the cardiothoracic ratio as a predictor of cardiac enlargement and dysfunction (abstract). *Acad Emerg Med* 2002;9:462.

McComb BL: The chest in profile. *J Thoracic Imaging* 2002;17:58–69.

Summers RL, Woodward LH, Kolb JC: Correlation of radiographic cardiothoracic ratio with cardiac function in patients with acute congestive heart failure. *Emerg Radiol* 1999;6;153–156.

Tarver RD: Radiology of community-acquired pneumonia. *Radiol Clin North Am* 2005;43:497–512.

Vilar J, Domingo ML, Soto C, Cogollos J: Radiology of bacterial pneumonia. *Europ J Radiol* 2004;51:102–113.

Whitten CR, Khan S, Munneke GJ, Grubnic S: A diagnostic approach to mediastinal abnormalities. *Radiographics* 2007;27:657–671.

Clinical Decision Rules for Chest Radiography

Roberts R, Schaider JJ, Reilley B, et al: Developing clinical decision rules to determine the need for chest radiographs in emergency department patients with chest pain (abstract). *Acad Emerg Med* 2001;8:504.

Rothrock SG, Green SM, Costanzo KA, et al: High yield criteria for obtaining non-trauma chest radiography in the adult emergency department population. *J Emerg Med* 2002;23:117–124.

High-Resolution CT

Gotway MB, Reddy GP, Webb WR, et al: High-resolution CT of the lung: Patterns of disease and differential diagnoses. *Radiol Clin North Am* 2005;43:513–542.

Kazerooni EA: High-resolution CT of the lungs. *AJR* 2001;177: 501–519.

Marchiori E, Souza AS, Franquet T, Muller NL: Diffuse high-attenuation pulmonary abnormalities: A pattern-oriented diagnostic approach on high-resolution CT. *AJR* 2005;184:273–282.

Chest Radiology: Patient 1

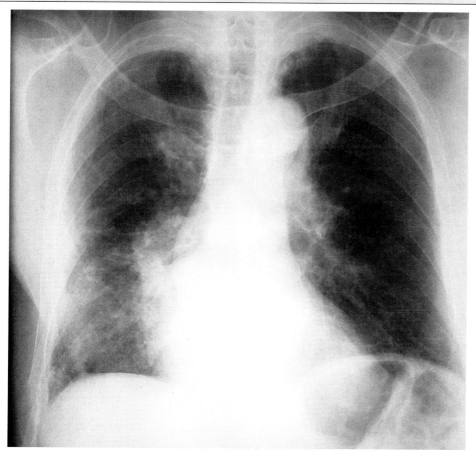

FIGURE 1

Cough and fever in an elderly man

A 78-year-old previously healthy man presented with two days of cough productive of thick purulent sputum, fever and dyspnea on exertion.

On examination, he was an elderly man who appeared acutely ill.

Vital signs—blood pressure 96/60 mm Hg, pulse 116 beats/min, respiratory rate 24 breaths/min, temperature 103.5°F rectal.

Lung examination revealed scattered ronchi, which were greater on the right than the left.

Blood tests and a chest radiograph were obtained and intravenous antibiotics were administered.

- What do the chest radiographs show (Figure 1)?

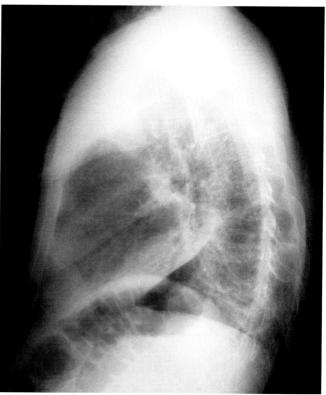

HOW TO READ A RADIOGRAPH

One of the primary roles of chest radiography in emergency department patients is to diagnose **pneumonia.** Although the chest radiograph is abnormal in nearly all cases, early in its course or with milder cases, the radiograph may be normal. Pneumonia is, therefore, a diagnosis based on clinical, not radiographic, findings. Radiography serves to confirm the diagnosis, to assess prognosis (e.g., poorer outcome with multilobar pneumonia), and to detect an underlying lesion such as a bronchogenic carcinoma causing postobstructive pneumonia.

Pathological Patterns of Pneumonia

There are **three pathological patterns** of pneumonia: **lobar pneumonia, bronchopneumonia** (lobular), and **interstitial pneumonia.** This classification is based on the pathogenesis of the infection and the histological appearance of infected lung tissue. Each pattern is associated with specific infecting organisms (Table 1).

Although these terms are often used to describe the radiographic appearance of pneumonia, there is only limited correlation between the infecting organism and radiographic pattern. For example, pneumococcal pneumonia can have a patchy radiographic appearance simulating bronchopneumonia; staphylococcal pneumonia can cause a relatively uniform segmental consolidation; and viral pneumonia often spreads to the airspaces and has an airspace-filling appearance. Radiographic findings are therefore not used to predict the infecting organism or to choose antibiotic therapy. Antibiotic therapy is based instead on clinical parameters such as severity of illness, host factors such as immunologic status, and clinical setting (community versus hospital acquired).

TABLE 1

Pathological Patterns of Pneumonia

	ORGANISMS	HISTOPATHOLOGY	CHARACTERISTIC RADIOGRAPHIC FINDINGS*
Lobar Pneumonia (segmental)	*Strep. pneumoniae, Klebsiella*	Alveoli filled with purulent exudate, alveolar walls not thickened	Focal airspace filling
Bronchopneumonia (lobular)	*Staph. aureus,* aspiration, *Pseudomonas,* tuberculosis	Infection in bronchus spreads distally to segmental airspaces; also may spread proximally to affect other lung segments	Patchy, airspace filling— involving one segment or multifocal; abscess or cavity formation
Interstitial Pneumonia	Viral, *Mycoplasma, Pneumocystis*	Alveolar walls thickened by inflammatory cells, spreads to adjacent airspaces	Reticular or reticulonodular pattern; diffuse, patchy, or focal airspace filling

*Radiographic pattern is variable; each infecting organism can produce various radiographic findings.

Lobar Pneumonia

The typical radiographic appearance of lobar pneumonia is **focal airspace filling** which creates an **ill-defined opacity** (Table 2). This is a reflection of its *pathogenesis* (Figure 2). Although commonly termed "lobar pneumonia," in most cases the infection is limited to one or two segments of the lung.

The infection begins within the alveolar airspaces and then spreads to adjacent airspaces via microscopic interconnecting channels (Figure 2). This results in relatively homogenous opacification of lung tissue (Figure 3). The margins of the infiltrate are ill defined (blurred) because the inflammatory exude spreads directly from airspace to airspace. The margin is sharp only where the pneumonia abuts an interlobar fissure. Often, some airspaces within the infiltrate remain aerated. Air-filled alveoli create a mottled appearance—an *air alveologram*. An air-filled bronchus within the infiltrate appears as a branching tubular structure—an *air bronchogram* (Figure 3B).

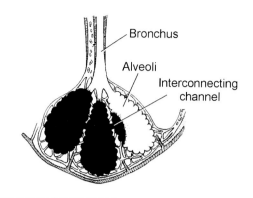

FIGURE 2   Pathogenesis of lobar pneumonia.

Infection begins within the alveolar airspaces and then spreads through microscopic interconnecting channels.

Bronchi often remain aerated, which, when surrounded by fluid-filled lung, creates air bronchogram.

The interconnecting channels serve to maintain alveolar aeration when a bronchus becomes obstructed.

From Fraser RS, Coleman N, Muller N, Paré PD: *Synopsis of Diseases of the Chest,* 3rd ed. Saunders, 2005, with permission.

TABLE 2

Radiographic Signs of Lobar Pneumonia—Focal Airspace Filling

1. Relatively homogeneous opacification of the lung

2. Ill-defined margins, except where the pneumonia abuts an interlobar fissure

3. Airspaces that remain aerated create a mottled appearance (air alveologram) or air bronchogram

4. Obliteration of a normal lung–soft tissue interface such as when the pneumonia lies adjacent to the heart or diaphragm—the "silhouette sign"

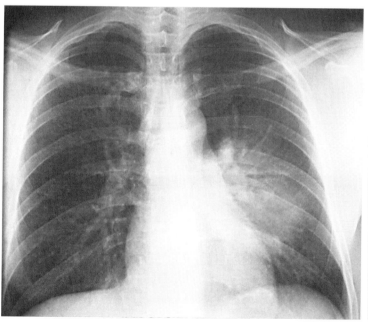

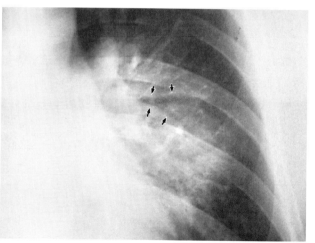

A   B

FIGURE 3   Lobar pneumonia localized to the middle region of the left lung.

It appears as an ill-defined opacity (indistinct margins) that has relatively homogeneous opacity. An air-bronchogram is visible (*arrows*).

• In which segment of the lung is this pneumonia located?

Lobar pneumonia usually involves a single segment of the lung. Its location can be determined by the radiographic findings. This serves both as an exercise in radiographic anatomy as well as an aide to identifying a pneumonia.

In Figure 4A, the pneumonia is located in the middle portion of the left lung and may therefore be in either the left upper lobe (lingular segments) or left lower lobe (superior segment) (Figure 4C). If the infiltrate were in the lingula, this would lie adjacent to the heart and obscure the left heart border. Obliteration of a normal air/fluid interface is known as a **silhouette sign.** However, because the left heart border is

visible in Figure 4A, the pneumonia must lie posterior to the heart in the superior segment of the left lower lobe. The lateral view confirms this localization (Figure 4B and D).

In patient 1's PA view, opacification of the lower portion of the right lung is seen (Figure 5A). This could be in either the right lower lobe or right middle lobe (Figure 5C). However, because the right heart border is obliterated, the pneumonia is anterior, i.e., located in the right middle lobe. On the lateral view, the pneumonia is seen anterior to the major fissure, which localizes it to the right middle lobe (Figure 5B and D).

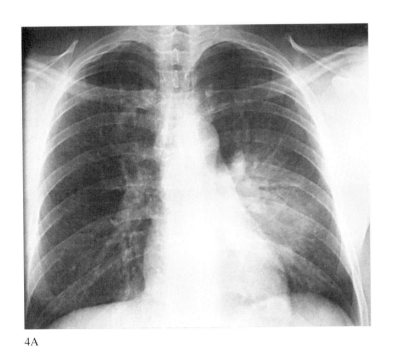

4A

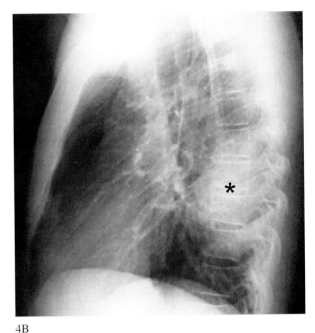

4B

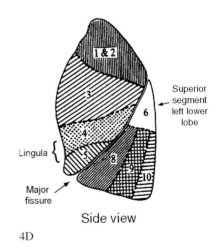

Frontal view
4C

Side view
4D

FIGURE 4   Lobar pneumonia—Superior segment of the left lower lobe.

A. The PA view shows the infiltrate in the middle of the left lung. The left heart border is preserved, meaning that the pneumonia lies behind the heart in the left lower lobe rather than in the upper lobe/lingula.

B. Lateral view confirms localization to the superior segment of the left lower lobe (*asterisk*).

C and D. Segments of the left lung.

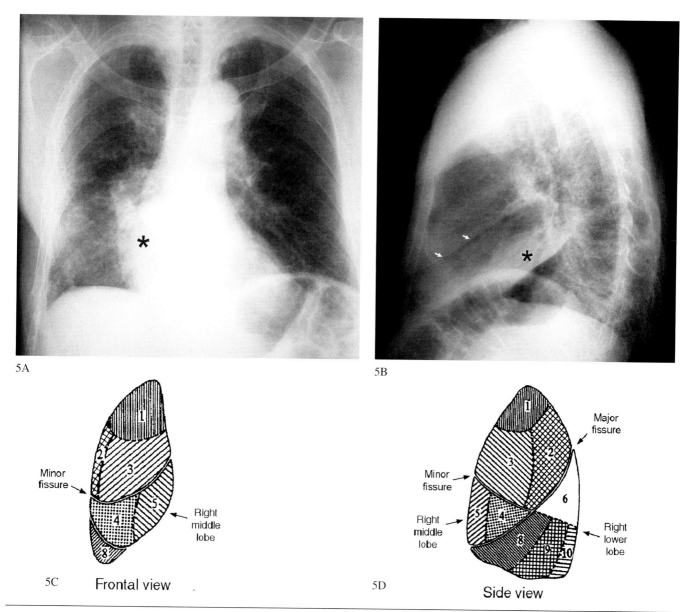

5A

5B

Minor fissure →

3

2

1

4

5

→ Right middle lobe

8

5C   Frontal view

Major fissure

1

2

3

6

Minor fissure →

Right middle lobe →

5

4

8

9 10

→ Right lower lobe

5D   Side view

FIGURE 5   Patient 1.

A. The PA view shows the infiltrate in the lower right lung. Because the right heart border is obscured (*asterisk*), the pneumonia lies anterior, adjacent to the heart in the right middle lobe, rather than posterior in the right lower lobe.

B. The lateral view confirms that the pneumonia is in the right middle lobe (*asterisk*). The inferior margin of the pneumonia is well-defined because it lies against the left major fissure. A second obliquely oriented shadow (*arrows*) represents the soft tissue of one of the patient's arms. The patient was too ill to raise his arms above his shoulders at the time the radiograph was exposed.

C and D. Segments of right lung

• An additionally clinically significant finding is present on these radiographs. What is it?

After a **targeted review** looking clinically suspected disorders, the radiographs should be examined **systematically** to avoid missing other important findings.

First, assess the technical **adequacy** of the image, considering penetration and level of inspiration and rotation. Next, look at each tissue type throughout the image. Begin with the **bones.** Look at each rib, the shoulders and clavicles, and vertebrae. Next, look at the **soft tissues** including the heart, mediastinum, and diaphragm. Finally, look at the air-filled

spaces of the **lungs.** Compare the lung at each rib interspace on the left to the same interspace on the right. Be sure to examine the lung behind the heart, the diaphragm (posterior costophrenic sulcus), and the clavicles where lesions can be overlooked without close inspection.

In a patient with pneumonia, signs of underlying illness that predispose to infection should be sought, such as a malignancy. Look for a mass causing bronchial obstruction, hilar adenopathy, or skeletal lesions.

In Patient 1, the important additional finding is an **expansile lesion of the right eighth rib** (Figure 6). Potential etiologies for this lesion include malignancy and infection such as tuberculosis.

Patient 1 Outcome

After the patient recovered from his pneumonia (blood cultures grew *Streptococcus pneumoniae*), an evaluation of the skeletal lesion was undertaken. A **skeletal survey** revealed collapse of the T10 vertebral body, a lytic lesion of the C2 spinous process,

and multiple punched-out lytic lesions of the skull (Figure 7). The **skull lesions** were typical of multiple myeloma. The bone scan was negative (aside from increased uptake at T10). This is characteristic of **multiple myeloma,** which causes bone lesions by osteolysis without new bone formation. New bone formation is responsible for the uptake of tracer on a bone scan. The urine was positive for Bence-Jones protein. The SPEP (serum protein electrophoresis) demonstrated an M-protein gamma globulin, and immunoelectrophoresis revealed a monoclonal IgG-kappa. Needle biopsy of T10 showed dense infiltration with malignant-appearing plasma cells confirming the diagnosis of multiple myeloma.

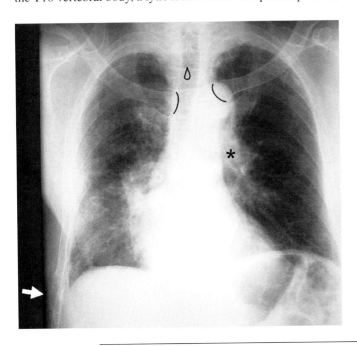
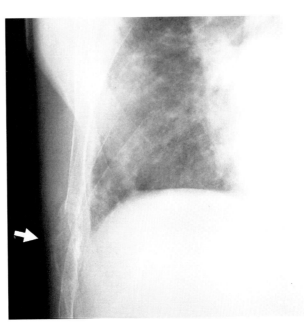

FIGURE 6   Patient 1—Initial PA view.

There is an expansile lytic lesion of the eighth rib (*arrow*).

The apparent enlargement of the left hilum simulating a hilar mass (*asterisk*) is actually due to rotated positioning of the patient. The patient is rotated to the left as indicated by the displacement of the medial clavicular heads (black lines) to the left relative to the spinous process (*black oval*).

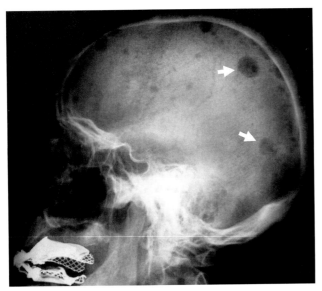
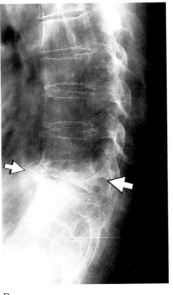

FIGURE 7 *A.* A skeletal survey revealed "punched-out" skull lesions that are pathognomonic for multiple myeloma (arrows). *B.* There was also pathological collapse of the T10 vertebral body (*arrows*).

A   B

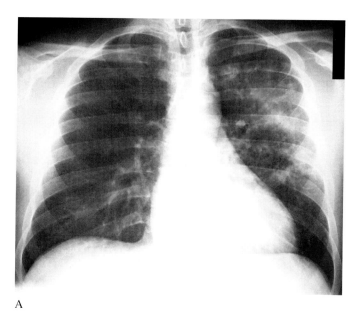

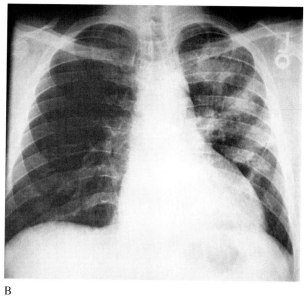

A   B

FIGURE 8   **Bronchopneumonia** *A.* Initial radiograph. *B.* Radiograph during ED visit one week later.

Bronchopneumonia

A 30-year-old man presented to the ED with persistent cough. He had been treated with oral azithromycin for 5 days for community acquired pneumonia. His initial chest radiograph showed patchy opacities in the left lung (Figure 8A). His cough had not improved and a second chest radiograph revealed progression of disease (Figure 8B).

There are three main **causes of treatment failure** in patients with community-acquired pneumonia. First, the infecting organism may not be responsive to the antibiotic prescribed, either due to **microbial resistance** or infection by an agent unresponsive to antibiotics such as a virus. Second, there may be infection with **unusual organisms** such as tuberculosis, fungi, or pneumocystis. Infection may be due to an unusual exposures such as during travel or animal exposure (tularemia, leptospirosis, psittacosis). Third, there may be a **noninfectious illness** that

can mimic pneumonia. These include pulmonary embolism, pulmonary edema, bronchial obstruction due to an endobronchial carcinoma, and a noninfections inflammatory disease (hypersensitivity pneumonitis, Wegener's granulomatosis, or eosinophilic pneumonia).

The radiograph reveals multiple patchy ill-defined opacities that can be categorized as a bronchopneumonia (Figure 8). The patient was hospitalized and evaluation revealed tuberculosis. His HIV test was negative.

Bronchopneumonia is a typical pattern of reactivation (postprimary) tuberculosis. The nidus of infection, usually in the upper lobe, ruptures into the bronchus and spreads endobronchially to other regions of the lung. Tuberculosis causes destruction of lung tissue with cavitation and heals with residual scarring (Figure 9).

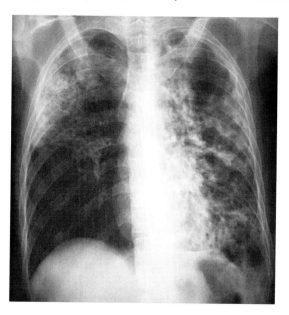

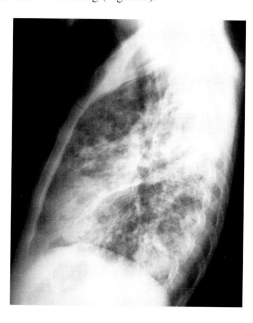

FIGURE 9   Extensive reactivation tuberculosis in another patient involving the entire left lung and right upper lobe.

There is pulmonary parenchymal destruction and cavitation including a large cavity in the apex of the left lung. The patient died despite aggressive in-hospital care.

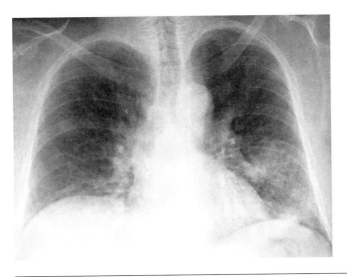
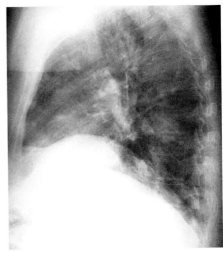

FIGURE 10   Varicella pneumonia

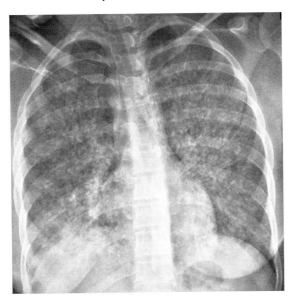
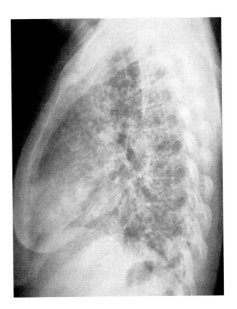

FIGURE 11   Varicella pneumonia

Interstitial Pneumonia—Varicella

Two young adults presented with typical cutaneous lesions of varicella and concomitant pulmonary infection. Neither patient had preexisting immunocompromise. Although pathologically, varicella pneumonia causes an interstitial pneumonitis, in the first case, only patchy airspace filling is present radiographically, simulating a bronchopneumonia (Figure 10).

In the second patient with varicella pneumonia, there is extensive involvement of both lungs. The diffuse **fine reticular pattern** is due to both interstitial infiltration and mottled, inhomogeneous airspace filling—a mix of aerated and fluid-filled alveoli (Figure 11).

SUGGESTED READING

Albaum MN, Hill LC, Murphy M, et al.: Interobserver reliability of the chest radiograph in community acquired pneumonia. *Chest* 1996; 110:343–350.

Gharib AM, Stern EJ: Radiology of pneumonia. *Med Clin North Am* 2001;85:1461–1491.

Metlay JP, Fine MJ: Testing strategies in the initial management of patients with community-acquired pneumonia. *Ann Intern Med* 2003; 138:109–118.

Kim EA, Lee KS, Primack SL: Viral pneumonias in adults: Radiographic and pathologic findings. *Radiographics* 2002;22:S137–S149.

Leung AN: Pulmonary tuberculosis: The essentials. *Radiology* 1999; 210:307–322.

Tarver RD: Radiology of community-acquired pneumonia. *Radiol Clin North Am* 2005;43:497–512.

Chest Radiology: Patient 2

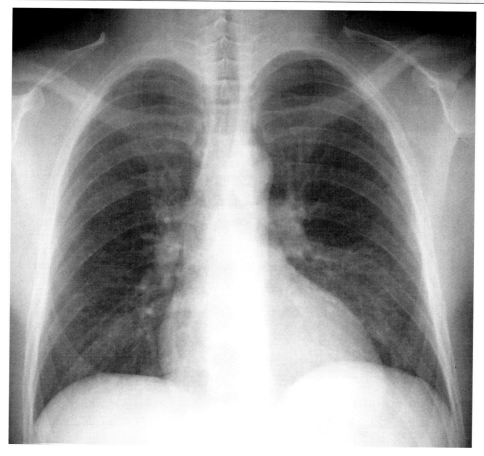

FIGURE 1

Cough and fever in a young man

A 34-year-old man presented with one day of fever and a cough productive of yellowish sputum. He complained of generalized myalgia and had vomited twice.

He had a history of intravenous drug use and had last injected drugs over one year earlier. He was tested and found to be PPD negative and HIV negative two months earlier.

On examination, he appeared healthy but had persistent cough. His vital sign were: blood pressure 118/78 mm Hg, pulse 88 beats/min, respiratory rate 24 breaths/min, temperature 100.8°F (oral), 103.4°F (rectal). Pulse oximetry oxygen saturation was 96% on room air.

Lung auscultation revealed bibasilar crackles. His neck was supple and oropharynx was clear. He was anicteric and had no rash, oral thrush, or lymphadenopathy. He had no heart murmur or hepatosplenomegaly.

A chest radiograph was obtained and interpreted as normal (Figure 1).

- Do you agree with this interpretation?

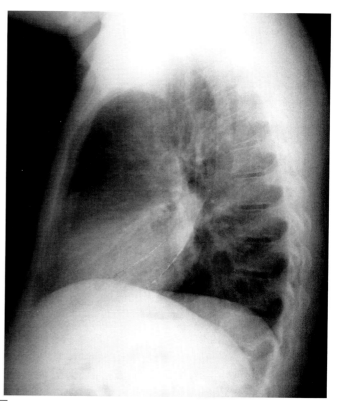

SILHOUETTES

In most patients, pneumonia is easy to detect. However, when the infiltrate is small or has only slightly greater opacity than adjacent normal lung, more subtle radiographic signs must be sought.

Silhouette signs occur when the airspaces of the lung are filled with fluid resulting in either the formation of a new abnormal air/fluid interface or obliteration of a normal air/fluid interface (loss of a silhouette). This silhouette effect, which occurs with pneumonia as well as other conditions that cause airspace filling, is one of the basic principles of chest radiography.

For an air/fluid interface to be visible on a radiograph (i.e., form a silhouette), it has to have a relatively sharp margin that is parallel to the direction of the x-ray beam. When the margin of a fluid collection is either gradual or not parallel to the x-ray beam, it appears indistinct (ill-defined) or may be completely invisible.

There are four types of silhouette signs (Table 1). The **first** and most well known is **loss of a normal air/fluid interface** that occurs when an abnormal fluid collection such as pneumonia lies adjacent to a soft tissue structure such as the heart or diaphragm. For example, a right middle lobe pneumonia obliterates the right heart border because the right middle lobe lies against the right atrium. This is often referred to as "the silhouette sign," although it is actually a misnomer because there is loss of a normal radiographic silhouette (air/fluid interface). In addition, a silhouette sign does not necessarily mean that the fluid collection is within the lung. A large pleural effusion can also obliterate the margin of the diaphragm.

A **second** silhouette sign is **obliteration of normal lung markings** (pulmonary blood vessels) when they are surrounded by fluid-filled lung. Because blood vessels are present throughout the lung, the usefulness of this silhouette sign is not limited to fluid collections that lie adjacent to the heart or diaphragm.

A **third** silhouette sign involves the formation of a new abnormal air/fluid interface where normally there are two adjacent air-filled structures. As pneumonia spreads, it may surround an aerated bronchus. The bronchus becomes visible and appears as an air-filled tubular structure within the infiltrate—an **air bronchogram** (see Patient 1, Figure 3 on page 17). Aerated alveolar air sacs surrounded by fluid-filled lung form an **air alveologram**, a 0.5–1-cm lucent area within a pulmonary opacity. Air alveolograms are responsible for the mottled, inhomogeneous appearance of many airspace-filling opacities. By contrast, a large pleural effusion is characterized by homogeneous radiographic opacification.

A **fourth** silhouette sign is due to the formation of an abnormal air/fluid interface at an **interlobar fissure.** A fissure nor-

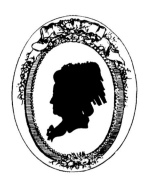

Elizabeth, Empress
of Russia, 1741
An early silhouette
portrait

mally appears as a fine white line, whereas an infiltrate adjacent to a fissure creates an abnormally sharp air/fluid silhouette. This can make an otherwise subtle infiltrate easier to detect because of the sharp border that occurs at the fissure.

Patient 2

In this patient, the pneumonia is easier to see on the **lateral view** than on the PA view-thanks to a silhouette sign. A portion of one of the major fissures is visible as a sharp air/fluid interface overlying the posterior portion of the heart just below the hilum (Figure 2). (A similar finding was present in Patient 1, Figure 5B on page 19.) The pneumonia is therefore either in the right middle lobe or the lingula of the left lung. By determining whether it is the right or left major fissure that is involved, the pneumonia can be localized to the right or left lung.

It is possible to differentiate the right and left major fissures on the lateral view by following the fissure down to its intersection with one of the domes of the diaphragm. There are four ways to distinguish the **left and right domes of the diaphragm** on a lateral radiograph. **First,** the right hemidiaphragm is usually higher than the left; however, this is not helpful in this patient. **Second,** if a gastric air bubble is present, it might be possible to identify the left hemidiaphragm by its proximity to the gastric air bubble—again, not possible in this case. **Third,** in a standard left lateral view, the right ribs are further from the imaging cassette and therefore appear larger and more posterior than the left ribs; the right hemidiaphragm can be followed to its intersection with the right ribs at the right costophrenic sulcus. However, the distinction is not clear in this case. The **fourth** criterion, useful in this patient, is the result of a silhouette effect. The anterior portion of the left hemidiaphragm lies against the heart, which "silhouettes out" the lung/diaphragm

---

TABLE 1

Four Silhouette Signs

1. Obliteration of a normal lung/soft tissue interface

2. Loss of normal lung markings

3. Air bronchogram or air alveologram

4. Accentuated interlobar fissure

interface, i.e., the left hemidiaphragm disappears anteriorly. The right hemidiaphragm is normally visible all the way to the anterior chest wall (Figure 2A).

In this patient's lateral view, the involved major fissure intersects with the left hemidiaphragm, i.e., the diaphragm that disappears anteriorly (Figure 2B). The infiltrate is anterior to the left major fissure and is therefore in the lingula of the left lung.

On the **PA view,** there is an ill-defined region of slightly increased opacity in the left mid-lung in the region of the lingula (Figure 3). A lingular infiltrate will often obliterate ("silhouette out") the left heart border because the lingula lies against the left ventricle. However, in this case, the infiltrate is relatively small and therefore does not cause a silhouette effect on the left heart border. In addition lung markings are not obliterated in the area because vascular markings are present in overlying aerated lung tissue.

Etienne de Silhouette

Etienne de Silhouette was the French Minister of Finance in 1759 under King Louis XV. It was a time of budgetary deficit, and he was appointed because he advocated a responsible fiscal policy. He initially enjoyed popular support because he proposed measures aimed at the wealthy, including taxation of the nobility. However, when his austerity measures became wider ranging, he was derided and forced out of office within months.

Black paper cutout portraits were becoming popular at that time. Etienne de Silhouette fancied these portraits and, as Finance Minister, he suggested that this cutout portraiture be substituted for more expensive portrait painting as a way for the nobility to reduce their expenditures. He was ridiculed by having his name associated with this lesser art form. The name took hold and, in 1835, the word "silhouette" was entered into the official dictionary of the French Academy.

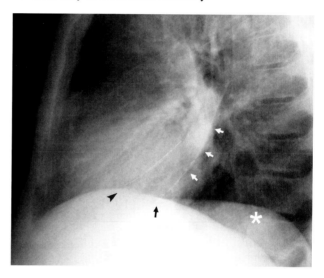

FIGURE 2B   Lateral view—detail.

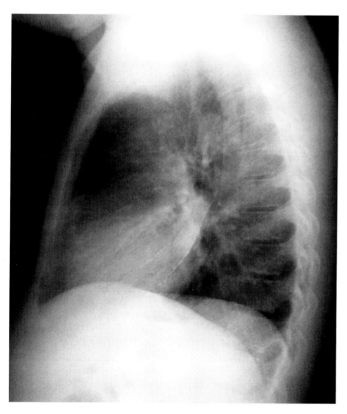

FIGURE 2A   Patient 2—Lateral view.

The lateral view shows an abnormal opacity just inferior to hilum (*asterisk*). Its posterior margin is sharp because it lies against one of the major fissures.

FIGURE 2B   Lateral view—detail.

The sharp posterior margin of the pneumonia highlights one of the major fissures (*white arrows*). The involved major fissure intersects the left hemidiaphragm (*black arrow*). The left hemidiaphragm (*asterisk*) disappears anteriorly because it lies against the heart rather than air-filled lung. The right hemidiaphragm, which intersects with the other major fissure (*arrowhead*), is visible to the anterior chest wall.

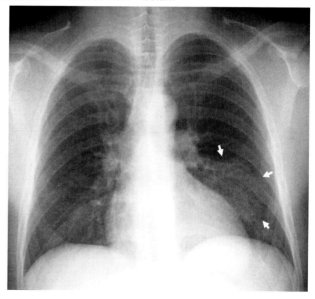

FIGURE 3   Patient 2—PA view.

A faint, ill-defined opacity is visible in the middle of the left lung, the lingular infiltrate (*arrows*).

Silhouette Signs Can Help Identify Subtle Pneumonias

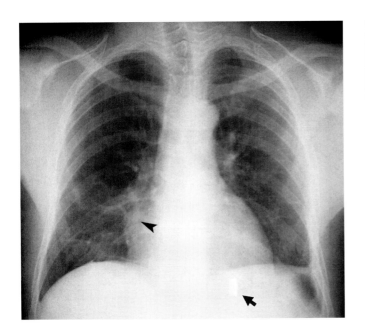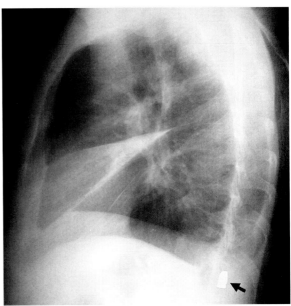

FIGURE 4   Silhouette sign—Right heart border.

On the PA view, the only clue to pneumonia is an indistinct right heart border (*arrowhead*). The left heart border, by contrast, is sharp.

The lateral view clearly shows the right middle lobe infiltrate. Its margins are well-defined because they abut the right major and minor fissures.

Incidentally, a bullet is seen embedded in the soft tissues of the back (*arrows*).

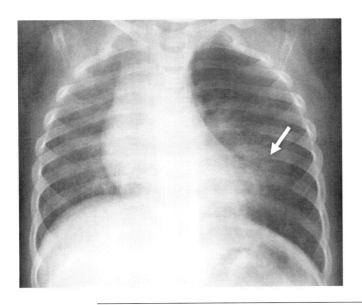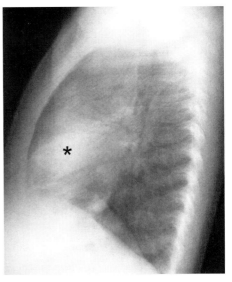

FIGURE 5   Silhouette sign—Left heart border.

A lingular pneumonia in a child is only evident on the frontal view by noting the indistinct left heart border (*arrow*).

On the lateral view, there is an ill-defined opacity overlying the heart (*asterisk*).

[From Schwartz DT, Reisdorff EJ: *Emergency Radiology.*
McGraw-Hill, 2000, with permission.]

Chest Radiology: Patient 3

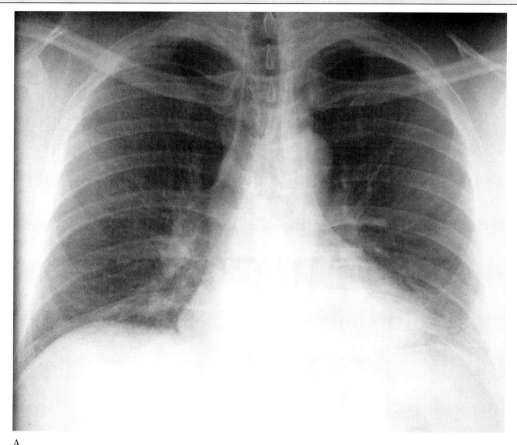

A

FIGURE 1

Non-productive cough, fever and myalgia in a young man

A 34-year-old man presented to the ED with a persistent non-productive cough, myalgias, coryza, and a low-grade fever that he had had for three days.

He was otherwise healthy, smoked half a pack of cigarettes per day, and had no history of asthma, pneumonia, or HIV risk factors.

On examination, he appeared well, and his vital signs were normal aside from a temperature of 100.4°F. He had a slight end-expiratory wheeze on lung auscultation. He was treated with an inhaled bronchodilator. His chest radiograph showed increased opacity in the lower portions of both lungs and indistinct lung markings (Figure 1). The lateral portion of the left heart border was obscured.

The radiograph was interpreted as showing bibasilar infiltrates.

• Do you agree with this interpretation?

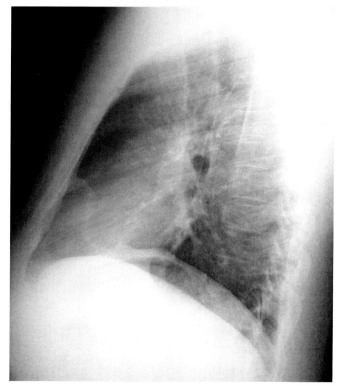

B

HIDDEN PNEUMONIAS AND PSEUDOINFILTRATES

Subtle radiographic signs of pneumonia (focal airspace filling) include indistinct pulmonary vascular markings and obliteration of a normal lung/soft tissue interface (the silhouette sign). Such findings seemed to be present in this patient. At the right base, there is increased opacity and indistinct lung marking. On the left, there is partial obliteration of the left heart border (Figure 1A).

However, the patient's clinical presentation was more consistent with an upper respiratory tract infection or bronchitis than a multilobar pneumonia. Furthermore, on the lateral view, there are no corresponding areas of increased lung opacity either overlying the heart in the lingula or right middle lobe, or behind the heart in the right or left lower lobes (Figure 1B). An additional finding on the PA view is an abnormally increased cardiothoracic ratio—the width of the heart is greater than half the width of the thorax, suggesting that the patient has an enlarged heart (Figure 1A).

The disparities between the patient's clinical and radiographic findings and between findings on the PA and lateral radiographs serve as a reminder that a systematic approach to radiograph interpretation should begin with an assessment of the technical **adequacy** of the radiographs. In this case, the x-ray penetration is correct (thoracic vertebral bodies are visible behind the heart) and the patient has been correctly positioned without rotation. However, the level of inspiration is inadequate—only the 9th rib is visible at the right cardiophrenic sulcus, whereas with a full inspiration, the 10th or 11th rib should be seen in this location (Figure 2).

The level of inspiration can also be assessed simply by noting the overall appearance of the radiograph. With incomplete inspiration, the vascular markings at the lung bases appear crowded and indistinct, and the heart appears more horizontally oriented and enlarged (Figure 2). In fact, using the overall appearance of the radiograph to assess the adequacy of inspiration can be more reliable than counting the ribs. For instance, in some patients with adequate inspiration, the 10th rib is at the right cardiophrenic sulcus, whereas in other patients, the 11th rib must be visible.

In this patient, the radiographs were repeated after the patient was instructed to take a complete inspiration. On the second PA view, the bibasilar "infiltrates" disappeared, the left heart border was clearly seen, and the heat size was normal (Figure 3). The magnitude of the effect caused by poor inspiration can be dramatic (Figure 4).

Several other radiographic findings can also be misinterpreted as abnormal intrapulmonary opacities—**pseudoinfiltrates** (Table 1). The lower lobe pulmonary arteries on both the frontal and lateral views can mimic a subtle infiltrate when the vessels are prominent. Questionable radiographic finding should therefore correlated with the patient's clinical presentation. For example, if the patient has cough and fever, increased opacity in the region of the lower lobe pulmonary arteries could represent a subtle pneumonia and the patient should be treated as such. When the questionable opacity could represent a malignancy, the patient should be referred for follow-up and repeat radiography or CT. Overlying soft tissues or skeletal structures can mimic a pulmonary lesion (Figure 5). On the other hand, intrapulmonary lesions can be obscured by superimposed bones, the heart, or diaphragm.

TABLE 1

Pseudoinfiltrates—Do not Mistake for Pulmonary Lesions

Poor inspiration	Crowding of lung marking at the lung bases
Lower lobe pulmonary arteries	On PA and lateral radiographs
Overlying soft tissue	Breast, pectoralis muscle, chest wall lesions, nipples, clothing
Skeletal lesions	Vertebral body osteophyte, healed rib fracture, crossing ribs, calcified costal cartilage

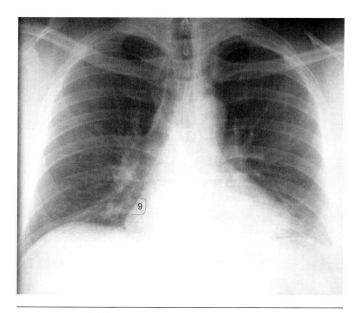

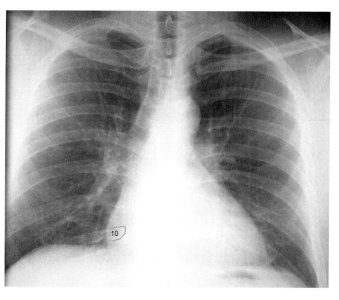

FIGURE 2   Initial PA view—Patient 3.

The vascular markings at both lung bases are crowded and indistinct. The left heart border is indistinct. The heart appears enlarged and has a horizontal orientation. These findings are due to the patient's incomplete inspiration—the ninth rib (9) lies just superior to the right cardiophrenic sulcus.

FIGURE 3   Repeat PA view—Patient 3.

With complete inspiration, the 10th rib (10) is seen above the cardiophrenic sulcus. The lung markings and cardiac borders now have a well-defined, normal appearance.

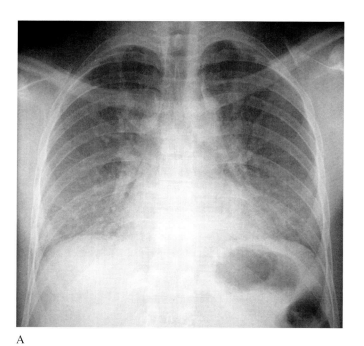

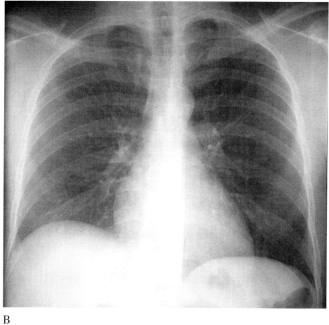

A   B

FIGURE 4   Pronounced effect of poor inspiration.

A young man who was infected with HIV presented to the ED with mild cough. The initial chest radiograph appeared to show bilateral airspace filling suggestive of pneumocystis pneumonia (A). However, the patient was well appearing, afebrile, had a normal oxygen saturation, and his CD4 T-cell count was greater than 200/mm^3. A repeat chest radiograph with compete inspiration showed that the lungs were, in fact, clear (B).

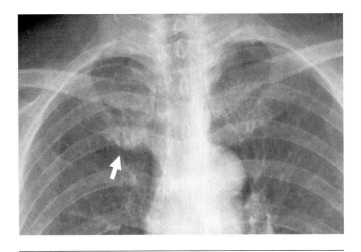

FIGURE 5   Calcified costal cartilage (*arrow*).

Costal cartilage calicification

Calcification of the first costal cartilage is common and should not be misinterpreted as a pulmonary lesion (Table 1). It can be recognized by its irregular appearance and location medial to the anterior end of the first rib (Figure 5). Costal cartilage calcification is usually bilateral.

When there is doubt as to the nature of the opacity, an apical lordotic chest radiograph can resolve the uncertainty. In this view, the clavicle and first ribs are projected above the apex of the lung and a lung lesion can be distinguished from rib calcification (Figure 6). The apical lordotic view can also be helpful when the costal calcification is overlying and obscuring a pulmonary lesion.

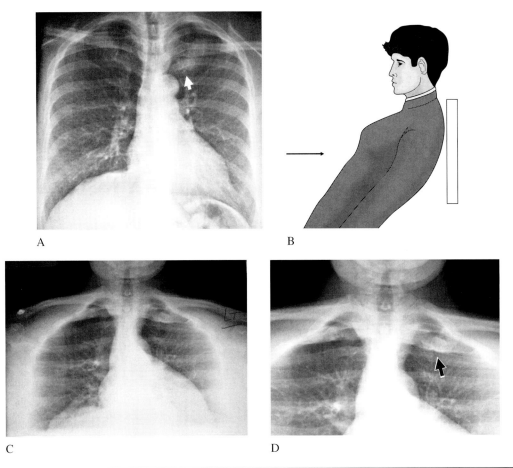

FIGURE 6   (*A*) Opacity in the region of the left lung apex (*arrow*). (*B*) Positioning of the apical lordotic view. (*C and D*) An apical lodotic view confirms that the opacity represents calcification of the first costal cartilage (*arrow*) and not a lesion the apex of the lung.

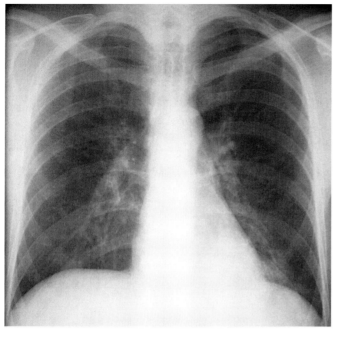

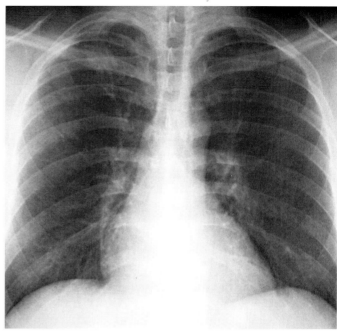

FIGURE 7   Patient 3B.

FIGURE 8   Patient 3C.

Two patients who presented to the ED with cough and fever.
• Where are their infiltrates?

HIDDEN INFILTRATES

Pulmonary lesions can be hidden by the heart, diaphragm, or ribs. The retrocardiac region is particularly difficult to assess on the frontal view (Figures 7 and 9A). Normally, pulmonary vascular markings and the diaphragm should be visible behind the heart (Figures 8 and 9B). When these are obscured, there may be a lesion in the left lower lobe.

The lateral view is helpful in detecting opacity in the retrocardiac region or in the left or right posterior costophrenic sulci (Figure 9C). When a patient is too ill to obtain a lateral view, the regions behind the heart and the domes of the diaphragms on the frontal view should be scrutinized for pulmonary lesions.

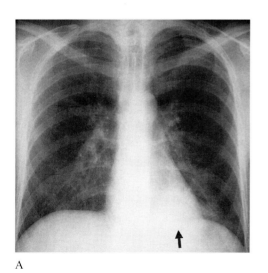

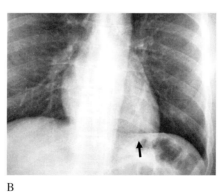

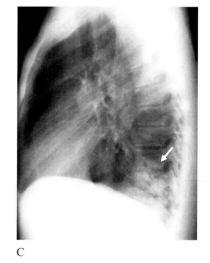

A

B

C

FIGURE 9   **Patient 3B.** (*A*) An abnormal opacity behind the heart obscures the vascular markings and the margin of the diaphragm (*arrow*). (*B*) In another patient, the retrocardiac region is normal—vascular markings and the diaphragmatic margin are visible (*arrow*). (*C*) In patient 3B, the lateral view shows pneumonia involving the posterior portion of the left lower lobe (*arrow*).

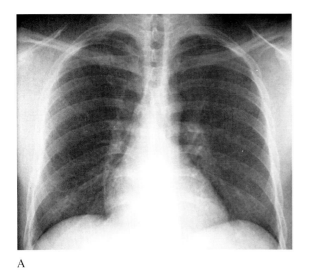

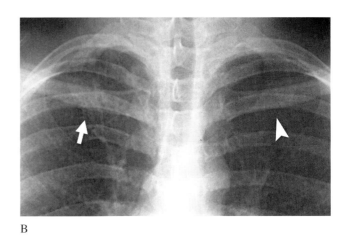

FIGURE 10   Patient 3C (see text for explanation).

Pulmonary lesions can also be missed in regions where there are overlapping skeletal structures (Table 2). In the region where the clavicle overlaps the anterior portion of the first rib and the posterior portion of the fourth rib, there is normally a region of increased opacity (Figure 10). In **Patient 3C,** the normal opacity where these three skeletal structures overlap is seen on the left (*arrowhead*). However, on the right, there is greater opacity in this region due to a superimposed lung lesion (*arrow*).

The patient had a persistent cough and was HIV positive. Even though the radiograph was interpreted as being normal, the patient was admitted to the hospital and found to have tuberculosis.

Cancers can also hide in the retroclavicular region (Figure 11). The lesion may initially be asymptomatic and incidentally discovered on a chest radiograph obtained for other reasons. If

the lesion is missed, the clinical outcome will be considerably worse when the patient returns weeks or months later with a larger symptomatic apical lung cancer. Calcification of the first costal cartilage can also cause an apparent opacity at the apex of the lung (Figure 5 and 6).

TABLE 2

Infiltrates that Can be Difficult to Find

Retrocardiac (left lower lobe)

Posterior costophrenic sulci—below and behind the left or right domes of the diaphragm

Retroclavicular

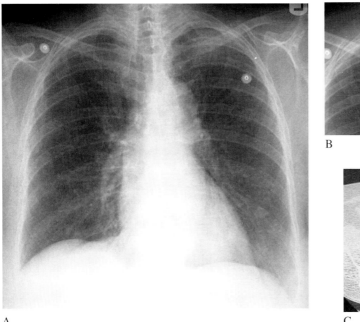

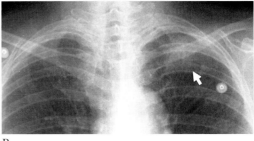

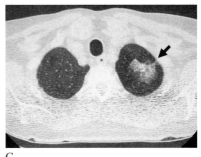

FIGURE 11   *A.* This chest radiograph was initially interpreted as normal. *B.* The patient was recalled to the ED the next day, when a retroclavicular lesion was recognized by the radiologist (*arrow*). *C.* CT revealed focal airspace filling (ground-glass opacification) due to a bronchoalveolar cell carcinoma (*arrow*).

Chest Radiology: Patient 4

Shortness of breath in a young woman

A 34-year-old woman presented to the ED with dyspnea that began three hours earlier.

The **ambulance call report** clearly captures the essence of the patient's clinical presentation (Figure 1).

Her chief complaint was: "I can't breathe." She had dull substernal chest pain. The ambulance crew noted that she was "hysterical and hyperventilating" and that she was taking birth control pills. During the previous month, she had had episodes of shortness of breath and dull chest pain.

She appeared ill, and the presumptive diagnosis was "rule-out myocardial infarction."

On arrival in the ED, she was anxious and in mild respiratory distress. Her vital signs were: blood pressure 120/80 mm Hg, pulse 104 beats/min, respiratory rate 24 breaths/min, and she was afebrile. Her oxygen saturation by pulse oxymetry was 88% on room air and 94% on 4 L/min oxygen administered by nasal cannula.

On examination, her lungs were clear to auscultation and her heart was rapid and regular without murmur, pericardial friction rub, or gallop. Her abdomen was not tender and there was no lower extremity edema or tenderness. She was overweight.

Blood tests, EKG, and chest radiographs were obtained. The EKG revealed sinus tachycardia and nonspecific T-wave flattening.

The chest radiographs were interpreted as being "normal" (Figure 2).

A bolus and infusion of heparin was administered by intravenous catheter.

- Should you order a chest radiograph in this patient?

- What are you looking for?

(There are three significant radiographic findings.)

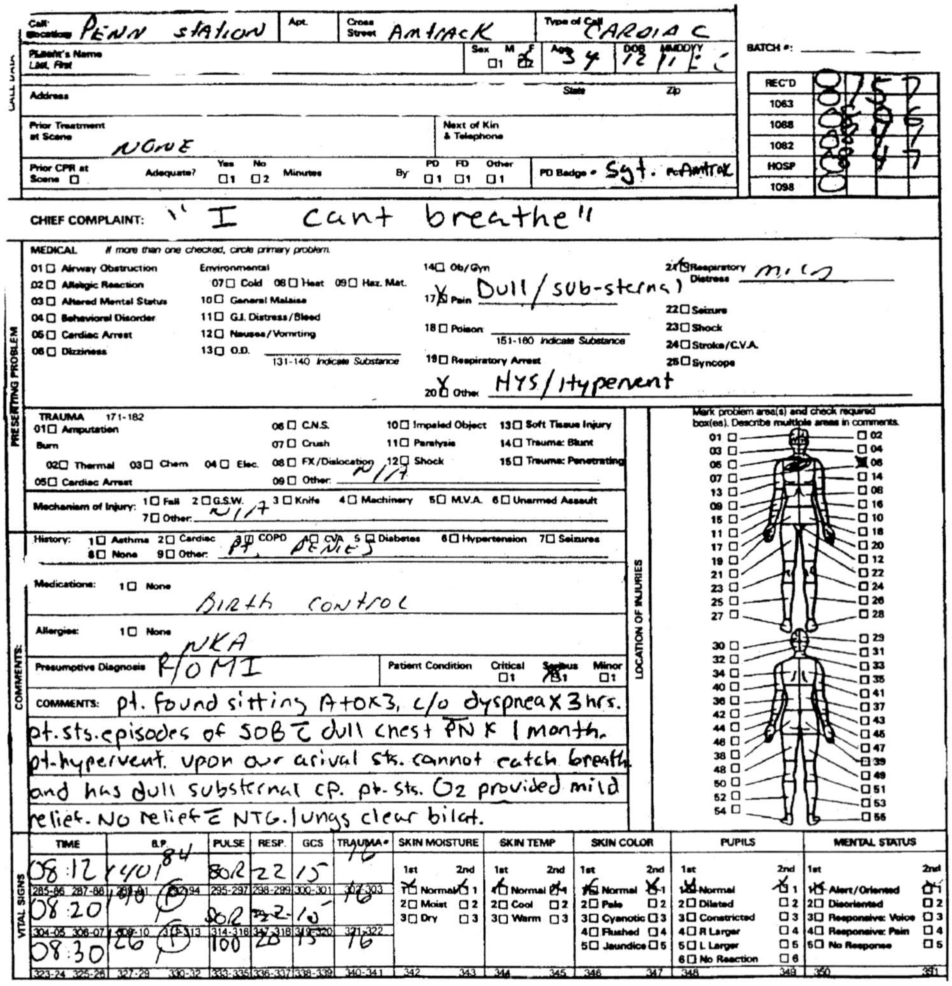

FIGURE 1

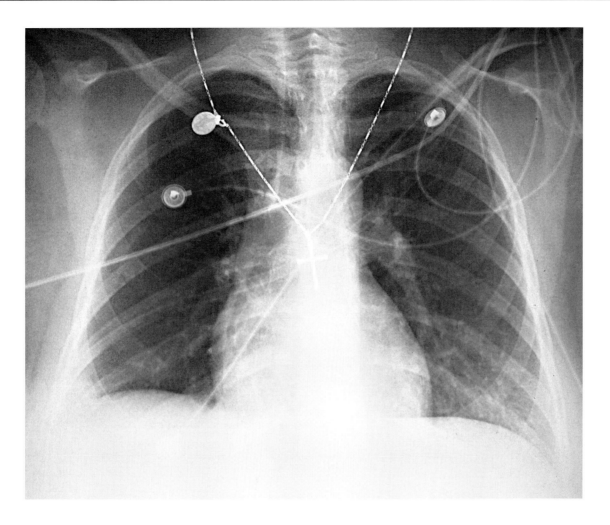

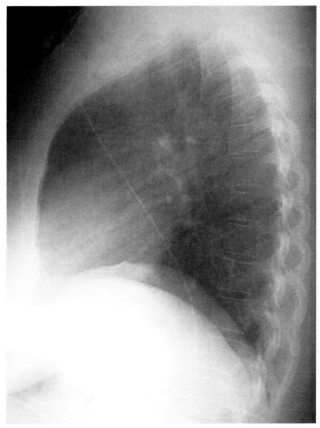

FIGURE 2

THINGS ARE NOT WHAT THEY APPEAR TO BE

Pulmonary embolism (PE) was the primary diagnostic consideration in this patient. Although the radiograph was initially interpreted as normal, there are three significant findings: (1) blunting of the right costophrenic sulcus; (2) relatively increased opacity at the left lung base; and (3) an enlarged left hilum (Figure 3).

Blunting of a costophrenic sulcus is most often due to a small pleural effusion, a finding that is sometimes seen in patients with PE (Figure 3, *arrowhead*). However, on the lateral view, the posterior costophrenic sulci are sharp rather than fluid-filled, as would be expected with a pleural effusion (Figure 4, *arrow*). In addition, pleural fluid generally creates a meniscus with a concave-up contour rather than convex, as seen on this patient's AP view. The opacity is therefore not a pleural effusion, but instead represents a peripheral region of airspace filling, i.e., an "infiltrate." It is not visible on the lateral view because it is small and has indistinct margins.

The **second** finding is **greater opacity of the left lung** compared to the right lung, particularly at the lung bases (Figure 3, *arrows*). Most often, focal increased pulmonary opacity is due to an infiltrate such as pneumonia. However, the lung markings on the left have a relatively normal appearance aside from some crowding of the vessels due to incomplete inspiration (only the ninth rib is visible at the right cardiophrenic sulcus). In addition, the lateral view does not show any increased opacity at the

lung bases as would be expected with an infiltrate (Figure 4). The difference in appearance of the left and right lung bases on the AP view in fact represents diminished lung markings on the right due to decreased blood flow to the right lung ("**oligemia**").

The **third** abnormality is **left hilar enlargement.** Hilar enlargement is most often due to a mass or lymphadenopathy. In this patient, however, the hilum has a tapering vascular appearance, rather than the rounded, lobular shape seen with hilar adenopathy (Figure 3, *asterisk*). This patient's hilar enlargement is due to increased blood flow to the left lung. In addition, the right hilum is nearly totally absent. This is due to markedly diminished blood flow to the right lung.

A **fourth** finding is also present. The **mediastinum is widened** and the **trachea is displaced** to the right—findings that are not expected with PE. Mediastinal widening is due to either enlargement of mediastinal structures such as the aorta or to increased mediastinal fluid, fat, or adenopathy. Mediastinal shift occurs either with loss of volume within the thorax on the side of displacement or with increased intrathoracic volume within the opposite side. However, **in this patient,** the apparent mediastinal widening and displacement are due simply to the patient's rotated positioning—the medial clavicular heads are displaced to the right of the spinous processes (Figure 3, *curved lines*). A **fifth** and final finding is that the patient is wearing a crucifix, a radiographic sign perhaps also of clinical significance.

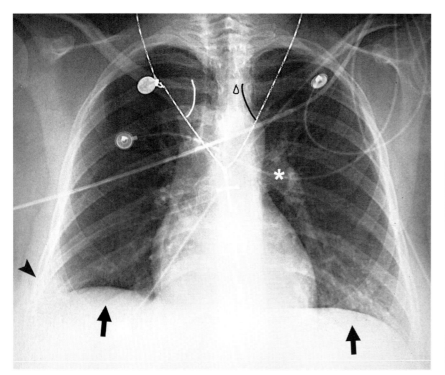

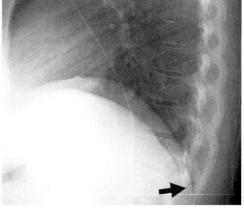

FIGURE 3   Patient 4—AP view (see text for explanation).

FIGURE 4   Lateral view.

How to Read a Chest Radiograph in Patients Suspected of Having a Pulmonary Embolism

Although chest radiography cannot establish the diagnosis of PE, it has several useful roles in patients suspected of having a PE (Table 1). When examining the radiographs, these findings should be sought (Table 2).

First, the classic finding is a relatively normal chest radiograph in a patient in "dire straits"—the presence of clear lungs is therefore suggestive of PE. **Second,** chest radiography can detect other conditions responsible for the patient's symptoms such as a pneumothorax, pulmonary edema, or pneumonia (although PE can cause focal airspace filling similar to pneumonia). **Third,** in some cases, there are radiographic abnormalities associated with PE, although most are nonspecific such as a small pleural effusion, plate-like atelectasis, or elevation of a hemidiaphragm (Table 2). A **fourth** role of chest radiography is to assist in the interpretation of lung scans, which are occasionally obtained instead of CT, or to select patients for lung scan rather than CT (see below).

Occasionally, there are radiographic findings that are characteristic of PE, although these may be subtle and difficult to identify with certainty (Table 2). Occlusion of a large pulmonary artery can produce **localized oligemia,** i.e., diminished lung markings in the region supplied by that vessel. In addition, the occluded pulmonary artery may be dilated proximally due to a large intraluminal thrombus, and then taper abruptly (the **knuckle sign**). Together, these two findings are termed the **Westermark sign.**

In this patient, there is oligemia of the right lung. This is most noticeable at the lung bases (in Figure 3, compare left to right). In addition, the left main pulmonary artery is markedly distended. Because the right pulmonary artery embolism was so massive, all of the blood flow was directed to the left pulmonary artery—a **"reversed Westermark sign."** (A pulmonary angiogram done later graphically demonstrates the reason for this finding.)

In some cases of PE, there is an area of **focal airspace filling.** This represents focal intraparenchymal hemorrhage due to ischemia or infarction of lung tissue that occurs distal to a large embolus. The area of hemorrhage is typically located at the lung periphery and appears as a wedge-shaped pleural-based opacity with its apex pointing toward the lung hilum (Figure 5). This has been termed "reversible infarction" because it clears rapidly over several days, reducing in size progressively like a "melting ice cube" without residual scarring. It is called a **Hampton's Hump** (Table 3) (AJR 1940;43:305).

In this patient, the opacity at the right costophrenic sulcus on the AP view is not visible on the lateral view and had a convex rather than concave-up contour. It is therefore not a pleural effusion, but instead is focal intraparenchymal hemorrhage—a Hampton's Hump (Figures 5 and 6).

TABLE 1

Role of Radiography in PE

1. Normal radiograph, patient in "dire straits"

2. Diagnose other disorders: pneumothorax, pulmonary edema, pneumonia*

3. Abnormalities suggestive of PE

4. Correlate with lung scan or assist in selecting lung scan versus CT**

*Focal airspace filling due to PE can mimic pneumonia

**Lung scan is more likely to be diagnostic in patients with normal chest radiographs

TABLE 2

Radiographic Findings in PE

- Normal
- Nonspecific abnormalities

    Small pleural effusion
    Plate like atelectasis
    Elevated hemidiaphragm

- Specific abnormalities

    Oligemia
    Pulmonary artery dilated } Westermark sign
    Hampton's hump

TABLE 3

Hampton's Hump

Peripheral—pleural-based opacity

Wedge-shaped—points to hilum

Homogenous—no air bronchogram

Resolves like a "melting ice cube," not patchy resolution, like pneumonia

Patient Outcome

Based on the patient's clinical presentation, intravenous heparin was administered. Her arterial blood gas on 4 L/min oxygen was pH 7.42, P_{CO_2} 28 mm Hg, and P_{O_2} 73 mm Hg. A **lung scan** was obtained and interpreted as "high probability" for PE. There was complete absence of perfusion of the right lung and relatively normal ventilation (a "super-high probability" lung scan) (Figure 7).

Pulmonary angiography was performed in anticipation of administering an intra-arterial thrombolytic agent. The pulmonary angiogram showed complete occlusion of the right main pulmonary artery and smaller emboli in the left (Figure 8). Because the patient remained hemodynamically stable and her

hypoxia was manageable using supplemental oxygen administered by nasal cannula, a thrombolytic agent was not administered. An **inferior vena cavagram** revealed a large thrombus in the left common iliac vein (Figure 9). Because this was a massive PE, an **inferior vena cava filter** was inserted to prevent another embolism, which could be fatal, before the iliac vein thrombus had time to stabilize.

The patient did well and was discharged from the hospital on coumadin anticoagulation. Her main risk factor was oral contraceptives that she had been taking for 13 years. A lung scan performed prior to discharge showed reperfusion of the right upper lobe.

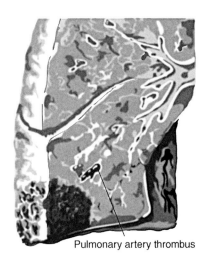

Pulmonary artery thrombus

FIGURE 5   Hampton's hump.
Intraparenchymal hemorrhage distal to an occluded pulmonary artery.

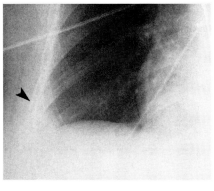

FIGURE 6   AP view detail.
Hampton's hump at right costophrenic sulcus (*arrow*).

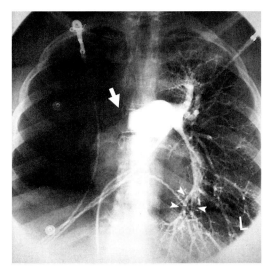

FIGURE 8   Pulmonary angiogram.
There is complete occlusion of the right main pulmonary artery (*arrow*) and multiple emboli in the left pulmonary arteries (*arrowheads*).

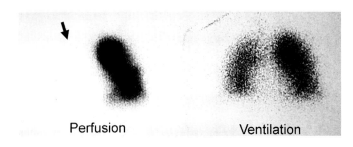

Perfusion   Ventilation

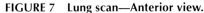

FIGURE 7   Lung scan—Anterior view.
There is no perfusion of the right lung (*arrow*), whereas ventilation is maintained—a ventilation/perfusion (V/Q) mismatch of the entire right lung.

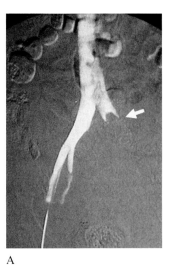

A

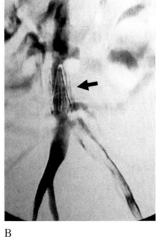

B

FIGURE 9   Inferior vena cavagram.
A. A thrombus occludes the left common iliac vein (*arrow*).
B. An inferior vena cava filter was inserted (*arrow*).

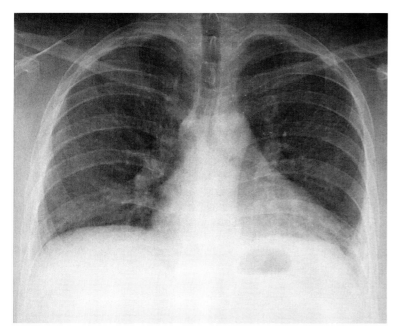 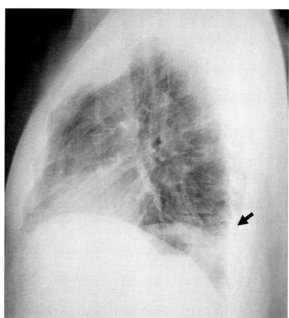

FIGURE 10   A   B

PATIENT 4B

A 30-year-old man presented to the ED with left upper back pain of 12 hours duration. It was sharp in quality and worse with inspiration. He had no cough or shortness of breath. He had a history of allergic asthma with exposure to cats and shrimp.

On examination, he was healthy appearing and in moderate distress due to his back pain. His blood pressure was 130/84 mm Hg, pulse 102 beats/min, respiratory rate 20 breaths/min, temperature 101.1°F (oral), and oxygen saturation 95% on room air. Inspiratory crackles were heard at the base of the left lung. He had left posterior thoracic and left costovertebral angle tenderness. Urinanalysis, which was performed because of the possibility of renal colic, showed no blood on dipstick analysis.

The **chest radiographs** showed a small infiltrate at the left base obscuring the posterior aspect of the left hemidiaphragm on the lateral view (Figure 10, *arrow*). The retrocardiac infiltrate was not visible on the AP view, but the patient had not taken a complete inspiration.

• **Should this patient be treated for community-acquired pneumonia with oral antibiotics and discharged from the ED?**

Although focal airspace filling is usually due to pneumonia, it may also represent focal intraparenchymal accumulation of blood or edema. Even though this patient had pleuritic chest pain and fever, which is suggestive of pneumonia, he did not have a cough productive of purulent sputum. Other disorders should be considered based on both the clinical and radiographic findings.

Further questioning revealed that four days earlier, the patient had driven his car from Georgia to New York City over the course of 24 hours, a risk factor for PE.

Because the patient had a history of an anaphylactic reaction to shell fish (facial swelling and wheezing), a **lung scan** rather than contrast CT was performed. The lung scan showed a single subsegmental perfusion defect with normal ventilation—a V/Q (ventilation/perfusion) mismatch in the left posterobasal segment. This was interpreted as "low probability" of PE.

• **Has PE been excluded in this patient?**

• **What should be done next?**

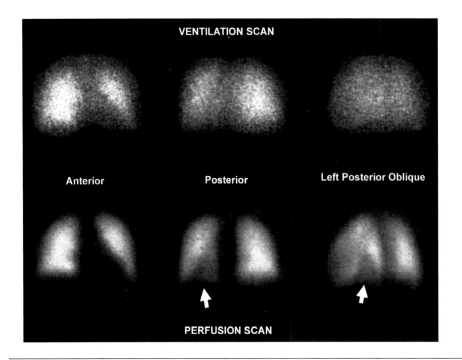

FIGURE 11   Lung scan (three views are shown).
A perfusion defect involves nearly the entire left posterobasal segment (*arrows*). Ventilation is normal.

One of the shortcomings of lung scan is that a "low probability" result has the connotation that PE is excluded. In fact, the incidence of PE in such patients is 16%—insufficient to exclude PE (PIOPED 1990). Only a normal perfusion scan can adequately exclude PE. In addition, lung scan interpretations can be variable. When this patient's scan was reread the next day, it was interpreted as "intermediate probability" because the V/Q mismatch involved nearly an entire segment (Figure 11). Furthermore, in patients without underlying lung disease, a V/Q mismatch is more predictive of PE than in patients with underlying lung disease in whom ventilation and perfusion defects are often due to the preexisting pulmonary disorder.

The patient was hospitalized and treated with heparin. To confirm the diagnosis of PE a **chest CT** was done following 12 hours of premedication with corticosteroids due to his history of anaphylactic-type allergies. The CT showed pulmonary emboli in the posterobasal and medial basal segmental pulmonary arteries (Figure 12A). The lung window images confirmed the airspace-filling infiltrate at the left lung base seen on the initial chest radiographs (Figure 12B and 10B).

Although **focal airspace filling** is usually due to pneumonia, it also occurs in patients with PE due to intraparenchymal hemorrhage. Therefore, finding what appears to be a pneumonia on chest radiography should not be considered as excluding PE, particularly when the infiltrate is peripheral (pleural based) and the patient's clinical presentation is not classic for pneumonia (cough productive of purulent sputum).

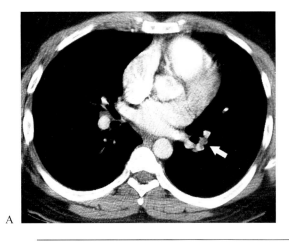

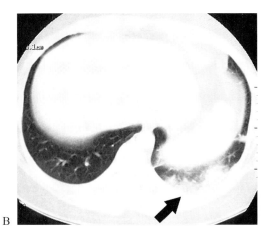

FIGURE 12   CT pulmonary angiogram.
A. Pulmonary emboli occlude left basal segmental pulmonary arteries (contrast-filling defects) (*arrow*).
B. A lung window image demonstrates the peripheral airspace-filling infiltrate which represents intraparenchymal hemorrhage in a patient with PE (*arrow*)—a "Hampton's hump." (Compare to Figure 10.)

Diagnostic Testing in Patients with Suspected Pulmonary Embolism

Lung scanning (ventilation/perfusion scintigraphy) was formerly the principal diagnostic test for PE. Its major shortcoming was that most patients (73%) had nondiagnostic results—low or intermediate probability (PIOPED 1990). One way to circumvent this is to combine clinical pretest probability of PE with lung scan results (i.e., a "low probability" lung scan would exclude PE in a patient with low pretest probability of PE). However, neither clinical assessment nor lung scan interpretation is sufficiently precise to reliably exclude PE.

Nonetheless, lung scans are useful in the 27% of patients who have either "high probability" or "normal" scans. Lung scans are currently obtained in patients who cannot undergo CT due to contrast allergy or renal insufficiency. In addition, in some protocols, lung scans are also used in patients with no underlying lung disease and normal chest radiographs, because lung scans are more likely to be diagnostic in these patients. In the absence of PE, the lung scan is likely to be "normal" (not "low probability"), which essentially excludes PE. In the presence of PE, the perfusion scan is likely to show a perfusion defect with normal ventilation (a V/Q mismatch), which is highly suggestive of PE, even when it involves only a single subsegmental region (Daftary et al. 2005).

DIAGNOSTIC TESTING STRATEGY   **Three recent developments** have advanced diagnostic testing in patients suspected of having PE: (1) **clinical prediction rules** to objectively assess pretest probability of PE; (2) sensitive *D-dimer assays* (rapid ELISA or immunoturbidimetric assays); and (3) helical **CT pulmonary angiography,** particularly using multirow detector CT (MDCT) (Figure 13).

The **diagnostic algorithm** begins with clinical assessment of the **pretest probability of PE.** One of three instruments (Wells, Geneva, or Carolinas criteria) can be employed (see Appendix), although they should be used in concert with the practitioner's clinical judgment.

If the clinical probability of PE is sufficiently low, then a normal **D-dimer** result excludes PE. However, the particular clinical prediction rule must be paired with the same D-dimer assay with which it was studied. This is because the frequency of PE in high-, medium-, and low-risk groups differs substantially among the different decision rules, and the sensitivity of the D-dimer assays also varies. For instance, patients with a high probability of PE using the Geneva criteria (original or revised) have a 70–80% incidence of PE, whereas using the Wells criteria, only 38% of high-probability patients have PE.

Using a highly sensitive D-dimer assay (rapid ELISA and possibly immunoturbidimetric), a negative D-dimer can exclude PE in low- and medium-risk patients (Perrier et al. 2005, Stein et al. 2007, van Belle et al. 2006). Whereas, using a lower sensitivity D-dimer assay (second-generation latex agglutination such as SimpliRED), a negative D-dimer can exclude PE only in low-risk patients (Brown et al. 2005, Kline et al. 2002, Wells et al. 2001). For example, lower sensitivity second-generation latex agglutination tests were used to exclude PE only in patients with a very low incidence of PE (1.3% in Wells et al. 2001, 4.6% in Kearon et al. 2006), or, in combination with a bedside

pulmonary function test in patients with a 12–13% incidence of PE (Brown et al. 2005, Kline et al. 2002, Rodger et al. 2006).

Use of highly sensitive D-dimer assays also varied among different investigators. Perrier (2005) used a rapid ELISA test to exclude PE in patients with up to 80% pretest probability of PE, whereas the Christopher investigators used the rapid ELISA or an immunoturbidimetric assay to exclude PE only in patients with up to a 37% pretest probability of PE (van Belle et al. 2006).

One additional question is whether the ready availability of highly sensitive but nonspecific D-dimer assays actually increases the use of diagnostic tests, namely CT, without increasing the number of cases of PE diagnosed (Kabrhel et al. 2006). Patients selected for D-dimer testing should therefore have at least a reasonable likelihood of having PE before D-dimer testing in initiated. A less sensitive but presumably more specific D-dimer assay, such as the Simpli-RED assay, would lead to fewer "false-positive" D-dimer results, but such a test could only be used to exclude PE in very low risk patients (<5% incidence of PE). In addition, D-dimer testing is more useful in relatively healthy outpatients seen in an ED setting. Debilitated, bed-bound, or hospitalized patients are likely to have a positive D-dimer assay simply on the basis of their underlying medical condition.

When the D-dimer assay is elevated or the patient's pretest probability of PE is too high to exclude PE using D-dimer alone, the patient should undergo **CT pulmonary angiography** (or lung scan). CT is highly effective at detecting PE, and the number of indeterminate (inadequate) studies is small (<5%). In some protocols, **CT venography** of the lower extremities and pelvis is included to increase the sensitivity of CT (Stern 2006, Loud 2001).

Whether a normal CT is adequate to exclude PE in all patients (i.e., CT sensitivity) has not been definitively established. Several studies have found that CT can miss pulmonary emboli that are limited to subsegmental pulmonary arteries, which occurs in approximately 6% of patients with PE (PIOPED 1990, Rathbun et al. 2000, van Strijen et al. 2005). However, these studies used single-detector helical CT scanners, and MDCT is better able to visualize subsegmental pulmonary arteries.

One way to assess CT's ability to exclude PE is by a "**clinical outcome trial.**" This differs from the traditional approach to evaluating a diagnostic test in which the test in question is

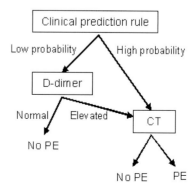

FIGURE 13 Diagnostic testing strategy for pulmonary embolism (Simplified; see text for explanation)

compared to a "gold standard" such as pulmonary angiography. In an *outcome trial,* patients whose CT scans do not show signs of PE are followed for a period of 3 months without being treated with anticoagulant medications. The absence of venous thromboembolic events, either PE or DVT, during follow-up means that a clinically significant PE had been excluded.

A number of studies found that fewer than 1% of patients with CT scans that are negative for PE had venous thromboembolic events on follow-up. This is equivalent to the results of pulmonary angiography, the traditional "gold standard." However, many of these studies had flaws that prevented definitive conclusions—too many patients were either lost to follow-up or excluded from the study, or too few patients were included to yield sufficiently narrow confidence intervals (Goodman et al. 2000, Qurioz et al. 2005).

More recent clinical outcome trials have used *MDCT* and incorporated diagnostic strategies that included clinical pretest probability assessment and D-dimer testing. Their results demonstrate the safety of withholding anticoagulation in patients with normal CT scans who are managed in accordance with the study protocol (Ghanima et al. 2005, Perrier et al. 2005, Stein et al. 2007, van Belle et at. 2006). However, one recent study (PIOPED II), found lower sensitivity for MDCT (90% for combined CT pulmonary angiography and lower extremity CT venography, and only 83% for chest CT alone), although reasons for this discrepancy are unexplained (Stein et al. 2006).

SUGGESTED READINGS

Chest Radiography for Pulmonary Embolism

Elliot CG, Goldhaber SZ, Visani L, DeRosa M: Chest radiographs in acute pulmonary embolism. *Chest* 2000;118:33–38.

Fraser RG, Paré JAP, Paré PD, Fraser RS, Genereux GP: *Diagnosis of Diseases of the Chest,* 4th ed. Saunders, 1999.

Stein PD, Terrin ML, Hales CA, et al.: Clinical, laboratory, roentgenographic, and electrocardiographic findings in patients with acute pulmonary embolism and no pre-existing cardiac or pulmonary disease. *Chest* 1991;100:598–603.

Tarleton GP, Manthey DE: The elusive Hampton's hump. *J Emerg Med* 2003;24:329–330.

CT for Pulmonary Embolism

Ghaye B, Nchimi A, Noukoua CT, Dondelinger RF: Does multi-detector row CT pulmonary angiography reduce the incremental value of indirect CT venography compared with single-detector row CT pulmonary angiography? *Radiology* 2006;240:256–262.

Goldhaber SZ: Multislice computed tomography for pulmonary embolism: A technological marvel. *N Engl J Med* 2005;352: 1812–1814.

Goodman LR, Lipchik RJ, Kuzo RS, et al.: Subsequent pulmonary embolism: Risk after a negative helical CT pulmonary angiogram: Prospective comparison with scintigraphy. *Radiology* 2000;215: 535–542.

Loud PA, Katz DS, Bruce DA, et al.: Deep venous thrombosis with suspected pulmonary embolism: Detection with combined CT venography and pulmonary angiography. *Radiology* 2001;219: 498–502.

Prologo JD, Gilkeson RC, Diaz M, Cummings M: The effect of single-detector CT versus MDCT on clinical outcomes in patients with suspected acute pulmonary embolism and negative results on CT pulmonary angiography. *AJR* 2005;184:1231–1235.

Quiroz R, Kucher N, Zou KH, et al.: Clinical validity of a negative computed tomography scan in patients with suspected pulmonary embolism: A systematic review. *JAMA* 2005;293:2012–2017.

Rathbun SW, Raskob GE, Whitsett TL: Sensitivity and specificity of helical computed tomography in the diagnosis of pulmonary embolism: A systematic review. *Ann Intern Med* 2000;132:227–232.

Stein PD, Fowler SE, Goodman LR, et al.: The PIOPED II Investigators: Multidetector computed tomography for acute pulmonary embolism. *N Engl J Med* 2006;354:2317–2327.

van Strijen MJL, de Monye W, Kieft GJ, et al.: Accuracy of single-detector spiral CT in the diagnosis of pulmonary embolism: A prospective multicenter cohort study of consecutive patients with abnormal perfusion scintigraphy. *J Thromb Haemost* 2005;3: 17–25.

Wittram C: How I do it: Ct pulmonary angiography. *AJR* 2007; 188:1255–1261

Protocols to Evaluate PE Using Clinical Probability Assessment, D-dimer assay and CT or Lung Scan

Anderson DR, Kovacs Mj, Dennie C, et al: Use of spiral computed tomography contract angiography and ultrasonography to exclude the diagnosis of pulmonary embolism in the emergency department. *J Emerg Med* 2005;29:399–404.

Brown MD, Vance SJ, Kline JA: An emergency department guideline for the diagnosis of pulmonary embolism: An outcome study. *Acad Emerg Med* 2005;12:20–25.

Daftary A, Gregory M, Daftary A, et al.: Chest radiograph as a triage tool in the imaging-based diagnosis of pulmonary embolism. *AJR* 2005;185:132–134.

Ghanima W, Almaas V, Aballi S, et al.: Management of suspected pulmonary embolism by D-dimer and multi-slice computed tomography in outpatients: An outcome study. *J Thromb Haemost.* 2005;3:1926–1932.

Kabrhel C, Matts C, McNamara M, Katz J, Ptak T: A highly sensitive ELISA D-dimer increases testing but not diagnosis of pulmonary embolism. *Acad Emerg Med* 2006;13:519–524.

Kearon C, Ginsberg JS, Douketis J, et al.: for the Canadian Pulmonary Embolism Diagnosis Study Group (CANPEDS): An evaluation of D-dimer in the diagnosis of pulmonary embolism: A randomized trial. *Ann Intern Med* 2006;144:812–821.

Musset D, Parent F, Meyer G, et al.: Diagnostic strategy for patients with suspected pulmonary embolism: A prospective multicentre outcome study. *Lancet* 2002;360:1914–1920.

Perrier A, Roy P-M, Sanchez O, et al.: Multidetector-row computed tomography in suspected pulmonary embolism. *N Engl J Med* 2005; 352:1760–1768.

Rodger MA, Bredeson CN, Jones G, et al.: The bedside investigation of pulmonary embolism diagnosis study (BIOPED). *Arch Intern Med* 2006;166:181–187.

Stein PD, Woodard PK, Weg JG, et al.: Diagnostic pathways in acute pulmonary embolism: Recommendations of the PIOPED II investigators. *Am J Med* 2006;119:1048–1055.

The PIOPED Investigators: Value of the ventilation/perfusion scan in acute pulmonary embolism: results of the Prospective Investigation of Pulmonary Embolism Diagnosis (PIOPED). *JAMA* 1990; 263:2753–2759.

van Belle A, Buller HR, Huisman MV, et al.: For the Writing Group for the Christopher Study Investigators: Effectiveness of managing suspected pulmonary embolism using an algorithm combining clinical probability, D-dimer testing, and computed tomography. *JAMA* 2006;295:172–179.

Clinical Decision Rules to Assess Probability of PE

Kline JA, Nelson RD, Jackson RE, Courtney DM: Criteria for the safe use of D-dimer testing in emergency department patients with suspected pulmonary embolism. *Ann Emerg Med* 2002;39:144–152.

Le Gal G, Righini M, Roy PM, et al.: Prediction of pulmonary embolism in the emergency department: The revised Geneva score. *Ann Intern Med* 2006;144:165–171.

Wells PS, Anderson DR, Rodger M, et al.: Excluding pulmonary embolism at the bedside without diagnostic imaging. *Ann Intern Med.* 2001;135:98–107.

Wells PS, Anderson DR, Rodger M, et al.: Derivation of a simple clinical model to categorize patients probability of pulmonary embolism. *Thromb Haemost* 2000;83:416–420.

Wicki J, Perneger TV, Junod AF, Bounameaux H, Perrier A: Assessing clinical probability of pulmonary embolism in the emergency ward: a simple score. *Arch Intern Med.* 2001;161:92–97.

Appendix: Clinical Prediction Rules for Pulmonary Embolism

Wells Criteria

Clinical signs of DVT	3
Alternate diagnosis less likely than PE	3
Heart rate >100	1.5
Immobilization or surgery within 4 weeks	1.5
Previous DVT/PE	1.5
Hemoptysis	1
Malignancy	1

Clinical probability:

Low	<2	1.3% PE
Moderate	2–6	16% PE
High	>6	38% PE

Used SimpliRED D-dimer assay to exclude PE in low-probability patients (Wells et al. 2001)

Unlikely	≤4	12% PE (van Belle) - 5% PE (Kearon)
Likely	>4	37% PE (van Belle) - 30% PE (Kearon)

Used rapid ELISA or immunoturbidimetric assay (van Belle et al. 2006), or SimpliRED (CANPEDS Kearon et al. 2006) to exclude PE in "PE unlikely" patients

Geneva Criteria

Age 60–79	1
Age (80	2
Previous PE or DVT	2
Recent surgery	3
Pulse >100	1
$PaCO_2$ <36 mm Hg	2
$PaCO_2$ = 36–39 mm Hg	2
PaO_2 <49 mm Hg	4
PaO_2 = 49–60 mm Hg	3
PaO_2 = 60–71 mm Hg	2
PaO_2 = 71–82 mm Hg	1
Platelike atelectasis	1
Hemidiaphragm elevation	1

Clinical probability:

Low	≤4	10% PE
Intermediate	5–8	38% PE
High	≥9	81% PE

(Wicki et al. 2001)

Low and intermediate risk patients are safe for exclusion of PE using rapid ELISA assay (Vidas D-dimer) (Perrier et al. 2005)

Revised Geneva Criteria

Age >65 years	1
Previous DVT or PE	3
Recent surgery or lower-limb fracture	2
Active malignancy	2
Unilateral lower-limb pain	3
Hemoptysis	2
Heart rate 75–94 beats/min	3
Heart rate ≥95	5
Signs of lower-limb DVT	4

Clinical probability:

Low	0–3	9% PE
Intermediate	4–10	28% PE
High	≥11	72% PE

(LeGal et al. 2006)

Carolinas Criteria (Kline)

Age >50 years or shock index (HR/SBP) >1
Unexplained hypoxemia (SO_2 <95%, nonsmoker, no asthma, no COPD)
Unilateral leg swelling
Recent surgery
Hemoptysis

Patients who are "safe" for D-dimer testing have none of the above criteria

Safe patients	13.3% PE
Unsafe patients	42% PE

Used bedside second-generation latex agglutination (SimpliRED) plus alveolar dead space measurement to exclude PE in "safe" patients.

(Brown et al. 2005, Kline et al. 2002)

Chest Radiology: Patient 5

Back pain in a middle-aged man

A 58-year-old man presented with back pain of two months' duration.

The back pain began after lifting heavy packages at the hotel where he worked as a porter. He had visited another doctor one month earlier for back pain, and naproxen was prescribed with some benefit.

Over the next two weeks, he noted difficulty walking due to weakness in his legs. He delayed coming to the hospital until a friend was able to drive him to the city from the upstate community in which he lived.

He had no prior history of low back pain. Five years earlier, he had a positive PPD skin test for tuberculosis, but was not treated. There was no history of intravenous drug use. He had no prior medical problems.

On examination, he was a slim but well-developed male in no distress (Figure 1). He was afebrile. Cardiac, pulmonary, and abdominal examinations were normal. On rectal examination, he had normal sphincter tone, his prostate was normal, and stool did not have occult blood.

On neurologic examination, there was mild wasting of his thigh muscles. Muscle strength testing showed 4+/5 hip flexion, 5−/5 knee flexion and extension, and 5/5 ankle plantar and dorsiflexion. On sensory examination, there was diminished light touch and pin prick below the waist and umbilicus. Position sense of his toes was normal. His reflexes were +3 patella and ankle bilaterally without clonus. Upper extremity reflexes were +2 bilaterally. His plantar reflex was flexion on the left, and withdrawal (or extension) on the right.

Chest, thoracic, and lumbar spine radiographs were obtained (Figures 2 and 3).

• What do they show?

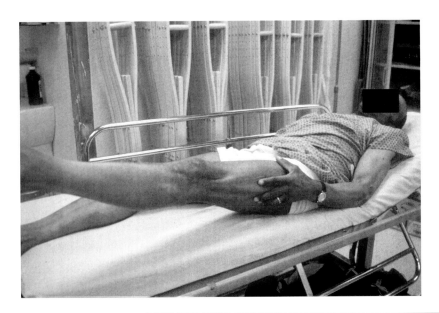
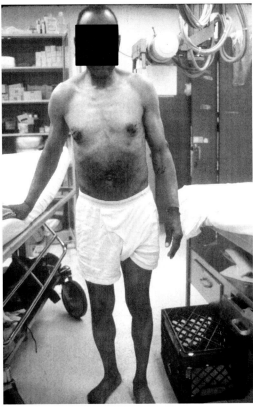

FIGURE 1   The patient had to use his hand to assist hip flexion. He could support his weight standing, but needed to hold on to a support while walking.

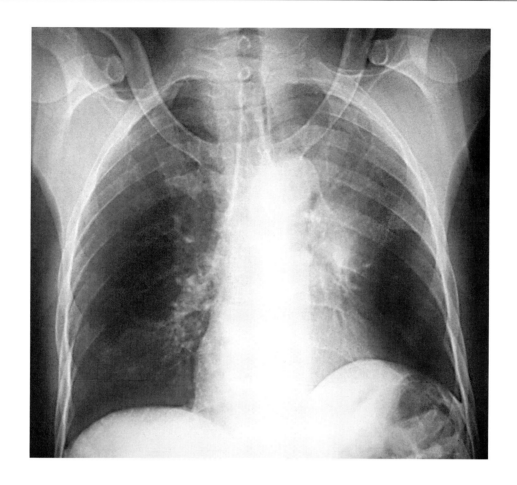

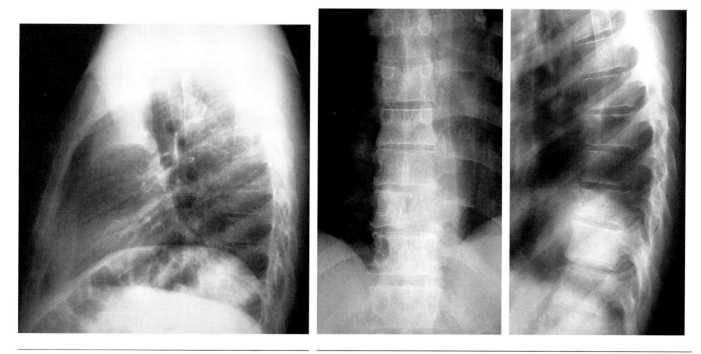

FIGURE 2 Chest radiographs.

FIGURE 3 Thoracic spine radiographs.

THE OWL'S EYES ARE CLOSED

This patient had bilateral lower extremity motor and sensory deficits indicative of a neurological lesion localized to the spinal cord. The brisk lower extremity reflexes reflect a spinal cord lesion (upper motor neuron), as opposed to a lumbar radicular or cauda equina syndrome (lower motor neuron). The loss of sensation below the T10–T11 dermatome suggests a lesion at this level of the spinal cord. (The associated vertebral lesion is located one or two levels above the spinal cord level).

The main diagnostic considerations include **spinal cord compression** due to a neoplasm (most likely metastatic) or infection (either pyogenic or tuberculous osteomyelitis) or, if an anatomical lesion is not found, transverse myelitis. The patient's spinal cord lesion is incomplete since it spares some sensory modalities, some muscle strength, and bowel and bladder function.

The **AP thoracic spine radiograph** shows a subtle but distinctive abnormality characteristic of metastatic vertebral disease, namely loss of the pedicles at T9. The normal appearance of a thoracic vertebra on a PA radiograph is likened to **an owl's face:** the pedicles being the **owl's eyes** and the spinous process the owl's beak. When the pedicles are eroded, the owl's eyes are missing (Figure 4).

The **lateral view** reveals erosion of the superior and inferior end-plates of T9. There is also loss of height of the T10 vertebral body with a bone outgrowth extending from the superior end-plate (Figure 5). The disk spaces are preserved. Lesions that are confined to the vertebrae and spare the disk are characteristic of **neoplastic disease.** In addition, neoplasia tends to involve noncontiguous vertebrae.

With **vertebral osteomyelitis,** infection begins in the intervertebral disk and adjacent vertebral body end-plates. Osteomyelitis therefore typically involves contiguous vertebrae and is associated with intervertebral diskspace narrowing (Figure 6). Nonetheless, definitive diagnosis usually requires a biopsy.

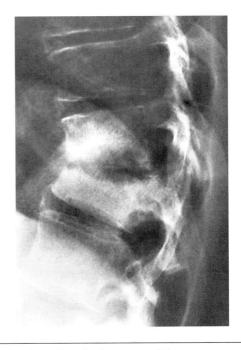

FIGURE 6   Vertebral osteomyelitis.

The intervertebral disk is eroded and there is involvement of adjacent vertebral body end plates.

[From Schwartz DT, Reisdorff EJ: *Emergency Radiolgy.* McGraw-Hill, 2000, with permission.]

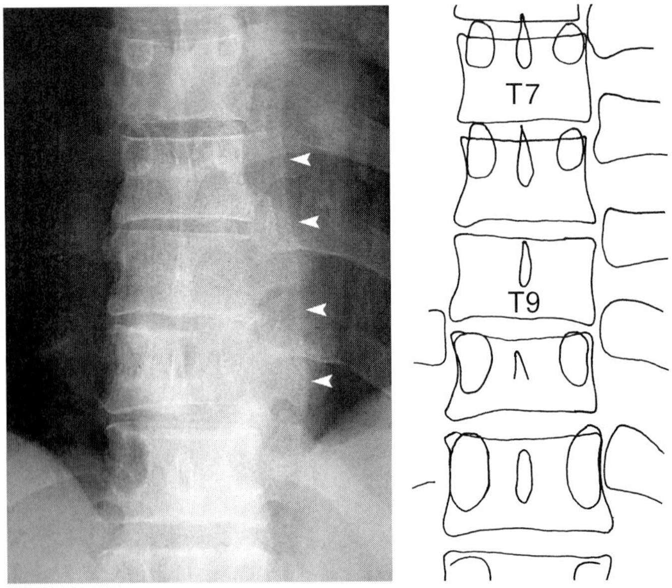

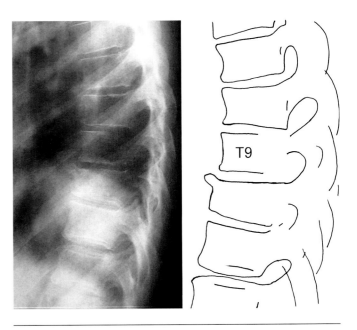

FIGURE 4   AP view of thoracic spine—Owl's face.

Normally, the pedicles and spinous process look like an owl's eyes and beak (T7 and T8). At T9, the pedicles are eroded—the "owl's eyes are closed." The left paraspinal line is visible and slightly displaced and convex due to a soft tissue mass adjacent to T9–10 *(arrowheads).*

FIGURE 5   Lateral view of thoracic spine.

There are erosions of the posterior portions of the superior and inferior end-plates of T9. At T10, there is slight loss of vertebral body height.

The patient's **chest radiograph** is notable for **increased opacity of the upper left lung** (Figure 2). Increased pulmonary opacity usually represents an "infiltrate" due to intraparenchymal fluid accumulation (e.g., purulent exudate in pneumonia). Since the left hilum appears prominent, this patient might have a postobstructive pneumonia due to a hilar mass. However, increased lung opacity may also be due to a reduction of intrapulmonary air, which is known as **atelectasis** (collapse of lung tissue).

Atelectasis has a variety of causes such as extrinsic compression of lung tissue adjacent to a mass or pleural effusion. However, the most clinically important cause of atelectasis results from obstruction of a major (lobar) bronchus by an endobronchial tumor, aspirated foreign body, or mucus plug. This is called **resorption atelectasis** because air trapped within the lung distal to the obstructed bronchus is eventually resorbed (Figure 7). Obstruction of a segmental or smaller bronchus usually does not result in atelectasis because interconnecting pores between airspaces maintain lung aeration.

Increased lung opacity does not always occur with lobar atelectasis. Instead, it depends on the quantity of retained fluid within the collapsed lung tissue. The radiographic hallmark of lobar atelectasis is **volume loss** (Table 1). The most direct sign of lobar atelectasis is the displacement of an interlobar fissure. Nonspecific signs of volume loss include shift of the mediastinum, elevation of the diaphragm, and compensatory hyperinflation of the remaining lung.

The margin of the collapsed lobe often has a sharp, well-defined border representing the displaced interlobar fissure. Upper and lower lobe collapse has typical radiographic appearances (see Figures 15 and 16 on p.50).

In this patient's radiographs, there are several indirect signs of volume loss: elevation of the left hemidiaphragm, shift of the trachea, and lateral and superior displacement of the left hilum (Figure 8). The opacity in the left perihilar region is not a hilar mass or adenopathy, but represents the displaced hilum and adjacent collapsed left upper lobe. No hilar mass is seen on the lateral chest radiograph (or subsequent CT).

The **lateral view** shows a well-defined triangular opacity at the anterior-superior mediastinum. This is the collapsed left upper lobe. Its well-defined margin represents the displaced left interlobar fissure (Figure 9).

Further imaging studies confirm these findings (Figures 10 to 13). Chest CT shows a collapsed left upper lobe due to obstruction of the left upper lobe bronchus. CT of the thoracic spine shows destruction of the 9th and 10th thoracic vertebral bodies and pedicles. A soft tissue mass extends from T8 to T10 with encroachment on the spinal canal. MRI reveals cord compression at T9. Abdominal CT reveals multiple metastatic nodules in the liver.

Bronchoscopy and biopsy revealed **non-small-cell lung carcinoma.** The patient was treated with radiation to the spine and lung. The left upper lobe reexpanded (Figure 14). Unfortunately, his lower extremity weakness did not improve.

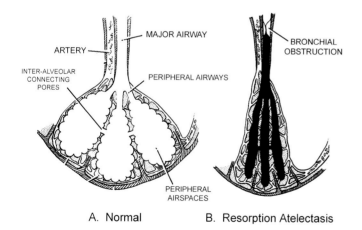

A. Normal   B. Resorption Atelectasis

FIGURE 7   Resorption atelectasis
Schematic representation of normal lung tissue (*A*) and the effect of obstruction of a major bronchus which causes *resorption atelectasis* (*B*).

Alveolar air is resorbed into the bloodstream and a small quantity of fluid remains in the collapsed airspaces.

[From: Fraser RS, Paré JAP, Fraser RG, Paré PD: *Synopsis of Diseases of the Chest*, 2nd ed. Saunders, 1994, with permission.]

TABLE 1

Radiographic Signs of Lobar Atelectasis

Displaced interlobar fissure (the principal sign)

Loss of aeration causing increased opacity (not always present)

Indirect signs of volume loss

   Elevated hemidiaphragm

   Mediastinal shift—trachea, heart, or hilum

   Rib cage narrowing

   Compensatory hyperinflation (of remaining lung)

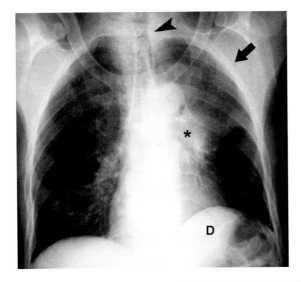

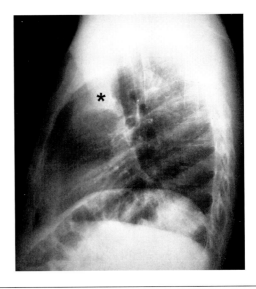

FIGURE 8   PA view showing left upper lobe atelectasis.
There is slightly increased opacity of collapsed left upper lobe (*arrow*). Signs of volume loss include tracheal shift (*arrowhead*), superior and lateral displacement of left hilum (*asterisk*), and elevated left hemidiaphragm (D).

FIGURE 9A   Lateral view.
The collapsed left upper lobe has a triangular shape (*asterisk*). The sharp inferior margin represents the displaced left major fissure.

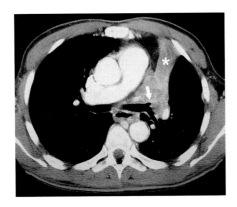

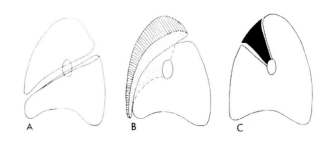

FIGURE 9B   Progressive collapse of the left upper lobe as seen on a lateral radiograph.
[From Felson B: *Chest Roentgenology*. Saunders, 1973, with permission.]

FIGURE 10   CT showing collapsed left upper lobe (*asterisk*) and occluded left upper lobe bronchus (*arrow*).

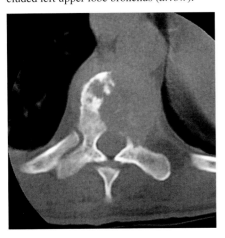

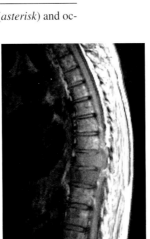

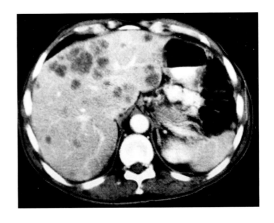

FIGURE 11   Erosion of T9 vertebral body and pedicle on CT correlates with the findings on the AP and lateral spine radiographs.

FIGURE 12   MRI showing spinal cord compression at T9 due to epidural extension of tumor. T10 vertebral body also has metastasis (decreased signal intensity).
Intervertebral disk spaces are preserved.

FIGURE 13   Multiple metastatic nodules in the liver.

In the vast majority of patients, low back pain following minor trauma such as lifting or bending is due to muscular strain or, occasionally, a herniated nucleus pulposus (intervertebral disk). Radiography is not needed in such cases.

Radiography is indicated if an underlying skeletal lesion such as malignancy or infection (osteomyelitis) is suspected. Patients at risk for such lesions include those with cancer known to metastasize to bone (lung, breast, prostate, renal, or thyroid), immunocompromised patients (AIDS), and injection drug users. Other patients at risk for osseous lesions include the elderly and patients with persistent pain of more that one or two

week's duration, fever, or any neurological signs or symptoms suggestive of spinal cord compression. Thoracic pain is more worrisome than lumbar pain because metastatic disease and infections tend to involve the thoracic region, whereas a muscular strain usually involves the lumbar region. If there are signs of spinal cord compression, emergency MRI and/or CT are indicated to assess the need for surgical decompression or radiation therapy.

Finally, nonmusculoskeletal causes of back pain must also be considered, including aortic dissection or aneurysm, renal diseases, or other intrathoracic or intra-abdominal disorders.

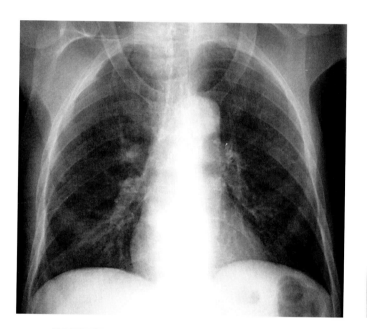 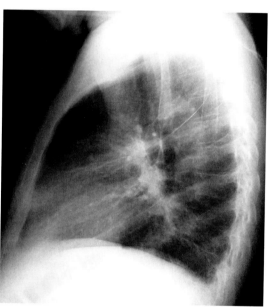

FIGURE 14 Follow-up chest radiograph after radiation therapy demonstrates re-expansion of the left upper lobe.

SUGGESTED READING

Spinal Cord Compression
Abdi S, Adams CI, Foweraker KL, O'Connor A: Metastatic spinal cord syndromes: Imaging appearances and treatment planning. *Clin Radiol* 2005;60:637–647.

Brandser EA, Burrows SL: Nontraumatic spine disorders: Part II. *Emerg Radiol* 2000;7:74–84.

Byrne TN: Spinal cord compression from epidural metastases. *New Engl J Med* 1992;327:614–619.

Darouiche RO: Spinal epidural abscess. *N Engl J Med* 2006;355:2012–2020.

De Michaelis BJ, El-Khoury GY: Nontraumatic spine disorders: Part I. *Emerg Radiol* 2000;7:65–73.

Jarvik JG: Imaging of adults with low back pain in the primary care setting. *Neuroimag Clin North Am* 2003;13:293–305.

Atelectasis
Felson B: *Chest Roentgenology.* Saunders,: 1973, pp:92–124.

Fraser RS, Paré JAP, Fraser RG, Paré PD: *Synopsis of Diseases of the Chest*, 2nd ed. Saunders, 1994, pp:165–198.

Gupta P: The Golden S sign. *Radiology* 2004;233:790–791.

Typical Patterns of Lobar Collapse (Atelectasis)

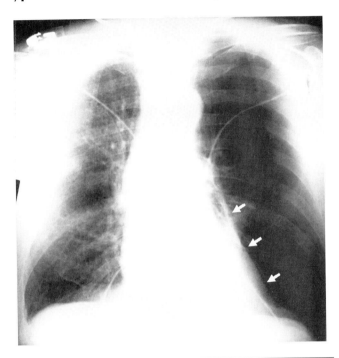

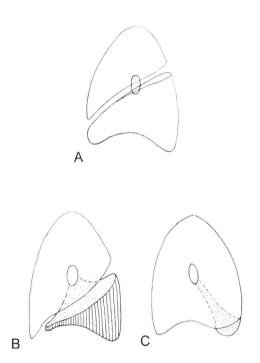

FIGURE 15A   Left lower lobe atelectasis.

The triangular-shaped collapsed lower lobe lies adjacent to the heart and mediastinum. Its sharp margin represents the displaced major fissure (*arrows*).

FIGURE 15B   Progressive lower lobe collapse as seen on a lateral view. The major (oblique) interlobar fissure migrates inferiorly and medially and thereby becomes visible on the frontal (PA) radiograph.

[From Felson B: *Chest Roentgenology*. Saunders, 1973, with permission.]

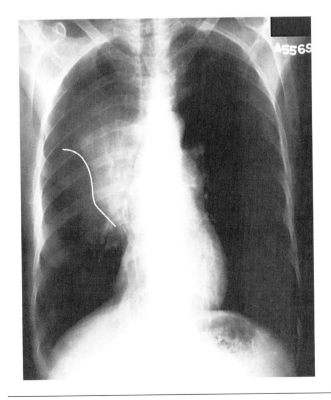

FIGURE 16   Right upper lobe atelectasis due to a hilar mass.

The concave lower margin of the collapsed right upper lobe and adjacent convex margin of the hilar mass form a reverse-S curve (*white line*). This is known as *Golden's reverse S sign*.

[From Schwartz DT, Reisdorff EJ: *Emergency Radilogy*. McGraw-Hill, 2000, with permission.]

Chest Radiology: Patient 6

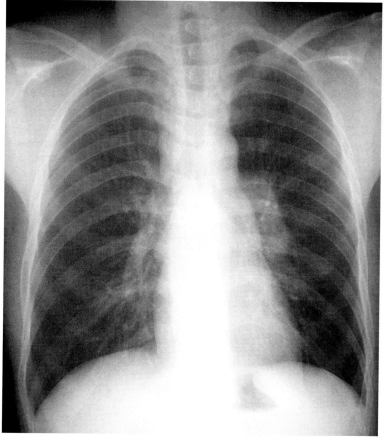 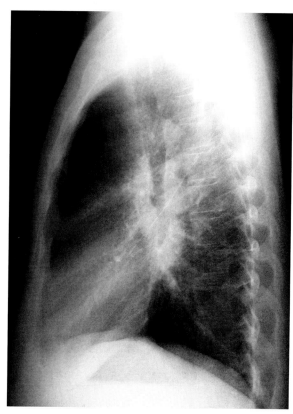

FIGURE 1

Cough and fever in young man

A 38-year-old man presented to the ED with fever, poor appetite, and a cough productive of yellowish sputum.

Over the previous two weeks, the patient noted progressive weakness and a 10-lb weight loss, worsening cough, and increasing fever and chills. He did not have chest pain or shortness of breath and had never previously been ill.

He smoked one pack of cigarettes per day and was formerly an alcoholic, but had not had a drink in over a month since being enrolled in a rehabilitation program. He had occasionally used cocaine in the past but had never used drugs intravenously. He also denied ever having had homosexual contacts. A tuberculin skin test two years earlier was positive, but he was not treated for this. He worked for a private refuse collecting company and, aside from a trip to North Carolina two years earlier,

had not traveled outside the New York metropolitan area. He had had no contact with wild or ill animals.

On **examination,** he was a slim young man in no acute distress. His vital signs were normal aside from a rectal temperature of 101.7°F. His oxygen saturation was 97% on room air. There were several nontender 1-cm lymph nodes in both axillae and inguinal regions. His lungs were clear and abdomen was nontender, without hepatosplenomegaly.

His white blood cell count was 6,000/mm^3, hematocrit 27.8% (MCV 88 μm^3) and platelet count 220,000/mm^3. Two hours after his arrival in the ED, his temperature rose to 104°F.

His chest radiographs are shown in Figure 1.

• What are the potential diagnoses in this patient?

THE ABNORMAL HILUM

In this patient's PA radiograph, you can compare an abnormal hilum on the left with a relatively normal hilum on the right (Figure 1). The hilum is often an area of difficulty in chest radiograph interpretation. Simply observing whether the hilum looks "big" is not a reliable means of determining whether it is normal or abnormal. Instead, accurate interpretation depends on an understanding of the normal anatomical features of the hilum and the changes that occur in various disease states.

The hila are composed of pulmonary arteries and veins, major bronchi, and lymph nodes. Normally, the *pulmonary arteries* make up most of the radiographic density of the hila (Figure 2). The *superior pulmonary veins* make a smaller contribution to hilar density, whereas the *inferior pulmonary veins* enter the left atrium inferior to the hilum and make no contribution to hilar density.

Although the absolute size of the hilum would seem to be a straightforward criterion of hilar enlargement, it is not reliable unless the enlargement is considerable. There are no definite measurements to use as a guide. When hilar enlargement is asymmetrical, one side can be compared to the other.

The **normal hilum** has a branching vascular appearance—successively dividing blood vessels gradually taper and diminish in radiopacity. The lower half of each hilum has greater vascular density than the upper half, in a proportion of two-thirds to one-third. This is because the lower halves of each lung are larger and receive more blood flow than the upper halves—a reflection of their conical shape (Figure 3).

There are thus **four criteria** used to access the hila: shape, radiopacity, proportunate size, and absolute size (Table 1).

Hilar abnormalities may be caused by vascular engorgement (arterial or venous), tumors, or enlarged lymph nodes (Table 2). When the hilum is enlarged by a **tumor** or **lymphadenopathy,** it has a rounded, lobular appearance and its radiopacity diminishes abruptly. Increased pulmonary vasculature causes hilar enlargement with a branching appearance. **Pulmonary venous distension** occurs with pulmonary venous hypertension due to left ventricular failure, mitral stenosis, or mitral regurgitation. In this case, the upper half of the hilum has greater than one-third of the vascular density because distended superior pulmonary veins contribute primarily to the upper zone of the hilum (Figure 2 and Figure 10 on p.57). **Pulmonary arterial distension** occurs with pulmonary artery hypertension (primary or secondary, e.g., COPD) in which the central pulmonary arteries are enlarged and then taper abruptly (see Figure 9 on p.56 and Introduction to Chest Radiology, Figure 6 on page 6).

Finally, **increased pulmonary blood flow,** which occurs with left-to-right intracardiac shunts (ventricular and atrial septal defects) and hyperdynamic circulation (high fever and pregnancy), causes enlarged hila in a branching vascular pattern associated with increased lung marking that extends to the lung periphery. Increased pulmonary blood flow must be two to three times greater than normal to be visible radiographically.

In Patient 6, the left hilum is enlarged and has a rounded lobular appearance with well-defined margins (Figure 4). This is due to *left hilar adenopathy*. The right hilum is normal. In addition, there is thickening of the right paratracheal stripe due to *right paratracheal adenopathy*. Normally, the right paratracheal stripe is less than 5 mm wide (Figures 3 to 5).

TABLE 1

Criteria Used to Evaluate the Hilum

1. **Shape**—A branching vascular appearance is normal

2. **Radiopacity**—Normally, gradually diminishes toward the periphery

3. **Proportionate size**—Two-third of the vascular density is in the lower portion of the hilum

4. **Absolute size**—Not reliable unless enlargement is considerable; compare left and right for symmetry

---

TABLE 2

Causes of Hilar Enlargement

Lymphadenopathy and tumors—Rounded, nonbranching structures in which the radiopacity abruptly diminishes at the margin of the tumor or lymph node

Pulmonary venous hypertension—Enlargement of the superior pulmonary veins causes increased vascular density in the upper half of the hilum; due to left ventricular failure, mitral stenosis or mitral regurgitation

Pulmonary arterial hypertension—Central pulmonary arteries are dilated and taper abruptly; due to primary pulmonary hypertension and lung diseases such as COPD

Increased pulmonary blood flow—Increased central and peripheral pulmonary vascular markings (peripheral lung markings become visible in the peripheral 1–2 cm of the lung); due to left-to-right intracardiac shunts and hyperdynamic circulation

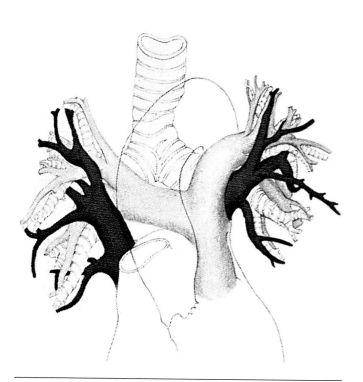

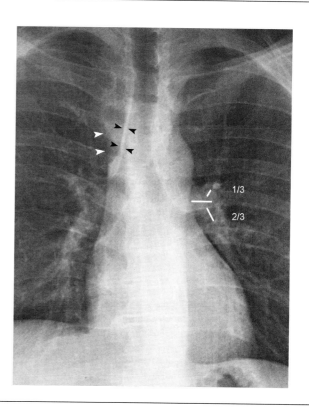

FIGURE 2   Hilar anatomy.
The pulmonary arteries (*light gray*) make up most of the hilar density. The superior pulmonary veins (*dark gray*) make a lesser contribution. The aorta is shown transparent and the superior vena cava (SVC) is cut away.
[From Novelline RA: *Squire's Fundamentals of Radiology,* 6th ed. Harvard University Press, 2004, with permission.]

FIGURE 3   Normal hila and mediastinum.
On the PA view, each hilum has a branching vascular appearance. One-third of the vascular density is in the upper half of the hilum and two-thirds in the lower half. This reflects the distribution of blood flow to the upper and lower halves of the lung.
The right paratracheal stripe is less than 5-mm wide (*black arrowheads*). The SVC casts a faint vertical shadow (*white arrowheads*).

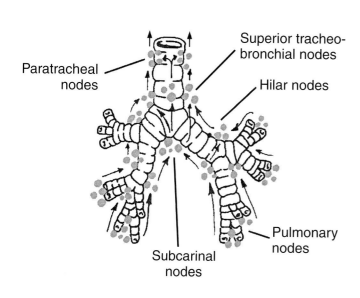

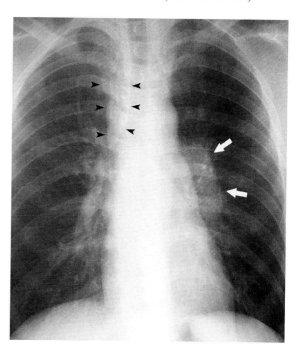

FIGURE 5   Tracheobronchial lymph node anatomy.
Patient 6 had enlarged left hilar lymph nodes as well as right paratracheal, subcarinal, and posterior tracheal adenopathy.
[From Pansky: *Review of Gross Anatomy,* 6th ed McGraw Hill, 1996, with permission.]

FIGURE 4   Hilar and mediastinal adenopathy—Patient 6.
The left hilum is enlarged and has a "lumpy" appearance (*white arrows*). In addition, right paratracheal adenopathy causes marked widening of the right paratracheal stripe (*black arrowheads*). (This widening is distinct from the shadow of the SVC, which is not visible here but is seen in Figure 3.)

Lateral Radiograph

The lateral view can be helpful in revealing hilar abnormalities, especially when the findings on the frontal view are equivocal. Correctly interpreting the lateral view requires knowledge of **normal hilar anatomy** (Figure 6).

The *trachea* is an air-filled structure that tapers and ends at the level of the hilum. The *right main pulmonary artery* is located anterior to the distal trachea. The *left mainstem bronchus* is seen end on as a round air-filled structure seen near the inferior end of the trachea. The *left main pulmonary artery* arches over the left mainstem bronchus and parallels the inferior border of the aortic arch. The *inferior pulmonary veins* enter the

left atrium just below the hilum. Normally, there is opacity anterior to the distal trachea (the right main pulmonary artery), but there should be aerated lung posterior and inferior to the distal trachea.

The lateral view is useful in confirming the presence of **hilar masses** or **adenopathy.** They appear as areas of increased opacity in locations where increased opacity is not normally seen, i.e., below the carina, posterior to the trachea, and anterior to the trachea above the hilum.

In Patient 6, the distal trachea and carina are encased in abnormal soft tissue—subcarinal and posterior paratracheal adenopathy (Figure 7).

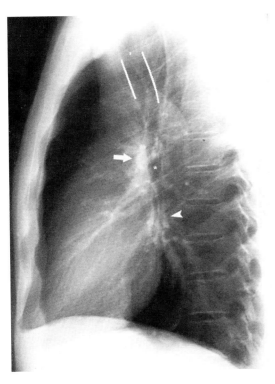

Figure 6A. Normal lateral view

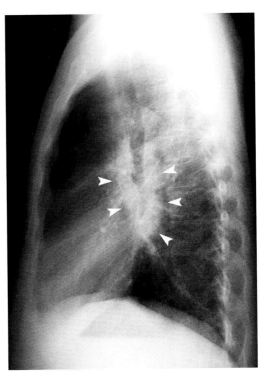

Figure 7. Patient 6—Lateral view

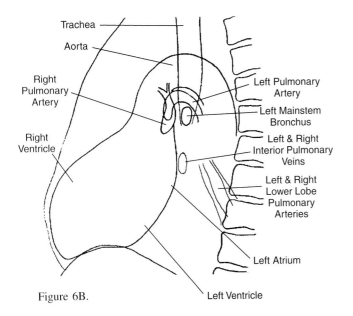

Figure 6B.

FIGURE 6   Normal hila and mediastinum—Lateral view.

The right pulmonary artery is anterior to the distal trachea (*arrow*). The left mainstem bronchus is seen end-on (*small asterisk*); its superior margin is highlighted by the arch of the left main pulmonary artery.

The inferior pulmonary veins are below the hila (*arrowhead*).

The tracheal walls are highlighted with white lines (A).

Posterior to the trachea are two vertically oriented lines —these are the bodies of the scapulae.

FIGURE 7   Hilar adenopathy—Lateral view—Patient 6.

The lateral view readily demonstrates hilar adenopathy which is seen as an area of increased opacity inferior, posterior, and anterior to the distal trachea encasing the distal trachea and carina (*white arrowheads*).

Differential diagnosis of hilar adenopathy

The differential diagnosis of **unilateral** or **asymmetric hilar adenopathy** includes infections (primary tuberculosis, fungi such as histoplasma, and bacteria such as tularemia or anthrax) and neoplasia (lymphoma or metastatic malignancy such as lung, breast, renal, melanoma) (Table 3).

Bilateral symmetrical hilar adenopathy is more likely sarcoidosis or viral infection (adenovirus or infectious mononucleosis), although the other disorders mentioned can also cause symmetrical hilar adenopathy (Figure 8).

Tuberculosis (TB) in adults is generally not associated with hilar adenopathy. In adults, TB is usually due to reactivation of prior disease and is characterized by multifocal cavitary infiltrates in the upper lobes, granuloma formation, and healing with fibrosis (see Patient 1, Figures 8 and 9 on page 21).

Primary TB, classically described in children, causes a lobar infiltrate indistinguishable from pyogenic pneumonia, and often hilar adenopathy. In this patient, the history of a positive tuberculin skin test two years earlier means that he had prior exposure to TB and reactivation TB would be expected. However, in patients with disorders of cell-mediated immunity such as AIDS, reactivation TB can have an appearance similar to primary TB (lobar infiltrate and hilar adenopathy).

In Patient 6, sputum specimens showed abundant acid fast bacilli. Despite his denying HIV risk factors, he was found to be infected with HIV and had a low CD4 T-cell count of 95/mm³. The patient was treated with a four-drug anti-TB regimen as well as antiretroviral medications. He became afebrile after four days of therapy.

TABLE 3

Hilar Adenopathy—Differential Diagnosis

BILATERAL ASYMMETRICAL AND UNILATERAL

Tuberculosis ("primary TB")

Fungal, atypical mycobacteria, viral, tularemia, anthrax

Metastatic or primary hilar tumor (bronchogenic carcinoma)

Lymphoma

Sarcoidosis, silicosis, drug reaction

BILATERAL SYMMETRICAL

Sarcoidosis—the prime diagnosis

Viral infection (adenovirus, mononucleosis)

Other causes mentioned above can be symmetrical

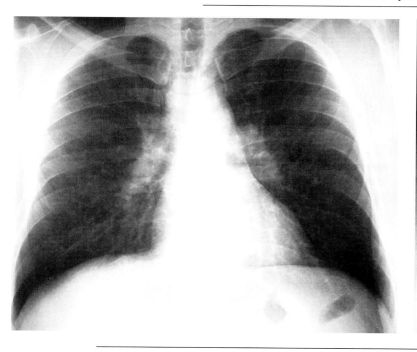
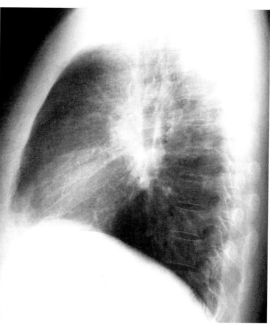

FIGURE 8   Bilateral symmetrical hilar adenopathy.

On the PA view, both hila have a lumpy, lobular appearance. The hilar abnormality can be more confidently identified on the lateral view, which shows the distal trachea surrounded by adenopathy.

This patient was a 25-year-old woman who presented to the ED with a persistent cough and low-grade fever. She was diagnosed with **sarcoidosis.**

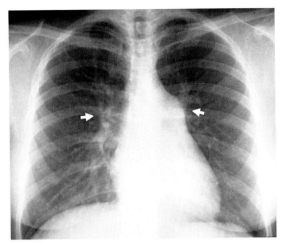

A. Initial PA view

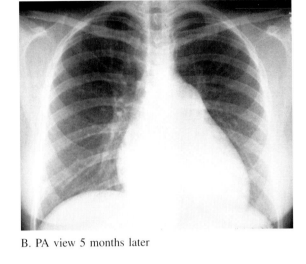

B. PA view 5 months later

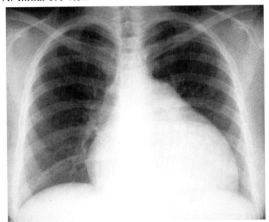

C. PA view 12 months later

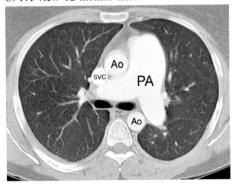

D. CT at time of initial admission

FIGURE 9   Primary pulmonary arterial hypertension.

A 24-year-old woman presented to the ED with exertional dyspnea, chest tightness, and lightheadedness for three weeks. She could walk an unlimited distance on the flat but became short of breath when walking up stairs. On the day of presentation, she nearly fainted while running up a flight of stairs.

On chest radiography (A), the central pulmonary arteries at the hila are prominent (*arrows*). The dilated left main pulmonary artery forms a bulge that obscures the aortic knob.

The patient was hospitalized. On further evaluation, there was no evidence of pulmonary emboli, valvular heart disease, or intracardiac shunts.

Over the subsequent year, there was progressive cardiomegaly (B and C), primarily due to right ventricular (RV) enlargement. The patient experienced increasing lower extremity edema due to RV failure. She was referred for heart/lung transplantation.

On CT (D), the main pulmonary artery is markedly dilated (PA). Normally, the diameter of the pulmonary artery is the same as the aorta (Ao). (SVC—superior vena cava).

On the lateral views (E–G), RV enlargement causes the heart to extend up more than half the anterior chest wall and progressively fill the retrosternal space (*asterisks*). The pulmonary arteries are prominent anterior to the distal trachea (*arrow*). The arch of the left main pulmonary artery is also markedly enlarged (*arrowhead*).

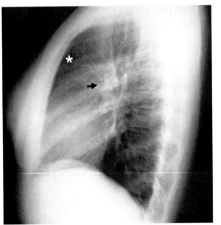

E. Initial lateral view

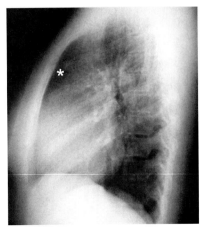

F. Lateral view 5 months later

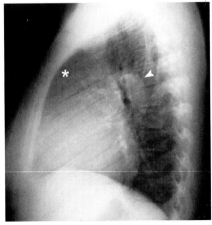

G. Lateral view 12 months later

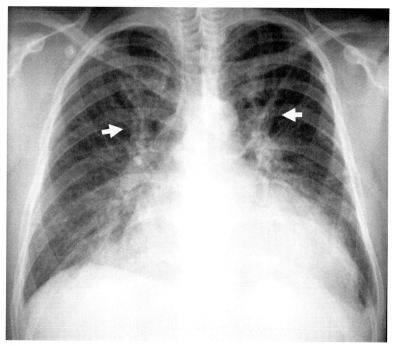

A

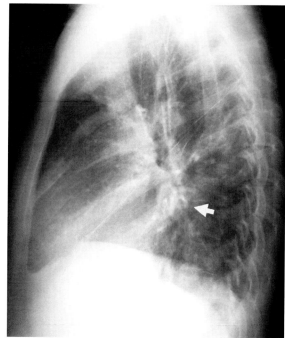

B

FIGURE 10   Pulmonary venous hypertension—Congestive heart failure.

(A) Left ventricular failure causes pulmonary edema in a patient with hypertensive heart disease. On the frontal (AP) view, hilar venous distension causes vascular prominence of the upper zones of the hila due to engorgement of the superior pulmonary veins (*arrows*).

(B) In another patient with mild congestive heart failure, increased opacity anterior to the distal trachea is due to hilar venous distension. The inferior pulmonary veins are distended and enter the left atrium inferior to the hila (*arrow*).

SUGGESTED READING

Busi Rizzi E, Schinina V, Palmieri F, et al.: Radiological patterns in HIV-associated pulmonary tuberculosis: Comparison between HAART-treated and non-HAART-treated patients. *Clin Radiol* 2003;58:469–473.

Earls JP, Cerva D, Berman E, et al.: Inhalational anthrax after bioterrorism exposure: Spectrum of imaging findings in two surviving patients. *Radiology* 2002;222:305–312.

Franquet T, Erasmus JJ, Giménez A, Rossi S, Prats R: The retrotracheal space: Normal anatomic and pathologic appearances. *Radiographics* 2002;22:S231–S246.

Goodman PC: Tuberculosis and AIDS. *Radiol Clin North Am* 1995; 33:707–717.

Harisinghani MG, McLoud TC, Shepard JO, et al.: Tuberculosis from head to toe. *Radiographics* 2000;20:449–470.

Havlir DV, Barnes PF: Tuberculosis in patients with human immunodeficiency virus infection. *N Engl J Med* 1999;340:367–373.

Jones BE, Ryu R, Yang Z, et al.: Chest radiographic findings in patients with tuberculosis with recent or remote infection. *Am J Respir Crit Care Med* 1997;156:1270–1273.

Keiper MD, Beumont M, Elshami A, Langlotz CP, Miller WT: CD4 T lymphocyte count and the radiographic presentation of pulmonary tuberculosis. *Chest* 1995;107:74–80.

McAdams HP, Erasmus J, Winter JA: Radiologic manifestations of pulmonary tuberculosis. *Radiol Clin North Am* 1995;33:655–678.

Miller WT, Miller WT, Jr: Tuberculosis in the normal host: Radiological findings. *Semin Roentgenol* 1993;28:109–118.

Perlman DC, El-Sadr WM, Nelson ET, et al.: Variation of chest radiographic pattern in pulmonary tuberculosis by degree of human immunodeficiency virus-related immunosupression. *Clin Infect Dis* 1997;25:242–246.

Saurborn DP, Fishman JE, Boiselle PM: The imaging spectrum of pulmonary tuberculosis in AIDS. *J Thoracic Imaging* 2002;17:28–33.

Chest Radiology: Patient 7

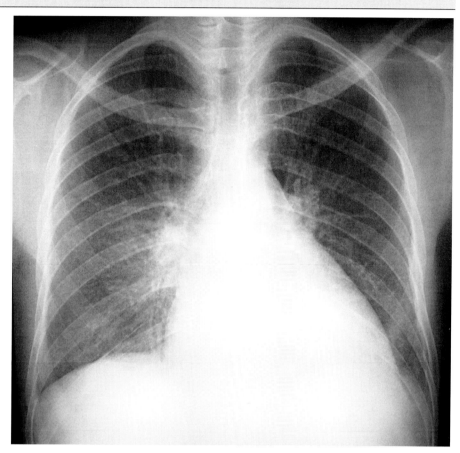

Cough with blood-tinged sputum in a young man with a history of alcoholism

A 36-year-old man presented to the ED complaining of a cough. He had been drinking heavily that night and did not have a place to stay.

On arrival in the ED, he was ill-kempt and lethargic, but arousable. His vital signs were normal: blood pressure 120/80 mm Hg, pulse 88 beats/min, respiratory rate 18 breaths/min, and temperature 98.8°F. His oxygen saturation was 97% on room air and finger stick blood glucose was 110 mg/dL. There was a laceration on his forehead that had been sutured two weeks ago, but no evident acute trauma. Because he had a cough that was productive of blood-tinged sputum, he was triaged to a respiratory isolation room. He stated that he had never had tuberculosis (TB), but a PPD tuberculin skin test had been positive in the past.

He was seen by a physician one hour later, at which time he was more alert. He stated that he had been assaulted with a stick two weeks previously and needed to have the sutures on his forehead removed. He also described a cough for about one week and shortness of breath when walking up stairs. He had similar symptoms several months earlier and had been prescribed medications that he was no longer taking. On examination, heart sounds were normal, and lungs were clear to auscultation.

For the past two months, he had been staying in a nearby homeless shelter or occasionally with a friend or on the street. He had had an HIV test in the past but did not know the result.

Chest radiographs were obtained (Figure 1).

FIGURE 1

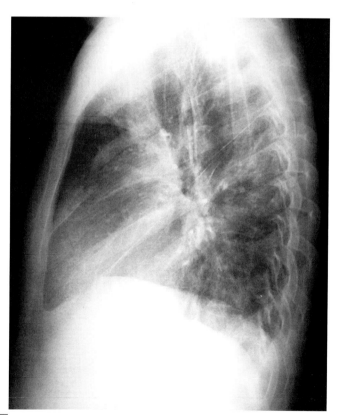

- What do they show?

WHEN THE HISTORY CAN HARM YOU

The major diagnostic concern in this patient, given his symptoms (cough and hemoptysis), history of a positive PPD skin test, and his social situation (alcoholism and homelessness), was tuberculosis (TB). With reactivation TB, the expected radiographic findings are an upper lobe infiltrate with cavitation and scarring. Alternatively, if the patient had primary TB or was immunocompromised, there could be segmental consolidation, **hilar adenopathy**, or a miliary pattern.

This case illustrates two problematic aspects of chest radiograph interpretation problematic—the **hila** and **lung markings**. There is great variation in the normal appearance of these structures, and detecting abnormalities can therefore be difficult.

Hilar Enlargement

In this patient, although the hila are prominent, they have a branching vascular appearance, not the "lumpy" appearance, characteristic of lymph node enlargement (Figure 2). In addition, the upper portions of the hila are enlarged relative to the lower portions. This is due to **pulmonary venous hypertension,** which causes dilation of the superior pulmonary veins. The enlarged *superior pulmonary veins* contribute mainly to the upper portions of the hila (Figure 3). The *inferior pulmonary veins* are also enlarged, but they enter the left atrium below the hila and therefore do not contribute to hilar density. They can be seen on the lateral view and appear as a region of increased opacity just inferior to the hila overlying the left atrium (the superior portion of the posterior heart border) (Figure 4). Pulmonary venous hypertension is usually due to left ventricular failure, mitral stenosis, or mitral regurgitation.

FIGURE 3   Hilar anatomy.

The superior pulmonary veins (dark gray) contribute to the vascular density of the upper zones of the hila. The pulmonary arteries are shown in light gray.

The superior vena cava is cut away. The aorta is shown as transparent.

[From Novelline RA: *Squire's Fundamentals of Radiology*, 6th ed. Harvard University Press, 2004, with permission.)

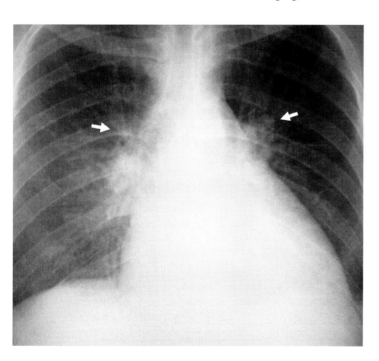

FIGURE 2   Upper zone hilar venous distension—Patient 7.

The superior pulmonary veins are distended, which causes vascular prominence in the upper zones of the hila (*arrows*).

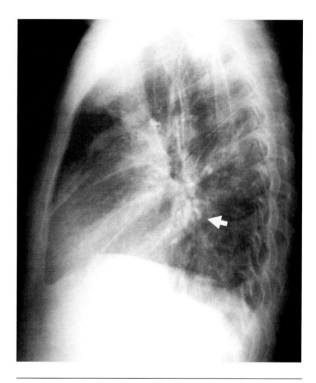

FIGURE 4   Lateral view—Patient 7.

Distended inferior pulmonary veins that enter the left atrium inferior to the hila (*arrow*).

Increased Interstitial Lung Markings

In this patient, the lung markings are abnormal. Normal lung markings are made up of pulmonary arteries and veins. The bronchi and interstitial connective tissues are not normally visible. In certain pulmonary disorders, the interstitial connective tissues are thickened by edema, inflammatory exudate, or neoplastic cells. When sufficiently thickened, interstitial tissues become visible on a chest radiograph.

Radiographically, **normal lung markings** appear as branching vascular structures with well-defined margins. They become finer and finer as they approach the lung periphery and disappear within 1 cm of the pleural surface. Because the lung is a three-dimensional structure, the branching blood vessels overlap and may appear to form a fine reticular pattern on a chest radiograph. In addition, a confluence of overlapping shadows can mimic a thin-walled cavity or cyst (Figure 5).

There is a wide range in the radiographic appearance of normal lung markings, and it can therefore be misleading to determine whether lung markings are abnormal based simply on whether they seem prominent or have a reticular appearance (Figure 5). To determine with greater assurance that the lung markings are abnormal, specific signs of abnormal interstitial tissues should be sought.

ANATOMY OF THE LUNG INTERSTITIAL TISSUES

Knowledge of the anatomy of the interstitial structures of the lung is necessary to identify abnormal lung markings. There are two main components: the **peribronchovascular tissues** that surround the bronchi (Figure 6) and pulmonary arteries, and the **septal connective tissues** that divide and support the lung parenchyma.

Septal tissues divide the lung into **lobules,** which are the smallest divisions of the lung that are completely surrounded by connective tissue. These lobules (formerly termed "secondary pulmonary lobules") are 1–2.5 cm in diameter and are most clearly delineated in the peripheral portions of the lung (Figures 7 and 8). The connective tissue walls of the pulmonary lobule are known as *interlobular septa*. The pulmonary veins and lymphatics course within the interlobular septa. The connective tissue surrounding the artery and bronchus within the lobule is known as *centrilobular connective tissue*. This later connective tissue component is continuous with the connective tissue that surrounds the large pulmonary blood vessels and bronchi—the *peribronchovascular connective tissue*.

The *alveolar walls* (also known as *intralobular septa*), are the third component of the lung interstitial tissues and are too small to be seen radiographically. However, thickened alveolar walls can sometimes be detected on CT, particularly high-resolution chest CT (HRCT).

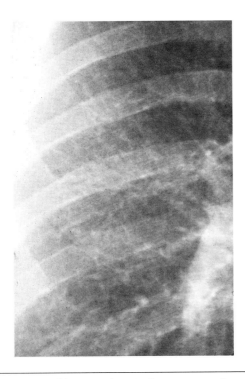

FIGURE 5   Normal but prominent pulmonary vascular markings.
Normal lung markings have a branching vascular appearance and disappear within 1 cm of the pleural surface. The overlap of blood vessels can have a reticular or cyst-like appearance.

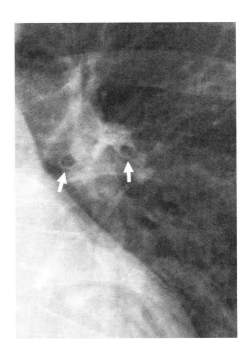

FIGURE 6   Normal bronchi seen on end.
The connective tissue making up the bronchial wall is normally "pencil-line" thin (*arrows*).

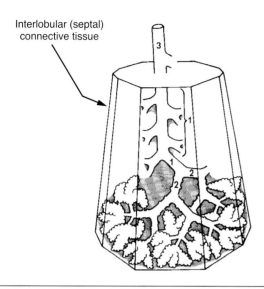

FIGURE 7 Components of a pulmonary lobule.

1. Terminal bronchioles
2. Respiratory bronchiole with surface alveoli
3. Lobular bronchus

Lung tissue distal to the *terminal bronchiole* (1) is an *acinus*. In this illustration, the *lobular bronchus* (3) gives off six terminal bronchioles, i.e., the lobule contains six acini. A pulmonary artery (not shown) accompanies the lobular bronchus.

[From Felson B: *Chest Roentgenology*. Saunders, 1973, with permission.]

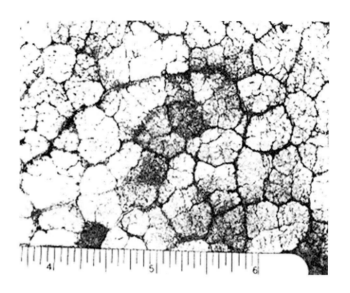

FIGURE 8 Surface of the lung showing pulmonary lobules.

[From Fraser RS, Colman N, Muller N, Paré PD: *Synopsis of Diseases of the Chest*, 3rd ed. Saunders, 2005, with permission.]

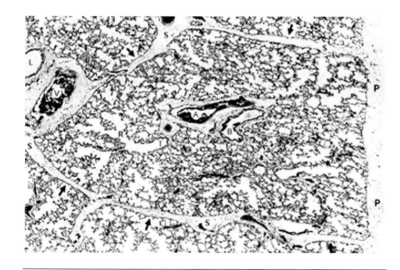

FIGURE 9 Histology of a pulmonary lobule.

Interlobular septal tissue (S, *arrows*) surrounds the parenchyma of the lobule and extends to the pleural surface (P).

In the center of the lobule is the *bronchovascular bundle* (lobular bronchus and artery, B and A) and the surrounding centrilobular connective tissue.

Venules (V) and lymphatics (L) are located within the interlobular septa. The terminal bronchioles (T) and respiratory bronchioles (R) lead to the alveolar air sacs.

[From Fraser RS, Colman N, Muller N, Paré PD: *Synopsis of Diseases of the Chest*, 3rd ed. Saunders, 2005, with permission.]

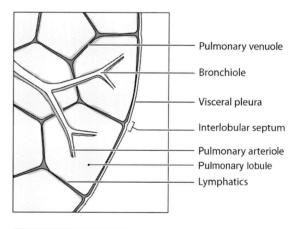

FIGURE 10 Schematic diagram of pulmonary lobular anatomy as depicted on CT.

Interlobular septa form the walls of the lobules.

At the center of each lobule are a bronchiole and pulmonary artery.

Peribronchovascular connective tissue surrounds the bronchi and pulmonary arteries extending into their divisions at the lobule where it forms the *centrilobular connective tissue*.

Pulmonary veins and lymphatics run within the interlobular septa.

(From Kazerooni EA: High-Resolution CT of the lungs. *AJR* 2001;177:501–519. Reprinted with permission from the American Journal of Roentgenology.]

RADIOGRAPHIC SIGNS OF THICKENED INTERSTITIAL TISSUES

To determine whether lung markings are abnormal, thickening of two specific structures should be identified—the **bronchovascular bundles** and the **connective tissue septa** (Table 1).

Thickening of connective tissues surrounding blood vessels makes the normally well-defined margins of lung markings appear indistinct and blurred. However, this radiographic finding can be difficult to identify with certainty.

Thickening of the connective tissues surrounding the bronchi is easier to recognize (Figure 6). When a bronchus is seen on end, thickening of the surrounding connective tissue appears as **peribronchial cuffing.** When seen from the side, thickened bronchial walls appear as two parallel lines that look like "tram tracks."

Thickening of the **septal connective tissues** has several radiographic appearances. **Thickened interlobular septa** are most readily seen at the lung periphery. They are perpendicular to the pleural surface and extend 1–2 cm inward from the pleura. These are known as **septal lines** or **Kerley B lines** (named after the radiologist who first described them).

Lung markings are normally not visible within 1 cm of the pleural surface. Lung marking that reach the pleural surface are therefore abnormal and represent thickened interlobular septa. Although usually associated with pulmonary edema, Kerley B lines also occur with other disorders that thicken the interlobular septa such as lymphangitic carcinomatosis (Figure 11).

When thickened interlobular septa (the same as Kerley B lines) are seen en-face, they form a **fine reticular pattern** and are referred to as **Kerley C lines.** Deeper within the lung, there are bands of connective tissue that radiate outward from the hila. When thickened, they become visible radiographically and are called **Kerley A lines.** These are usually seen in the upper lung zones.

Lastly, infiltration or edema of subpleural connective tissues appears as **thickening of the interlobar fissures.** This is usually best seen on the lateral view because both major (oblique) fissures as well as the minor (horizontal) fissure are visible. On the frontal view, only the minor fissure is visible. Thickening of the interlobar fissures is sometimes incorrectly referred to a "fluid in the fissures," even though, the fluid is subpleural in location.

In summary, when lung markings appear abnormally prominent, you should look for specific signs of interstitial lung tissue thickening to accurately identify increased interstitial markings. These signs are peribronchial cuffing, blurred vascular markings, thickened interlobular septa (Kerley B lines), a fine reticular pattern (Kerley C lines), Kerley A lines, and thickening of the interlobar fissures (Table 1; Figures 12 and 13).

TABLE 1

Signs of Increased Interstitial Markings

1. Peribronchovascular connective tissue thickening

   - Peribronchial cuffing (bronchus on-end)

   - "Tram tracks" (side view of bronchus)

   - Blurred vascular markings (indistinct margins)

2. Septal connective tissue thickening

   - Thickened interlobular septa (called Kerley B or septal lines)

   - Fine reticular pattern (Kerley C lines = superimposed Kerley B lines)

   - Kerley A lines (thickened deep intraparenchymal septal bands that radiate from the hilum in the upper lungs)

3. Thickened interlobar fissures (subpleural connective tissue thickening)

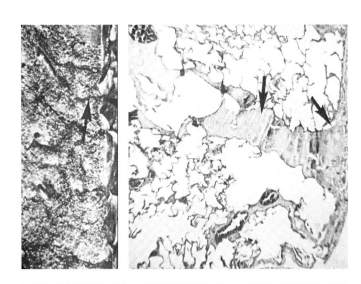

FIGURE 11   Thickened interlobular septa.

Thickened interlobular septa (*arrows*) in a patient who died of acute pulmonary edema—gross and microscopic anatomy.

[From Heitzman ER: *The Lung: Radiologic-Pathologic Correlations*, 2nd ed., Mosby-Year Book, 1984, with permission.]

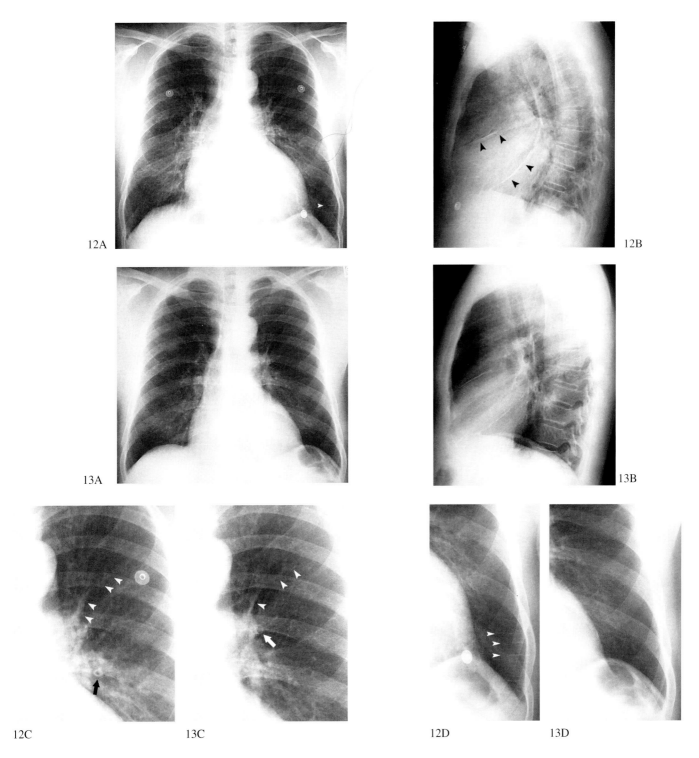

12A

12B

13A

13B

12C   13C   12D   13D

Mild interstitial pulmonary edema in a patient with poorly controlled hypertension and hypertensive cardiomyopathy

FIGURE 12 (A-D)   Initial radiographs showed subtle signs of interstitial pulmonary edema (increased interstitial markings).

FIGURE 13 (A-D)   Pulmonary edema resolved after several days treatment with diuretic medications.

Peribronchovascular edema—

      Blurred vascular margins (12C, *arrowheads*), later resolved (13C, *arrowheads*).

      Peribronchial cuffing (12C, *black arrow*), also resolved (13C, *white arrow*).

Septal lines (Kerley B lines) were present initially (12A and 12D, *arrowheads*), later resolved (13A and 13D).

Cardiac enlargement and **hilar venous distension** (upper zone vascular prominence) (12A), improved in 13A.

Cephalization—upper zone blood vessels were slightly distended (12C, *arrowheads*).

Lateral radiograph— Thickened interlobar fissures (subpleural edema) (12B, *black arrowheads*), later resolved (13B).

PATHOLOGY OF INTERSTITIAL LUNG DISEASES

Thickening of the interstitial tissues may be either smooth (linear) or nodular. **Smooth interstitial thickening** is seen radiographically as a *fine reticular pattern* and exhibits the radiographic findings mentioned above. It is usually due to interstitial edema, lymphangitic carcinomatosis or interstitial pneumonitis.

Nodular interstitial thickening creates a *nodular or reticulonodular pattern* on the chest radiograph. Nodular thickening is due to granulomatous or other inflammatory conditions or neoplastic infiltration (which usually forms large nodules or masses).

Finally, destruction of lung parenchyma can result in thin-walled cysts, large emphysematous bullae, or scarring and pulmonary fibrosis causing a *coarse reticular pattern* or *honeycomb pattern*.

CT, particularly HRCT using thin sections (1.5-mm slice thickness), can more reliably distinguish smooth from nodular interstitial thickening and localize nodules to the interlobular septa (perilymphatic nodules) or peribronchovascular tissues (centrilobular nodules). HRCT can also visualize other pulmonary parenchymal disorders including airspace disease and cysts. HRCT is used in patients with chronic diffuse lung diseases and can detect changes even when the chest radiograph is normal. Nonetheless, chest radiology is the mainstay in patients with acute illnesses such as pneumonia and pulmonary edema (Gotway et al. 2005, Kazerooni 2001).

DIFFERENTIAL DIAGNOSIS OF A FINE RETICULAR PATTERNS

There are many causes of **increased interstitial lung markings** (a fine reticular pattern). However, only two diseases are **acute**: interstitial pulmonary edema and interstitial pneumonitis (e.g., viral or mycoplasma pneumonia). Both of these disorders can also cause airspace filling. The clinical presentation generally helps differentiate these two disorders—cough and fever with pneumonia versus dyspnea and underlying cardiac disease with pulmonary edema.

Among the many causes of **chronic** increased interstitial marking, lymphangitic carcinomatosis, pulmonary lymphoma, collagen-vascular disorders, sarcoidosis, interstitial fibrosis, and pneumoconiosis (Table 2).

TABLE 2

Causes of Increased Interstitial Markings (Fine Reticular Pattern)

- Acute—often associated with airspace filling

    Interstitial pulmonary edema
    Interstitial pneumonitis—viral, mycoplasma

- Chronic interstitial lung diseases

    Neoplastic infiltration (lymphangitic carcinomatosis, lymphoma)
    Sarcoidosis
    Collagen-vascular diseases
    Interstitial pneumonitis
    Idiopathic pulmonary fibrosis
    Pneumoconiosis (silicosis, asbestosis)

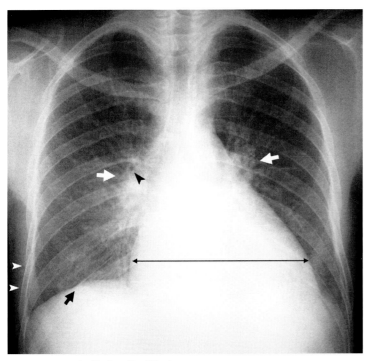

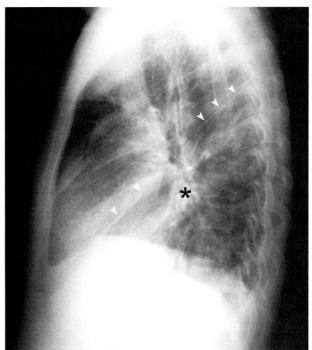

A. Patient 7—PA view   B. Patient 7—Lateral view

FIGURE 14   Patient 7—Interstitial pulmonary edema due to mild congestive heart failure.

A. PA view—There is perihilar haze and upper zone hilar venous distension (*white arrows*). Thickening of the peribronchial tissues causes peribronchial cuffing (*black arrowhead*). Faint septal lines (Kerley B lines) are visible at the lung periphery (*white arrowheads*). Thickening of subpleural connective tissues is seen in the inferior accessory fissure, an anatomical variant (*black arrow*). The heart is enlarged (*double headed arrow*).

B. Lateral view—The inferior pulmonary veins are dilated (*asterisk*). The right major (oblique) interlobar fissure is slightly thickened (*white arrowheads*).

Patient 7 Outcome

In this patient, there are several specific signs of **increased interstitial markings.** These include: peribronchial cuffing, blurred vascular markings, faint Kerley B lines and thickened interlobar fissures. This, in concert with moderate **cardiac enlargement** and upper-zone hilar venous distension, suggests that the patient has **interstitial pulmonary edema** due to mild CHF (Figure 14). In addition, there is increased opacity of the lung adjacent to the hila. This "*perihilar haze*" represents central perivascular edema and incipient airspace pulmonary edema. More pronounced airspace-filling edema causes the classic "*bat-wing*" pattern.

When the patient's medical record was reviewed, it was discovered that he had been admitted to the hospital two months earlier for dyspnea and was diagnosed as having CHF, presumably due to alcoholic cardiomyopathy. An echocardiogram showed severe diffuse left ventricular hypokinesis. Digoxin and furosemide were prescribed. During that admission, three sputum samples were collected that were negative for tuberculosis. When questioned about this, the patient stated that he had stopped his medications and did not keep his clinic appointment because he was feeling better. Because the patient was having only mild symptoms at the time of the current ED visit, his medications were restarted and he was encouraged to return for his clinic appointment. His scalp sutures were removed, thiamine was administered and he was referred to a program for alcoholism.

Summary

This case illustrates two fundamental points. First, it can be useful to review radiographs "objectively," without allowing their interpretation to be influenced by the clinical presentation of the patient. The initial reason for obtaining a chest radiograph in this patient was to diagnose tuberculosis. By considering only that diagnosis, the correct interpretation of the radiograph could be missed.

Second, a thorough history and physical examination are always essential, even when the patient is not forthcoming with the necessary information. One cannot rely on a cursory clinical evaluation because the patient's symptoms seem inconsequential or because he is "just drunk" or "only looking for a place to stay"—otherwise, it could be the history that harms you.

RADIOGRAPHIC STAGES OF CONGESTIVE HEART FAILURE

A sequence of radiographic findings occurs with progressively more severe CHF. There are **three stages** (Table 3). The heart is usually enlarged, although in a patient with acute myocardial infarction and no prior cardiac disease, the heart may be normal in size.

Cephalization

In very mild CHF (either acute or chonic), a subtle radiographic finding is *cephalization* of pulmonary blood flow. Normally, due to the effect of gravity, the blood vessels in the upper portions of the lungs are narrower than those in the lower portions of the lungs (on an upright chest radiograph). In mild CHF, there is a relative thickening of the upper lung vasculature known as cephalization (Figure 12C).

This finding can be difficult to identify with certainty. One technique is to look at the radiograph upside-down. Because we are accustomed to seeing the lower lung markings appear thicker than the upper lung markings, the disparity in caliper between the upper and lower vessels may be more apparent when the radiograph is viewed upside-down. When there is cephalization, abnormal thickening of the upper lobe blood vessels will make the lung markings in the upside-down radiograph seem to have a normal appearance in which thicker vessels are seen in the lower portion of the radiograph. When there is no cephalization, the small caliber of normal apical blood vessels will be even more apparent.

The pathophysiology of cephalization is uncertain.

Interstitial Pulmonary Edema

Increasing left ventricular failure and the concomitant rise in pulmonary venous pressure causes *interstitial pulmonary edema*. Radiographic manifestations include peribronchovas-cular and septal connective tissue thickening as illustrated above (Table 1 and Figures 12–14).

The **lateral view** can be helpful in identifying interstitial pulmonary edema when the findings on the frontal view are equivocal. Thickening of the **interlobar fissures** (subpleural edema) can be an important clue to the presence of CHF (Figure 12B). In addition, a small pleural effusion may be better seen on the lateral view in the posterior costophrenic sulcus.

Pulmonary venous hypertension also causes enlargement of the superior pulmonary veins in the upper portions of the hilum. Upper zone hilar venous distention should not be equated with "cephalization" (upper zone pulmonary vascular distension). Although both occur with CHF, cephalization represents abnormal thickening of the lung markings in the superior portions of the lungs on an upright radiograph.

Airspace-Filling Pulmonary Edema

With worsening left ventricular failure, pulmonary venous pressure increases and edema leaks into the alveoli, resulting in *airspace-filling pulmonary edema*. Classically, airspace filling in CHF has a central distribution that results in a "bat-wing" or "butterfly" patterns of pulmonary opacity (Figure 15). However, alveolar edema can also be diffuse, patchy, or even asymmetrical, like a pneumonia. Mild airspace filling appears as a "perihilar haze" (Figure 14).

In a patient with emphysema, pulmonary edema can look like pulmonary fibrosis (a coarse reticular pattern) because edema fills only the lung tissue remaining between enlarged emphysematous airspaces (see Figures 17 and 18 on p.70).

On physical examination, a patient with airspace-filling pulmonary edema will have râles on auscultation of the lungs. With interstitial edema, the lungs are clear to auscultation. Therefore, a chest radiograph can be more sensitive than physical examination at detecting pulmonary edema (see Patient 7 examination, page 59).

TABLE 3

Stages of Pulmonary Edema due to Congestive Heart Failure

1. Cephalization of pulmonary blood flow—Abnormal thickening of the upper lung vascular markings relative to the lower lung vasculature (PCWP 12–17 mm Hg)

2. Interstitial pulmonary edema (PCWP 18–24 mm Hg)

   Increased interstitial markings (see Table 1)
   Pulmonary venous hypertension—upper zone hilar venous distension

3. Airspace (alveolar) pulmonary edema (PCWP ≥ 25 mm Hg)
   Air-space filling—diffuse or patchy distribution
   "Bat-Wing" (central) distribution is typical
   Perihilar haze (early airspace edema)

PCWP = pulmonary-capillary wedge pressure (normal 5–11 mm Hg)

CLASSIFICATION OF AIRSPACE-FILLING PULMONARY EDEMA

Left ventricular failure causes **hydrostatic pulmonary edema.** Hydrostatic pulmonary edema can also be due to fluid overload such occurs as in patients with oliguric renal failure.

Permeability pulmonary edema (also termed "noncardiogenic pulmonary edema") is due to increased permeability of the alveolar-capillary membrane. This may occur either with or without **diffuse alveolar damage** (Gluecker et al. 1999, Ware and Matthay 2005). Permeability edema associated with diffuse alveolar damage is also known as "acute lung injury." It is due to either direct exposure of lung tissue to toxic agents or to circulating mediators of systemic inflammation. Permeability pulmonary edema without diffuse alveolar damage occurs with heroin-induced pulmonary edema and high-altitude pulmonary edema, both of which can resolve rapidly once the inciting agent is removed.

Permeability pulmonary edema causes diffuse or patchy airspace filling that is *not* central in distribution. The heart size is usually normal. In addition, the clinical scenario is also usually substantially different in patients with cardiogenic versus non-cardiogenic pulmonary edema (Figure 16) (Ware and Matthay 2005).

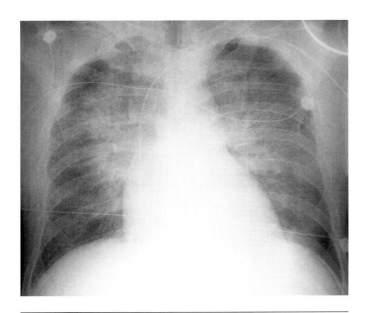

FIGURE 15   Cardiogenic pulmonary edema—Bat wing pattern.
The classic bat-wing appearance of airspace filling due to congestive heart failure has a central distribution.
[From Schwartz DT, Reisdorff EJ: *Emergency Radiology*. McGraw-Hill, 2000, with permission].

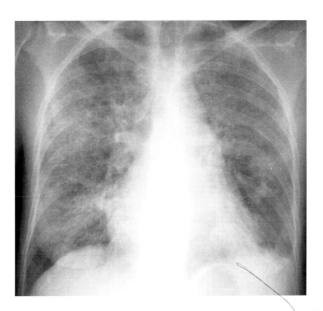

FIGURE 16   Noncardiogenic pulmonary edema.
Diffuse airspace edema without a central distribution in a patient following an overdose of heroin.

SUGGESTED READING

Brady WJ, Aufderheide T, Kaplan P: Cardiovascular Imagin. In Schwartz DT, Reisdorff EJ, eds *Emergency Radiology*, McGraw-Hill, 2000.

Felson B: *Chest Roentgenology*. Saunders, 1973.

Fraser RS, Colman N, Muller N, Paré PD: *Synopsis of Diseases of the Chest*, 3rd ed. Saunders, 2005.

Groskin SA: *Heitzman's the Lung Radiologic-Pathologic Correlations*, 3rd ed. Mosby-Year Book, 1993.

Hansell DM, Armstrong P, Lynch DA, McAdams P: *Imaging of Diseases of the Chest*, 4th ed. Mosby, 2005.

Muller NL, Colman NC, Paré PD, Fraser RS: *Fraser and Paré's Diagnosis of Diseases of the Chest, 4th ed.* Saunders, 2000.

Reed JC: *Chest Radiology: Plain Film Pattern and Differential Diagnosis*, 5th ed. Elsevier, 2003.

Wagner MJ, Wolford R, Hartfelder B, Schwartz DT: Pulmonary chest radiology. In Schwartz DT, Reisdorff EJ, eds. *Emergency Radiology*. McGraw-Hill, 2000.

Pulmonary Edema

Gluecker T, Capasso P, Schnyder P, et al.: Clinical and radiologic features of pulmonary edema. *Radiographics* 1999;19:1507–1531.

Ware LB, Matthay MA: Acute pulmonary edema. *N Engl J Med* 2005; 353: 2788–2796.

High-Resolution CT

Gotway MB, Reddy GP, Webb WR, et al.: High-resolution CT of the lung: Patterns of disease and differential diagnoses. *Radiol Clin North Am* 2005;43:513–542.

Kazerooni EA: High-resolution CT of the lungs. *AJR* 2001;177: 501–519.

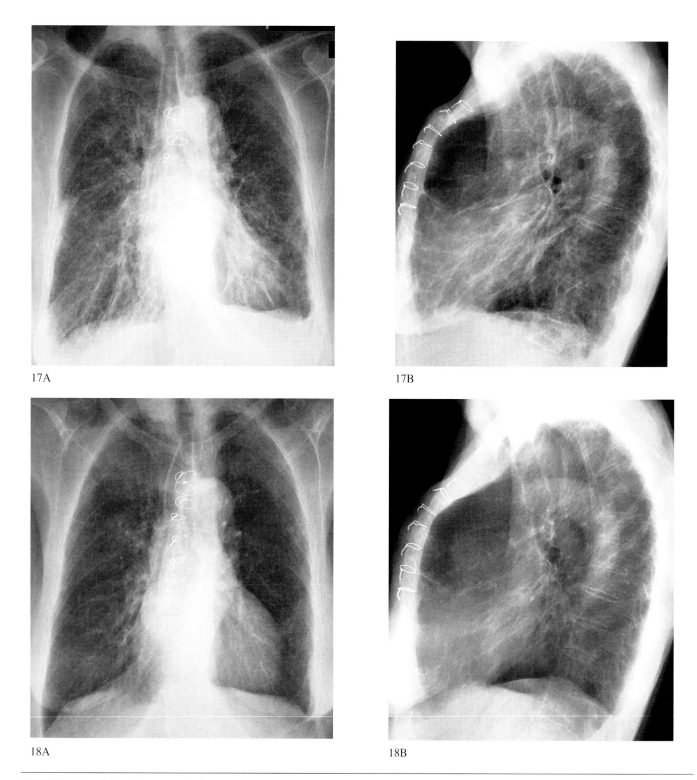

17A

17B

18A

18B

FIGURES 17 and 18   Coarse reticular pattern

A 73-year-old woman presented to the ED with progressive
dyspnea for two days. She had previously had coronary artery
bypass surgery.

The **initial chest radiographs** (Figure 17) show a **coarse
reticular pattern** suggestive of pulmonary fibrosis. There are
sternotomy wires from the patient's prior cardiac surgery. However, she also had a history of COPD. In patients with underlying emphysematous lung disease, pulmonary edema can produce a coarse reticular pattern.

Several days after being treated for CHF with diuretic medications, the coarse reticular pattern has largely resolved (Figure 18).

The underlying COPD is evident both before and after treatment. On the PA views (*A*), the lungs are hyperexpanded. On
the lateral views (*B*), the diaphragm is flattened and the AP
chest diameter is increased.

Chest Radiology: Patient 8

Weakness and nausea in a woman with a history of breast cancer

A 43-year-old woman with a history of metastatic breast cancer presented to the ED with three days of nausea, weakness, and abdominal discomfort.

Adenocarcinoma of the breast had been diagnosed two years earlier. At the time, she was treated with a mastectomy and adjuvant chemotherapy. Two months ago, the patient was found to have multiple nodular pulmonary metastases. She declined additional chemotherapy.

Over the past month, she noted an occasional nonproductive cough and dyspnea on exertion. Over the past three days, she had intermittent nausea, vomiting, and epigastric discomfort associated with poor oral intake. There was no fever, chills, chest pain, diarrhea, or constipation.

On examination, she was a well-developed and well-nourished female who appeared weak, but in no acute distress.

Her vital signs were—blood pressure 80/50 mm Hg, pulse 120 beats/min (irregular on palpation), respirations 24 breaths/min, temperature 99.2°F (rectal), SO_2 96% on room air; when standing, the patient felt lightheaded and her blood pressure was 75/50 mm Hg and pulse 130 beats/min

There were scattered râles on lung examination. The heart was normal, abdomen non-tender and stool was negative for occult blood. There was no edema of the lower extremities.

Two liters of normal saline were administered by intravenous infusion over two hours. Afterwards, the patient stated that she felt better and was able to tolerate oral liquids. Repeat vital signs showed her blood pressure to be 110/70 mm Hg, pulse 90 beats/min (irregular), respirations 20 breaths/min. There were no orthostatic changes.

Blood tests including complete blood count, electrolytes, renal and liver functions were normal.

Her chest radiograph and EKG are shown (Figures 1 and 2).

After intravenous rehydration, she felt well enough to go home.

• What would you do?

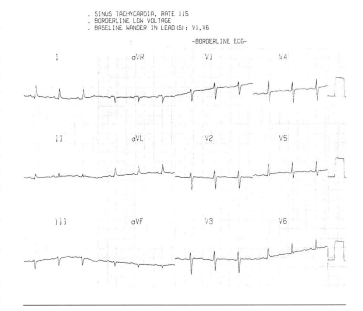

FIGURE 1

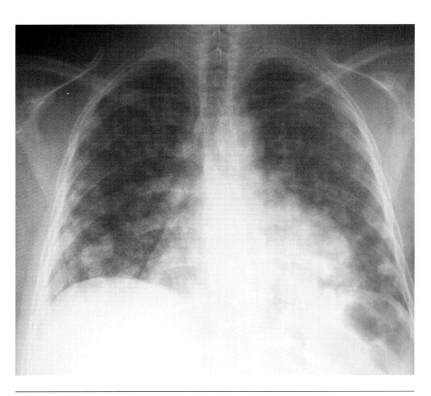

FIGURE 2

71

KUSSMAUL'S PULSE

This patient, with a known malignancy, presented with nonspecific abdominal symptoms. These were accompanied by hypotension and tachycardia which were felt to have been caused by dehydration from poor oral intake. The patient improved with intravenous rehydration.

The **chest radiograph** shows multiple nodular opacities scattered throughout both lungs (Figure 1). These metastases were noted on a chest CT performed one month earlier (Figure 3). However, finding one radiographic abnormality should not distract you from noticing others. A *systematic approach* to radiograph interpretation can help to prevent such an error (see Introduction to Chest Radiology). Her heart is significantly enlarged (see Figure 4). Cardiac enlargement can be due to either a dilated cardiomyopathy or a pericardial effusion. Although an effusion is often described as producing a globular-shaped heart, it is usually not possible to differentiate a pericardial effusion from cardiac enlargement on a chest radiograph. An echocardiogram can readily make this distinction.

A pericardial effusion does not generally cause symptoms unless it is at elevated pressure and impedes cardiac output, i.e., tamponade. The diagnosis of cardiac tamponade rests on clinical findings. Beck (1935) described a triad of signs consisting of (1) systemic hypotension, (2) elevated systemic venous pressure, and (3) muffled heart sounds. **Beck's triad** is typical of acute tamponade which may be due to abrupt intrapericardial hemorrhage from penetrating trauma, invasive cardiac procedures, or rupture of an ascending aortic dissection or myocardial infarction. The complete triad is rarely present.

When tamponade develops gradually, the presentation is different and often less dramatic. **Dyspnea** may be the predominant symptom. This is believed to be due to lung stiffening caused by interstitial edema perhaps at a microscopic level since the chest radiograph generally does not show pulmonary

edema. Hypotension may not be present; the patient may even be hypertensive. Tamponade thus has a spectrum of presentations ranging from circulatory collapse to mildly reduced cardiac output with symptoms of dyspnea and chest or abdominal discomfort.

The characteristic **chest radiographic appearance** of tamponade is an enlarged heart with clear lungs. When a pericardial effusion develops rapidly, as with penetrating or blunt trauma causing acute hemopericardium, the heart size may be normal (200 mL of fluid must accumulate before the heart would appear enlarged). However, most nonhemorrhagic subacute or chronic pericardial effusions causing tamponade are moderate to large (300–600 mL).

Jugular venous distension is a characteristic clinical finding and is important in distinguishing tamponade from hypovolemia as a cause of hypotension. However, neck vein distension might not be present with tamponade when there is concomitant hypovolemia. **Pulsus paradoxicus** is one key to the diagnosis of tamponade, and should be tested whenever tamponade is suspected. There is an accentuated fall in the systolic pulse pressure (>10 mm Hg) during inspiration. Nonetheless, pulsus paradoxicus is not present in one-quarter of patients with tamponade, particularly patients who are hypotensive.

Patient outcome

In this patient, pulsus paradoxicus was not tested, although it was likely present. The irregular pulse palpated in this patient (noted in the initial vital signs) was in fact due to disappearance of the radial pulse during inspiration—the *paradoxical pulse* described by Kussmaul in 1873. The pulsus paradoxicus is "paradoxical" not because of the fall in systolic blood pressure during inspiration but because the palpated pulse disappears or diminishes despite the continued presence of auscultated heart sounds.

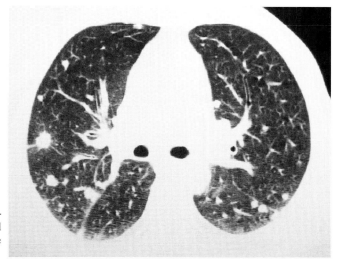

FIGURE 3 Chest CT performed one month earlier showing multiple pulmonary metastases.

The **EKG** showed sinus rhythm with "borderline" low voltage (QRS amplitude in the limb leads was <5 mm) suggestive of a pericardial effusion. *Electrical alternans*, a more specific sign of tamponade, was not clearly present. It occurs when there is a very large pericardial effusion in which the heart swings during cardiac contraction causing a beat-to-beat variation in the EKG axis (QRS amplitude). An EKG after pericardiocentesis showed increased voltage (Figure 5).

This patient's clinical presentation was initially felt to be due simply to dehydration; she did improve with rehydration. However, hypotension due to cardiac tamponade will also temporarily improve after fluid administration. Hemodynamic compromise would have recurred had her tamponade not been definitively treated by removing the pericardial effusion. Her abdominal symptoms remained unexplained although abdominal discomfort can occur with tamponade (Famularo 2005). In fact, her poor oral intake and hypovolemia were probably responsible for unmasking the underlying tamponade.

Echocardiography showed a moderate-size pericardial effusion (Figure 6). There was diastolic collapse of the right atrium and right ventricle indicative of tamponade. During pericardiocentesis, 600 mL of bloody fluid was removed. The systolic pressure increased from 80 to 110 and heart rate decreased from 120 to 70. The effusion reaccumulated the next day and surgery was performed to create a pericardial window. Biopsy and cytology showed adenocarcinoma.

The patient was treated with chemotherapy. She did well until five months later when the pericardial effusion reaccumu-lated, causing tamponade. The patient expired during that hospitalization.

Diagnosis of Pericardial Tamponade

Tamponade should be suspected in patients with hypotension or dyspnea, particularly patients at risk for pericardial effusions due to cancer, especially breast and lung cancer, uremia, rheumatologic disorders such as systemic lupus erythematosus or rheumatoid arthritis, and penetrating or blunt chest trauma. Suggestive clinical signs should be sought including jugular venous distension and pulsus paradoxicus, although these are not always present. The chest radiograph usually shows an enlarged heart. However, small effusions (100–200 mL) may not cause cardiomegaly even though they can cause tamponade when they accumulate rapidly or when the pericardial membrane is stiffened from fibrosis.

Echocardiography is the test of choice to detect a pericardial effusion and can also show signs indicative of tamponade (right ventricular and right atrial diastolic collapse). CT can detect a pericardial effusion and might be performed as the initial test when tamponade is not suspected and other disorders are being investigated such as pulmonary embolism or aortic dissection.

Treatment consists of emergency pericardiocentesis when there is hemodynamic compromise. Intravenous fluid administration can often be used as an initial temporizing measure.

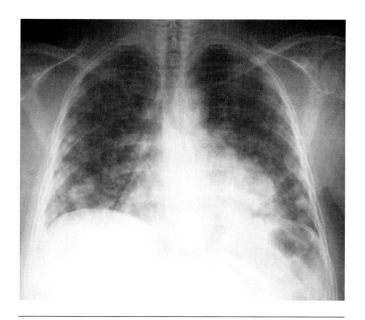

FIGURE 4A Initial chest radiograph showing multiple pulmonary metastases and an enlarged heart (cardiothoracic ratio >50%). The patient is rotated slightly to the right, which makes the right side of the heart appear larger.

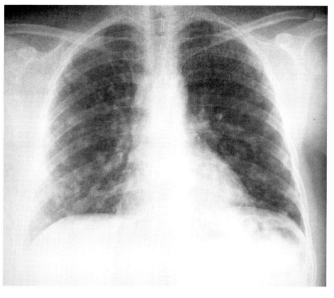

FIGURE 4B Chest radiograph 1 month before presentation showing a normal heart size. Pulmonary metastases were present.

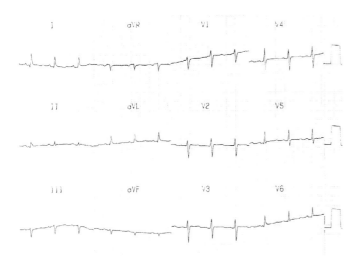

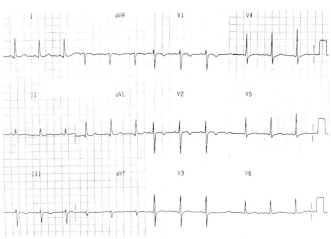

FIGURE 5A   Initial EKG showing low voltage in the limb leads (<5 mm). There is slight beat-to-beat variation in the QRS amplitude of leads V1, V4 and V5 (*electrical alternans*).

FIGURE 5B   EKG after pericardiocentesis and drainage of the pericardial effusion showing increased QRS amplitude.

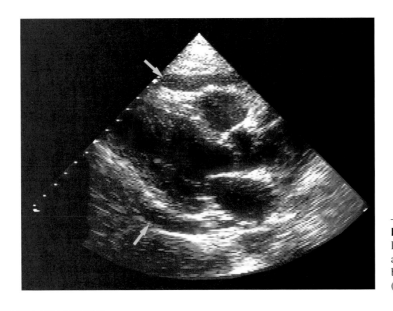

FIGURE 6   Echocardiogram (long axis left parasternal view) showing a moderate pericardial effusion (1 cm thickness) both anterior and posterior to the heart (*arrows*).

SUGGESTED READINGS

Beck CS: Two cardiac compression triads. *JAMA* 1935;104:714–716.

Blaivas M, Graham S, Lambert MJ: Impending cardiac tamponade, an unseen danger? *Am J Emerg Med.* 2000;18:339–340.

Brown J, MacKinnon D, King A, Vanderbush E: Elevated arterial blood pressure in cardiac tamponade. *New Engl J Med* 1992;327: 463–466.

Eisenberg MJ, Dunn MM, Kanth N, et al.: Diagnostic value of chest radiology for pericardial effusion. *J Am Coll Cardiol* 1993;22: 588–593.

Eisenberg MJ, Romeral LM, Heidenreich PA, et al.: The diagnosis of pericardial effusion and cardiac tamponade by 12-lead ECG. *Chest* 1996;110:318–324. Comment: 308–310.

Famularo G: Atypical cardiac tamponade mimicking acute abdomen. *Am J Emerg Med* 2005;23:706–707.

Jabr FI: Intractable vomiting as the initial presentation of pericardial effusion. *Am J Emerg Med* 2004;22:624.

Jang T, Aubin C, Naunheim R, Char D: Letter. *Ann Emerg Med* 2005; 45:460.

Longo MJ, Jaffe CC: Electrical alternans. *New Engl J Med* 1999;341: 2060.

Paelinck B, Dendale A: Cardiac tamponade in Dressler's syndrome. *New Engl J Med* 2003;348:e8.

Piskoti EI, Adams CP: The utility of ultrasound in a case of pericardial tamponade. *J Emerg Med* 2002;22:411–414.

Price AS, Leech SJ, Sierzenski PR: Impending cardiac tamponade: A case report highlighting the value of bedside echocardiography. *J Emerg Med* 2006;30:415–419.

Roy CL; Minor MA; Brookhart MA; Choudhry NK; Does this patient with a pericardial effusion have cardiac tamponade? *JAMA* 2007;297:1810–1818.

Spodick DH: Acute cardiac tamponade. *New Engl J Med* 2003;349: 684–690.

Wu LA, Nishimura RA: Pulsus paradoxicus. *New Engl J Med* 2003; 349:666.

Zahger D, Milgalter E: A broken heart. *New Engl J Med* 1996;334: 319–321.

Chest Radiology: Patient 9

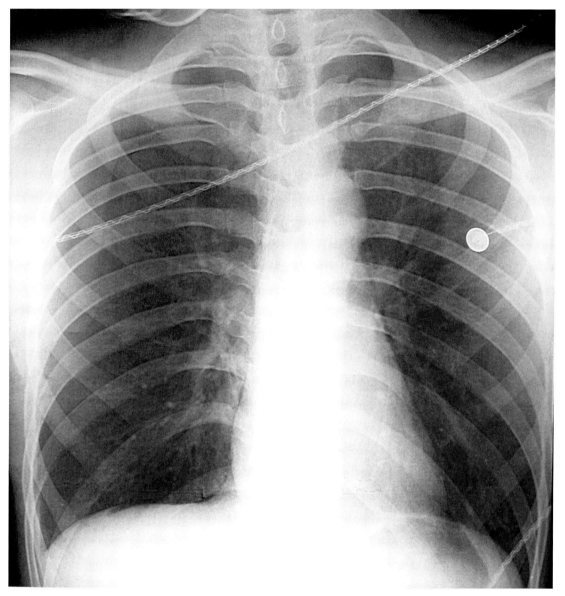

FIGURE 1

Chest pain of sudden onset in a young man

A 24-year-old man presented to the ED with unilateral chest pain that began about six hours earlier.

The pain was initially "sharp" in quality and began abruptly. The pain had been persistent since it began and was now dull and aching. It was worse with deep inspiration. There was no associated shortness of breath, diaphoresis, nausea, cough, fever, or chills. The pain was not relieved by ibuprofen.

The patient had no risk factors for coronary artery disease aside from a history of smoking one pack of cigarettes per day for the past six years. He denied using cocaine or other drugs.

On examination, he was a healthy appearing young man in no apparent distress.

Vital signs—blood pressure 120/80 mm/Hg, pulse 84 beats/ min, respirations 18 breaths/min, temperature 99.°F rectal, SO_2 97% on room air

Lungs—equal bilateral breath sounds without wheeze or râles; there was no chest wall tenderness

Heart—regular rhythm without murmur, rub, or gallop.

Abdomen—soft and nontender

• What does his chest radiograph show (Figure 1)?

A FINE LINE

Chest radiography is often not a helpful test in the evaluation of patients with chest pain; however, when pneumonia, malignancy, thoracic aortic aneurysm, or pneumothorax is suspected, radiography can be diagnostic. An upright chest radiograph can confirm or exclude a pneumothorax in nearly all patients, although in some cases, the findings can be subtle and must be specifically sought when examining the chest radiograph.

A **spontaneous pneumothorax** (not due to trauma or iatrogenic) can be either primary or secondary, i.e., associated with an underlying pulmonary disorder. Such disorders include chronic obstructive pulmonary disease (COPD), cysts or cavities due to necrotizing pneumonia (staphylococcus aureus), malignancies, tuberculosis, or pneumocystis pneumonia, and interstitial lung diseases such as sarcoidosis, collagen vascular diseases, pneumoconiosis, or idiopathic pulmonary fibrosis.

Primary spontaneous pneumothorax occurs in patients without underlying lung disease. It is most common in young adults, predominantly males in their third or fourth decades, who almost invariably have histories of cigarette smoking. There is rupture of an apical bleb (air-containing cyst within the visceral pleura) or subpleural bulla (enlarged airspace due to degeneration of alveoli). The precipitating event may be increased intrathoracic pressure due to physical exertion, although most cases occur at rest.

Clinical Manifestations

Chest pain is the primary symptom, occurring in 90% of cases. It is usually of abrupt onset, "sharp" in quality, localized to one side of the thorax, and worse with deep inspiration (pleuritic). The chest pain may become "dull and aching" over the subsequent 1–2 days. Dyspnea is present in 80% of patients, although it may abate over time. Severe dyspnea is uncommon and, when present, is often a sign of a tension pneumothorax. Severe dyspnea can also occur with a relatively small pneumothorax in patients who have significant underlying lung disease such as COPD. On physical examination, unilateral absent breath sounds are found only when the pneumothorax is large.

Radiography

The radiographic findings are usually striking. The collapsed lung is displaced medially and inferiorly, and the surrounding pneumothorax is radiolucent and devoid of lung markings. Occasionally, however, the radiographic signs are subtle. The key radiographic finding is the **fine line of visceral pleura** which parallels the inner margin of the thoracic wall (Figure 2).

Contrary to what would be expected, the radiopacity of the collapsed lung is often not greater than the radiopacity of the normal lung (Figure 1). This is because pulmonary blood flow (normal lung markings are pulmonary blood vessels) diminishes in the collapsed lung in proportion to the extent of collapse, except when there is nearly total collapse.

In patients whose radiographic findings are equivocal, an **expiratory radiograph** can make a small pneumothorax more conspicuous. Expiration compresses the lung and increases the relative size of the pneumothorax (Figure 3).

Whenever possible, the radiograph should be taken with the patient in an upright position. When the patient is **supine,** a pneumothorax collects anteriorly and may be impossible to detect. A large pneumothorax may widen the costophrenic sulcus—the "deep sulcus" sign (Figure 4) (Kong 2003). However, even a large pneumothorax can be completely invisible on a supine AP portable view—an occult pneumothorax. It may be detected on CT of the chest or upper abdomen (Figure 5) (Ball et al. 2006).

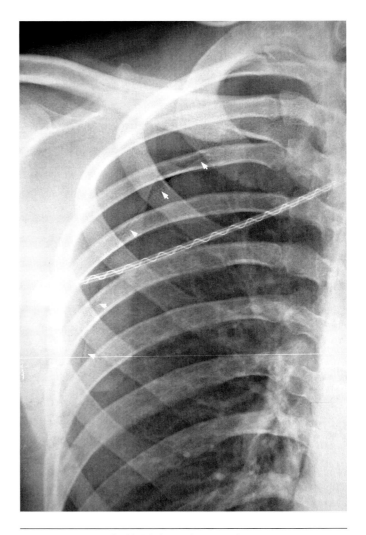

FIGURE 2   Detail of initial PA view—Patient 9.
The visceral pleura at the edge of the collapsed lung is barely visible. It can be identified by looking for a fine line that parallels the curve of the lateral chest wall (*arrows*).

Bedside **ultrasonography** has been used to rapidly detect pneumothoraces in trauma patients and can be incorporated into the FAST exam (Rowan 2002). In one study, the sensitivity of sonography was 98% compared to 75% for supine AP chest radiography, whereas a second study found only 60% sensitivity, similar to that of supine radiography (Blavias et al. 2005, Kirkpatrick et al. 2004).

Radiographic findings that can mimic a pneumothorax include large emphysematous bullae usually in the apex of the lung (Waseem et al. 2005). When there is uncertainty, a CT of the chest should be obtained. A fold of overlying skin, clothing, or a bed sheet can mimic the visceral pleural line of a medium-sized pneumothorax. However, if the line is followed, it will extend outside of the thorax.

In this patient, there is thin lucent band adjacent to the heart border (Figure 1). This should not be misinterpreted as a pneumomediastinum or pneumopericardium. It is due to an optical edge enhancement phenomenon known as a *Mach band*.

Patient Outcome

This patient was admitted to the hospital for observation and treated with 10 L/min oxygen per nasal cannula. He was discharged the following day after repeat radiography showed no increase in the size of his pneumothorax. He was referred for later follow-up care in the medical clinic and strongly advised to stop smoking.

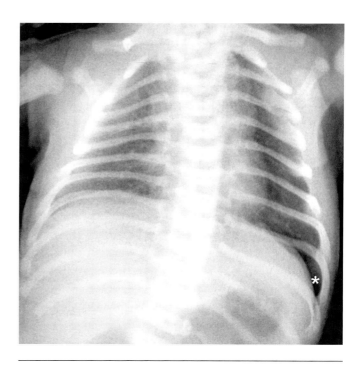

FIGURE 4   Deep sulcus sign.
Supine chest radiograph of a neonate illustrates the deep sulcus sign with abnormal deepening and lucency of the left lateral costophrenic angle (*asterisk*). Findings on right lateral decubitus chest radiograph (not shown) confirmed the presence of a pneumothorax on the left side.
[From Kong A: The deep sulcus sign. Radiology. 2003;228:415, with permission.]

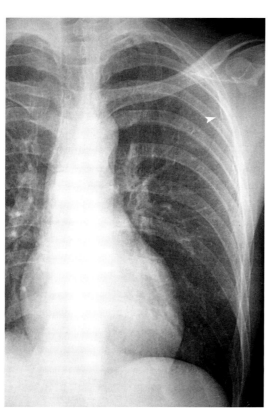

A. Inspiratory view

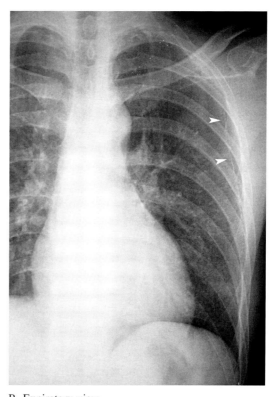

B. Expiratory view

FIGURE 3   Expiratory radiography.
When there are questionable findings of a pneumothorax (*A, arrowhead*), repeat radiography during expiration (*B*) can more clearly reveal a pneumothorax (*arrowheads*).

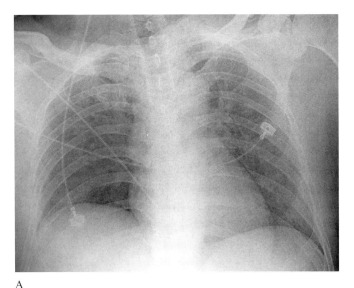

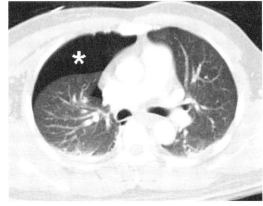

A   B

FIGURE 5   Occult pneumothorax.

A 40-year-old man was hit on his right shoulder and right posterior thorax by falling debris from a construction site. He was hemodynamically stable and in no respiratory distress. There was marked soft tissue swelling over the area of impact. The initial AP portable supine chest radiograph was normal (*A*).

Because of the mechanism of injury, a chest CT was obtained (*B*). This revealed a moderate-sized pneumothorax in the anterior portion of the right side of the chest (*asterisk*). A chest tube was inserted that reexpanded his right lung. There was also a right fifth rib fracture.

This moderately large pneumothorax was invisible on the supine AP portable chest radiograph because the collapsed lung occupied the entire width of the right hemithorax.

ESTIMATING THE SIZE OF A PNEUMOTHORAX

The size of a pneumothorax has implications with regard to patient care, i.e., a "small" primary spontaneous pneumothorax in a mildly symptomatic patient can be managed by observation alone without inserting a chest tube or other drainage procedure.

Traditionally, pneumothorax size is expressed as a percentage of thoracic volume. This may be based on the subjective impression of the person interpreting the radiographs, although such interpretations are subject to considerable interobserver variability (Rhea et al. 1981). Various formulae have been devised to assess pneumothorax size, although they are cumbersome to use and can be inaccurate (Engdahl et al. 1993). Even though an exact percentage can be calculated, it is only a rough approximation (Figure 6).

A **qualitative classification scheme** is easier to apply. Three sizes of pneumothorax can be distinguished: small, medium, and large (Henry et al. 2003, Miller 1993). A **small** pneumothorax is confined to the apex of the thorax and a thin rim around the lung (less than 1 or 2 cm) (Figure 7). A **medium** pneumothorax occupies up to one-half of the thoracic diameter. With a **large** pneumothorax, the lung is completely or nearly completely collapsed (Figure 8).

In one **quantitative scheme**, three measurements of interpleural distance are made on an upright chest radiograph—one at the lung apex and two at the upper and lower halves of the thorax (Figure 6). The *average interpleural distance*

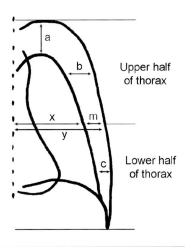

FIGURE 6   Pneumothorax size calculations.

Average interpleural distance (AID) = $(a + b + c) / 3$

Rhea (1981): Ptx % = $(5 + 9) \times$ AID (after Choi 1998)

Collins (1995): Ptx % = $(4 + 14) \times$ AID

Light formula: Ptx % = $(1 - x^3/y^3) \times 100$

ACCP (2001): "small" $a < 3$ cm; "large" $a \geq 3$ cm

BTS (2003): "small" $m < 2$ cm; "large" $m \geq 2$ cm

Measurements in centimeters. Ptx = pneumothorax. m, x, y = average (or midthoracic) widths (Henry et al. 2003, Light et al. 2005)

(AID) is then used in a nomogram or formula to determine pneumothorax size (Choi et al. 1998, Rhea et al.1981). However, when compared to direct volumetric measurements made using helical CT, these calculations were found to underestimate pneumothorax size. These formulae were therefore revised based on CT measurements (Collins et al. 1995).

An alternative method (the *Light formula*) uses the cube of the "average" diameters of the lung and thorax (an approximation of volume) to calculate pneumothorax size (Noppen et al. 2001). However, these three formulae produce disparate results (Table 1). For instance, a measured pleural space of 2 cm is calculated as a 23% pneumothorax using Rhea's formula, 32% using Collins', and 42% using Lights'.

TABLE 1

Calculated pneumothorax size (%)

AID = 1 cm ⇒ 15% (Rhea)

AID = 1 cm ⇒ 20% (Collins)

m = 1 cm (y = 12 cm; x = 11 cm) ⇒ 23% (Light)

AID = 2 cm ⇒ 23% (Rhea)

AID = 2 cm ⇒ 32% (Collins)

m = 2 cm (y = 12 cm; x = 10 cm) ⇒ 42% (Light)

AID = Average interpleural distance

More **recent guidelines** have proposed using single measurements to determine patient care. Only two sizes of pneumothorax are distinguished: small and large. **Small** pneumothoraces can be managed by observation, as long as the patient is stable, has only mild symptoms, and has no underlying lung disease. **Large** pneumothoraces need chest tube or catheter aspiration to reexpand the lung.

The American College of Chest Physicians (ACCP) proposed using an apex to cupola distance of 3 cm to distinguish small from large pneumothoraces (*a* in Figure 6) (Baumann et al. 2001). The British Thoracic Society (BTS) uses an average pneumothorax width of 2 cm to distinguish large from small pneumothoraces, although the exact method of measurement is not specified (Chan et al. 2004, Henry et al. 2003).

The ACCP criterion for a small pneumothorax (<3 cm at the lung apex) would appear similar to the BTS criterion. However, one study classified patients by both criteria and found that the BTS criterion rated 50% more patients as having small pneumothoraces that could be managed by observation alone without chest tube drainage (Marquette et al. 2006). ACCP criterion is therefore more conservative in rating pneumothorax size as small. Both guidelines are based on the consensus of a panel of experts and not objective data from high-quality clinical studies.

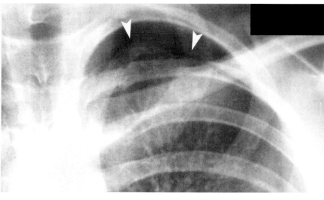

B

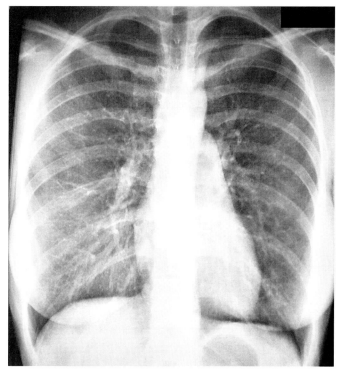

A

FIGURE 7 Small (apical) pneumothorax.

A 27-year-old woman with a small pneumothorax (A and B) was followed as an outpatient with resolution of her pneumothorax.

Seven months later, she had a contralateral large pneumothorax treated with chest tube. One year later, she had a second large recurrent pneumothorax on the right treated by chest tube and chemical pleurodesis. Current management of recurrent pneumothorax would instead entail thoroscopic bullectomy and mechanical abrasion pleurodesis.

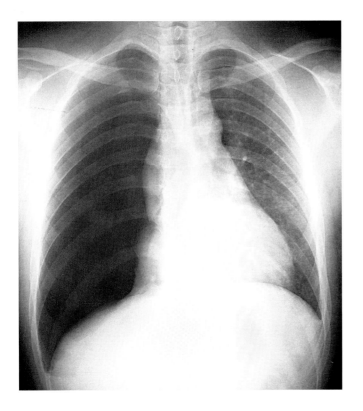

FIGURE 8   Extra-large pneumothorax.

A 22-year-old man presented with an abrupt onset of right-sided chest pain and mild dyspnea. His vital signs were normal and breath sounds were absent on the right.

The chest radiograph showed complete collapse of the right lung. Using a three-tiered classification of pneumothorax size (small, medium, and large), this is a large pneumothorax.

In addition, there is shift of the heart and trachea to the left, and depression of the right side of the diaphragm—radiographic signs of a tension pneumothorax (an "extra-large" pneumothorax). However, radiographic signs of tension pneumothorax do not equate with clinical signs, i.e., hypotension and shock. The patient remained hemodynamically stable during his time in the ED.

A chest tube was inserted, reexpanding the right lung. There was a persistent air leak through the chest tube over the next four days. This required thoroscopic surgery to excise the bleb and close the defect in the apex of his right lung.

MANAGEMENT OF PATIENTS WITH SPONTANEOUS PNEUMOTHORAX

Treatment decisions are based on the clinical status of the patient, the size of the pneumothorax (large or small), and the presence of underlying lung disease.

Small Pneumothoraces

Patients with no underlying lung disease who have only mild symptoms and normal vital signs can be managed with observation alone. The criteria for a "small" pneumothorax can be based on ACCP or BTS guidelines, a pneumothorax size of less than 15% or 20% (although not all published studies state their method of measurement), or the simple assessment that the pneumothorax is limited to the lung apex or a thin layer adjacent to the lung.

If this is the patient's *first primary spontaneous pneumothorax* and the patient is reliable and able to return promptly to the ED if symptoms worsen, the patient may be discharged home and scheduled for a return visit with repeat radiography in 12–48 hours. Prior to discharge, the ACCP recommends observation in the ED for 3–6 hours and repeat radiography to assure that the pneumothorax size has not increased. When there is concern about the ability of the patient to return promptly to the hospital if his or her condition were to worsen, admission to the hospital is warranted. Hospitalization is obligatory in patients

with *underlying lung disease* because there is greater potential for rapid deterioration.

Oxygen should be administered while the patient is in the hospital since this will hasten resorption of the pneumothorax. A small pneumothorax may require 1–2 weeks to resolve and therefore additional follow-up visits and radiography should be arranged.

Large Pneumothoraces

Patients with large pneumothoraces require catheter or chest tube placement to reexpand the lung. The method of treatment is a subject of controversy. Several small clinical trials and the BTS guidelines suggest attempting aspiration via a small catheter when the patient is clinically stable (Ayed et al. 2006, Chan and Lam 2005, Light 2002, Miller 2001, Noppen et al. 2002). This is successful in 50–60% of cases in reported series, but has not gained wide acceptance. The ACCP guidelines do not recommend catheter aspiration, but instead advise inserting a small bore pigtail catheter (7–14 F) or standard chest tube (16–22 F) for stable patients, and larger chest tube (24–28 F) for unstable patients or those who may require positive-pressure ventilation (Henry 2006, Marquette et al. 2006).

Recurrent Pneumothorax

There is a 30% recurrence rate following a primary spontaneous pneumothorax, most occurring within one year. The rate of subsequent recurrence is 50%. Therefore, patients with a second spontaneous pneumothorax should be hospitalized and referred to a surgeon for thoracoscopy or thoracotomy to staple or over-sew any remaining bullae or blebs and perform upper thoracic pleural symphysis using parietal pleural abrasion (Ng et al. 2006, Sawada et al. 2005). When surgery cannot be performed due to a patient's underlying medical conditions, instillation of a sclerosing agent, either talc slurry or doxycycline, is an alternative procedure for pleurodesis that will also reduce the frequency of recurrence (Figure 9).

Tension Pneumothorax

A tension pneumothorax is a life-threatening emergency in which air progressively enters the pleural space with each successive breath but cannot escape due to a one-way valve phenomenon at the lung surface. Intrapleural pressure rises, which eventually impedes systemic venous return resulting in diminished cardiac output, hypotension, and shock. Whenever tension pneumothorax is suspected, catheter aspiration should be performed immediately. A rapid egress of air and rise in blood pressure will confirm the diagnosis. Treatment should not be delayed while awaiting chest radiography (Figure 10).

Clinically, the patient is hypotensive or pulseless, or has severe dyspnea. Breath sounds are absent on the involved side, and the trachea may be deviated to the opposite side. Tension pneumothorax commonly occurs in patients who are intubated and receiving positive-pressure ventilation, although it can occur in nonintubated patients. The lung is usually totally collapsed. However, when the lung is noncompliant (stiffened by underlying disease such as COPD or interstitial lung disease), there may be only partial collapse (Figure 11). The radiographic hallmark of a tension pneumothorax is mediastinal shift to the side opposite the pneumothorax (Figure 8).

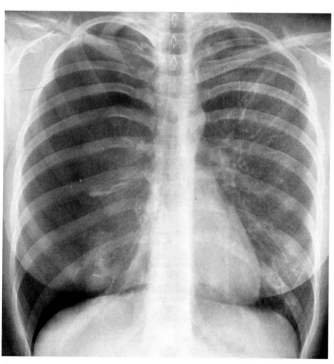

A

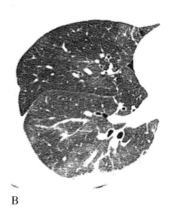
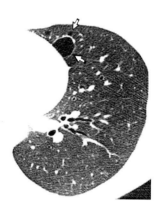

B

FIGURE 9 **Recurrent pneumothorax: Is it a primary or secondary pneumothorax?**

A 21-year-old woman presented with cough and chest pain of two days duration. She had had a spontaneous pneumothorax nine months earlier. She smoked one half a pack of cigarettes per day for seven years and had "quit smoking" two days ago.

The **chest radiograph** revealed a large right pneumothorax (A). A chest tube was inserted with successful re-expansion of the lung. The patient was admitted to the thoracic surgery service for her recurrent, presumably primary, spontaneous pneumothorax. The plan was to perform video-assisted thoracoscopic surgery (VATS) to resect blebs or bullae at the lung apex.

A **chest CT** was done to define the pulmonary lesions prior to thoracoscopy. However, instead of revealing apical bullae or blebs associated with "primary" spontaneous pneumothorax, it revealed numerous pulmonary parenchymal cysts ranging from 2 mm to 15 mm in diameter (B, arrows). This was suspicious for lymphangioleiomyomatosis, a potentially fatal progressive pulmonary disorder (although the cysts are usually of more uniform size).

During VATS, a right apical bleb resection, right lower lobe biopsy and pleurodiesis were performed. Histopathological examination and immunochemical stains were consistent with emphysema. She was strongly advised to continue smoking cessation and follow up with a pulmonologist.

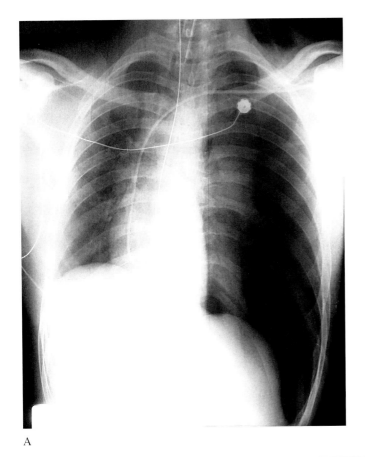

A

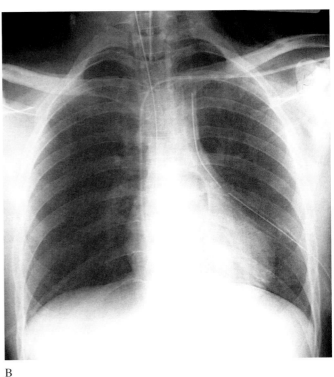

B

FIGURE 10   Tension pneumothorax—The radiograph that should never be taken.

A 28-year-old man with apparently isolated head trauma, and alcohol and cocaine intoxication required sedation and endotracheal intubation in the ED. He was stabilized and then admitted for observation to the surgical intensive care unit. Due to poor venous access, a left large-bore subclavian intravenous catheter was inserted. A chest radiograph obtained after intubation and line placement did not disclose a pneumothorax.

One hour later, his blood pressure suddenly dropped to 70 mm Hg and intravenous fluid resuscitation was begun. A diagnostic peritoneal lavage (DPL) did not reveal intra-abdominal bleeding. A chest radiograph was then obtained which revealed that the cause of hypotension was a tension pneumothorax (A). There is marked shift of the mediastinum to the right and depression of the left side of the diaphragm.

The tension pneumothorax was iatrogenic in origin, due to placement of a central venous catheter and then positive pressure ventilation. A chest tube was inserted, which lead promptly to hemodynamic stabilization (B).

A tension pneumothorax should have been suspected based on the clinical scenario and the absence of breath sounds on the left. Emergency needle decompression was warranted without delaying for radiography.

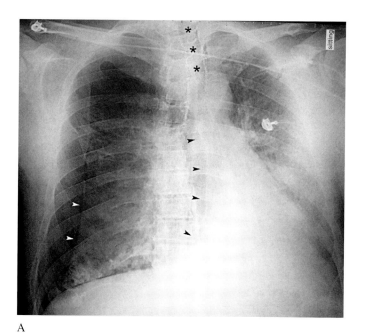

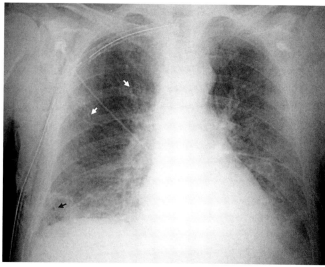

A   B

FIGURE 11   Tension pneumothorax without complete lung collapse—non-compliant lungs.

A 43-year-old man with a history of AIDS, pneumocystis pneumonia and deep vein thrombosis (DVT) presented to the ED with an abrupt onset of shortness of breath and chest pain. He had had a non-productive cough for the preceding two days.

On examination, he was cachectic and in moderate respiratory distress but was able to speak in complete sentences. His blood pressure was 110/72 mm Hg, pulse 146 beats/minute, respirations 50 breaths/minute, temperature 101° F and SO_2 82% on 10 liters/minute oxygen administered by face mask. He had diminished breath sounds on the right. Potential diagnoses included pneumonia, pneumothorax or pulmonary embolism.

A portable chest radiograph showed mild diffuse bilateral airspace-filling consistent with pneumocystis pneumonia, a medium-sized right pneumothorax (*white arrowheads*) and mediastinal shift to the left (*A*). The trachea is deviated to the left

(*asterisks*) and the medial portion of the right lung has herniated across the midline (*black arrowheads*). A 28-French chest tube was inserted on the right which released a rush of air and the patient's dyspnea and tachycardia rapidly improved. Repeat chest radiography confirmed re-expansion of the right lung (*B*).

This was a **secondary spontaneous pneumothorax**, i.e., due to underlying lung disease. Pneumocystis pneumonia often causes cyst formation within the lung parenchyma, which predisposes to the development of pneumothoraces. Multiple cysts were evident on the post-thoracostomy radiograph in this patient (*arrows in B*).

The patient's underlying lung disease (multiple episodes of pneumocystis pneumonia) resulted in non-compliant—lungs the explanation for a tension pneumothorax without total lung collapse.

FIGURE 12   Spontaneous hemopneumothorax.

In this patient, there is a medium-sized pneumothorax (*white arrowheads*). The pleural fluid collection on this upright chest radiograph has a straight superior margin (*black arrowheads*) rather than the concave-upwards meniscus usually seen with a pleural effusion. Surface tension forces that normally exist between closely opposed visceral and parietal pleural surfaces are responsible for the meniscus formation seen with simple pleural effusions. When there is a concomitant pneumothorax, such surface tension forces are lacking and the superior surface of pleural fluid collection is flat.

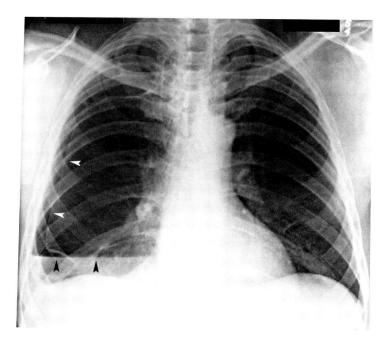

Hemopneumothorax

Spontaneous hemopneumothoraces (not due to trauma) are uncommon. They occur when there is a vascular injury associated with rupture of a bleb or bulla. Irrespective of the size of the pneumothorax, it requires drainage by chest tube. A large-bore chest tube should be used (32–36 F) to assure adequate drainage of the hemothorax (Figure 12).

SUGGESTED READING

Baumann MH, Strange C, Heffner JE, et al.: Management of spontaneous pneumothorax: An American College of Chest Physicians Delphi consensus statement. *Chest* 2001;119:590–602.

Henry M, Arnold T, Harvey J: BTS guidelines for the management of spontaneous pneumothorax. *Thorax* 2003;58 (Suppl 2): ii39–ii52. www.chestnet.org/education/cs/pneumothorax/interactive/toc.php www.chestnet.org/education/cs/pneumothorax/qrg/index.php

Light RW, Lee YCG: Pneumothorax, chylothorax, hemothorax, and fibrothorax. In Mason RJ, Murray JF, Broaddus VC, Nadel JA, eds.: *Murray & Nadel's Textbook of Respiratory Medicine*, 4th ed. Saunders, 2005, 1961–1986.

Sahn SA, Heffner JE: Spontaneous pneumothorax. *New Engl J Med* 2000;342:868–874.

Chest radiology

Chan SS, Henry M, Arnold T, Harvey J: Estimation of size of pneumothorax under the new BTS guidelines. *Thorax* 2004; 59: 356–357.

Choi BG, Park SH, Yun EH, et al.: Pneumothorax size: Correlation of supine anteroposterior with erect posteroanterior chest radiographs. *Radiology* 1998;209:567–569.

Collins CD, Lopez A, Mathie A, et al.: Quantification of pneumothorax size on chest radiographs using interpleural distances: Regression analysis based on volume measurements from helical CT. *AJR* 1995;165:1127–1130.

Engdahl O, Toft T, Boe J. Chest radiograph—a poor method for determining the size of a pneumothorax. *Chest* 1993;103:26–29.

Kong A: The deep sulcus sign. *Radiology* 2003;228:415–416.

Noppen M, Alexander P, Driesen P, et al.: Quantification of the size of primary spontaneous pneumothorax: Accuracy of the Light index. *Respiration* 2001;68:396–399.

O'Connor AR, Morgan WE: Radiological review of pneumothorax. *BMJ* 2005;330;1493–1497

Rhea JT, DeLuca SA, Greene RE: Determining the size of pneumothorax in the upright patient. *Radiol* 1981;144:733–736.

Waseem M, Jones J, Brutus S, et al.: Giant bulla mimicking pneumothorax. *J Emerg Med* 2005;29:155–158.

Occult pneumothorax

Ball CG, Kirkpatrick AW, Laupland KB, et al.: Incidence, risk factors and outcomes for occult pneumothoraces in victims of major trauma. *J Trauma* 2005;59:917–925.

Ball CG, Kirkpatrick AW, Fox DL, et al.: Are occult pneumothoraces truly occult or simply missed? *J Trauma* 2006; 60:294–299.

Gilligan P, Hegarty D, Hassan TB: The point of the needle. Occult pneumothorax: A review. *Emerg Med J* 2003; 20: 293–296.

Henderson SO, Shoenberger JM: Anterior pneumothorax and a negative chest x-ray. *J Emerg Med* 2004;26:231–232.

Ultrasonography

Blaivas M, Lyon M, Duggal S: A prospective comparison of supine chest radiography and bedside ultrasound for the diagnosis of traumatic pneumothorax. *Acad Emerg Med* 2005;12:844–849.

Kirkpatrick AW, Sirois M, Laupland KB, et al.: Hand-held thoracic sonography for detecting post-traumatic pneumothoraces: The Extended Focused Assessment with Sonography for Trauma (EFAST). *J Trauma* 2004;57:288–295.

Aspiration of pneumothoraces

Ayed AK, Chandrasekaran C, Sukumar M: Aspiration versus tube drainage in primary spontaneous pneumothorax: A randomized study. *Eur Respir J* 2006;27:477–482.

Chan SSW, Lam PKW: Simple aspiration as initial treatment for primary spontaneous pneumothorax: Results of 91 consecutive cases. *J Emerg Med* 2005;28:133–138.

Henry MT: Simple sequential treatment for primary spontaneous pneumothorax: One step closer. *Eur Respir J* 2006;27:448–450.

Light RW: Manual aspiration—The preferred method for managing primary spontaneous pneumothorax? *Am J Resp Crit Care Med* 2002;165:1202–1203.

Liu CM, Hang LW, Chen WK, et al.: Pigtail tube drainage in the treatment of spontaneous pneumothorax. *Am J Emerg Med* 2003;21: 241–244.

Marquette CH, Marx A, Leroy S, et al.: the Pneumothorax Study Group: Simplified stepwise management of primary spontaneous pneumothorax: A pilot study. *Eur Respir J* 2006;27:470–476.

Miller AC, Baumann MH, Strange C, Heffner JE: Pneumothorax—What's wrong with simple aspiration? *Chest* 2001;120:1041–1042

Noppen M, Alexander P, Driesen P, et al.: Manual aspiration versus chest tube drainage in first episodes of primary spontaneous pneumothorax—A multicenter, prospective, randomized pilot study. *Am J Resp Crit Care Med* 2002;165:1240–1244.

Video assisted thoracic surgery

Ng CSH, Lee TW, Wan S, Yim APC: Video assisted thoracic surgery in the management of spontaneous pneumothorax: The current status. *Postgrad Med J* 2006;82:179–185.

Sawada S, Watanabe Y, Moriyama S: Video-assisted thoracoscopic surgery for primary spontaneous pneumothorax: Evaluation of indications and long-term outcome compared with conservative treatment and open thoracotomy. *Chest* 2005;127:2226–2230.

Chest Radiology: Patient 10

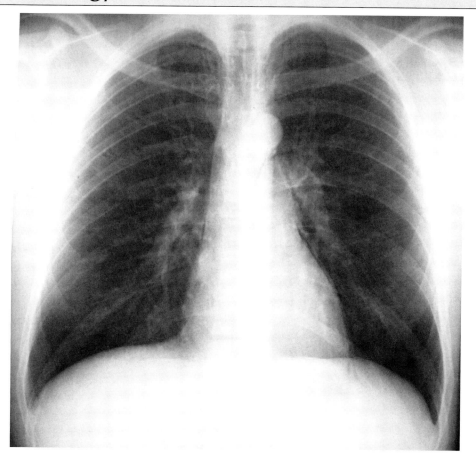

FIGURE 1

Chest pain in a young man after receiving a blow to the chest

A 25-year-old man was in an altercation while smoking "crack" cocaine. He was punched in his back, the left side of his chest, and his neck. He was taken to the hospital where no significant injury was found. The next day, his chest radiograph was re-read and the patient was recalled.

The patient appeared well, with only mild tenderness at the above-mentioned areas of injury. He was otherwise asymptomatic.

- What is the cause of the abnormalities seen in these radiographs (Figure 1)?

- Should you admit this patient to the hospital?

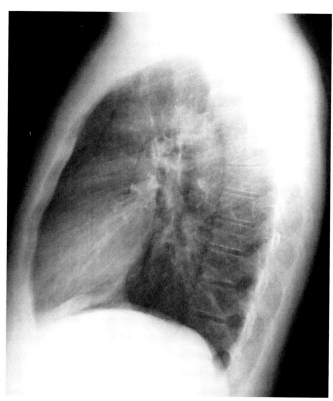

THE MACKLIN EFFECT

Occasionally, it is unclear whether a patient has sustained a traumatic injury or has a nontraumatic disorder. The abnormality in this patient—pneumomediastinum—could potentially be due to either of the two.

The PA chest radiograph shows **linear air collections** adjacent to the mediastinum (heart and aorta) and an associated fine white line representing the displaced mediastinal pleura (Figure 2A). In addition, linear air collections extend up the mediastinal fascial planes into the neck. On the lateral view, there is air surrounding mediastinal structures, particularly the aorta (Figure 2B). The lateral cervical spine radiograph, obtained because the patient had neck pain following trauma, shows air within the prevertebral soft tissues (Figure 2C).

Pneumomediastinum can occur following blunt or penetrating **trauma**, often, but not always, major trauma, or can occur **"spontaneously,"** without evident trauma.

There are three potential sources of mediastinal air: the esophagus, the tracheobronchial tree, and the lung. Injury to each of these structures should be suspected in patients with pneumomediastinum. The clinical scenario usually provides evidence as to which organ is the site of air leak into the mediastinum.

The most frequent source of mediastinal air is the **lung.** Pneumomediastinum occurs in clinical settings associated with alveolar hyperinflation and high intrapulmonary pressure such as asthma, forceful inhalation followed by breath holding (as occurs during use of illicit drugs such as crack cocaine), positive pressure ventilation (especially in patients with noncompliant lungs, e.g., ARDS), and a rapid ascent during scuba diving. Alveolar air ruptures into the adjacent interstitial lung tissues and then dissects along the bronchovascular connective tissues to the hilum and then into the mediastinum. This is known as the **Macklin effect** (Wintermark and Schnyder 2001, Smith and Ferguson 1991). Blunt trauma such as a direct blow to the chest or abrupt deceleration in a motor vehicle collision can also cause alveolar rupture and pneumomediastinum.

The patient with pneumomediastinum presents with chest pain (90% of cases), dyspnea (50% of cases), and occasionally

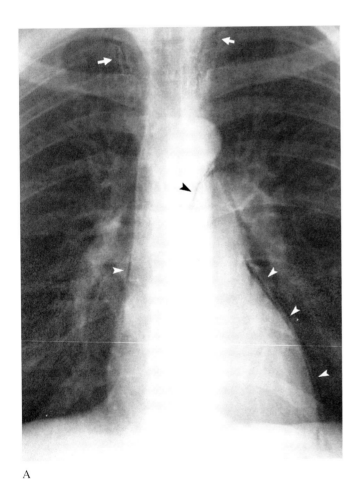
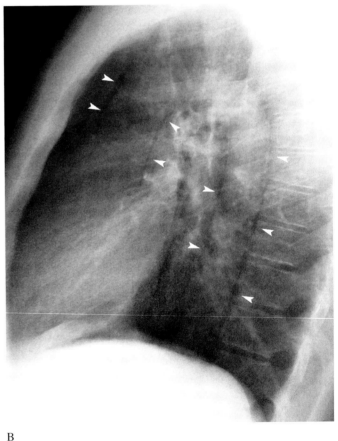

A   B

FIGURE 2 Initial radiographs—Patient 10.

(A) The PA view shows a thin layer of air is adjacent to the left and right heart borders and the fine white line of the raised parietal pleura (*white arrowheads*). Air outlines the lateral margin of the descending aorta (*black arrowhead*) and tracks into the soft tissues of the superior mediastinum and base of the neck (*arrows*).

(B) On the lateral view, a thin layer of air outlines the ascending and descending aorta (*arrowheads*).

neck pain or dysphagia. On physical examination, cardiac auscultation may reveal a crunching or cracking sound synchronous with cardiac contractions, known as *Hammond's sign*. Air that has migrated into the subcutaneous tissues of the neck and chest wall causes palpable crepitus and swelling, which may be considerable.

Esophageal perforation can result from blunt or penetrating trauma, including iatrogenic trauma (medical instrumentation). It can also occur following vomiting, usually forceful vomiting (**Boerhaave's syndrome**). Esophageal perforation leads to mediastinitis and sepsis. The clinical picture of esophageal rupture is usually sufficiently distinctive to prevent misdiagnosis as a more benign form of pneumomediastinum, although missed ED cases have been reported (Howton 2004). When pneumomediastinum occurs in association with vomiting, esophageal perforation should always be suspected. With the possible exception of a small esophageal puncture due to endoscopy and biopsy, esophageal rupture is usually accompanied by considerable mediastinal inflammation and edema. Clinically, the patient

has fever and systemic toxicity, although initially the patient may appear well. Radiographically, there may be mediastinal widening due to fluid accumulation within the mediastinum as well as pneumomediastinum. However, the radiographic findings are often nonspecific—a pleural effusion, infiltrate or atelectasis, and early on the radiograph may be normal. Esophageal perforation is diagnosed by a contrast esophagram or CT (Ghanem et al. 2003, Fadoo et al. 2004). Water-soluble contrast material should be used because it is not irritating to mediastinal tissues if extravasation occurs (Keberle et al. 2000) (see Figures 6 and 7 on p. 90).

Tracheobronchial rupture occurs with penetrating trauma or forceful abrupt deceleration as in a motor-vehicle collision. It is a catastrophic injury usually associated with a pneumothorax and other major thoracic injuries such as pulmonary contusions and laceration (Lin et al. 1995). Distal airways injury due to laceration of the pulmonary parenchyma is most often caused by penetrating thoracic trauma. A pneumothorax with persistent air leak is the usual clinical presentation, not pneumomediastinum.

Lastly, pneumomediastinum can result from air tracking inferiorly from the head and neck (following a retropharyngeal infection or surgical procedure), air tracking superiorly from an abdominal or retroperitoneal source, or from a gas-forming infection within the mediastinum itself.

Management

Esophageal and tracheobronchial injuries generally require surgical treatment. The clinical course of **spontaneous pneumomediastinum** (from intraparenchymal alveolar rupture) is relatively benign, although this has not been rigorously studied except in several small case series (Newcomb and Clarke 2005, Weissberg and Weissbeg 2004, Smith and Ferguson 1991, Abolnik et al. 1991). Potential complications include rupture of the mediastinal air across the parietal pleura, causing a pneumothorax, or expansion of the pneumomediastinum leading to respiratory compromise ("tension pneumomediastinum"). However, respiratory compromise is rare because the mediastinal air can usually decompress into the soft tissues of the neck. An occult injury to the esophagus or proximal airways should always be considered, although such injuries are usually evident on clinical grounds. Antecedent vomiting should prompt consideration of esophageal rupture (Howton 2004).

One retrospective series of patients with spontaneous pneumomediastinum (17 patients, 13 associated with inhalation of illicit drugs) found that all patients had benign clinical courses. There were no complications such as respiratory decompensation, pneumothorax or occult esophageal perforation. The authors suggest that these patients do not necessarily need to be hospitalized. However, the number of patients studied was too small to reach definitive conclusions (Panacek et al. 1992). Other authors recommend 24 hours of observation, although the data to support this are scant.

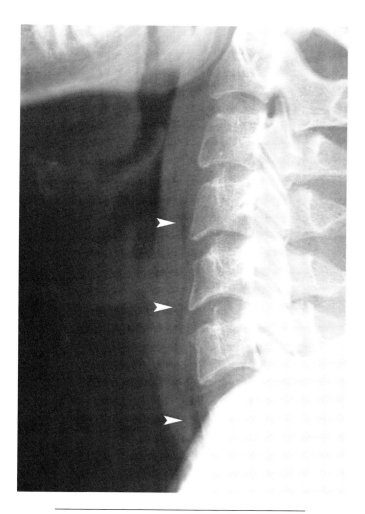

FIGURE 2C The cervical spine radiograph shows air within the prevertebral soft tissues (*arrowheads*).

Radiography

Chest radiography is the principal diagnostic test for pneumomediastinum, although small amounts of air may only be detected by CT (Bejvan and Godwin 1996, Zylak et al. 2000, Kaneki et al. 2000). The chest radiograph shows a thin layer of air adjacent to the heart or aorta separated from the lung by a fine line representing the displaced mediastinal parietal pleura (Figure 3).

Air that collects inferiorly between the heart and diaphragm outlines the medial surface of the diaphragm creating the "continuous diaphragm sign" (Figure 4A). The left side of the descending aorta may also be outlined by air, which, where it intersects the medial portion of the left hemidiaphragm, forms a radiolucent V— "Naclero's V sign." Air often tracks into the prevertebral and subcutaneous soft tissues of the neck, and, when considerable, may extend into the subcutaneous tissues of the chest wall (Figure 4).

On the **lateral view**, a thin layer of air may be seen outlining the aorta (Figure 2B), the anterior extent of the left hemidiaphragm (Figure 4B), the retrosternal space, and surrounding the origin of the right main pulmonary artery (the "ring around the artery sign").

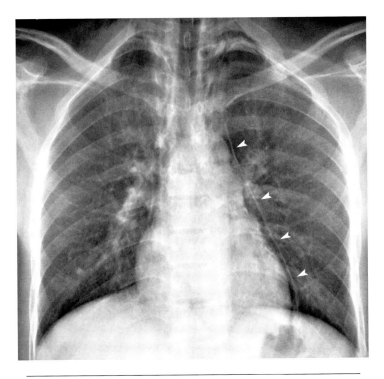

FIGURE 3 Pneumomediastinum in a 20-year-old man with an asthma exacerbation.

A thin white line representing the medial surface of the parietal pleura is raised from the left heart border and aortic arch (*arrowheads*).

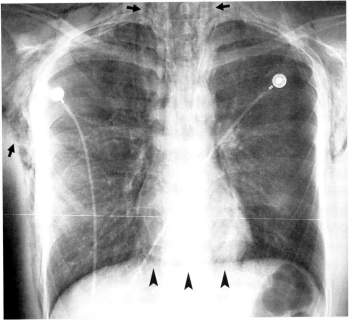 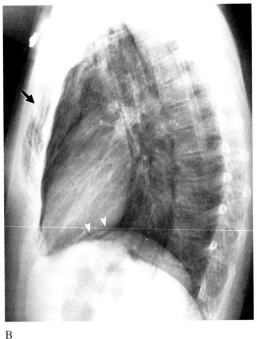

A   B

FIGURE 4 Massive pneumomediastinum.

A 14-year-old boy with an asthma exacerbation developed marked swelling and palpable crepitus of the soft tissues of his upper chest wall and neck.

(A) The PA view shows extensive subcutaneous emphysema (*arrows*). Air in the mediastinum outlines the normally invisible inferior margin of the heart—the "continuous diaphragm sign" (*arrowheads*).

(B) The lateral view shows subcutaneous air in the anterior chest wall (*arrow*) and air between the heart and left hemidiaphragm—the "continuous left hemidiaphragm sign" (*arrowheads*).

Pneumomediastinum can be mimicked by a **Mach band** adjacent to the left or right heart border (Figure 5). A Mach band is an optical illusion that results from the tendency of visual perception to accentuate or enhance edges between regions of moderately or slightly different optical density. (No Mach effect occurs between areas of great density difference, i.e., black and white.) A dark Mach band appears adjacent to such radiopaque structures as the heart (Chasen 2001, Friedman et al. 1981, Lane et al. 1976). When the lower lobe pulmonary artery parallels the heart border, this effect is increased. A Mach band can be distinguished from pneumomediastinum by the absence of the fine line of displaced parietal pleura seen with pneumomediastinum (Figures 2A and 3). Extension of air into the neck and abnormalities on the lateral view (air adjacent to the aorta) are also not seen with a Mach band pseudo-pneumomediastinum.

Patient Outcome

This patient was admitted to the hospital and observed for 24 hours. He remained asymptomatic. A contrast esophagram did not show perforation. Additional testing (esophagoscopy or bronchoscopy) was deemed not to be necessary. The etiology of his pneumomediastinum was likely either forceful inhalation of crack cocaine or the blunt chest trauma. In patients who have used cocaine and present to the ED with chest pain, myocardial ischemia and aortic dissection must also be considered.

Pneumopericardium

Air adjacent to the heart may also be due to pneumopericardium (air within the pericardial sac). However, pneumopericardium has different causative mechanisms and different potential complications. These two conditions can usually be distinguished clinically and radiographically. In a patient with pneumomediastinum, the air adjacent to the heart is located in the virtual space between the parietal pleura and parietal pericardium. The thin membrane seen parallel to the heart is therefore the parietal pleura, not the pericardium.

Pneumopericardium is rare in adults. It is more common in infants who are being treated for respiratory distress syndrome with mechanical ventilation. In infants, the pericardial sac is not completely closed at the origins of the great vessels, allowing for entry of air.

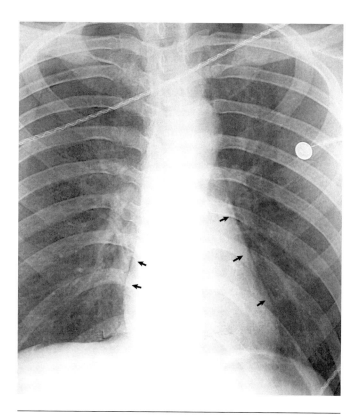

FIGURE 5 Pseudo-pneumomediastinum—Mach band.
The edge-enhancement property of visual perception creates an illusory dark band adjacent to the heart borders, particularly the left heart border (*arrows*).

In adults, pneumopericardium occurs with penetrating or, less commonly, blunt trauma that tears the thick fibrous pericardium. It is often associated with concurrent cardiac injury. Medical instrumentation, e.g., pericardiocentesis, can cause iatrogenic pneumopericardium. Pneumopericardium can also occur with gas-forming infections of the pericardium. When the pericardial sac is markedly distended, it can impede cardiac output in a fashion similar to tamponade (**tension pneumopericardium**). This requires emergency treatment with needle decompression (Shorr et al. 1987, Spotnitz and Rautman 1987, Demetriades 1990).

Radiographically, pneumopericardium can be distinguished from pneumomediastinum in two ways: (1) the pericardium is considerably thicker than the parietal pleura and is seen as a thick gray line between the air surrounding the heart and the lung and (2) air within the pericardial sac does not extend superiorly to the proximal ascending aorta. CT can more readily distinguish pneumopericardium from pneumomediastinum (Ladurner 2005).

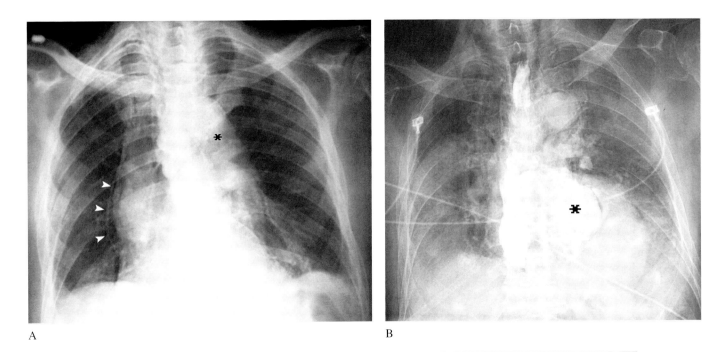

A

B

FIGURE 6   Boerhaave's syndrome—Esophageal rupture.

An 80-year-old man presented with chest and upper back pain that began after an episode of vomiting.

(A) The chest radiograph showed pneumomediastinum, particularly along the right heart border (*arrowheads*). The mediastinum appears widened, but this is due largely to the tortuous aorta (*asterisk*), which is common in the elderly, and rightwards rotated positioning of the patient.

(B) An esophagram showed extravasation and a large extraluminal collection of water-soluble contrast (*asterisk*) due to esophageal rupture. Emergency surgery was performed to close the esophageal defect. No underlying esophageal cancer or other lesion was found. The patient was discharged three weeks later in good clinical condition.

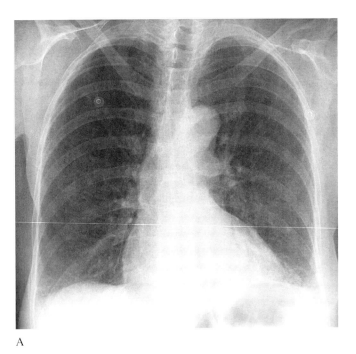

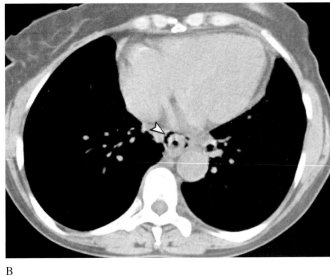

A

B

FIGURE 7   Pneumomediastinum due to esophageal perforation with negative radiography.

An 70-year-old woman presented with vomiting and upper abdominal pain after taking four bisacodyl tablets in preparation for colonoscopy. She felt better after being treated with intravenous fluids, morphine, and metoclopramide. Her chest radiograph was normal (*A*).

Her abdomen was nontender, but because of persistent pain and malaise, she underwent an abdominal CT. The upper CT slices (*B*) revealed air adjacent to the esophagus (*arrowhead*). An esophageal tear was confirmed by a contrast esophagram. The patient was taken to the operating room for repair of her esophageal perforation.

SUGGESTED READING

Park DR, Vallières E: Pneumomediastinum and mediastinitis. In Mason RJ, Murray JF, Broaddus VC, Nadel JA, eds. *Murray & Nadel's Textbook of Respiratory Medicine,* 4th ed. Saunders, 2005: 2039–2064.

Wintermark M, Schnyder P: The Macklin effect: A frequent etiology for pneumomediastinum in severe blunt chest trauma. *Chest* 2001; 120:543–547.

Newcomb AE, Clarke CP: Spontaneous pneumomediastinum: A benign curiosity or a significant problem? *Chest* 2005;128:3298–3302.

Weissberg D, Weissberg D: Spontaneous mediastinal emphysema. *Europ J Cardiothor Surg* 2004;26:885–888.

Abolnik I, Lossos IS, Breuer R: Spontaneous pneumomediastinum: A report of 25 cases. *Chest* 1991;100:93–95.

Smith BA, Ferguson DB: Disposition of spontaneous pneumomediastinum. *Am J Emerg Med* 1991;9:256–259.

Panacek EA, Singer AJ, Sherman BW, et al: Spontaneous pneumomediastinum: Clinical and natural history. *Ann Emerg Med* 1992; 21:1222–1227.

Bratton SL, O'Rourke PP: Spontaneous pneumomediastinum. *J Emerg Med* 1993;11:525–529.

Caraballo V, Barish RA, Floccare DJ: Pneumomediastinum presenting as acute upper airway obstruction. *J Emerg Med* 1996;14:159–162.

Lin MY, Wu MH, Chan CS, et al: Bronchial rupture caused by blunt chest injury. *Ann Emerg Med* 1995;25:412–415.

Baumann MH, Sahn SA: Hamman's sign revisited. Pneumothorax or pneumomediastinum? *Chest* 1992;102:1281–1282.

Illicit Drug Use

Brody SL, Anderson GV, Gutman JB: Pneumomediastinum as a complication of "crack" smoking. *Am J Emerg Med* 1988;6:241–243.

Fajardo LL: Association of spontaneous pneumomediastinum with substance abuse. *West J Med* 1990;152:301–304.

Riccio JC, Abbott J: A simple sore throat? Retropharyngeal emphysema secondary to free-basing cocaine. *J Emerg Med* 1990;8:709–712.

Seaman ME: Barotrauma related to inhalational drug abuse. *J Emerg Med* 1990;8:141–149.

Radiography

Agarwal PP: The ring-around-the-artery sign. *Radiology* 2006; 241: 943–944.

Bejvan SM, Godwin JD: Pneumomediastinum: Old signs and new signs. *AJR* 1996;166:1041–1048.

Kaneki T, Kubo K, Kawashima A, et al. Spontaneous pneumomediastinum in 33 patients: Yield of chest computed tomography for the diagnosis of the mild type. *Respiration* 2000;67:408–411.

Wintermark, M, Wicky, S, Schnyder, P, et al: Blunt traumatic pneumomediastinum: Using CT to reveal the Macklin effect. *AJR* 1999; 172:129–130.

Zylak CM, Standen JR, Barnes GR, Zylak CJ: Pneumomediastinum revisited. *RadioGraphics* 2000;20:1043–1057.

Mach Bands

Chasen MH: Practical applications of Mach band theory in thoracic imaging. *Radiology* 2001;219:596–610.

Friedman AC, Lautin EM, Rothenberg L: Mach bands and pneumomediastinum. *J Can Assoc Radiol* 1981;32:232–235.

Lane EJ, Proto AV, Phillips TW: Mach bands and density perception. *Radiology* 1976;121:9–17.

Boerhaave's Syndrome (Esophageal Perforation)

Fadoo F, Ruiz DE, Dawn SK, et al: Helical CT esophagography for the evaluation of suspected esophageal perforation or rupture. *AJR* 2004;182:1177–1179.

Ghanem N, Altehoefer C, Springer O, et al: Radiological findings in Boerhaave's syndrome. *Emerg Radiol* 2003;10:8–13.

Howton JC: Boerhaave's syndrome in a healthy adolescent male presenting with pneumomediastinum. *Ann Emerg Med* 2004;43:785. (Initially misdiagnosed as benign pneumomediastinum, the patient returned 10 hours later, critically ill.)

Keberle M, Wittenberg G, Trusen A, Hoppe F, Hahn D: Detection of pharyngeal perforation: Comparison of aqueous and barium containing contrast agents. *AJR* 2000;175:1435–1438.

Vial CM: Boerhaave's syndrome: diagnosis and treatment. *Surg Clin North Am* 2005;85:515–524.

Pneumopericardium

Capizzi PJ, Martin M, Bannon MP: Tension pneumopericardium following blunt injury. *J Trauma* 1995;39:775–780.

Demetriades D, Charalambides D, Pantanowitz D, Lakhoo M: Pneumopericardium following penetrating chest injuries. *Arch Surg* 1990;125:1187–1189.

Demetriades D, Levy R, Hatzitheofilou C, Chun R: Tension pneumopericardium following penetrating trauma: case report. *J Trauma* 1990;30:238–239.

Hernandez-Luyando L, Gonzalez de las Heras E, Calvo J, et al: Posttraumatic tension pneumopericardium. *Am J Emerg Med* 1997;15:686–687.

Hudgens S, McGraw J, Craun M: Two cases of tension pneumopericardium following blunt chest injury. *J Trauma* 1991;31:1408–1410.

Ladurner R: Pneumopericardium in blunt chest trauma after high-speed motor vehicle accidents. *Am J Emerg Med* 2005;23:83–86.

Shorr RM, Mirvis SE, Indeck MC: Tension pneumopericardium in blunt chest trauma. *J Trauma* 1987;27:1078–1082.

Spotnitz AJ, Kaufman JL: Tension pneumopericardium following penetrating chest injury. *J Trauma* 1987;27:806–808.

Chest Radiology: Patient 11

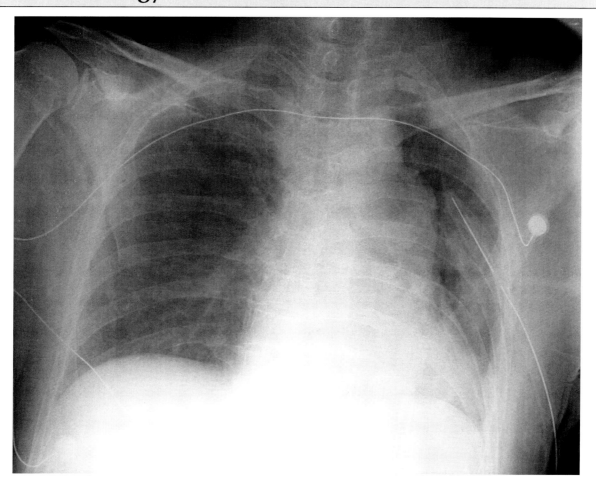

FIGURE 1   Patient 11A

A pedestrian struck by a motor vehicle

A 49-year-old man was struck by a van that was turning a street corner. He had a transient loss of consciousness.

In the trauma resuscitation area, the patient was awake and alert, but would repeatedly ask what had happened despite being told this information on several occasions. He complained of left hip and left-sided chest pain.

His vital signs were: blood pressure 110/70 mmHg, pulse 110 beats/min, respiratory rate 28 breaths/min, SO_2 100% on 10 L/min O_2. His physical examination was remarkable for contusions to the left side of his face and head, palpable tenderness and crepitus over the left lateral chest wall with diminished breath sounds on the left, and tenderness, swelling, and inability to move the left hip due to pain.

A chest tube was inserted on the left without return of blood or air. One liter of normal saline and 8 mg morphine sulfate were administered intravenously. Repeat vital signs were as follows: blood pressure 120/88 mm/Hg, pulse 88 beats/min, respirations 18 breaths/min.

Radiographs of the cervical spine, chest, and pelvis revealed a left chest tube, a left sixth rib fracture, and a left proximal femoral fracture. Bedside sonography was negative for intraperitoneal or pericardial blood.

The trauma service brought the patient to the radiology suite. A head CT revealed a small traumatic subarachnoid hemorrhage. An abdominal CT revealed a small splenic laceration and adjacent peritoneal blood without active arterial extravasation of contrast. Cervical spine CT was normal. An intertrochanteric femoral fracture was seen on left hip radiographs. Left hand and wrist radiographs revealed a fifth metacarpal shaft fracture.

The patient remained stable and was admitted to the surgical intensive care unit for monitoring and eventual repair of his orthopedic injuries.

His chest radiograph is shown in Figure 1.

- Are any additional tests needed?

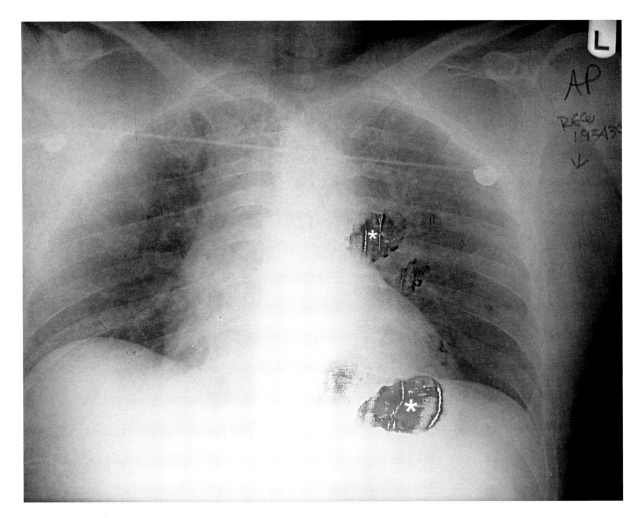

FIGURE 2   Patient 11B

A driver in a motor vehicle collision

A 45-year-old man who was driving a small car struck a slow moving vehicle that had stopped short in front of him while he was going at approximately 30 miles per hour. He was wearing a seatbelt and his air bag deployed. The front end of his car was crushed inwards but there was no intrusion into the vehicle's front passenger compartment.

There was no loss of consciousness. He complained of pain in the anterior chest, but had no shortness of breath.

His vital signs were as follows: blood pressure 120/70 mm/Hg, pulse 84 beats/min, and respiratory rate 20 breaths/ min. On examination, his anterior chest wall was mildly tender, without crepitus. His breath sounds were normal. He had mild upper abdominal tenderness. There were superficial abrasions of his right eyebrow and nose.

The patient remained stable.

His chest radiograph is shown in Figure 2. (*Asterisks* denote defects in x-ray film.)

• Are any additional tests needed?

WHY ORDER CHEST RADIOGRAPHS IN PATIENTS WITH BLUNT TRAUMA TO THE CHEST?

For many types of traumatic injuries to the thorax, the diagnosis is evident based on clinical examination-radiography serves mainly to confirm the clinical impression (e.g., a large pneumothorax, hemothorax, or rib fractures). However, a traumatic tear of the aorta is a life-threatening injury that does not produce characteristic clinical findings. In fact, up to one-quarter of patients with aortic injury have no external signs of thoracic trauma. Chest radiography can provide indirect evidence of an aortic injury, and the detection of signs of aortic injury is therefore, one of the most important roles of chest radiography in victims of blunt chest trauma.

In 85% of cases, the aortic wall is completely torn ("aortic rupture"), which is an immediately fatal exsanguinating injury (Figure 3A). Patients who survive to reach medical care have an incomplete aortic tear in which the hemorrhage is temporarily contained by the outer layers of the aortic wall, forming a *pseudoaneurysm* (Figure 3B). This is an unstable condition, which, if untreated, leads to aortic rupture and fatal exsanguination in nearly all patients—40% within the first 24 hours. With prompt surgical treatment, survival is expected in a large majority of cases. It is therefore essential to consider this diagnosis in all patients who have sustained severe traumatic injuries. On the other hand, aortic injuries are uncommon, occurring in less than 1% of patients admitted to trauma centers.

The mechanism of injury causing blunt traumatic aortic tears is an abrupt deceleration such as occurs during a motor vehicle collision, a fall from significant height, or a forceful direct blow to the chest. Aortic injuries occur most commonly at the *aortic isthmus*, which is located just distal to the origin of the left subclavian artery. This is the region between the fixed descending aorta and the more mobile aortic arch. Significant bending and shear forces occur in this region during trauma (Figure 4).

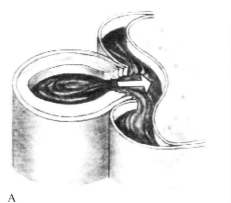 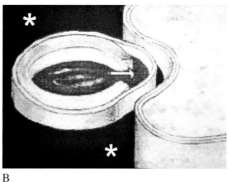

A   B

FIGURE 3   Acute traumatic aortic injuries.

(*A*) Complete aortic rupture with exsanguination into the pleural space – a rapidly fatal injury.

(*B*) Incomplete aortic tear—a focal intramural hematoma is contained by the outer portions of the aortic wall. Mediastinal blood (*asterisks*) surrounds the aorta and displaces the pleural surface. The source of the mediastinal blood is *not* the aorta itself, but smaller branch vessels such as the intercostal arteries that are torn at the time of injury.

[From Hood RM, Boyd AD, Culliford AT: *Thoracic Trauma*. Saunders, 1990, with permission.]

FIGURE 4   Mechanism of injury causing aortic tear.

Shear and bending forces at the junction between the relatively fixed descending aorta and more mobile aortic arch cause most aortic injuries. A small number are due to torsional forces at the ascending aorta.

The great vessels of the aortic arch (innominate, left carotid or left subclavian artery) may also be torn during blunt chest trauma.

Smaller branch vessels such as the intercostal arteries are almost always torn and are the source of mediastinal hemorrhage in patients with incomplete aortic tears.

[From Symbas PN: *Cardiothoracic Trauma*. Saunders, 1989, with permission.]

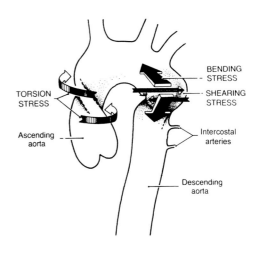

DIAGNOSTIC IMAGING FOR AORTIC INJURY

Chest Radiography

An AP portable chest radiograph is the initial imaging test in patients with blunt chest trauma. The chest radiograph, however, does not visualize the aortic injury directly; rather it detects **hemorrhage into the mediastinum**. The source of mediastinal blood is *not* the injured aorta itself because patients who survive the initial aortic injury have sustained only incomplete aortic tears (Figure 3). The mediastinal blood comes instead from torn smaller branch vessels such as the intercostal arteries, internal mammary artery, or corresponding veins. These vessels can be injured either with or without a concomitant aortic injury. Therefore, in patients with hemomediastinum, a definitive diagnostic test (aortography or MDCT) must be obtained. In fact, only 30% of patients with mediastinal blood have aortic injuries.

Although mediastinal blood is present in more than 90% of patients with aortic injury, the radiographic technique is frequently suboptimal making it difficult or impossible to detect hemomediastinum (Cleverley et al. 2002). Furthermore, in 5–10% of patients with aortic injuries, the radiographic findings can be subtle or even normal. Therefore, patients at high risk of aortic injury due to severe mechanisms of injury, particularly when there are other significant thoracic injuries, should undergo further testing for aortic injury when the radiographs are normal, equivocal, or suboptimal.

Aortography

Aortography is traditionally the definitive test since it directly visualizes the aortic injury. However, in patients undergoing aortography based on chest radiographic and clinical criteria (severity of trauma), only about 15% of patients will have an aortic injury. Nonetheless, obtaining a large number of negative aortograms is necessary in order to avoid missing this highly lethal but treatable injury. Currently, CT has largely replaced aortography as a screening tool and, more recently, as a definitive test for aortic injury.

Computed Tomography

The evolution of CT technology has advanced its role in the diagnosis of aortic injuries.

CT is highly sensitive at detecting **mediastinal blood** and is therefore useful when the chest radiograph is equivocal or suboptimal (Figure 6). CT with an intravenous contrast bolus can detect an **aortic injury directly**—a pseudoaneurysm or intimal flap (Figure 7). However, single-detector helical CT cannot detect every small aortic injury, nor can it define the full anatomical extent of the injury, which is necessary in planning surgery. Furthermore, some CT signs of aortic injury are nonspecific (contour abnormality) and confirmation by aortography may be necessary. Therefore, aortography is still needed when the CT

shows periaortic mediastinal blood alone or a nonspecific aortic contour abnormality. On the other hand, a CT showing no periaortic blood and no aortic contour abnormality is generally considered sufficient to exclude aortic injury. Mediastinal blood that is in an anterior or posterior location and not periaortic is associated with either sternal, vertebral, or rib fractures and not aortic injury (Dyer et al. 2000, Mirvis et al. 1998, Gavant et al. 1996, Gavant 1999).

Multidetector CT (MDCT) can produce thin-section (<1 mm) images through the entire chest with optimal aortic contrast opacification (CT aortogram) and may be capable of definitively detecting or excluding an aortic injury. A CT that does not show an aortic wall injury, even when periaortic blood is present, would, in centers with expertise in CT interpretation, definitively exclude aortic injury. In addition, high-resolution multiplanar (two-dimensional) and three-dimensional reformatted CT images may be adequate for planning surgery (see Figure 15B on p. 100). MDCT can potentially replace aortography as the definitive diagnostic test except in the few cases with equivocal MDCT results (Mirvis 2006).

CT can detect very small intimal tears that cannot be visualized by aortography. Such minimal aortic injuries probably do not require surgical treatment, although long-term study of this condition is not yet available (Holmes et al. 2002, Malhotra et al. 2001).

CT Trauma Protocols

In trauma patients, chest CT is often performed in conjunction with CT of other regions. The sequence of CT scans in such cases is as follow: first, noncontrast CT of the head and cervical spine, then chest CT angiography beginning early after the start of the contrast bolus (15–20 seconds), followed by abdominal and pelvic CT either continuing in the arterial phase or slightly delayed for optimal parenchymal enhancement (90 seconds after the start of the contrast bolus). If a bladder injury is suspected, a CT cystogram is performed with the bladder distended with contrast (contrast either excreted after a 3–5 minute delay or instilled via a Foley catheter).

Transesophageal Echocardiography

Transesophageal echocardiography (TEE) can directly visualize the aortic intimal flap (Figure 8). Although an initial study demonstrated very high sensitivity, this was not confirmed on a subsequent report (Smith et al. 1995, Minard et al. 1996). TEE can play a role in an unstable patient requiring emergency laparotomy for intraabdominal hemorrhage. An intraoperative TEE can be used to identify an aortic injury that could then be repaired during the surgical procedure. TEE would be indicated in patients whose initial chest radiograph shows mediastinal hemorrhage or in whom there is a high clinical suspicion of aortic injury due to the presence of other severe chest injuries.

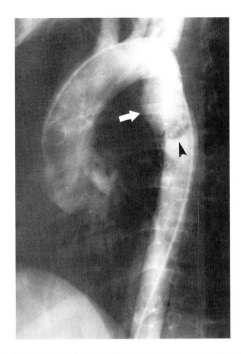

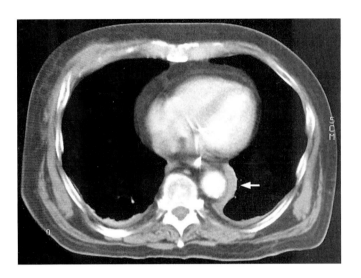

FIGURE 5   An aortogram showing an intimal flap displaced into the aortic lumen (*arrowhead*), and a pseudoaneurysm contained by the intact outer aortic wall (*arrow*).

Note that there is no extravasation of contrast from the aorta, i.e., the mediastinal blood associated with aortic injury does not originate from the aorta itself.

[From Schwartz DT, Reisdorff EJ: *Emergency Radiology*. McGraw-Hill, 2000.]

FIGURE 6   **Contrast CT showing periaortic blood** (*arrow*).

An aortic injury was not visible on this CT scan and aortography was needed to visualize the aortic injury.

[From Schwartz DT, Reisdorff EJ: *Emergency Radiology*. McGraw-Hill, 2000.]

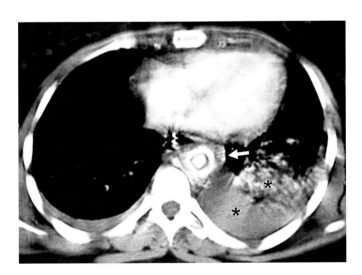

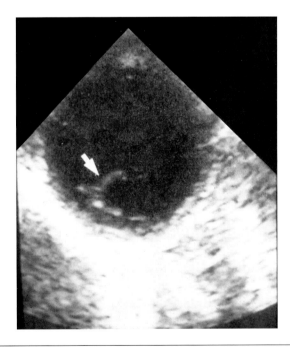

Figure 7   Contrast CT showing an acute aortic injury.

There is a circumferential traumatic dissection of the aorta forming an inner true lumen and an outer false lumen that is contained by the intact outer portion of the aortic wall. There is a small amount of periaortic blood (*arrow*) as well as a left hemothorax and pulmonary contusion (*asterisks*).

FIGURE 8   Transesophageal echocardiogram showing an aortic intimal tear (*arrow*).

[From Smith MD et al: *New Engl J Med* 1995;332: 356–362, with permission.]

CHEST RADIOGRAPHIC SIGNS OF AORTIC INJURY

Radiographic findings associated with aortic injury are due to the presence of mediastinal blood (Table 1). The radiographic hallmark is **widening of the mediastinum** (Figure 9). Various criteria have been used to assess mediastinal widening: more than 8 cm on a supine radiograph, more than 6 cm on an upright radiograph, greater than 25% of the thoracic width at the aortic knob, or the "subjective impression" of an experienced observer.

The second most frequent sign of mediastinal hemorrhage is an **indistinct or distorted aortic contour** (aortic knob or proximal descending aorta).

The major problem with these two radiographic signs is that they may also be the result of the **suboptimal radiographic technique** which is frequently seen with supine portable chest radiographs, especially if the patient has not taken a full inspiration (Figure 10). If a good quality chest radiograph cannot be obtained, chest CT is effective at detecting mediastinal hemorrhage. Furthermore, 10% of patients with aortic injury do *not* have a widened mediastinum. These patients often have more subtle radiographic manifestations of mediastinal blood (White 1994) (see Figures 14 and 15A on p. 100).

Other signs of mediastinal hemorrhage are less dependent on radiographic technique. **Mediastinal pleural reflection lines** may be distorted by blood in the mediastinum (Figure 11). These signs include:1) widened right paratracheal stripe; 2) opacified aorticopulmonary window; 3) displacement of the left or right paraspinal line; and 4) spread of the mediastinal blood over the apex of the left lung forming a left apical pleural cap (Figures 12 and 13). The left paraspinal line parallels the vertebral bodies inferior to the aortic arch. Although its position adjacent to the vertebral bodies is variable, it normally disappears at and above the aortic knob. With mediastinal blood, the left paraspinal line may become

visible superior to the aortic knob and may extend to the apex of the lung forming a left apical pleural cap.

Finally, blood surrounding the aortic isthmus may displace adjacent structures such as the trachea, left mainstem bronchus, and esophagus (with nasogastric tube). To best show these mediastinal details, the chest radiograph should be slightly over-penetrated (dark). These mediastinal abnormalties are also of value in patients with nontraumatic thoracic disorders such as mediastinal lymphadenopathy (see Chest Radiology Patient 6, Figure 4 on Page 53).

TABLE 1

Radiographic Signs of Traumatic Aortic Injury

Mediastinal hematoma

   Wide mediastinum

   Indistinct or distorted aortic knob or proximal descending aorta

   Opacification of the aorticopulmonary window

   Wide right paratracheal stripe

   Left paraspinal line displaced and extending superior to aortic knob

   Left apical pleural cap

   Right paraspinal line displaced

   Mass effect due to periaortic blood at the aortic arch

      Trachea or nasogastric tube displaced to the right

      Depressed left mainstem bronchus

Signs of severe chest trauma

   Rib fractures—especially first or second ribs

   Pulmonary contusion

   Hemothorax, pneumothorax

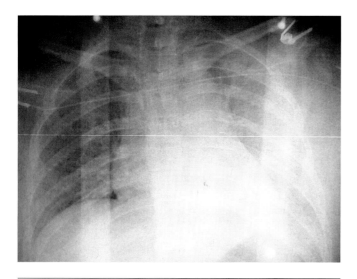

FIGURE 9   Featureless widening of the mediastinum in a patient with hemomediastinum and aortic injury.

In addition, the trachea is deviated to the right. This is not due to rotated positioning of the patient, but is due to the aortic injury. Opacification of the left hemithorax is due to a hemothorax and pulmonary contusion as confirmed by CT. (The CT of this patient is shown in Figure 7.)

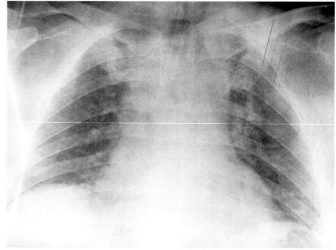

FIGURE 10   Mediastinal widening due to incomplete inspiration.

Further imaging revealed that there was no mediastinal hematoma or aortic injury. An endotracheal tube is present.

[From: Schwartz DT, Reisdorff EJ: *Emergency Radiology*. McGraw-Hill, 2000.]

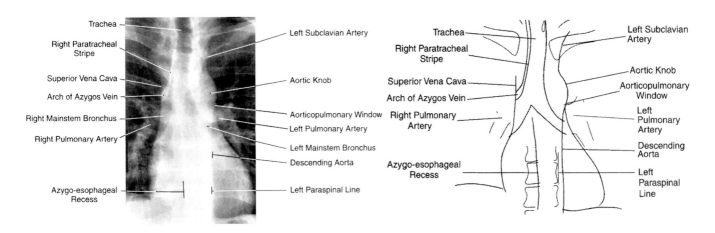

FIGURE 11   Mediastinal pleural reflection lines.

Left subclavian artery—a curved shadow that disappears at the superior border of the clavicle.

Right paratracheal stripe—normally < 5 mm wide; terminates inferiorly at the *arch of the azygos vein.*

Aorticopulmonary window—space between aortic arch and superior border of left pulmonary artery.

Left paraspinal line—adjacent to vertebral bodies; normally disappears above the aortic knob.

Azygo-esophageal recess—inferior to the arch of the azygos vein, the medial surface of the right lung extends into the mediastinum and lies against the esophagus (this is not the right side of the descending aorta).

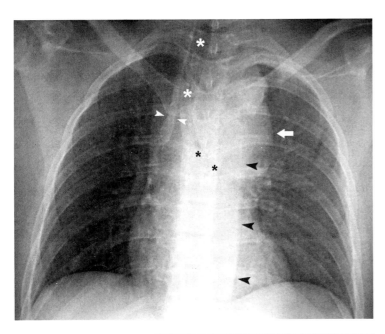

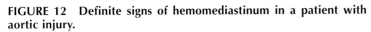

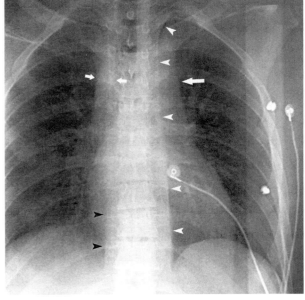

FIGURE 12   Definite signs of hemomediastinum in a patient with aortic injury.

The mediastinum is widened and the aortic knob is distorted by surrounding blood (*arrow*).

Mediastinal blood causes widening of the **right paratracheal stripe** (*white arrowheads*) and displacement of the **left paraspinal line** (*black arrowheads*), which extends up to the aortic knob.

The **trachea** is displaced to the right (*white asterisks*) and the left mainstem bronchus is displaced inferiorly (*black asterisks*). This is due to blood surrounding the aorta. The faint shadow of the SVC is visible to the right of the paratracheal stripe. (The aortogram of this patient is shown in Figure 5.)

[From: Schwartz DT, Reisdorff EJ: *Emergency Radiology.* McGraw-Hill, 2000.]

FIGURE 13   Definite signs of hemomediastinum in a patient with aortic injury.

The **right paratracheal stripe** is widened (*small white arrows*). The SVC is not visible.

The **left paraspinal line** is displaced laterally and extends above the aortic arch to the apex of the lung, forming a small left apical pleural cap superiorly (*white arrowheads*). The **right paraspinal line** is also displaced (*black arrowheads*).

The **aortic knob** is indistinct (*large white arrow*).

[From: Schwartz DT, Reisdorff EJ: *Emergency Radiology.* McGraw-Hill, 2000.]

Radiographic (and clinical) findings of **other severe thoracic injuries** such as multiple rib fractures (particularly the first and second ribs), hemothorax, or pulmonary contusion are also important in deciding to order an aortogram, CT, or TEE. Although they are only indirectly related to aortic injury, their presence should heighten the suspicion of aortic injury. Furthermore, a large hemothorax or pulmonary contusion can obscure the mediastinum and make it impossible to detect signs of mediastinal hemorrhage.

Whether a **normal chest radiograph** excludes an aortic injury is a matter of controversy. One careful review of radiographs in patients with aortic injury did not find any normal radiographs. However, this study excluded technically suboptimal radiographs, was conducted by expert trauma radiologists, and the radiographic findings were subtle (Figures 14 and 15) (White et al. 1994). In two large clinical series, 5–7% of aortic injury cases had radiographs that were interpreted as negative

for aortic injury (Fabian et al. 1997, Hunt et. al. 1996). However, the quality of the radiographic technique in these cases was not mentioned, and the radiographic criteria used to assess aortic injury were not stated. Several other case series also report normal mediastinal appearance in patients with aortic injury (Exadaktylos et al. 2001, Woodring 1990). Only when a chest radiograph is of sufficient quality to clearly determine that the mediastinal contours are normal could it be considered adequate to exclude a mediastinal hematoma (Mirvis 2006). However, in one study, 10% of aortic injury cases do not have a mediastinal hematoma on CT and so even a normal, technically optimal chest radiograph should not be used alone to exclude aortic injury (Cleverley et al. 2002).

Although of limited value in excluding aortic injury, the chest radiographic signs of mediastinal blood should be recognized and, when present, should prompt a rapid definitive investigation for aortic injury.

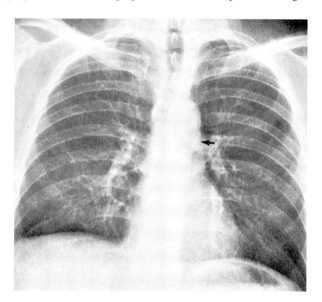

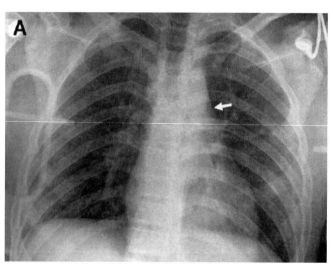

FIGURE 14   Hemomediastinum without a widened mediastinum.

This erect AP radiograph shows fluid filling the aorticopulmonary window, a subtle radiographic sign of hemomediastinum (*arrow*). The patient had a traumatic aortic tear during a motor vehicle collision.

[From White CS, Mirvis SE, Templeton PA: Subtle chest radiographic abnormalities in patients with traumatic aortic rupture. *Emerg Radiol* 1994;1:73, with permission.]

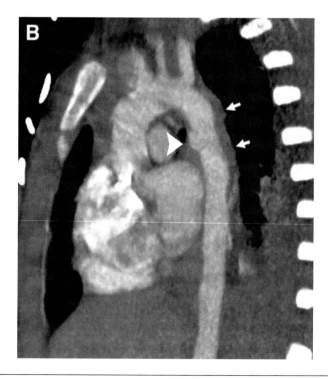

FIGURE 15   Nearly normal chest radiograph in a patient with an aortic injury.

(*A*) An AP supine radiograph shows a nearly normal mediastinal contour. The aortic knob and aorticopulmonary window are (*arrow*).

(*B*) MDCT oblique sagittal reformatted image shows a pseudoaneurysm (*arrowhead*). Mediastinal blood surrounds the aorta (*arrows*).

[From: Mirvis SE: Thoracic vascular injury. Radiol Clin North Am 2006;44:181–197, with permission.]

PATIENT 11A OUTCOME

The following day, the patient developed increasing chest pain and dyspnea. Upon review of the initial chest radiograph, the widened mediastinum was noted (Figure 16). An aortogram was performed that revealed an injury of the proximal descending aorta (Figure 17). The patient underwent emergency thoracotomy and aortic replacement. His recovery was uneventful.

Although the chest radiographic findings were, in retrospect, obvious, the clinicians caring for the patient were distracted by the presence of other serious injuries and perhaps attributed the widened mediastinum to suboptimal radiographic technique (Willemsen et al. 2001, Savitt 1999) (Table 2).

Had there been doubt about the chest radiographic findings or the need for aortography, CT of the chest could have been performed at the time of the abdominal CT. This would have confirmed the presence of mediastinal blood and possibly identified the aortic injury.

Review of the patient's abdominal CT revealed periaortic blood on the most superior slices at the diaphragmatic crura that should have served as a clue to the presence of an aortic injury (Wang 2004).

TABLE 2

Reasons That the Diagnosis of Traumatic Aortic Injury Is Missed

1. Lack of external signs of thoracic trauma

2. Clinicians distracted from considering aortic injury by other more common or obvious injuries—abdominal, pelvic, extremity, or craniofacial injuries

3. Failure to appreciate the radiographic signs of aortic injury, particularly subtle signs

4. Attributing a widened or indistinct mediastinum to the AP supine technique

5. Suboptimal radiographic technique obscures signs of hemomediastinum

6. Not obtaining a portable chest radiograph with the best possible technique (full inspiration)

7. "Normal" chest radiograph (seen in 5-7% of cases)

8. Not obtaining CT of the chest in patients at high risk based on the mechanism of injury or the presence of other serious thoracic injuries

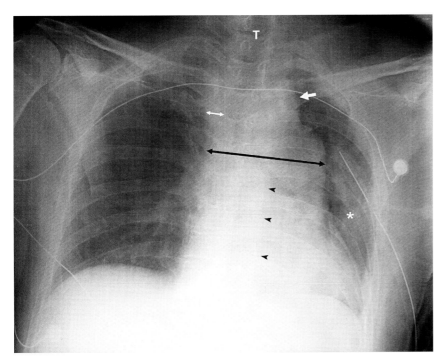

FIGURE 16 The chest radiograph revealed marked widening of the mediastinum (11 cm) (*black double-headed arrow*).

There are three other signs of hemomediastinum:

• Abnormal contour above the aortic knob (*white arrow*).

• Wide right paratracheal stripe (20 mm) (*white double-headed arrow*).

• Displaced left paraspinal line (*arrowheads*).

The trachea (T) is displaced to the left due to rotated positioning of the patient. Opacification of the left lung is due to pulmonary contusion (*asterisk*).

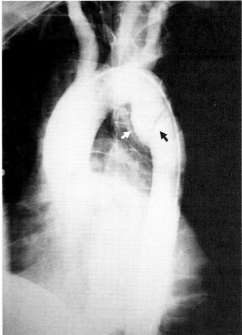

FIGURE 17 Aortogram showing intimal flap (*black arrow*) and contained hematoma—pseudoaneurysm (*white arrow*).

The aorta itself is of normal size demonstrating that the apparently enlarged aortic knob on the chest radiograph is caused by blood adjacent to the aorta and not the aortic pseudoaneurysm itself.

PATIENT 11B OUTCOME

Despite the description of a dangerous mechanism of injury, the patient appeared well—he had probably slowed his car considerably by the time of impact. Although the chest radiograph showed marked mediastinal widening (11 cm) and an indistinct contour, it was an AP supine view with poor inspiration (Figure 18).

The patient was sufficiently stable to have a **repeat AP chest radiograph** while sitting upright and with more complete inspiration (Figure 19). The mediastinum was normal. Because of the mechanism of injury and upper abdominal tenderness, the patient had a CT scan looking for intra-abdominal injuries. Several CT slices of the chest were taken which confirmed the absence of mediastinal hemorrhage and excluded aortic injury.

There are several factors that contribute to the apparent mediastinal widening often seen on AP supine chest radiographs (Table 3). A shallow level of inspiration is the major factor and can often be corrected by instructing the patient inspire fully.

TABLE 3

Causes of Mediastinal Widening on Portable Radiographs

1. AP versus PA technique enlarges anterior structures because they are further from the imaging cassette

2. Short distance between imaging cassette and x-ray source further magnifies anterior structures

3. Supine versus upright positioning causes mediastinal soft tissues to flatten and become broader and the superior vena cava to become distended

4. Shallow inspiration

5. Rotated positioning of the patient

6. Lordotic projection magnifies anterior structures

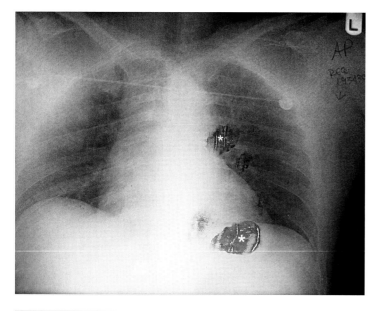

FIGURE 18   Initial radiograph—Patient 11B.

The mediastinum is markedly widened (>11 cm) and indistinct. However, the radiographic technique is suboptimal—incomplete inspiration and rotated positioning—which accounts for these findings. A normal right paratracheal stripe can be seen despite the suboptimal radiographic technique (*arrowheads*).

The trachea (T) is displaced to the right. Although this finding is associated with aortic injury, the patient was positioned with rightward rotation, which accounts for the tracheal deviation (asterisks—defects in x-ray film).

There were no other clinical or radiographic signs of thoracic trauma such as rib fractures, pulmonary contusion or hemothorax, which makes an aortic injury less likely.

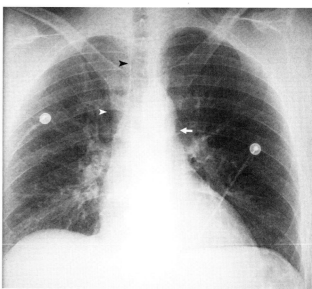

FIGURE 19   Repeat radiograph with upright positioning and full inspiration.

The mediastinum now appears normal, although not as well delineated as on a PA radiograph. Normal features that can be identified include the aorticopulmonary window (*white arrow*) and the right paratracheal stripe (*black arrowhead*). The mediastinal width is <6 cm. Measurement of mediastinal width should not include the superior vena cava (*white arrowhead*).

Summary

An aortic injury is a potentially fatal but survivable condition if promptly diagnosed and treated. The chest radiograph has a limited but potentially important role in the diagnosis of aortic injury. The key radiographic findings are signs of mediastinal hemorrhage. When there are definite signs of mediastinal blood (Figures 12 and 13), a definitive diagnostic test should be perfomed, either catheter aortography or MDCT aortography.

In most patients, however, the chest radiograph is less helpful. In some case, the mediastinum appears indistinct or wiedened which could simply be due to the AP supine radiographic technique (Figures 9, 10, 18 and 19). In other cases, the chest radiograph may be normal or nearly normal (Figures 14 and 15).

When the mechanism of injury is sufficiently severe to have caused an aortic injury, chest CT should be performed. The absence of mediastinal blood or an aortic contour abnormality effectively excludes aortic injury. Definitive signs of aortic injury should prompt surgical treatment (Figure 7). Nonspecific signs such as periaortic blood or an aortic contour abnormality (Figure 6) may necessitate a second definitive test-aortography.

In institutions that have **MDCT** readily available, thin section CT with intravenous contrast can be used as an initial screening test for hemodynamically stable major trauma victims. This is usually performed in concert with abdominopelvic CT as well as head and cervical spine CT. Although the frequency of aortic injury is as low as 5% (Mirvis 1998), this approach is justified to identify a potentially fatal but treatable injury. Although this is lower than the 15% yield that is accepted for catheter aortography, MDCT is noninvasive and therefore should be more widely used. In addition, CT can detect other thoracic injures that can be missed on chest radiography such as a pneumothorax (see Patent 9, Figure 5 on page 78), pulmonary contusion or thoracic spine fracture.

SUGGESTED READING

Brady WJ, Aufderheide T, Kaplan P: Cardiovascular imaging. In Schwartz DT, Reisdorff EJ: *Emergency Radiology*. McGraw-Hill, 2000.

Cisek J, Wilkinson K: Radiographic Priorities in Trauma. In Schwartz DT, Reisdorff EJ: *Emergency Radiology*. McGraw-Hill, 2000.

Harris JH, Harris WH: *The Radiology of Emergency Medicine*, 4th ed. Williams and Wilkins, 2000 496–529. Describes alterations in mediastinal lines that occur with aortic injuries.

Moore EE, Feliciano DV, Mattox KL: *Trauma* 4th ed. McGraw-Hill, 2003.

Chest Radiography

Cook AD, Klein JS, Rogers FB, et al.: Chest radiographs of limited utility in the diagnosis of blunt traumatic aortic laceration. *J Trauma* 2001;50:843–847.

Creasy JD, Chiles C, Routh WD, Dyer RB: Overview of traumatic injury of the thoracic aorta. *Radiographics* 1997;17:27–45.

Exadaktylos AK, et al.: Do we really need routine computed tomographic scanning in the evaluation of blunt chest trauma in patients with "normal" chest radiograph? *J Trauma* 2001;51:1173–1176. (Yes, in major trauma.)

Ho RT, Blackmore CC, Bloch RD, et al.: Can we rely on mediastinal widening on chest radiography to identify subjects with aortic injury? *Emerg Radiol* 2002;9:183–187.

Lee FT, Katzberg RW, Gutierrez OH, et al.: Re-evaluation of plain radiographic findings in the diagnosis of aortic rupture: The role of inspiration and positioning on mediastinal width. *J Emerg Med* 1993;11:289–296.

Mehta SG, Meyermann M: Images in Emergency Medicine: Traumatic aortic transection. *Ann Emerg Med* 2007;49:408–419.

Mirvis SE, Bidwell JK, Buddemeyer EU, et al.: Value of chest radiography in excluding traumatic aortic rupture. *Radiology* 1987;163: 487–493.

Schwab CW, Lawson RB, Lind JF, Garland LW: Aortic injury: Comparison of supine and upright portable chest films to evaluate the widened mediastinum. *Ann Emerg Med* 1984;13:896–899.

White CS, Mirvis SE, Templeton PA: Subtle chest radiographic abnormalities in patients with traumatic aortic rupture. *Emerg Radiol* 1994;1:72–77.

Thirteen (12%) of 107 aortic injury cases had subtle CXR findings. All of these patients except one had *normal* mediastinal width (<8 cm), although the mediastinal to chest width ration was >25% in six cases. All had an abnormal aortic contour, loss of the aortic silhouette, and/or other subtle signs.

Woodring JH: The normal mediastinum in blunt traumatic rupture of the thoracic aorta and brachiocephalic arteries. *J Emerg Med* 1990;8:467–476. (7.3% had a normal mediastinum on their chest radiograph.)

MDCT

Alkadhi H, Wildermuth S, Desbiolles L, et al.: Vascular emergencies of the thorax after blunt and iatrogenic trauma: Multidetector row and three-dimensional imaging. *Radiographics* 2004;24:1239–1255.

Mirvis SE: Thoracic vascular injury. *Radiol Clin North Am* 2006;44:181–197.

Rivas LA, Fishman JE, Múnera F, Bajayo DE: Multislice CT in thoracic trauma. *Radiol Clin North Am* 2003;41:599–616.

Helical CT

Bruckner BA, DiBardino DJ, Cumbie TC, et al.: Critical evaluation of chest computed tomography scans for blunt descending thoracic aortic injury. *Ann Thorac Surg* 2006;81;1339–1346. (55% of CT indeterminate)

Cleverley JR, Barrie JR, Raymond GS, et al.: Direct findings of aortic injury on contrast-enhanced CT in surgically proven traumatic aortic injury: A multi-centre review. *Clin Radiol* 2002;57: 281–286.

Collier B, Hughes KM, Mishok K, et al.: Is helical computed tomography effective for diagnosis of blunt aortic injury? *Am J Emerg Med* 2002;20:558–561.

Demetriades D, Gomez H, Velmahos GC, et al.: Routine helical computed tomographic evaluation of the mediastinum in high-risk blunt trauma patients. *Arch Surg* 1998;133:1084–1088.

Dyer DS, Moore EE, et al.: Can chest CT be used to exclude aortic injury? *Radiology* 1999;213:195–202.

Dyer DS, Moore EE, Ilke DN, et al.: Thoracic aortic injury: How predictive is mechanism and is chest computed tomography a reliable screening tool? A prospective study of 1,516 patients. *J Trauma* 2000; 48:673–683.

Fabian TC, David KA, Gavant ML, et al.: Prospective study of blunt aortic injury: Helical CT is diagnostic and antihypertensive therapy reduces rupture. *Ann Surg* 1998;227:666–677.

Fishman JE, Nunez D, Kane A, et al.: Direct versus indirect signs of traumatic aortic injury revealed by helical CT. *AJR* 1999;172: 1027–1031.

Fishman JE: Imaging of blunt aortic and great vessel trauma. *J Thor Imag* 2000;15:97–103.

Gavant ML, Flick P, Menke P, Gold RE: CT aortography of thoracic aortic rupture. *AJR* 1996;166:955–961.

Gavant ML: Helical CT grading of traumatic aortic injuries: impact on clinical guidelines for medical and surgical management. *Radiol Clin North Am* 1999;37:553–574.

Malhotra AK, Fabian TC, Croce MA, et al.: Minimal aortic injury: A lesion associated with advancing diagnostic techniques. *J Trauma* 2001;51:1042–1048.

Malloy PC, Richard HM: Thoracic angiography and intervention in trauma. *Radiol Clin North Am* 2006;44:239–249.

Mirvis SE, Shanmuganathan K, Buell J, Rodriguez A: Use of spiral computed tomography for the assessment of blunt trauma patients with potential aortic injury. *J Trauma* 1998;45:922–930.

Mirvis SE, Shanmuganathan K, Miller B, et al.: Traumatic aortic injury: Diagnosis with contrast enhanced thoracic CT: Five year experience at a major trauma center. *Radiology* 1996;200: 413–422.

Parker MS, Matheson L, Rao AV, et al.: Making the transition: The role of helical CT in the evaluation of potentially acute thoracic aortic injuries. *AJR* 2001;176:1267–1272.

Patel NH, Stephens KE, Mirvis SE, et al.: Imaging of acute thoracic aortic injury due to blunt trauma: A review. *Radiology* 1998; 209:335–348.

Scaglione M, Pinto A, Pinto F, et al.: Role of contrast-enhanced helical CT in the evaluation of acute thoracic aortic injuries after blunt chest trauma. *Eur Radiol* 2001;11:2444–2448.

Shiau YW, Wong YC, Ng CJ, et al.: Periaortic contrast medium extravasation on chest CT in traumatic aortic injury: A sign for immediate thoracotomy. *Am J Emerg Med* 2001;19:229–231.

Wintermark M, Wicky S, Schnyder P: Imaging of acute traumatic injuries of the thoracic aorta. *Eur Radiol* 2002;12:431–442.

Wong YC, Wang LJ, Lim KE, et al.: Periaortic hematoma on helical CT of the chest: A criterion for predicting blunt traumatic aortic rupture. *AJR* 1998;170:1523–1525.

Clinical Studies of Blunt Aortic Trauma

Blackmore CC, Zweibel A, Mann FA: Determining risk of traumatic aortic injury: How to optimize imaging strategy. *AJR* 2000;174: 343–347. (Derived clinical prediction rule)

All aortic injury cases had at least one of the seven of criteria: age >50 years, unrestrained vehicle occupant, hypotension, thoracic injury, abdominopelvic injury, extremity fracture, or head injury.

Cook J, Salerno C, Krishnadasan B, et al.: The effect of changing presentation and management on the outcome of blunt rupture of the thoracic aorta. *J Thoracic Cardiovascular Surgery* 2006;131: 594–600.

Fabian TC, Richardson JD, Croce MA, et al.: Prospective study of blunt aortic injury: Multicenter trial of the AAST. *J Trauma* 1997;42:374–80. (7% of patients had "normal" chest radiographs.)

Holmes JHT, Bloch RD, Hall RA, et al.: Natural history of traumatic rupture of the thoracic aorta managed nonoperatively: A longitudinal analysis. *Ann Thorac Surg* 2002;73:1149–1154.

Hunt JP, Baker CC, Lentz CW, et al.: Thoracic aorta injuries: management and outcome of 144 patients. *J Trauma* 1996;40:547–555. (5% of patients had "normal" chest radiographs.)

McGwin G, Metzger J, Moran SG, Rue LW: Occupant- and collision-related risk factors for blunt thoracic aorta injury. *J Trauma* 2003;54:655–662.

Nagy K, Fabian T, Rodman G, et al.: Guidelines for the diagnosis and management of blunt aortic injury. *J Trauma* 2000;48:1128–1143.

Pate JW, Gavant ML, Weiman DS, et al. Traumatic rupture of the aortic isthmus: Program of selective management. *World J Surg* 1999;23:59.

Pretre R, Chilcott M: Blunt trauma to the heart and great vessels. *New Engl J Med* 1997;336:626–632.

Savitt DL: Traumatic aortic rupture: Delayed presentation with a normal chest radiograph. *Am J Emerg Med* 1999;17:285–287. (A missed case resulted in litigation; chest radiograph was suboptimal.)

Willemsen HW, Bakker FC, Patka P, Haarman HJ: Traumatic rupture of the thoracic aorta: time to diagnosis and treatment. *Eur J Emerg Med* 2001;8:39–42. (Three of the six cases had delayed diagnosis.)

TEE

Minard G, Schurr MJ, Croce MA, et al.: A prospective analysis of transesophageal echocardiography in the diagnosis of traumatic disruption of the aorta. *J Trauma* 1996;40:225–230. (Not 100% reliable.)

Smith MD, Cassidy JM, Souther S, et al.: Transesophageal echocardiography in the diagnosis of traumatic rupture of the aorta. *New Engl J Med* 1995;332:356–362.

Chest Radiology: Patient 12

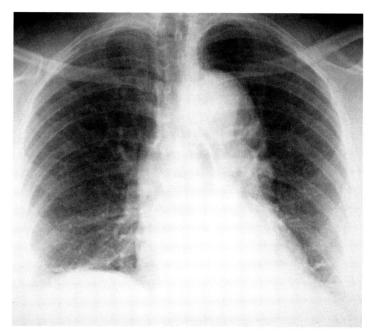 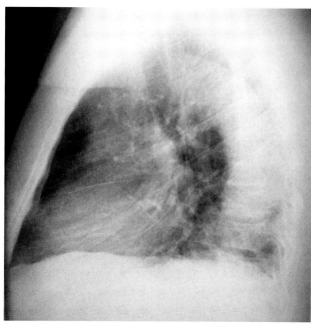

FIGURE 1

Abdominal pain in a middle-aged man

A 56-year-old man presented to the ED with abdominal pain that began several hours earlier.

He had locked himself out of his house and was crawling through the window when he experienced an abrupt onset of abdominal pain. He felt something "pop" as he slid over the window sill and stood up. The pain was periumbilical in location and radiated to the middle of his back. He described it as a dull "gas" pain. He felt slight nausea, but had no vomiting, diarrhea, constipation, fever, or difficulty urinating. There was no chest pain or shortness of breath. He had never experienced similar pain in the past.

The patient had no prior medical problems aside from an elevated blood pressure that had been noted one year earlier. However, he did not follow up or receive antihypertensive medications. He smoked one-half a pack of cigarettes per day. He did not drink alcohol or use illicit drugs. He worked as an electrician for the municipal transit authority.

On examination, he was overweight and appeared comfortable, but periodically was in distress when the abdominal pain recurred. His blood pressure was 156/90 mm Hg, pulse 94 beats/min, respirations 18 breaths/min, temperature 99.2°F, and oxygen saturation 95% while breathing room air. His lungs were clear. His heart had a regular rhythm without murmur, gallop, or rub. His abdomen was obese but not distended. There was mild diffuse tenderness, but no focal tenderness, rebound tenderness, or palpable mass. Bowel sounds were normal and there were no bruits. The right flank was tender.

The **EKG** showed left ventricular hypertrophy with strain (lateral T wave inversions). **Blood test results** showed a leukocyte count of 12,300 cells/mm^3, hematocrit 41.5%, normal electrolytes, and normal renal and liver values. A urinalysis showed 1+ blood and 10–20 RBC/high power field.

The **chest radiograph** was interpreted as showing a tortuous aorta (Figure 1).

- Is the chest radiograph normal?

- Which disorders should be suspected in this patient?

- Is further diagnostic imaging needed?

THE TORTUROUS AORTA

Bedside **abdominal ultrasonography** showed no abdominal aortic aneurysm, gallstones or hydronephrosis. An **abdominal CT** with oral and intravenous contrast was performed. When the emergency physician called the radiologist for a preliminary report, he was first told that the CT was normal. Shortly thereafter, the radiologist called back and reported that there was an aortic dissection on the most superior slices. A faint intimal flap separated the aorta into a true and a false lumens, which were equally opacified by the intravenous contrast material (Figure 2).

Upon reassessment, the patient's blood pressure was markedly elevated to 220/140 mm Hg and heart rate was 104 beats/min. A second EKG showed no acute ischemic changes. The hypertension was treated with intravenous labetalol and an infusion of nitroglycerine.

To determine the proximal extent of the dissection, i.e., whether it involved only the descending aorta or extended into the aortic arch and ascending aorta, additional imaging was necessary. Because the patient had just received a dose of intravenous contrast, a second dose for a chest CT would have increased the risk of contrast-induced nephrotoxicity. A **transesophageal echocardiogram** (TEE) was therefore performed, which revealed dissection of the descending aorta originating at an intimal tear just distal to the left subclavian artery (Figure 3). There was no involvement of the aortic arch or ascending aorta and no pericardial effusion.

The aortic dissection was managed with careful control of the patient's blood pressure. After 24 hours in the intensive care unit, oral antihypertensive medications were started. The patient was discharged from the hospital 10 days later. His aortic dissection remained stable on subsequent clinic visits. He was monitored with serial CT scans at 6 and 12 months. Over time there was thrombosis of the false lumen and no increase in aortic diameter.

- **Was there any evidence on the initial chest radiograph that the patient was having an aortic dissection?**

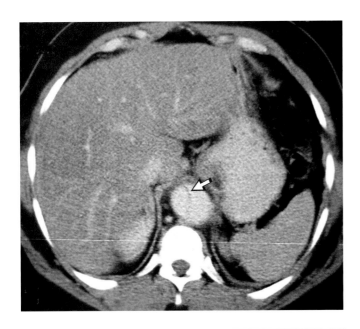

FIGURE 2 Superior CT slice shows an intimal flap (*arrow*) spanning the aortic lumen.

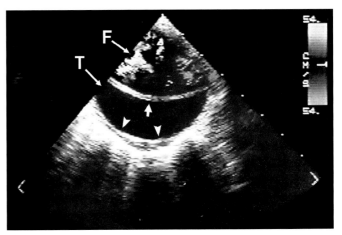

FIGURE 3 TEE of the descending thoracic aorta.

The intimal flap (*arrow*) separates the true lumen (T) from the false lumen (F). The true lumen is completely surrounded by intima (*arrowheads*). There is turbulent flow within the false lumen (F) as indicated by the superimposed color Doppler signal (shades of gray in this image).

AORTIC DISSECTION—PATHOPHYSIOLOGY

Understanding the radiographic manifestions of aortic dissection requires knowledge of its pathophysiology and pathologic anatomy.

The aortic wall is composed of three concentric layers: the *intima* which lines the aortic lumen; the relatively thick elastic *media;* and the outer *adventitia.* In patients with aortic dissection, the media is weakened by *degeneration of its elastin fibers.* This is associated with aging, chronic hypertension, and a congenital or acquired defect in elastin such as Marfan syndrome. Hemodynamic stresses on the inner surface of the aortic wall tear the intima and allow blood from the aortic lumen to enter and split the aortic into two layers. The hematoma dissects along the length of the aorta forming a *false lumen,* which is separated from the *true lumen* by an *intimal flap* (Figure 4).

The intimal tear occurs most often either at the midportion of the ascending aorta, which is subjected to the full force of left ventricular ejection, or at the proximal descending aorta, where there are sheer stresses between the more mobile aortic arch and relatively fixed descending aorta. Blood flowing into the false lumen may either reenter the true lumen forming a "double-barreled" aorta or rupture through the adventitia causing fatal exsanguination. Over time the false lumen may eventually thrombose and stabilize.

Ascending versus descending aortic dissection

The prognosis, potential complications and treatment differ significantly depending on whether the dissection involves the ascending or descending aorta.

Ascending dissection poses a greater threat because it may extend into the aortic valve causing acute aortic insufficiency and congestive heart failure, or may rupture into the pericardial sac causing tamponade. Because of these potentially fatal complications, surgery is needed for ascending aortic dissection, unless the patient is too debilitated or has substantial comorbidities (28% of cases). The in-hospital mortality rate is 35%. In the IRAD series, 62% of dissections were ascending (Hagan et al. 2000).

Descending aortic dissection can usually be managed medically by controlling blood pressure and reducing the force of ventricular contraction using β-adrenergic blocking agents and, secondarily, vasodilating medications. Surgery is needed when there is progressive extension of the dissection, occlusion of a major branch vessel such as the superior mesenteric artery or renal arteries, or leakage with impending rupture (20% of cases). A descending dissection that extends proximally into the aortic arch, but not to the ascending aorta, can generally be managed nonoperatively. In-hospital mortality is 15%.

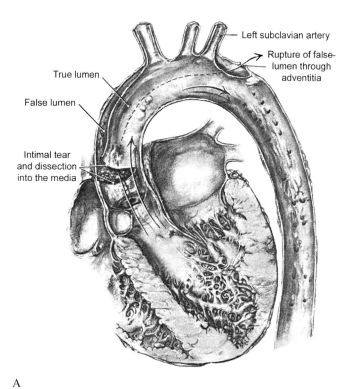

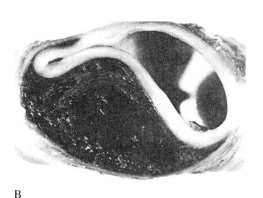

B   A

FIGURE 4 Pathologic anatomy of aortic dissection.

(*A*) A postmortem specimen of aortic dissection. An intimal tear of the ascending aorta allowed blood to enter and split the aortic wall forming a false lumen. The dissection propagated along the aortic arch and then ruptured through the outer portion of the aortic wall causing fatal exsanguination. Note that the cross-sectional diameter of the aorta remain unchanged by the dissection.

(*B*) Dissection shown in cross-section. The hematoma splits the media and displaces the intima and adjacent media into the aortic lumen. Thrombus fills the false lumen.

[From: Lindsay J, Hurst JW: *The Aorta.* Grune and Stratton, 1979, with permission.]

There are two **classification systems** for aortic dissection. In the **Stanford classification,** type A involves the ascending aorta and type B involves only the descending aorta. This relates to the differences in management described above. In the **De-Bakey system,** type 1 involves both the ascending and descending aorta, type 2 involves only the ascending aorta and type 3 involves only the descending aorta (Figure 5).

The older term **"dissecting aortic aneurysm"** is misleading and should be avoided because, although the aorta is invariably dilated in patients with aortic dissection, the dilation is not always to an amount considered aneurysmal (5 cm diameter at the ascending aorta and 4 cm at the descending thoracic aorta). In addition, many large aortic aneurysms, particularly those associated with atherosclerosis (thoracic, thoracoabdominal, and abdominal aortic aneurysms), are prone to leakage and rupture rather than to dissection.

A variant of aortic dissection is an **intramural hematoma** (IMH). The vasa vasorum within the diseased aortic media are torn resulting in hemorrhage into the media. The hematoma may then split the media in a fashion similar to aortic dissection. An IMH may rupture across the intima, producing a condition indistinguishable from aortic dissection. Other "acute aortic syndromes" that can present similarly to aortic dissection include a *penetrating atherosclerotic ulcer* and *leaking thoracic aortic aneurysm* (Haro 2005, Tsai et al. 2005).

WHAT ARE THE CHEST RADIOGRAPHIC FINDINGS OF AORTIC DISSECTION?

Many texts state that the chest radiograph is abnormal in up to 90% of patients with aortic dissection (Braunwald 2005, Hagan et al. 2000, Klompas 2002, Rosen 2006, Slater 1976, Tintinalli 2004). However, this is potentially misleading because it implies that there are useful radiographic findings in a large majority of patients. In most cases, the radiographic abnormalities are nonspecific and of limited diagnostic utility. In addition, because the chest radiograph is normal in 10% of patients, a normal chest radiograph alone should not be used to exclude the diagnosis of aortic dissection, although the criteria used to determine whether a chest radiograph is "normal" are not clearly defined. In some circumstances, however, the radiographic findings can serve as a clue to the presence of aortic dissection.

Radiographic findings that are associated with aortic dissection include (1) enlargement of the aorta (the principal sign), (2) enlargement of one aortic segment in comparison to the others (ascending aorta, aortic knob, or descending aorta), (3) progressive enlargement of the aorta compared to prior radiographs, (4) widening of the mediastinum, (5) a pleural effusion (usually left-sided), and (6) displacement of the calcified intima into the lumen of the aorta—the "calcium sign" (Table 1).

With the **calcium sign**, aortic intimal calcification is displaced 1 cm or more from the outer margin of the aorta. Although uncommon (5–8% of cases of aortic dissection), it is the most specific radiographic finding of aortic dissection because it directly visualizes displacement of the intimal flap into the aortic lumen (Klompas 2000, Luker et al. 1994, Spittell et al. 1993). However, due to the oblique orientation of the aortic arch, calcification of a portion of the aortic wall may appear to be displaced into the aortic lumen when it is simply in a more medially located segment of the aortic arch. The calcium sign is therefore more reliable in the ascending or descending aorta (Figure 6).

Aortic enlargement and mediastinal widening

The radiographic signs most often associated with aortic dissection are aortic enlargement and mediastinal widening. They are present in 70–80% of patients with aortic dissection (Hagan et al. 2000, Klompas 2002, von Kodolitsch et al. 2000 and 2004).

TABLE 1
Radiographic Findings in Aortic Dissection
Aortic enlargement (ascending, arch, descending)
Progressive enlargement compared to prior images
Mediastinal widening (= aortic enlargement)
Pleural effusion (left-sided)
Calcium sign—displaced intimal calcification

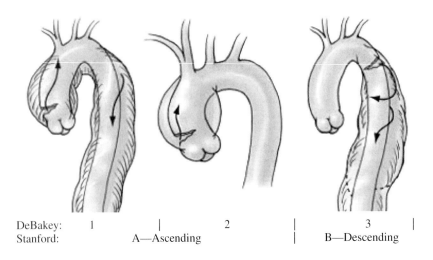

DeBakey: 1 | 2 | 3 |
Stanford: A—Ascending | B—Descending

FIGURE 5   Classification of aortic dissection.

[From Brunicardi FC, Andersen DK, et al.: *Schwartz's Principles of Surgery,* 8th ed. McGraw-Hill, 2005, with permission.]

MEDIASTINAL WIDENING   "Mediastinal widening" is a nonspecific term that refers to an increase in any of soft tissue component of the mediastinum.

In patients with **aortic dissection,** mediastinal widening is due to **aortic enlargement.**

Mediastinal widening also occurs in patients with **blunt traumatic aortic injury.** However, with aortic trauma, mediastinal widening is due to hemorrhage within the mediastinum. Forceful blunt chest trauma causes an aortic intimal tear forming a pseudoaneurysm, i.e., a focal hematoma contained by the adventitia (see Patient 11, Figures 3–5 on p 96–97). The mediastinal hemorrhage results from torn smaller branch vessels and not from the aorta itself. The pseudoaneurysm is not visible on chest radiography.

The pathologic anatomy and radiographic findings for aortic dissection and blunt aortic trauma are therefore substantially different, even though both result in "mediastinal widening." Occasionally, trauma may precipitate aortic dissection, presumably in patients with a pre-existing weakened aortic wall (see Patient 11, Figures 9–13 on p 98–99).

AORTIC ENLARGEMENT   Some degree of aortic enlargement is almost invariably present in patients with aortic dissection. However, aortic enlargement is due to *chronic* weakening of the aortic wall–the weakened aortic wall is predisposed to dissection.

Aortic enlargement does not occur acutely at the time of dissection. Aortic dissection is an *entirely intraluminal event*—the intimal flap and intramural hematoma are not visible radiographically. (The *calcium sign* is the one exception in which the displaced calcified intima is visible on a chest radiograph.)

The common misimpression that aortic enlargement is a direct sign of acute aortic dissection is due to the way that aortic dissection is usually, although incorrectly, depicted. Many illustrations of aortic dissection show the outer layer of the aortic wall displaced outward by the dissecting hematoma (Figures 5 and 7A). A more accurate representation of acute aortic dissection shows the intimal flap displaced into the aortic lumen, while the outer diameter of the aorta remains largely unchanged (Figures 7B and 4). CT and TEE confirm that this is anatomically correct (Figures 2 and 3).

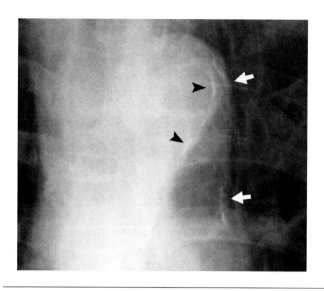

FIGURE 6   Pseudo-calcium sign.

Displacement of the calcified intima more that 1 cm inwards from the aortic margin is indicative of aortic dissection. However, due to the oblique orientation of the aortic arch, calcification of the aortic arch may normally appear separated from the aortic wall (*black arrowheads*).

White arrows indicate calcification of the posterior portion of the aortic arch and the descending aorta.

The calcium sign is therefore more useful in the descending or ascending aorta.

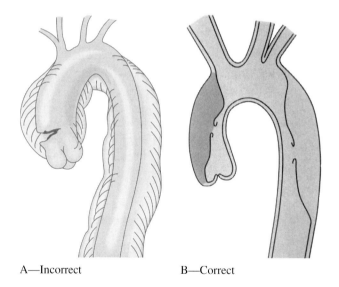

A—Incorrect   B—Correct

FIGURE 7   Schematic depictions of aortic dissection.

(*A*) The common erroneous depiction of acute aortic dissection shows displacement of the outer portion of the aortic wall by the dissecting hematoma. This implies incorrectly that with acute aortic dissection the aorta enlarges abruptly.

(*B*) An anatomically correct illustration shows that with aortic dissection the inner layer of the aortic wall is displaced into the aortic lumen. The outer diameter of the aorta is largely unchanged. Acute aortic dissection is therefore not visible on chest radiography.

Over time (weeks or months), the outer portion of the aortic wall may weaken allowing the aorta to dilate.

[*B* from Creager MA: *Vascular Disease* (Atlas of Heart Disease, vol. 7). Mosby, 1996, with permission.]

A second problem with aortic enlargement as a sign of acute aortic dissection is that **aortic enlargement occurs normally in older persons.** Due to weakening of the aortic wall with aging, the aorta gradually becomes dilated (ectatic) and elongated (uncoiled)—this is known as a **tortuous aorta**–"having many twists and turns". (Figure 8) An enlarged aorta could therefore be considered "normal" in an older individual, even though aortic enlargement is also a "sign" of aortic dissection.

When **prior radiographs** are available, progressive aortic enlargement can be considered a sign of aortic dissection. In Luker's series (Luker 1994), this was seen in a number of cases of aortic dissection. However, progressive aortic enlargement occurs gradually and is not abruptly at the time of dissection. In addition, lack of progressive aortic enlargement does not exclude the diagnosis of aortic dissection.

RADIOGRAPHIC TECHNIQUE   Many patients with aortic dissection have AP portable radiographs and the radiographic technique is often suboptimal, particularly when the patient is supine, has not taken a full inspiration or has rotated positioning. With suboptimal radiographs, the mediastinum may appear indistinct and widened (see Patient 11, Figures 18 and 19 on page 102). Aortic enlargement can thereby be mimicked by poor radiographic technique. Nonetheless, despite suboptimal technique, an enlarged aorta can often still be identified and should not be mistakenly attributed solely to the suboptimal radiographic technique (see Patients 12F, 12G, and 12H). Whenever possible, the chest radiograph should be obtained with the patient sitting upright, with full inspiration and minimal rotation.

Is Chest Radiography Useful in the Diagnosis of Aortic Dissection?

Numerous case series have been published that evaluate the radiographic findings of patients with aortic dissection. Klompas (2002) performed a meta-analysis of 13 published studies (1337 patients) and found the sensitivity of an *abnormal aortic contour* was only 71% (i.e., 29% of patients with aortic dissection had a "normal" aortic contour). Combining the results of the three studies that included patients *without* aortic dissection (170 patients), the sensitivity of an abnormal arotic contour was 82%, specificity 59%, negative likelihood ratio (LR−) 0.3, and positive likelihood ratio (LR+) 2.1.

Von Kodolitsch et al. (2004) studied chest radiography in 216 patients with suspected aortic dissection, of whom 109 (50%) had aortic dissection or other aortic pathology. A *widened aortic contour* (based on the radiologist's report) was present in 69% of patients with acute aortic syndromes (i.e., not present in 31% of cases) and was present in 21% of patients without aortic syndromes, yielding a sensitivity of 69%, specificity of 79%, LR− 0.4, and LR+ 3.2.

It was therefore concluded that due to its modest sensitivity and specificity, **chest radiography is of "limited value"** in the diagnosis of aortic dissection. The absence of a widened aortic contour will decrease the likelihood of aortic dissection slightly, but generally not by an amount sufficient to allow the diagnosis of aortic dissection to be excluded without a definitive imaging test.

These studies have several **shortcomings.** First, criteria used to determine aortic abnormality were not explicitly defined but based simply on the radiologist's report. This is particularly problematic in the elderly because aortic enlargement is commonly present and it is uncertain whether aortic enlargment should be interpreted as normal or abnormal (Figure 8). Second, patients were not stratified by their age, and age is a major factor in determining normalcy of the aorta. Finally, interobserver variability of interpretation among radiologists was not studied.

Although it was reasonable for the authors to conclude that the role of chest radiography is limited, helpful information can, in some cases, be gained by considering the **degree of aortic enlargement** and the **age of the patient.**

Aortic enlargement can be viewed as a continuum (mild, moderate or marked), rather than simply normal or abnormal (Figures 9 and 10). Although there are no criteria to precisely differentiate mild, moderate, and marked aortic enlargement, these three degrees of aortic enlargement can generally be distinguished. Even in an older individual, a markedly enlarged aorta can usually be differentiated from a normal but tortuous aorta.

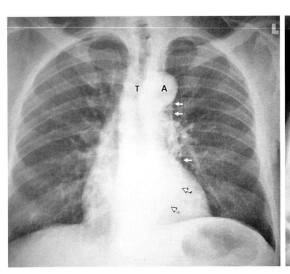
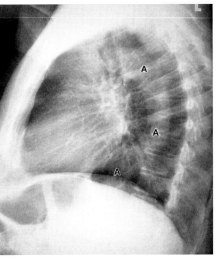

FIGURE 8   Tortuous aorta.
On the PA view, the aortic knob is moderately dilated (A), which is "normal" in this 74-year-old male. The descending aorta is displaced laterally (below the aortic knob) and then curves medially to cross the diaphragm (*arrows*). The trachea (T) is displaced to the right by the enlarged aortic knob.

On the lateral view, the aorta is dilated and elongated such that it is displaced posteriorly and lies adjacent to the thoracic vertebral bodies   (A). The descending aorta is visible because it is surrounded by the left lung.

Second, aortic size must also be assessed in relation to the **age of the patient.** In the **elderly,** a mildly or moderately enlarged aorta can be a normal finding, i.e., a tortuous aorta. However, a *markedly* enlarged aorta is abnormal and this finding can provide a clue to the presence of aortic dissection (Figures 9 and 10F). This is most useful when the clinical presentation is atypical and aortic dissection is not the primary diagnostic consideration. Nonetheless, aortic dissection can occur in patients with only mild or moderate aortic dilation and these cases likely account for the 20–30% of patients with aortic dissection who have chest radiographs in which the aorta appears aorta appears "normal for age" (Figures 10D and E).

In **younger individuals** (age ≤40 years), chest radiography is potentially more useful. Any degree of aortic dilation is abnormal and indicates an increased risk of aortic dissection (Figure 10G). On the other hand, a truly normal narrow aortic contour substantially reduces the likelihood of aortic dissection (Figure 10A). Because aortic dissection is rare in young persons and a narrow aortic contour is present in most young individuals, the finding of an enlarged aorta can be an important clue that aortic dissection may be present.

Because the radiologist's report may not convey the magnitude or even the presence of aortic enlargement, clinicians should examine the radiographs themselves to assess aortic size. For example, a moderately enlarged aorta might be described as "torturous" or might not be commented upon because this could be considered normal in an older individual. A markedly enlarged aorta might also be described simply as "tortuous" even though this should be considered abnormal even in an older patient (Figure 9). In a young person, an enlarged or "tortuous aorta" should always be considered abnormal and should prompt consideration of aortic dissection, if it were not already a diagnostic consideration (Figure 10G).

CONCLUSION   Whenever the clinical findings suggest aortic dissection, the diagnosis should be pursued with a confirmatory imaging test regardless of the chest radiographic findings. However, when the patient's clinical presentation is atypical and not suggestive of aortic dissection, radiography is potentially helpful by calling attention to the possibility of an aortic disorder. This is especially true in **young individuals** because any aortic enlargement is abnormal and suggestive of an aortic disorder, whereas a normal narrow aortic contour substantially reduces the likelihood of dissection. In the **elderly,** chest radiography is less useful because mild or moderate aortic dilation is common and could be considered normal, even though dissection may be

present. However, marked aortic enlargement is abnormal and should prompt consideration of aortic dissection, if not already suspected.

Patient 12 Outcome

This patient had relatively nonspecific abdominal pain and appeared comfortable during most of his time in the ED. His clinical presentation was not typical for aortic dissection, although it did have some suggestive features—the pain began abruptly and radiated to his back. However, its onset was associated with minor trauma and therefore the pain could have been mistakenly attributed to a muscle strain.

Other clues to the serious nature of the patient's pain were that it was persistent and he appeared in distress when the pain recurred. An abdominal CT was warranted, although a specific disorder was not suspected prior to the CT scan.

The markedly dilated aorta on chest radiography could have served a clue to the presence of aortic dissection (Figure 9). Had aortic dissection been suspected, the CT protocol would have been modified to include images of the chest to determine the proximal extent of the dissection. This information is needed to determine treatment, although it was provided by a subsequent TEE. In addition, a rapid bolus of intravenous contrast and timing the scan for maximal aortic opacification would have been used—a CT angiogram.

Because the patient had flank pain and hematuria, renal colic might have been suspected and a noncontrast CT performed. This would have missed the diagnosis of aortic dissection entirely. However, the clinical presentation (periumbilical abdominal pain) was not consistent with renal colic. In this patient, the correct diagnosis was made using the correct, if not optimal, test.

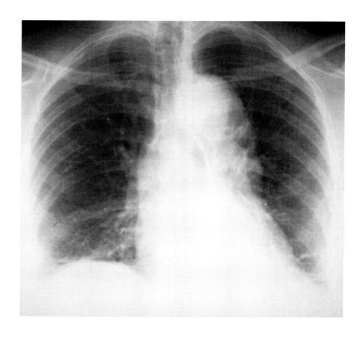

FIGURE 9   Chest radiograph—Patient 12.
The radiograph was interpreted simply as showing a "tortuous aorta." However, the aortic knob and descending aorta were markedly enlarged, particularly for a 56-year-old man. Although this finding was longstanding and not a direct sign of an acute aortic dissection, it was indicative of aortic wall weakening and an increased risk for dissection. This should prompt consideration of an aortic disorder as a cause of a patients's chest or abdominal pain.

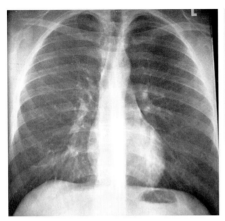

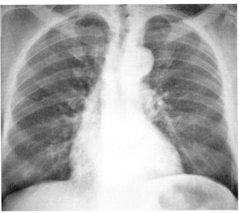

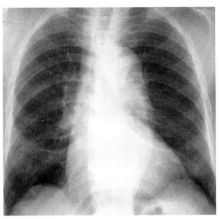

A. **Normal aorta** in a 27-year-old man—Dissection is unlikely

B. Moderately dilated **tortuous aorta** in a 74-year-old man is "normal for age," although dissection could be present

C. Markedly dilated and elongated, **tortuous aorta** in an 81-year-old man is suspicious for dissection. Chest CT showed no dissection

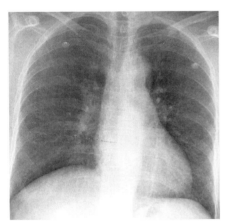

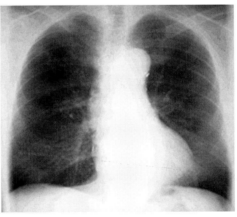

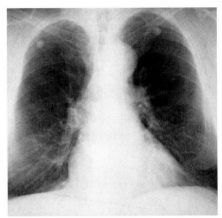

D. **Aortic dissection** in a 58-year-old woman. The aorta is only mildly dilated aorta and is "normal for age"

E. **Aortic dissection** in a 61-year-old man. The moderately dilated aorta is indistinguishable from a tortuous aorta that is "normal for age"

F. **Aortic dissection** in a 63-year-old man. The aortic knob is markedly dilated, which is suspicious for dissection

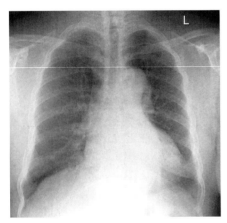

G. **Aortic dissection** in a 40-year-old man. The moderately dilated aorta is clearly "abnormal for age" and suggests that aortic pathology is present

FIGURE 10   Radiographic appearances of the aorta.
Aortic enlargement can be graded as mild, moderate or severe and is shown in young (age ≤ 40 years), middle-aged and older individuals.

Elderly persons with markedly dilated aortas are at increased risk of dissection (C and F), although dissection can occur in patients with only mildly or moderately dilated aortas (D and E), which are "normal" in the elderly (B).

In a **young person** with chest, back, or abdominal pain, any aortic dilation is abnormal and should prompt consideration of aortic dissection (G). A normal narrow aortic contour in a young person substantially reduces the likelihood of dissection (A).

AORTIC DISSECTION—DIAGNOSIS

The diagnosis of aortic dissection rests primarily on a careful clinical evaluation and confirmatory imaging tests, usually CT. Chest radiography plays, at most, a secondary role as described above.

There is a wide range of clinical presentations. The diagnosis is relatively straightforward when there is an abrupt onset of severe pain that migrates from the anterior chest to the back, has a tearing or ripping quality, or is associated with signs of branch vessel occlusion such as pulse deficits, neurological or extremity ischemia, or a murmur of aortic insufficiency.

When the patient presents solely with chest, back, or abdominal pain and the pain is not typical for aortic dissection, the diagnosis can be delayed or missed entirely. Such clinical presentations are, in fact, common (Hagan et al. 2000, Klompas 2002). In 84% of cases, the pain begins abruptly, and this feature should be noted when questioning patients about their pain. However, the pain has a tearing or ripping in quality in only 50% of cases, and is migratory in only 31% of cases. Dissection causing nonmigratory chest, back, or abdominal pain is frequently misdiagnosed. Although aortic dissection is generally considered a disorder causing chest pain, the pain is localized to the anterior chest in only 60% of cases.

Pain associated with signs or symptoms of aortic branch vessel occlusion is a hallmark of aortic dissection, although this is present in only a minority of cases. These include deficits in the carotid or femoral pulses or a discrepancy in blood pressure of more than 20 mm Hg as measured in upper extremities (31% of cases), neurological symptoms or stroke (17% of cases), and mesenteric or renal ischemia (Patient 12I). A murmur of aortic insufficiency is present in 28% of cases. The blood pressure is often, although not always, elevated (50% of cases).

Hypertension is present in 70% of patients with descending dissection, but only 36% of those with isolated ascending dissection. The blood pressure elevation reflects chronic hypertension, which underlies most cases of aortic dissection, as well as catecholamine release at the time of dissection. Hypotension is due to either leakage into the pericardial sac and tamponade, acute aortic valve insufficiency, or rupture into the chest or abdomen.

The **EKG** is normal in 22% of cases or, more commonly, shows nonspecific ST segment and T-wave changes. In 3–7% of cases, the EKG shows changes suggestive of an acute myocardial infarction.

Most cases of aortic dissection occur in middle-aged or elderly persons and chronic hypertension is the most common **risk factor** (70% of cases). Young persons (≤40 years of age) constitute only 7% of cases (Januzzi et al. 2004). Risk factors for dissection in young persons include Marfan syndrome (50% of cases), hypertension (34% of cases), a bicuspid aortic valve, prior aortic valve surgery, pregnancy, and cocaine use.

AORTIC DISSECTION—MISDIAGNOSIS

Among all patients that present to the ED with chest, back, or abdominal pain, aortic dissection is uncommon. However, among ED patients with aortic dissection, misdiagnosis or delayed diagnosis is, unfortunately, common. In Sullivan's series (Sullivan et al. 2000), 25 of 44 cases of aortic dissection (57%) were misdiagnosed during their initial ED evaluation.

In some patients, aortic dissection is diagnosed when an imaging test, usually CT, is obtained for reasons other than suspected aortic dissection. In these cases, the clinical consequences of diagnostic delay are usually limited (Patients 12A, 12C, and 12D). However, clinically significant problems occur when misdiagnosis leads either to the patient being inappropriately discharged from the ED with a mistaken impression of a benign disorder (Patient 12F), or when a patient is hospitalized and treated for another disease such as an acute coronary syndrome, stroke, or abdominal disorder (Patients 12G and 12H).

Location of pain is a major determinant in the frequency of misdiagnosis. In Sullivan's series, misdiagnosis occurred in 2 of 14 patients (14%) with chest and back pain, 6 of 11 patients (55%) with chest pain alone, and 12 of 13 patients (92%) with abdominal pain alone.

Misdiagnosis is especially common in young patients (less than age 40 years), although they constitute only a small minority of cases of aortic dissection (7%). In Sullivan's series, three of the four young patients with aortic dissection (41 years of age or less) were initially misdiagnosed. All three patients were discharged from the ED and one died at home. Aside from being attentive to the details of the clinical presentation, consideration of chest radiographic findings can be helpful in young patients. An enlarged aortic contour is not expected in a young person and, when present, should prompt further investigation for aortic dissection (Figure 10G and Patients 12C and 12F).

In older or middle-aged individuals, aortic dissection is often missed when the patient is hospitalized with a presumptive diagnosis of another disorder, most commonly an acute coronary syndrome. When heparin or a thrombolytic agent is administered, the consequences can be disastrous. This, too, is not uncommon. In Davis' series (Davis 2005), 9 of 44 patients with aortic dissection (21%) had heparin or a thrombolytic agent administered and two of these patients died. Misdiagnosed patients had a higher incidence of chest pain without back pain, non-specific ST segment changes on EKG, and lacked mediastinal widening on radiography. Clinical details of the cases were not provided so it is uncertain whether these misdiagnoses could have been avoided.

Conclusion

Several steps can be taken to avoid misdiagnosis of aortic dissection. These include: (1) considering the diagnosis of aortic dissection in all patients with chest, back, or abdominal pain, (2) noting clinical features suggestive of dissection such as an abrupt onset or migration of pain, (3) looking for subtle clinical signs of aortic dissection such as a blood pressure differential or murmur of aortic valve insufficiency, (4) not using clinical parameters that have limited sensitivity to exclude aortic dissection (e.g., the absence of pulse deficits or lack of a markedly enlarged aortic contour on chest radiography), and (5) considering aortic dissection as a cause of cerebral, mesenteric, renal, or extremity ischemia (Rogers and Mc-Cormack 2004).

Chest radiography plays a secondary role in the diagnosis of aortic dissection. Patients with clinical presentations suggestive of aortic dissection should have definitive testing regardless of their chest radiographic findings. In patients with atypical clinical presentations in whom aortic dissection is not a primary or even suspected diagnosis, an enlarged aortic contour should raise the suspicion of aortic dissection. However, middle-aged or older individuals with aortic dissection often have only mild or moderate aortic enlargement that is "normal for age." A markedly enlarged aorta is clearly abnormal and should prompt consideration of aortic dissection. Chest radiography is potentially most useful in young individuals, because any aortic enlargement is abnormal and this can provide an important clue to the presence of an aortic disorder. A normal narrow aortic contour, on the other hand, argues against aortic dissection (Figure 10A).

Because aortic dissection is such a serious disorder, a low threshold must be maintained to pursue definitive diagnostic testing. This is particularly true now that highly accurate, noninvasive tests are readily available in the emergency department, namely helical CT. Nonetheless, aortic dissection is an uncommon disorder and excessive testing of patients with chest, back, or abdominal pain should be avoided. A careful clinical examination should be used to appropriately select patients for further testing.

CONFIRMATORY TESTING FOR AORTIC DISSECTION

Various imaging modalities are available to confirm or exclude aortic dissection—helical CT, transesophageal echocardiography (TEE), MRI, and catheter angiography. In addition to establishing the diagnosis of aortic dissection, information is needed regarding the location of the dissection (ascending or descending aorta), major branch vessel involvement, aortic valve insufficiency, and the presence of blood in the pericardial sac (Nienaber et al. 1993).

In the past, **aortography** was the gold standard diagnostic test. However, aortography is now rarely used because it is invasive and has limited sensitivity (only 88%). All of the currently available imaging modalities (CT, MRI, and TEE) are highly accurate for aortic dissection: sensitivity 98–100% and specificity 95–98% (Shiga et al. 2006).

Helical CT is readily available in the ED and therefore most widely used. It reliably detects aortic dissection, can define its extent, and detect branch vessel involvement and a

pericardial effusion. CT cannot detect aortic valvular insufficiency and therefore must be supplemented by echocardiography in cases of ascending aortic dissection. Multidetector CT (**MDCT**) offers greater anatomical detail and can better define the extent of dissection and the presence of branch vessel involvement (Patients 12B to 12F, and 12I). Earlier reports of CT found a lower sensitivity (94%); however, these studies did not use helical CT or a rapid bolus of intravenous contrast (Nienaber et al. 1993).

The **CT protocol** for aortic dissection employs a rapid intravenous contrast and scans at the time of maximal aortic opacification—CT angiography (Patients 12B–12F). This is preceded by a noncontrast CT to detect an intramural hematoma. On a noncontrast CT, an intramural hematoma has greater attenuation (appears lighter) than the nonopacified aortic lumen or an atherosclerotic mural thrombus. The CT should include both chest and abdomen.

Transesophageal echocardiography (TEE) can accurately detect aortic dissection and define its extent. It is used in patients who are too unstable to be transported to the CT scanner or who have contraindications to intravenous contrast. TEE can also detect aortic valve insufficiency and hemopericardium, but not aortic branch vessel involvement (Figure 11 and Patients 12A and 12G).

Transthoracic echocardiography (TTE) may, in some cases, be able to identify an intimal flap in the ascending aorta. TTE can detect a pericardial effusion as a complication of an ascending aortic dissection. This is particularly useful in a patient with shock of unknown etiology. Abdominal ultrasonography can occasionally visualize an intimal flap in the descending aorta (Piskoti and Adams 2002, Sherman and Cosby 2004, Sierzenski et al. 2004). Sensitivity ranges from 60% to 85%.

MRI is highly accurate at detecting aortic dissection although it is often not readily available for ED patients. It can be used in stable patients who have contraindications to intravenous contrast. Its capabilities are similar to helical CT–aortic valvular insufficiency cannot be detected (Patient 12B).

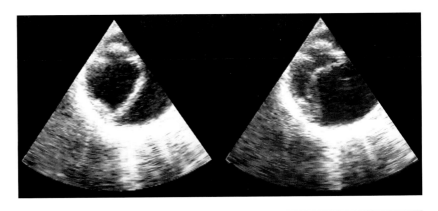

FIGURE 11   Transesophageal Echocardiogram (TEE) of aortic dissection.
Two images show the mobile intimal flap oscillating with each cardiac contraction. This aortic dissection involves most of the aortic circumference. The more centrally located true lumen is completely surrounded by intima. The false lumen can also be distinguished by the acute angle that the intima makes where it contacts the outer portion of the aortic wall.

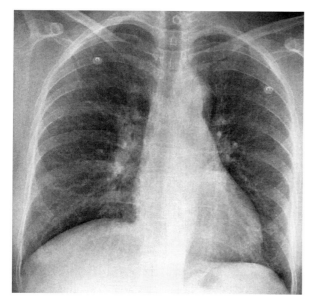
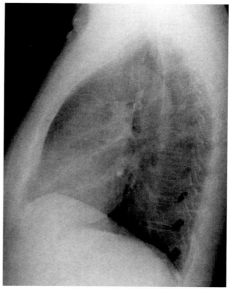

FIGURE 12

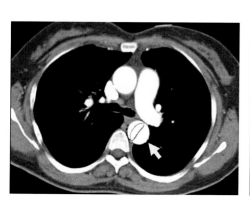
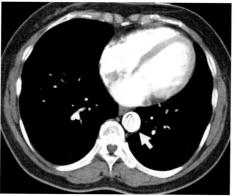
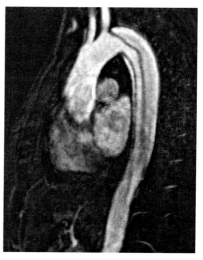

FIGURE 13   CT Angiogram

FIGURE 14   MRI six month later.

PATIENT 12B: DESCENDING AORTIC DISSECTION—MILDLY DILATED AORTA—NORMAL FOR AGE

A 58-year-old woman presented to the ED with a complaint of chest pain that began suddenly while she was swimming. It was 10/10 in severity and radiated to the epigastric region and lower back. She had no prior medical problems. She stated that both her mother and brother had died suddenly in their 50s from "aortic aneurysms."

On examination, she was in moderate distress due to her chest pain. Her blood pressure was 175/68 mm Hg in the right arm and 171/72 mm Hg in the left arm, and her heart rate was 70 beats/min. The remainder of her physical examination was normal. Her chest pain was treated with intravenous morphine. An EKG showed non-specific flattening of the T-waves in the lateral and inferior leads.

PA and lateral **chest radiographs** were interpreted as normal without mediastinal widening or cardiac enlargement (Figure 12). The aorta was only mildly dilated and elongated, which was normal for her age.

A **CT angiogram** performed within 1 hour of her arrival revealed aortic dissection beginning at the origin of the left subclavian artery and extending through the descending thoracic and abdominal aorta to the iliac arteries (Figure 13, *arrows*). The dissection involved nearly the entire aortic circumference. The outer diameter of the aorta was normal. Perfusion of the celiac, superior, and inferior mesenteric arteries, and renal arteries was well maintained.

The patient's blood pressure was managed with intravenous labetalol and then oral medications. The dissection remained stable, as shown by MRI six months later (Figure 14).

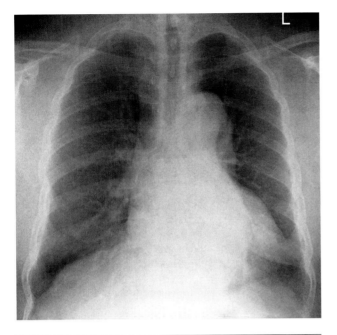

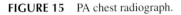

FIGURE 15   PA chest radiograph.

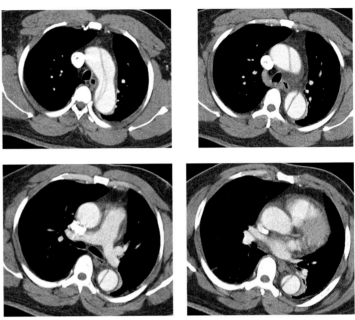

FIGURE 16   Axial CT images showing aortic dissection involving the aortic arch and descending aorta, but not the ascending aorta.

PATIENT 12C: DESCENDING AORTIC DISSECTION INVOLVING THE AORTIC ARCH IN A YOUNG MAN— AORTA IS MODERATELY DILATED—ABNORMAL FOR AGE

A 40-year-old man who had been diagnosed with hypertension two months earlier (although it was likely longstanding) presented to an ED with two days of periumbilical and midepigastric abdominal pain. An abdominal CT was performed, which revealed dissection of the abdominal aorta and the patient was transferred to a tertiary medical center for cardiovascular consultation. He was pain free on transfer.

Upon arrival at the second hospital, his blood pressure was 180/114 mm Hg and pulse 97 beats/min. His abdomen was obese but nontender. An EKG showed left ventricular hypertrophy by voltage criteria with lateral T-wave inversions. His hypertension was treated with intravenous nitroprusside and labetolol.

Chest radiography revealed a dilated aortic arch and elongated descending aorta, which is clearly abnormal given his relatively young age (Figure 15). This reflected his longstanding hypertension and risk for aortic dissection.

A **CT angiogram** of the chest and abdomen was performed which revealed aortic dissection of the descending thoracic aorta that extended proximally into the aortic arch and distally through the entire abdominal aorta to the left common iliac artery (Figure 16).

The ascending aorta was not involved. However, to confirm this, a TEE was performed. This demonstrated that the proximal extent of the dissection involved the aortic arch, but not the ascending aorta. The patient was managed nonoperatively.

TTE revealed severe left ventricular hypertrophy, which was likely due to his longstanding hypertension, a left ventricular ejection fraction of 70%, a dilated aortic root (4.2 cm) and ascending aorta (4 cm), and no aortic valve insufficiency or pericardial effusion. He was managed with antihypertensive medications including β-adrenergic blocking agents and serial CT scans.

In a young person with chest, back, or abdominal pain, a moderately dilated aorta on chest radiography strongly suggests aortic dissection as a potential diagnosis (Figure 15).

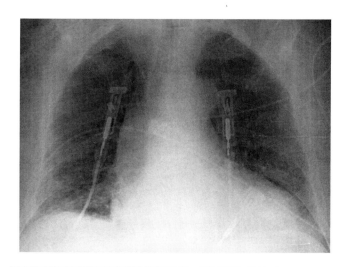

FIGURE 17   Initial AP view (suboptimal technique).

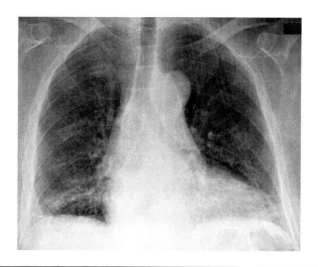

FIGURE 18   Repeat AP view using better technique.

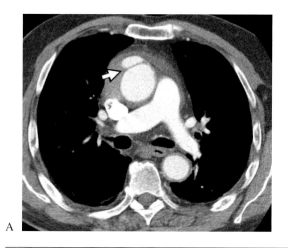

FIGURE 19

PATIENT 12D: ASCENDING AORTIC DISSECTION—MODERATELY DILATED AORTA—NORMAL FOR AGE

A 77-year-old man was brought to the ED by ambulance for a complaint of chest pain that began while he was watching television. The pain had a dull, pressure-like quality, was 5/10 in severity, worse with deep inspiration, and associated with shortness of breath. It was mid-sternal in location and did not radiate. He had no history of heart disease or hypertension. Aspirin and nitroglycerine were administered in the ambulance.

In the ED, he was in no apparent distress. His blood pressure was 140/80 mm Hg, pulse 90 beats/min, respirations 20 breaths/min, and O$_2$ saturation 95% while breathing room air. An EKG showed no acute ischemic changes. His chest pain resolved with sublingual nitroglycerine.

An **AP chest radiograph** was interpreted as showing bibasilar patchy atelectasis, an enlarged heart, but no mention was made of an abnormal mediastinum (Figure 17). A second AP view confirmed that the aorta was moderately enlarged, but not by an amount unexpected for his age (Figure 18).

His serum troponin level was normal and **D-dimer assay** was positive (>1000 ng/mL). A **chest CT** was ordered for suspected pulmonary embolism. The chest CT revealed dissection limited

to the ascending aorta (Figure 19A, *arrow*) and a moderate-sized **pericardial effusion** (Figure 19B, P). There was no pulmonary embolism.

The patent was treated with intravenous labetolol to lower his systolic blood pressure to 110 mm Hg. A TTE revealed an intimal flap in the ascending aorta, no aortic valve insufficiency, a pericardial effusion without signs of tamponade, and normal left ventricular function.

He was taken to the operating room for supracoronary graft replacement of the ascending aorta. The aortic valve was normal. A small tear was found in the anterior wall of the ascending aorta that accounted for the hemopericardium. His graft remained stable on follow-up CT scans over the subsequent 2 years.

Although a CT pulmonary angiogram is timed for maximal opacification of the pulmonary arteries, there is generally sufficient opacification of the aorta to detect aortic dissection. However, abdominal images are not included in a CT pulmonary angiogram and these are needed if the descending thoracic and abdominal aorta is involved.

PATIENT 12E:
DESCENDING DISSECTION—MODERATELY DILATED AORTA

A 62-year-old man presented to the ED with "sharp" pain of acute onset that began in his posterior thorax and extended to his anterior chest. His blood pressure was 150/100 mm Hg in the right arm and 130/90 mm Hg in the left. His EKG was normal.

A portable **chest radiograph** was interpreted as showing a normal heart and mediastinal structures (Figure 20). However, his aortic knob was moderately dilated. This could be considered normal for age, but is also suspicious for an aortic dissection.

An emergency **CT** of the chest and abdomen was performed using a 16-slice multidetector CT with multiplanar reformatted images. It revealed aortic dissection originating at the left subclavian artery and extending throughout the entire descending thoracic and abdominal aorta (Figures 21 and 22). The dissection flap extended into the superior mesenteric artery, but there was no CT evidence of bowel ischemia.

The patient was managed medically with control of his blood pressure.

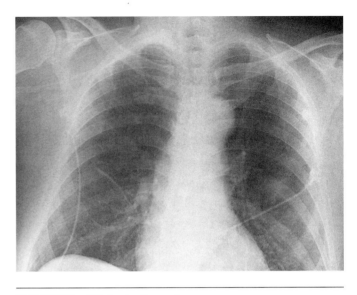

FIGURE 20   AP chest radiograph.

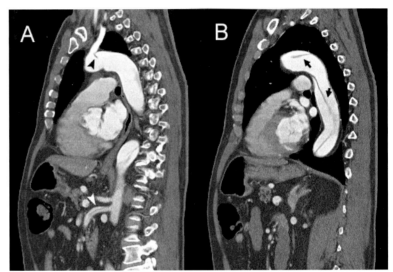

FIGURE 21   Sagittal CT images.

The dissection originated at the base of the left subclavian artery (*black arrowhead*). The intimal flap extended the entire length of the descending aorta (*black arrows*) and into the superior mesenteric artery (*white arrowhead* in A).

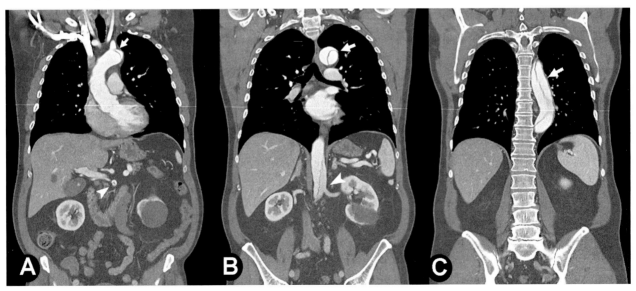

FIGURE 22   Coronal CT images.

The dissection extended from the left subclavian artery through the descending aorta (*arrows*) and involved the superior mesenteric artery (*arrowhead* in A). The left renal artery is supplied by the true lumen (*arrowhead* in B). The left kidney inferior pole has a simple cyst.

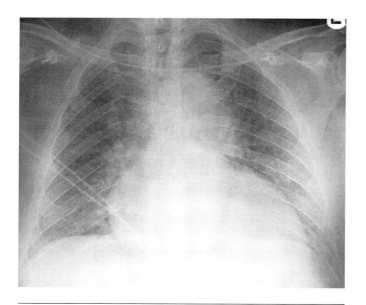

FIGURE 23   Initial AP radiograph.

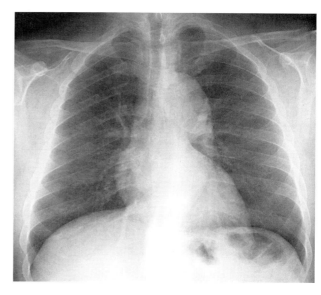

FIGURE 24   PA radiograph.

PATIENT 12F: DESCENDING DISSECTION—AORTA MARKEDLY DILATED FOR AGE

A 45-year-old man developed upper abdominal pain one week before presenting to the ED. Pain was present in his back and he felt constipated. There was no chest pain. He had a ten-year history of hypertension, but had not taken antihypertensive medications for the past two years.

He visited his physician five days earlier for abdominal discomfort and constipation. His blood pressure was noted to be 210/130 mm Hg. He was treated as an outpatient with oral antihypertensive medications and laxatives. His abdominal pain persisted and an abdominal CT was ordered. The CT revealed abdominal aortic dissection, and he was referred to the ED of a tertiary care medical center.

An AP portable **chest radiograph** was interpreted as showing a "widened mediastinum" (Figure 23). A PA radiograph (Figure 24) confirmed that the "widened mediastinum" was due to a markedly dilated aorta and should not be attributed to suboptimal radiographic technique. In a relatively young patient, such a dilated aorta is a sign of aortic pathology (Figure 25).

An **MDCT** of the chest and abdomen revealed a type B aortic dissection beginning at the origin of the left subclavian artery and extending to the infrarenal aorta above the aortoiliac bifurcation (Figure 26). He was treated with an intravenous infusion of esmolol.

A **TTE** revealed moderate left ventricular hypertrophy and a markedly decreased left ventricular ejection fraction of 20% due to hypertensive cardiomyopathy. Multiple medications were needed to control his blood pressure. The aortic dissection remained stable with medical management.

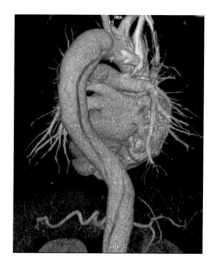

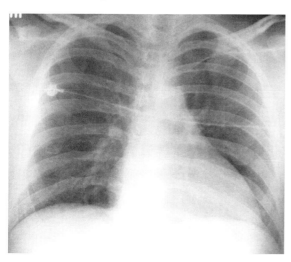

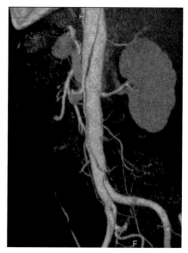

FIGURE 25   For comparison, an AP supine radiograph in a 30-year-old male shows that the superior mediastinum at the level of the aortic knob normally appears relatively narrow. Therefore, the wide mediastinum seen in Figure 23 should not be attributed to the AP spine radiographic technique, but is in fact due to an enlarged aorta.

FIGURE 26   16-slice MDCT.
Three-dimensional images viewed from posterior show aortic dissection of the descending thoracic and abdominal aorta.

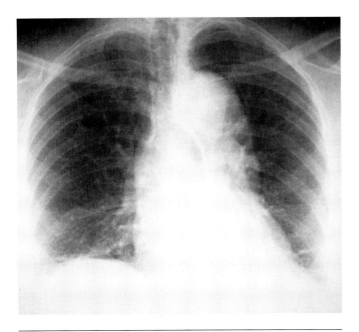

FIGURE 27 AP portable supine chest radiograph.

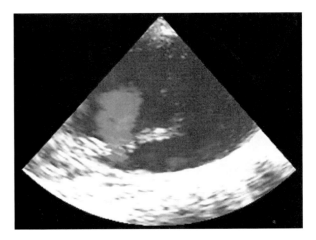

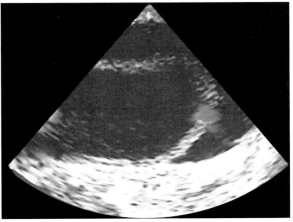

FIGURE 28 TEE of aortic dissection.
Flow through the intimal tear is seen as a gray shade in this color Doppler TEE image. Most of the flow through the aorta is perpendicular to the ultrasound transducer and therefore does not produce a Doppler signal.

PATIENT 12G: ASCENDING DISSECTION AND SHOCK IN A YOUNG WOMAN—AORTA DILATED FOR AGE

A 41-year-old woman presented to the ED with midepigastric pain that radiated to the back and chest. It was associated with nausea and shortness of breath, but no vomiting, diaphoresis, or radiation to her arms or jaw. The patient had no prior medical problems and took no medications.

On examination, she was overweight and appeared uncomfortable due to her epigastric and back pain. Her blood pressure was 220/114 mm Hg and pulse 84 beats/min. There was tenderness in the midepigastrium.

EKG showed symmetrical T-wave inversions in leads V2 to V6 and II, III, and aVF. Intravenous morphine was administered to treat the patient's pain. Her blood pressure gradually diminished over one hour to 156/78 mm Hg.

A portable **chest radiograph** was interpreted as showing a normal heart and pulmonary vasculature and clear lungs (Figure 27). Despite the suboptimal technique, the superior mediastinum was widened, although this was not commented on in the radiologist's report. Her serum troponin level was normal.

An **abdominal ultrasound** examination was performed and showed a normal gallbladder. During sonography, the patient became lightheaded and her blood pressure decreased to 60/30 mm Hg. After a bolus of 500 mL normal saline, her blood pressure was 84/46 mm Hg and pulse 90 beats/min. A second EKG showed T-wave inversions with additional 1 mm ST-segment

depressions in leads V2–V5. Intravenous heparin was administered for a possible acute coronary syndrome.

The cardiac catheterization service was called. They performed a **bedside TTE**, which revealed a moderate pericardial effusion, normal aortic valve, and a dissection flap in the proximal ascending aorta. The heparin infusion was stopped.

A **bedside TEE** confirmed the presence of an ascending aortic dissection not involving the aortic valve and a moderate-sized pericardial effusion (Figure 28). The dissection extended distally through the entire descending thoracic aorta to the level of the diaphragm. The intimal tear was in the midaortic arch.

The patient was taken directly to the operating room for repair of her ascending aortic dissection. There was rupture through the aortic adventitia posteriorly causing tamponade. The aortic valve was not involved. The ascending aorta was replaced with a Dacron graft.

One clue to the aortic dissection was the **widened mediastinum** on chest radiography. This was due to an aorta that was excessively dilated given her relatively young age. The EKGs were suggestive of an acute coronary syndrome, although the changes were nonspecific and could be chronic or due to the aortic dissection. During abdominal sonography, examination of the patient's heart, particularly when she became hypotensive, might have revealed a pericardial effusion and treatment with heparin would have been avoided.

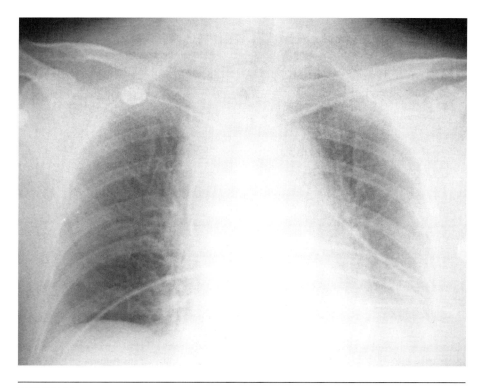

FIGURE 29

PATIENT 12H: AORTIC DISSECTION MISDIAGNOSED AS AN ACUTE CORONARY SYNDROME

A 69-year-old woman presented to the ED with crushing, "vice-like" chest pain that began 40 minutes earlier. It was substernal, did not radiate, and was associated with nausea, diaphoresis, and a bloated feeling. She had a history of hypertension treated with enalapril, hypercholesterolemia, and had smoked half a pack of cigarettes per day for many years. She had no history of cardiac disease.

On physical examination, she appeared in moderate distress due to her chest pain. Her blood pressure was 130/80 mm Hg and pulse 71 beats/min. Her lungs, heart, and abdomen were normal. Her EKG was normal aside from small Q-waves in leads II and III.

Aspirin, sublingual nitroglycerine, and morphine were administered, resulting in relief of her chest pain over 30 minutes. An intravenous bolus of heparin and infusions of heparin and nitroglycerine were begun to treat a possible acute coronary syndrome. Blood test results were normal aside from a white blood cell count of 16,500 cells/mm^3.

An AP portable **chest radiograph** was interpreted as showing cardiomegaly and "possibly a prominent mediastinal shadow," but this could not be fully evaluated due to the patient's positioning and shallow level of inspiration (Figure 29). A repeat radiograph showed a "tortuous aorta." In the medical resident's admission note, it is stated that this was "not consis-

tent with aortic dissection." Two sets of cardiac enzymes were negative.

Eight hours after admission, the chest pain recurred and the patient became markedly short of breath, requiring endotracheal intubation. An EKG was unchanged. Following intubation, the patient's blood pressure dropped to 80/50 mm Hg. This responded to fluid resuscitation. The initial clinical suspicion was a pulmonary embolism, and a bedside TTE was performed to look for right heart strain suggestive of a massive pulmonary embolism. Instead, a moderate-sized pericardial effusion was found. The heparin infusion was stopped. A TEE was then performed, which showed an ascending aortic dissection. The patient became progressively hypotensive and could not be taken to the operating room. She expired shortly thereafter.

Clues to the presence of aortic dissection rather than an acute coronary syndrome were the lack of ischemic EKG changes and cardiac enzyme elevations despite the patient's relatively severe symptoms. The patient was not specifically questioned about whether the pain began abruptly and the blood pressure was not checked in both arms. The chest radiograph did show a markedly enlarged tortuous aorta desite the AP supine radiographic technique. This could be considered "normal" in an elderly person, especially one with hypertension, but should not be interpreted as reducing the likelihood of aortic dissection.

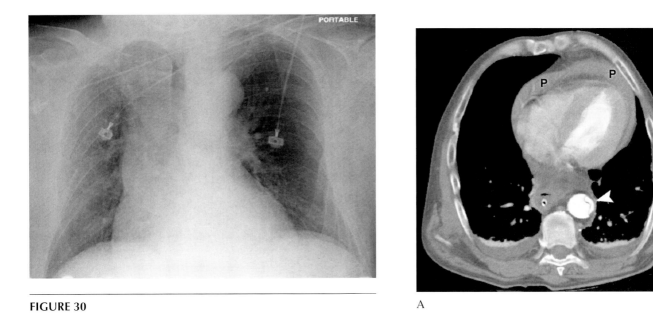

FIGURE 30   A

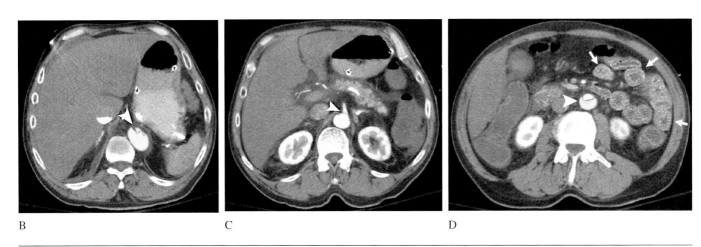

B   C   D

FIGURE 31   CT Angiogram of the Abdomen

PATIENT 12I: AORTIC DISSECTION PRESENTING AS AN ABDOMINAL CATASTROPHE

A 48-year-old man presented to the ED with gastrointestinal bleeding. He had had two episodes of hematemesis and one large bloody bowel movement during the preceding hour. His initial blood pressure was 80/50 mm Hg and pulse 120 beats/min. He appeared acutely ill and complained of nausea and mild abdominal pain, but no chest or back pain. His abdomen had mild diffuse tenderness without rebound tenderness.

His hypotension was unresponsive to vigorous fluid resuscitation. His **chest radiograph** was interpreted as being normal aside from suboptimal radiographic technique (Figure 30). A bedside sonogram revealed a 2-cm diameter abdominal aorta (an intraluminal flap was not noted). Views of the heart were not obtained. The patient was intubated and sent for an abdominal CT angiogram for possible acute mesenteric ischemia (Figure 31).

CT revealed aortic dissection with an intimal flap extending across the ostium of the superior mesenteric artery (Figure 31C, *arrowhead.*) Bowel wall thickening with target signs was indicative of mesenteric ischemia involving most of the small bowel (Figure 31D, *arrows*). Slices through the inferior thorax

revealed a pericardial effusion (Figure 31A, P). His hypotension and mesenteric ischemia could therefore have been due to both occlusion of the SMA and to pericardial tamponade. Surgery was not undertaken due to the expected high mortality and he expired soon after being transferred to the intensive care unit.

Review of the initial **chest radiograph** shows a widened mediastinum (Figure 30). Much of this widening is due to his rightward rotated positioning, although had the patient not been rotated, his markedly enlarged aorta would have been more evident. During abdominal sonography, a subxyphoid view of the heart would have revealed the pericardial effusion. Both of these factors would have prompted consideration of aortic dissection, and a chest CT would have been performed in addition to the abdominal CT. The dissection presumably involved the ascending aorta, although in this patient, the information would not have changed the outcome. TEE could have been used after abdominal CT if the patient had survived long enough to undergo surgery.

SUGGESTED READING

Ankel F: Aortic dissection. In Marx JA, Hockberger RS, Walls RM, et al., eds. *Rosen's Emergency Medicine: Concepts and Clinical Practice*, 5th ed. Mosby, 2002.

Creager MA, Braunwald E: *Atlas of Heart Diseases*, 2nd ed. Current Medicine Group, 2003.

Creager MA, Dzau VJ, Loscalzo J: *Vascular Medicine: A Companion to Braunwald's Heart Disease.* Saunders, 2006.

Doroghazi RM, Slater EE: *Aortic Dissection.* McGraw-Hill, 1983.

Halperin JL, Olin JW: Diseases of the aorta. In Fuster V, Alexander RW, O'Rourke RA, eds. *Hurst's The Heart*, 11th ed. McGraw-Hill, 2004.

Isselbacher EM: Diseases of the aorta. In Zipes DP, Libby P, Bonow RO, Braunwald E, eds. *Braunwald's Heart Disease: A Textbook of Cardiovascular Medicine*, 7th ed. Saunders 2005:1403–1436.

Lindsay J, Hurst JW: *The Aorta.* Grune and Stratton, 1979.

Loscalzo J, Creager MA, Dzau VJ: *Vascular Medicine: A Textbook of Vascular Biology and Diseases*, 2nd ed. Lippincott Williams and Wilkins, 1996.

Prince LA, Johnson GA: Aortic dissection and aneurysms. In *Tintinalli's Emergency Medicine: A Comprehensive Study Guide*, 6th ed. McGraw-Hill, 2004.

Reviews

Coady MA, Rizzo JA, Goldstein LJ, Elefteriades JA: Natural history, pathogenesis, and etiology of thoracic aortic aneurysms and dissections. *Cardiol Clin* 1999;17:615–635.

Haro LH: Challenges, controversies, and advances in aortic catastrophes. *Emerg Med Clin North Am* 2005;23:1159–1177.

Khan IA, Nair CK: Clinical, diagnostic, and management perspectives of aortic dissection. *Chest* 2002;122:311–328.

Nienaber CA, Eagle KA: Aortic dissection: New frontiers in diagnosis and management. Part I: From etiology to diagnostic strategies. *Circulation* 2003;108:628–635.

Nienaber CA, Eagle KA: Aortic dissection: New frontiers in diagnosis and management. Part II: Therapeutic management and follow-up. *Circulation* 2003;108:772–778.

Pretre R, Von Segesser LK: Aortic dissection. *Lancet* 1997;349:1461–1464.

Rogers RL, McCormack R: Aortic disasters. *Emerg Med Clin North Am* 2004;22:887–908.

Tsai TT, Nienaber CA, Eagle KA: Acute aortic syndromes. *Circulation* 2005;112:3802–3813.

Clinical Features

Altman LK: The man on the table devised the surgery: Dr. Michael E. DeBakey. New York Times, Dec. 25, 2006.

Bushnell J, Brown J: Clinical assessment for acute thoracic aortic dissection. *Ann Emerg Med* 2005; 46:90–92. (commentary on JAMA review)

Eagle KA, Quertermous T, Kritzer GA, et al.: Spectrum of conditions initially suggesting acute aortic dissection but with negative aortograms. *Am J Cardiol* 1986;57:322–326.

Hirst AE, Johns VJ, Kime SW: Dissecting aneurysm of the aorta: A review of 505 cases. *Medicine (Baltimore)* 1958;37:217–279.

Klompas M: Does this patient have an acute thoracic aortic dissection? *JAMA* 2002;287:2262–2272.

Mészáros I, Mórocz J, Szlávi J, et al.: Epidemiology and clinicopatholology of aortic dissection. A population-based longitudinal study over 27 years. *Chest* 2000;117:1271–1278.

O'Gara PT, Greenfield AJ, Afridi NA, Houser SL: Case 12-2004: A 38-year-old woman with acute onset of pain in the chest. *New Engl J Med* 2004;350:1666–1674.

Rosman HS, Patel S, Borzak S, et al.: Quality of history taking in patients with aortic dissection. *Chest* 1998;114:793–795.

Sarasin FP, Louis-Simonet M, Gaspoz JM, Junod AF: Detecting acute thoracic aortic dissection in the emergency department: time constraints and choice of the optimal diagnostic test. *Ann Emerg Med* 1996;28:278–288.

Wolfson AB, Bessen HA: Thoracic aortic dissection: Ruling in and ruling out [editorial]. *Ann Emerg Med* 1996;28:349–351.

Slater EE, DeSanctis RW: The clinical recognition of dissecting aortic aneurysm. *Am J Med* 1976;60:625–633.

Spittell PC, Spittell JA, Joyce JW, et al.: Clinical features and differential diagnosis of aortic dissection: Experience with 236 cases (1980–1990). *Mayo Clin Proc* 1993;68:642–651.

von Kodolitsch Y, Schwartz AG, Nienaber CA: The clinical prediction of acute aortic dissection. *Arch Intern Med* 2000;160:2977–2982.

Young J, Herd AM: Painless acute aortic dissection and rupture presenting as syncope. *J Emerg Med* 2002;22:171–174.

International Registry of Acute Aortic Dissection (IRAD)— Clinical Features

Hagan PG, Nienaber CA, Isselbacher EM, et al.: The International Registry of Acute Aortic Dissection (IRAD): New insights into an old disease. *JAMA* 2000;283:897–903.

Januzzi JL, Isselbacher EM, Fattori R, et al.: Characterizing the young patient with aortic dissection: Results from the International Registry of Aortic Dissection (IRAD). *J Am Coll Cardiol* 2004;43: 665–669.

Mehta RH, O'Gara PT, Bossone E, et al.: Acute type A aortic dissection in the elderly: Clinical characteristics, management, and outcomes in the current era. *J Am Coll Cardiol* 2002;40:685–692.

Suzuki T, Mehta RH, Ince H, et al.: Clinical profiles and outcomes of acute type B aortic dissection in the current era: Lessons from the International Registry of Aortic Dissection (IRAD). *Circulation* 2003;108 (Suppl II): s312–s317.

Upchurch GR, Nienaber C, Fattori R, et al.: Acute aortic dissection presenting with primarily abdominal pain: A rare manifestation of a deadly disease. *Ann Vasc Surg* 2005;19:367–373.

Misdiagnosis—Heparin, rt–PA administration

Davis DP, Grossman K, Kiggins DC, et al.: The inadvertent administration of anticoagulants to ED patients ultimately diagnosed with thoracic aortic dissection. *Am J Emerg Med* 2005;23:439–442.

Khoury NE, Borzak S, Gokli A, et al.: "Inadvertent" thrombolytic administration in patients without myocardial infarction: Clinical features and outcome. *Ann Emerg Med* 1996;28:298–293. One case of aortic dissection.

Marian AJ, Harris SL, Pickett JD, et al.: Inadvertent administration of rtPA to a patients with type 1 aortic dissection and subsequent cardiac tamponade. *Am J Emerg Med* 1993;11:613–615.

Rogers RL, McCormack R: Aortic disasters. *Emerg Med Clin North Am* 2004;22:887–908.

Sullivan PR, Wolfson AB, Leckey RD, Burke JL: Diagnosis of acute thoracic aortic dissection in the emergency department. *Am J Emerg Med* 2000;18:46–50.

Chest Radiography

Earnest F, Muhm JR, Sheedy PF: Roentgenographic findings in thoracic aortic dissection. *Mayo Clin Proc* 1979;54:43–50.

Gupta R, Gernsheimer J: Acute aortic dissection shown on lateral chest x-ray film. *J Emerg Med* 2002;23:285–286.

Hartnell GG, Wakeley CJ, Tottle A, et al.: Limitations of chest radiography in discriminating between aortic dissection and myocardial infarction: Implications for thrombolysis. *J Thorac Imaging* 1993; 8:152–155.

Hogg K, Teece S: Best evidence topic report: The sensitivity of a normal chest radiograph in ruling out aortic dissection. *Emerg Med J* 2004;21:199–200.

Jaeschke R, Guyatt G, Sackett DL: Users' guides to the medical literature. III. How to use an article about a diagnostic test. A. Are the results of the study valid? Evidence-Based Medicine Working Group. *JAMA* 1994;271:389–391.

Jagannath AS, Sos TA, Lockhart SH, Saddekni KW: Aortic dissection: A statistical analysis of the usefulness of plain radiographic findings. *AJR* 1986;147:1123–1126.

Luker G, Glazer HS, Eagar G, et al.: Aortic dissection: Effect of prospective chest radiographic diagnosis on delay to definite diagnosis. *Radiology* 1994;193:813–819.

von Kodolitsch Y, Nienaber CA, Dieckmann C, et al.: Chest radiography for the diagnosis of acute aortic syndrome. *Am J Med* 2004; 116:73–77.

MDCT

Gotway MB, Dawn SK: Thoracic aorta imaging with multislice CT. *Radiol Clin North Am* 2003;41:521–543.

Hayter RG, Rhea JT, Small A, et al.: Suspected aortic dissection and other aortic disorders: Multi-detector row CT in 373 cases in the emergency setting. *Radiology* 2006;238:841–852.

White CS, Kuo D, Kelemen M, et al.: Chest pain evaluation in the emergency department: Can MDCT provide a comprehensive evaluation? *AJR* 2005;185:533–540.

Wintersperger BJ, Nikolaou K, Becker CR: Multidetector-row CT angiography of the aorta and visceral arteries. *Seminar Ultrasound CT MRI* 2004;25:25–40.

CT, MRI, TEE

Batra P, Bigoni B, Manning J, et al.: Pitfalls in the diagnosis of thoracic aortic dissection at CT angiography. *Radiographics* 2000;20: 309–320.

Castaner E, Andreu M, Gallardo X, et al.: CT in nontraumatic acute thoracic aortic disease: Typical and atypical features and complications. *Radiographics* 2003;23:93–110.

Cigarroa JE, Isselbacher EM, DeSanctis RE, Eagle KA: Diagnostic imaging in the evaluation of suspected aortic dissection. *New Engl J Med* 1993;328:35–43.

Jeudy J, Waite S, White CS: Nontraumatic thoracic emergencies. *Radiol Clin North Am* 2006;44:273–293.

Ledbetter S: Helical CT in the evaluation of emergent thoracic aortic syndromes: Traumatic aortic rupture, aortic aneurysm, aortic dissection, intramural hematoma, and penetrating atherosclerotic ulcer. *Radiol Clin North Am* 1999;37:575–589.

Moore A, Eagle KA, Bruckman D, et al.: Choice of computed tomography, transesophageal echocardiography, magnetic resonance imaging, and aortography in acute aortic dissection: International Registry of Acute Aortic Dissection (IRAD). *Am J Cardiol* 2002;89:1235–1238.

Nienaber CA, von Kodolitsch Y, Nicolas V, et al.: The diagnosis of thoracic aortic dissection by noninvasive imaging procedures. *New Engl J Med* 1993;328:1–9.

Sebastià C, Pallisa E, Quiroga S, et al.: Aortic dissection: Diagnosis and followup with helical CT. *Radiographics* 1999;19:45–60.

Shiga T, Wajima Z, Apfel CC, et al.: Diagnostic accuracy of transesophageal echocardiography, helical computed tomography, and magnetic resonance imaging for suspected thoracic aortic dissection: Systematic review and meta-analysis. *Arch Intern Med* 2006;166:1350–1356.

Sommer T, Fehske W, Holzknecht N, et al.: Aortic dissection: A comparative study of diagnosis with spiral CT, multiplanar transesophageal echocardiography, and MR imaging. *Radiology* 1996;199:347–352.

Yee J, Hung RK: Spiral CT angiography of aortic dissection. *Emerg Radiol* 1999;6:24–31.

Yoshida S, Akiba H, Tamakawa M, et al.: Thoracic involvement of type A aortic dissection and intramural hematoma: Diagnostic accuracy: Comparison of emergency helical CT and surgical findings. *Radiology* 2003;228:430–435.

Transthoracic Echocardiography

Blaivas M, Sierzenski PR: Dissection of the proximal thoracic aorta: A new ultrasonographic sign in the subxiphoid view. *Am J Emerg Med* 2002;20:344–348.

Fojtik JP, Costantino TG, Dean AJ: The diagnosis of aortic dissection by emergency medicine ultrasound. *J Emerg Med* 2007;32: 191-196.

Piskoti EI, Adams CP: The utility of ultrasound in a case of pericardial tamponade. *J Emerg Med* 2002;22:411–414.

Sherman SC, Cosby K: Emergency physician ultrasonography: Aortic dissection. *J Emerg Med* 2004;26:217–218.

Sierzenski PR, Dickman E, Leech SJ, et al.: Emergency physician ultrasound decreases physician times to diagnosis, beta-blocker therapy, and operative repair in patients with acute aortic dissection. *Acad Emerg Med* 2004;11:580–581.

Intramural Hematoma (IMH)

Coady MA, Rizzo JA, Elefteriades JA: Pathologic variants of thoracic aortic dissections: Penetrating atherosclerotic ulcers and intramural hematomas. *Cardiol Clin* 1999;17:637–657.

Evangelista A, Mukherjee D, Mehta RH, et al.: Acute intramural hematoma of the aorta: A mystery in evolution. *Circulation* 2005;111:1063–1070.

Ganaha F, Miller DC, Sugimoto K, et al.: Prognosis of intramural hematoma with and without penetrating atherosclerotic ulcer: a clinical and radiological analysis. *Circulation* 2002;106:342–348.

Isselbacher EM. Intramural hematoma of the aorta: Should we let down our guard? *Am J Med* 2002;113:244–246.

Macura KJ, Corl FM, Fishman EK, et al.: Pathogenesis in acute aortic syndromes: Aortic dissection, intramural hematoma, and penetrating atherosclerotic aortic ulcer. *AJR* 2003;181:309–316.

Maraj R, Rerkpattanapipat P, Jacobs LE, et al.: Meta-analysis of 143 reported cases of aortic intramural hematoma. *Am J Cardiol* 2000;86:664–668.

Nienaber CA, et al.: Aortic intramural haematoma: Natural history and predictive factors for complications. *Heart* 2004;90:372–374.

Nienaber CA, Sievers HH: Intramural hematoma in acute aortic syndrome: More than one variant of dissection? *Circulation* 2002; 106:284–285.

Sawhney N, DeMaria AN, Blanchard DG: Aortic intramural hematoma: An increasingly recognized and potentially fatal entity. *Chest* 2001;120:1340–1346.

Song J-K, Kim H-S, Song J-M, et al.: Outcomes of medically treated patients with aortic intramural hematoma. *Am J Med* 2002;113: 181–187.

von Kodolitsch Y, Csösz SK, Koschyk DH, et al.: Intramural hematoma of the aorta: Predictors of progression to dissection and rupture. *Circulation* 2003;107:1158–1163.

Chest Radiology: Patient 13

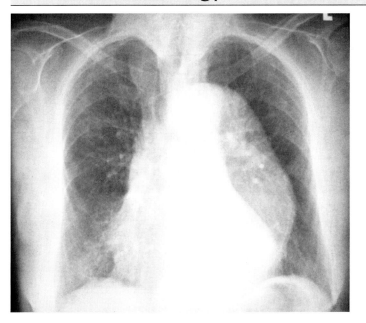
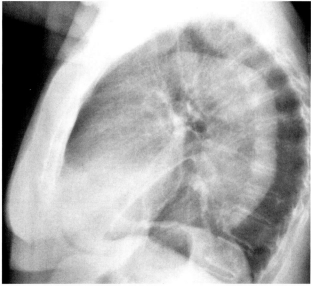

FIGURE 1

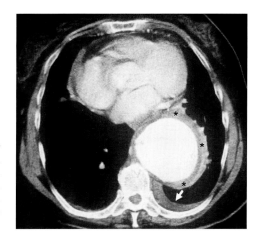

FIGURE 2 CT showing a markedly enlarged arota with surrounding mutal thrombus (*asterisks*) and a small pleural effusion (*arrow*). There was no aortic dissection.

Chest pain and dyspea in an elderly woman with COPD

A 73-year-old woman presented to the ED complaining of chest pain and shortness of breath. The pain was in the left anterior chest and left flank. She had a nonproductive cough and slight wheezing. She had had the pain intermittently for 1 week. It had become more severe in the past few hours and was associated with vomiting. She had a history of COPD.

On examination, she was a frail, slender female who was in distress when the chest pain was present, but comfortable when it abated. Her blood pressure was 140/80 mm/Hg, pulse 104 beats/min, respirations 20 breaths/min, temperature 100.0°F (rectal), and O_2 saturation 96% on 2 L/min of oxygen. Breaths sounds were diminished bilaterally and there were faint wheezes at both lung apices.

EKG showed voltage criteria for left ventricular hypertrophy and no acute ischemic changes. Morphine and albuterol were administered with improvement of her symptoms.

A chest radiograph revealed a massively dilated ascending, transverse, and descending thoracic aorta. The lungs were hyperexpanded and clear (Figure 1).

Her internist was contacted, who stated that she had a thoracic aortic aneurysm but because of her COPD, a cardiovascular surgeon felt that the operative risk for elective repair was too high.

A CT scan of the chest and abdomen was interpreted as showing a large thoracoabdominal aneurysm extending from the ascending aorta to the suprarenal abdominal aorta. Its widest dimension was 8.5 cm at the descending thoracic aorta. There was no evidence of aortic dissection. A small left pleural effusion was also noted that was not visible on the chest radiograph (Figure 2).

A cardiovascular consultant recommended administering analgesic medication. The plan was to admit the patient to the hospital for continued observation.

• Do you agree with this management?

ATHEROSCLEROTIC AORTIC ANEURYSMS

The second common disorder associated with dilation of the thoracic aorta, aside from aortic dissection, is an atherosclerotic thoracic aortic aneurysm. Atherosclerotic aortic aneurysms, both abdominal and thoracic, are complicated by leakage and rupture and are not generally associated with dissection (Table 1). In one series, thoracic aortic aneurysms were as common as aortic dissection (Clouse et al. 2004).

Atherosclerotic aortic aneurysms are most common in the infra-renal abdominal aorta (the typical location of an abdominal aortic aneurysm). Atherosclerotic aortic aneurysms in the thoracic aorta can involve the ascending aorta, aortic arch, or descending thoracic aorta. They may extend into the abdomen forming a thoracoabdominal aortic aneurysm (Figure 3).

Aneurysmal dilation of the aorta is defined as being greater than 5 cm in diameter in the ascending aorta, 4 cm in the descending thoracic aorta, and 3 cm in the abdominal aorta as measured by cross-sectional imaging (CT, MRI, or TEE). The average normal aortic width is 3.5 cm in the ascending aorta, 2.5 cm in the aortic arch, and 2 cm in the descending thoracic aorta.

The underlying pathogenesis of atherosclerotic aortic aneurysms is not completely understood. It is uncertain whether the atherosclerotic plaque causes weakening of the aortic wall and secondary aortic distention or whether the plaques form preferentially in regions where the aortic wall is weakened and the aorta is already dilated. It is also unknown why atherosclerosis that affects the aorta is associated with vascular dilation, whereas in large muscular arteries, such as the carotid or coronary arteries, atherosclerosis causes luminal narrowing and occlusion.

Gradual leakage often precedes fatal rupture of an atherosclerotic aortic aneurysm. Thickening of the aortic wall by the atheromatous plaque and the associated mural thrombus is protective of the aneurysm wall and allows leakage to occur in advance of fatal aneurysm rupture and exsanguination (Figure 4). In addition, the plaque causes sclerosis of the aortic wall and prevents the splitting of the aortic wall that occurs with aortic dissection.

The greater the diameter of the aortic aneurysm, the more likely it is to rupture. This is due to the increased wall tension that occurs in tubular structures of enlarged diameter (Laplace's law). Therefore, elective repair of a thoracic aortic aneurysm is recommended when its diameter exceeds 6.5-7 cm. This is analogous to the situation with infra-renal abdominal aortic aneurysms in which elective repair is recommended when the aneurysm diameter is 5.5 cm or more.

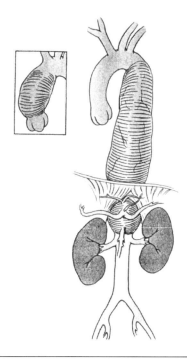

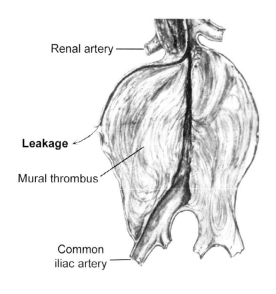

FIGURE 3 Atherosclerotic thoracoabdominal aneurysm that involves the descending thoracic aorta and suprarenal abdominal aorta.

The inset shows an isolated ascending aortic aneurysm.

An aneurysm may involve both the ascending and descending aorta, as in Patient 13.

[From Crawford ES, Coselli JS: Thoraco-abdominal aortic aneurysms. *Semin Thorac Cardiovasc Surg* 1991;3:302, with permission.]

FIGURE 4 An infrarenal atherosclerotic abdominal aortic aneurysm that is nearly completely filled by mural thrombus.

The mural thrombus protects the aneurysm wall and allows gradual leakage to occur before exsanguinating rupture. The same principle pertains to a thoracic aortic aneurysm.

[From Lindsay J, Hurst JW: *The Aorta.* Grune and Stratton, 1979, with permission.]

Although the initial presentation of a thoracic aortic aneurysm may be rupture, fifty percent are discovered incidentally on chest radiographs obtained for reasons other than suspected aortic pathology. In some cases, the patient may experience chest discomfort, sometimes described as "pulsating," or symptoms due to compression of adjacent structures such as the larynx causing hoarseness (see Patient 13C).

Penetrating Atherosclerotic Ulcers

A penetrating atherosclerotic ulcer (PAU) can form in the atherosclerotic plaque. When it penetrates deeply into the aortic wall, it can lead to aneurysm leak and rupture. A patient with a PAU may present with chest or back pain and the lesion can be detected by CT, MRI, or TEE.

Treatment recommendations for PAU vary considerably. Some authors recommend conservative management with risk factor reduction including blood pressure control and cholesterol lowering medications. Other authors consider PAU to be a lesion that precedes aortic rupture and should therefore be treated surgically either with replacement of the aneurysm with a synthetic graft or by endovascular placement of a stent-graft.

A PAU can lead to formation of an **intramural hematoma** (IMH)—a sign of impending rupture that requires surgical treatment. An IMH appears on CT as a high-attenuation crescent within the thickened aortic wall. It is often visualized better by a noncontrast CT. Noncontrast CT should therefore be performed prior to a contrast CT when an acute aortic syndrome is suspected, either aortic dissection or a leaking aneurysm, to identify an IMH.

Patient Outcome

Two hours after being admitted, while awaiting a hospital bed, the patient suddenly became acutely short of breath and hypotensive. An EKG was unchanged. She was intubated, but then suffered a cardiac arrest and could not be resuscitated. The cardiac arrest was likely due to rupture of her thoracic aortic aneurysm.

Although the initial interpretation of the CT as not showing an aortic dissection was considered reassuring that an aortic catastrophe was not imminent, the small pleural effusion, represented leakage from the aneurysm and was a sign of impending rupture. Due to her severe COPD, she may not have survived emergency aortic surgery; however, her medical condition was more precarious than initially believed.

TABLE 1

Distinguishing Aortic Disorders

Traumatic aortic injury

Shearing forces at the aortic isthmus during blunt trauma cause an intimal tear.

A localized intramural hematoma at the site of injury is contained by the adventitia (a *pseudoaneurysm*).

Chest radiography—Wide mediastinum due to mediastinal blood, not an enlarged aorta. Mediastinal blood is from torn branch vessels, not the aorta itself.

Aortic dissection

Aortic wall is split length-wise by a hematoma that enters the media through an intimal tear.

Chronic hypertension is the most common risk factor. In younger persons, a connective tissue disorder is usually present such as Marfan syndrome.

Chest radiography—Wide mediastinum due to a dilated aorta is seen in most, but not all, cases. Dissection itself is not visible; it is an entirely intraluminal event. Aortic dilation is chronic, due to a weakened aortic wall, and not due to acute aortic expansion at the time of dissection.

Aortic dilation is common in the elderly (tortuous aorta) and is a nonspecific finding. The larger the aorta, the more likely that a dissection is present, but an aorta that is "normal-sized" for a middle-aged or elderly person may be harboring a dissection.

Thoracic aortic aneurysm

Aortic atherosclerosis associated with aortic dilation. Aortic dilation is often marked.

Complicated by leakage and rupture, not dissection—Atherosclerotic plaque and mural thrombus causes aortic wall fibrosis which "protects" the aortic wall from dissection.

Chest radiography—Markedly widened mediastinum due to aneurysmal aortic dilation.

Half are asymptomatic at time of discovery, i.e., an incidental finding on chest radiography obtained for other reasons.

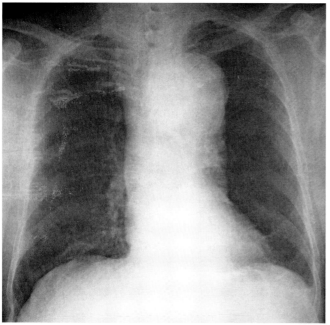

FIGURE 5A   Initial chest radiograph.

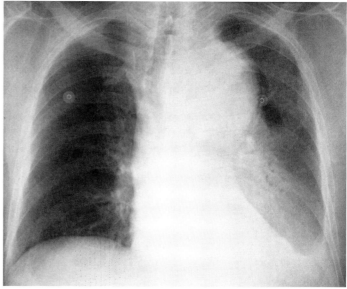

FIGURE 5B   Chest radiograph in the ED. several hours later

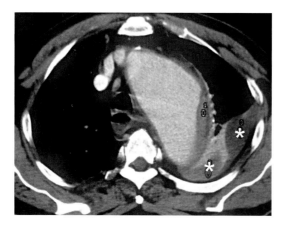
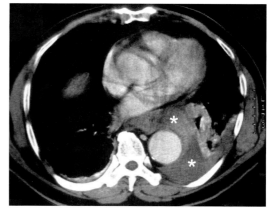

FIGURE 6   CT showing a large leaking atherosclerotic thoracic aortic aneurysm.

Patient 13B: A leaking thoracic aortic aneurysm

A 61-year-old man presented to the ED with "sharp" pain in the left side of his back and left shoulder for 2 days. Earlier that day, he went to his doctor's office, where a chest radiograph was obtained that showed a "wide mediastinum" (Figure 5A). He was told to go to the hospital, but instead went home. The chest pain recurred shortly thereafter and he called for an ambulance.

In the ED, he was in no acute distress. His blood pressure was 140/90 mm/Hg in both arms, and his pulse was 110 beats/minute. He did not have any prior medical problems. A chest radiograph showed a massive thoracic aortic aneurysm. There was a left pleural effusion that was not present on the radiograph obtained several hours earlier in his doctor's office (Figure 5B).

An emergency chest and abdominal CT showed a large thoracic aortic aneurysm that was 6.5 cm at the aortic arch and tapered to 4 cm at the descending thoracic aorta (Figure 6). There was fluid suggestive of blood in the mediastinum surrounding the aorta and a left pleural effusion (*asterisks*). This was consistent with a leaking thoracic aortic aneurysm. The site of disruption could not be located.

The patient was taken immediately to the operating room and underwent repair of the thoracic aortic aneurysm and replacement of the descending thoracic aorta from the left subclavian artery to the diaphragm with a Dacron graft. He made a good postoperative recovery.

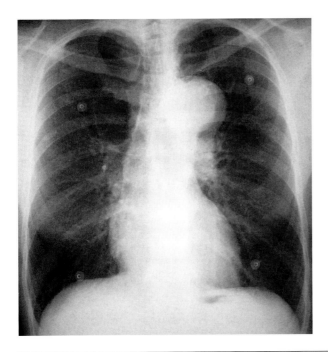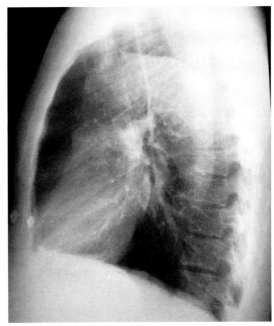

FIGURE 7

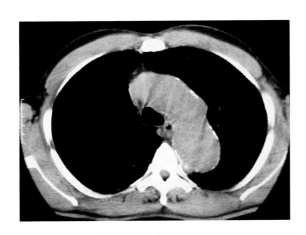

FIGURE 8   CT.

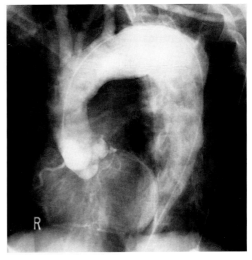

FIGURE 9   Aortogram

Patient 13C A nonleaking thoracic aortic aneurysm

A 41-year-old man presented to the ED with mild intermittent chest pain that he had had for the past 6 weeks, but had become more persistent over the past several days. It was left sided and associated with a slight cough, but no shortness of breath. He also noted hoarseness for the past 2 weeks. He had a history of hypertension and was taking antihypertensive medications. Eight months earlier, he had been in a motor vehicle collision in which he hit his chest on the steering wheel. He was seen at another ED, but was not hospitalized. He was HIV positive and his most recent CD4 count was 280 cells/mm^3.

A chest radiograph revealed aneurysmal dilation of the aortic arch (Figure 7). A chest CT confirmed an aneurysm of the aortic arch and proximal descending aorta that was 6.5 cm in its greatest diameter (Figure 8). There was no evidence of leakage,

ulceration, or dissection. An aortogram performed in preparation for surgery demonstrated that the aneurysm involved primarily the proximal descending thoracic aorta distal to the origin of the left subclavian artery (Figure 9). The differential diagnosis included atherosclerosis, a posttraumatic chronic aortic pseudoaneurysm and, given the patient's HIV infection, a syphilitic aortic aneurysm.

Serologic tests for syphilis were negative. He was scheduled for elective surgery the following week. He underwent successful repair with graft replacement of his proximal descending aorta and adjacent portion of the aortic arch. At operation, the aorta had extensive atheromatous changes. Histopathology showed "cystic medial necrosis." Histological stains and cultures for infective organisms were negative.

SUGGESTED READING

Creager MA, Braunwald E: *Atlas of Heart Diseases*, 2nd ed. Current Medicine Group, 2003.

Creager MA, Dzau VJ, Loscalzo J: *Vascular Medicine: A Companion to Braunwald's Heart Disease.* Saunders, 2006.

Halperin JL, Olin JW: Diseases of the aorta. In Fuster V, Alexander RW, O'Rourke RA, eds. *Hurst's The Heart*, 11th ed. McGraw-Hill, 2004.

Isselbacher EM: Diseases of the aorta. In Braunwald E, Zipes DP, Libby P, Bonow R, eds. *Braunwald's Heart Disease: A Textbook of Cardiovascular Medicine*, 7th ed. Saunders, 2005: 1403–1436.

Clinical and Radiographic Features

Clouse WD, Hallett JW, Hartzell HV, et al.: Acute aortic dissection: Population-based incidence compared with degenerative aortic aneurysm rupture. *Mayo Clin Proceed* 2004;79:176–180.

Coady MA, Rizzo JA, Goldstein LJ, Elefteriades JA: Natural history, pathogenesis, and etiology of thoracic aortic aneurysms and dissections. *Cardiol Clin* 1999;17:615–635.

Coady MA, Rizzo JA, Hammond GL, et al.: What is the appropriate size criterion for resection of thoracic aortic aneurysms? *J Thorac Cardiovasc Surg* 1997;113:476–491; discussion 489–491

Elefteriades JA: Natural history of thoracic aortic aneurysms: Indications for surgery, and surgical versus nonsurgical risks. *Ann Thorac Surg* 2002;74(suppl):s1877–s1880.

Fultz PJ, Melville D, Ekanej A, et al.: Nontraumatic rupture of the thoracic aorta: Chest radiographic features of an often unrecognized condition. *AJR* 1998;171:351–357.

Kawasaki S, Kawasaki T: Evolution of a thoracic aortic aneurysm. *New Engl J Med* 2007;356:1251.

Macura KJ, Corl FM, Fishman EK, Bluemke DA: Pathogenesis in acute aortic syndromes: Aortic aneurysm leak and rupture and traumatic aortic transection. *AJR* 2003;181:303–307.

Tsai TT, Nienaber CA, Eagle KA: Acute aortic syndromes. *Circulation* 2005;112:3802–3813.

Penetrating Atherosclerotic Ulcer

Cho KR, Stanson AW, Potter DD: Penetrating atherosclerotic ulcer of the descending thoracic aorta and arch. *J Thorac Cardiovasc Surg* 2004;127:1393–1401.

Coady MA, Rizzo JA, Elefteriades JA: Pathologic variants of thoracic aortic dissections: Penetrating atherosclerotic ulcers and intramural hematomas. *Cardiol Clin* 1999;17:637–657.

Coady MA, Rizzo JA, Hammond GL, et al.: Penetrating ulcer of the thoracic aorta: What is it? How do we recognize it? How do we manage it? *J Vasc Surg* 1998;27:1006–1016.

Hayashi H, Matsuoka Y, Sakamoto I, et al.: Penetrating atherosclerotic ulcer of the aorta: Imaging features and disease concept. *Radiographics* 2000;20:995–1005.

Kazerooni EA, Bree RL, Williams DM: Penetrating atherosclerotic ulcers of the descending thoracic aorta: Evaluation with CT and distinction from aortic dissection. *Radiology* 1992;183:759–765.

Macura KJ, Corl FM, Fishman EK, et al.: Pathogenesis in acute aortic syndromes: Aortic dissection, intramural hematoma, and penetrating atherosclerotic aortic ulcer. *AJR* 2003;181:309–316.

Quint LE, Williams DM, Francis IR, et al.: Ulcer-like lesions of the aorta: Imaging features and natural history. *Radiology* 2001; 218:719–723.

Stanson AW, Kazmier FJ, Hollier LH, et al.: Penetrating atherosclerotic ulcers of the thoracic aorta: Natural history of clinicopathologic correlations. *Ann Vasc Surg* 1986;1:15–23.

Computed Tomography

Gotway MB, Dawn SK: Thoracic aorta imaging with multi-slice CT. *Radiol Clin North Am* 2003;41:521–543.

Hayter RG, Rhea JT, Small A, et al.: Suspected aortic dissection and other aortic disorders: Multi-detector row CT in 373 cases in the emergency setting. *Radiology* 2006;238:841–852.

Jeudy J, Waite S, White CS: Nontraumatic thoracic emergencies. *Radiol Clin North Am* 2006;44:273–293.

Ledbetter S: Helical CT in the evaluation of emergent thoracic aortic syndromes: Traumatic aortic rupture, aortic aneurysm, aortic dissection, intramural hematoma, and penetrating atherosclerotic ulcer. *Radiol Clin North Am* 1999;37:575–589.

Schwartz S, Taljanovic M, Smyth S, et al.: CT findings of rupture, impending rupture, and contained rupture of abdominal aortic aneurysms. *AJR* 2007;188:57–62.

Sharma U, Ghai S, Paul SB, et al.: Helical CT evaluation of aortic aneurysms and dissection—A pictorial essay. *Clinical Imaging* 2003;27:273–280.

Chest Radiology: Patient 14

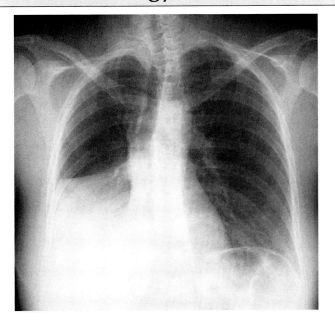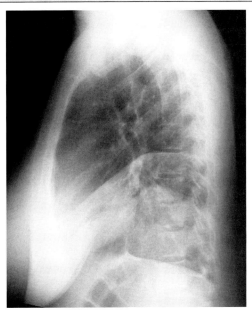

FIGURE 1   Patient 14A

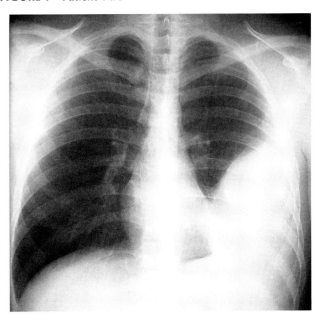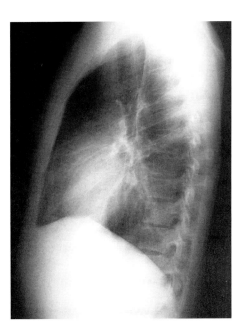

FIGURE 2   Patient 14B

Partial opacification of the thorax in two patients

Two patients with opacification of the lower portion of one lung. Despite the similar radiographic appearance of the PA views, the cause of the opacification is quite different. This is reflected by the differences in their lateral views.

Patient 14A. A 32-year-old woman was hospitalized for an asthma exacerbation. She also had a history of alcoholism and was intoxicated at the time of her presentation to the ED (Figure 1).

Patient 14B. A 32-year-old man complained of left-sided pleuritic chest pain (Figure 2).

- **What is the explanation of the radiographic findings in these patients?**

WHITE-OUT

What Is the Differential Diagnosis of Opacification of the Lower Portion of a Hemithorax?

Patient 14A

The first possibility is consolidation due to **pneumonia.** Although this is consistent with the patient's clinical presentation, several radiographic findings argue against this diagnosis. First, it is unusual for pneumonia to cause such homogeneous opacification of the lung. With pneumonia there usually are aerated alveoli and bronchi interspersed within the infiltrate (air-alveolograms and air bronchograms) that gives pneumonia a mottled appearance (inhomogeneous opacification).

Second, pneumonia usually has ill-defined margins. An infiltrate can have a well-defined margin when it is adjacent to an interlobar fissure. In this patient's PA view, the upper margin of the opacity is sharp (Figure 3A). This sharp horizontal margin seems as though it would represent the minor fissure (horizontal fissure) as would occur with consolidation of the right middle lobe. However, on the lateral view, the corresponding horizontal line lies posterior to the hilum, not anterior as would be expected if it were the minor fissure (Figure 3B).

A **second** possible diagnosis is a **pleural effusion.** A pleural effusion does cause homogeneous opacification, as is seen in this patient. In addition, on an upright chest radiograph, a pleural effusion characteristically has a sharp superior margin. However, the effusion's upper margin usually curves upward at the lateral chest wall, forming a *meniscus.* In this patient, there is no meniscus. In addition, a right lateral decubitus chest radiograph (right-side down) was obtained, which did not show layering as would be expected with a pleural effusion (Figure 4).

A **third** possibility is that the opacity is due to **decreased aeration of the lung.** Diminished aeration causes loss of lung volume and is known as **atelectasis** or **collapse.** The most clinically important cause of atelectasis is obstruction of a major (lobar) bronchus, which causes collapse of an entire lobe of the lung. Bronchial obstruction may be caused by an endobronchial tumor, a hilar mass, an aspirated intraluminal foreign body, or mucus plug. Obstruction of a smaller bronchus (segmental or subsegmental peripheral airway) does not cause atelectasis because alveolar aeration is maintained by innumerable interalveolar connecting pores (Figure 5A).

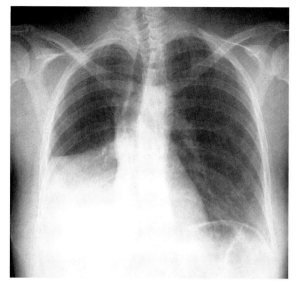

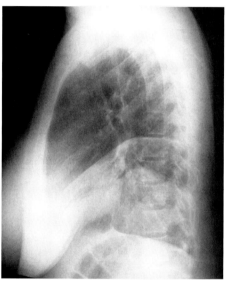

FIGURE 3   PA and lateral views—Patient 14A.

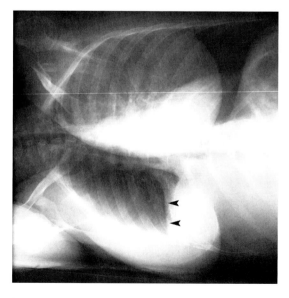

FIGURE 4   Right lateral decubitus view.
No layering was seen (*arrowheads*).

When a lobar bronchus is obstructed, the air within the obstructed lobe is gradually resorbed into the blood stream, resulting in collapse of the entire lobe. For this reason, obstructive atelectasis is also known as **resorption atelectasis** (Figure 5B). Radiographically, atelectasis is characterized by signs of volume loss (Table 1). The principal radiographic feature is shift of an interlobar fissure. There are often also nonspecific signs of volume loss such as shift of the trachea, heart, or mediastinum, an elevated hemidiaphragm, rib cage narrowing, and compensatory hyperinflation of adjacent lung tissue. Finally, the collapsed lobe is usually radiopaque, although this may not occur when there is only a small amount of retained fluid within the collapsed lobe.

Collapse of each lobe has a characteristic radiographic appearance. The margin of the collapsed lobe is well defined because it is formed by an interlobar fissure (Figure 6).

Collapse of the **lower lobe** creates an elongated triangle adjacent to the mediastinum extending from the hilum to the diaphragm. Its sharp lateral border is the major (oblique) fissure that is displaced inferiorly and medially. Collapse of an **upper lobe** creates a triangular or concave opacity extending from the hilum to the apex of the lung (see Patient 5, Figures 8, 15, and 16, on pages 48–50). Collapse of the **right middle lobe** creates an ill-defined opacity on the PA radiograph. On the lateral radiograph, it forms a wedge-shaped opacity extending anteriorly from the hilum. With combined **right middle and lower lobe** atelectasis, the opacity slopes down from the hilum and extends to the lateral chest wall.

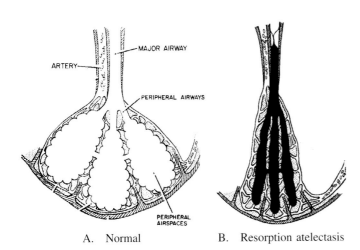

A. Normal   B. Resorption atelectasis

FIGURE 5   Schematic diagram of normal lung tissue (*A*) and the changes seen with obstruction of a lobar bronchus causing *resorption atelectasis* (*B*).

[From Fraser RS, Colman N, Muller N, Paré PD: *Synopsis of Diseases of the Chest*, 3rd ed. Saunders, 2005, with permission.]

TABLE 1

Radiographic Signs of Lobar Atelectasis

1. Displaced interlobar fissure (the principal sign)

2. Non-specific signs of volume loss

   Elevated hemidiaphragm
   Shift of the trachea, heart, or hilum
   Rib cage narrowing
   Compensatory hyperinflation

3. Loss of aeration causing increased opacity (not always present)

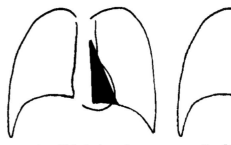

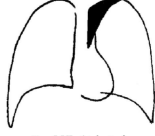

A. LLL Atelectasis   B. LUL Atelectasis

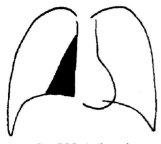

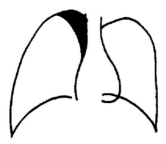

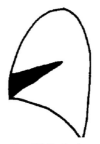

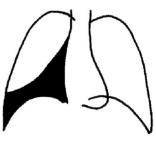

C. RLL Atelectasis   D. RUL Atelectasis   E. RML Atelectasis   F. RLL + RML Atelectasis

FIGURE 6   **Characteristic patterns of lobar atelectasis.**

In this patient, there are several **signs of volume loss.** The trachea is displaced to the right (Figure 7, *asterisk*). There is also displacement of the interlobar fissures—the primary sign of atelectasis. On the PA view, the well-defined superior margin of the opacity is *not* the minor fissure (Figure 7, *arrowheads*). The explanation is evident on the lateral view. Posterior to the hilum, the major fissure is pulled downward and assumes a horizontal position (Figure 8A, *arrows*). On the PA view, the horizontal border of the opacity is, therefore, the displaced posterior portion of the *major fissure* (Figure 7).

On a normal lateral view, the *minor fissure* extends horizontally anterior to the hilum. In this patient, the minor fissure is not in its expected location. Anterior to the hilum, the margin of the opacity slopes inferiorly in the expected location of the major fissure (Figure 8A, *arrowheads*). This, however, is the dis-

placed minor fissure, not the major fissure. Both the right minor and major fissures are displaced inferiorly. The anterior portion of the major fissure in not visible because it is embedded within the opacity (Figure 8B).

These radiographic findings are indicative of **combined right middle and lower lobe collapse** (Figure 6F). However, in this patient, there is only a moderate loss of lung volume, as well as the dense opacification of the collapsed lobes. This occurs when the obstructed lobes contain a considerable amount of fluid. The fluid cannot be resorbed after the bronchus is obstructed, but remain trapped within the obstructed airspaces (Figure 9).

Combined collapse of the right middle and lower lobes occurs because the right middle lobe and lower lobe bronchi are joined proximally to form the *bronchus intermedius*, the first division of the right mainstem bronchus.

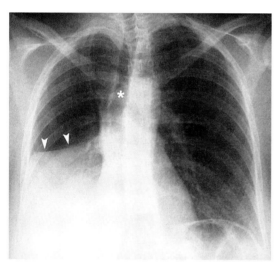

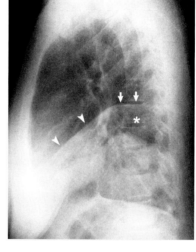

FIGURE 7   PA view showing RML and RLL collapse.

The trachea is deviated to the right due to volume loss (*asterisk*). The sharp superior margin of the opacity is the retracted posterior margin of the major fissure (*arrowheads*).

FIGURE 8   Lateral view showing RML and RLL collapse.

The posterior portion of the major fissure is horizontal (*arrows*). The minor fissure slopes downward anterior to the hilum (*arrowheads*).

The anterior portion of the major fissure is embedded within the collapsed right middle and lower lobes.

The *superior segment* of the RLL remains partly aerated. This accounts for the relatively lucency seen just inferior to the posterior portion of the major fissure (*asterisk*).

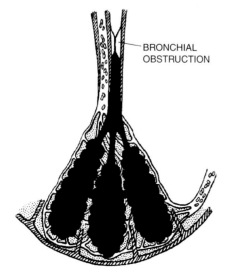

FIGURE 9   Resorption atelectasis in a patient with considerable bronchial and alveolar secretions.

There is less volume loss and greater opacification of the collapsed lobe due to retained secretions.

[From Fraser RS, Colman N, Muller N, Paré PD: *Synopsis of Diseases of the Chest*, 3rd ed. Saunders, 2005, with permission.]

Patient 14A Outcome

The etiology of this patient's bronchial obstruction can be surmised from her clinical presentation. Her asthma exacerbation caused increased bronchial secretions. Alcohol intoxication decreased her ability to clear secretions by coughing. She developed bronchial obstruction due to a mucus plug. The copious bronchial secretions that were retained within the obstructed right middle and lower lobes account for the relatively slight loss of lung volume, as well as the dense opacification of the collapsed lobes.

A CT scan obtained soon after her admission confirmed the diagnosis of right middle and lower lobe atelectasis due to a mucus plug in the bronchus intermedius (Figure 10). The patient was treated with chest percussion to clear the mucus plug and bronchial secretions. Her atelectasis gradually resolved over the next 4 days (Figure 11).

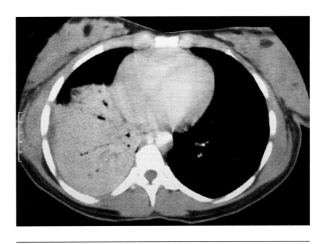

FIGURE 10 CT showing consolidation of the collapsed RML and RLL distal to a mucus plug in the *bronchus intermedius*. Considerable secretions are retained in the obstructed lung. A small amount of air remains entrapped within bronchi forming small air bronchograms.

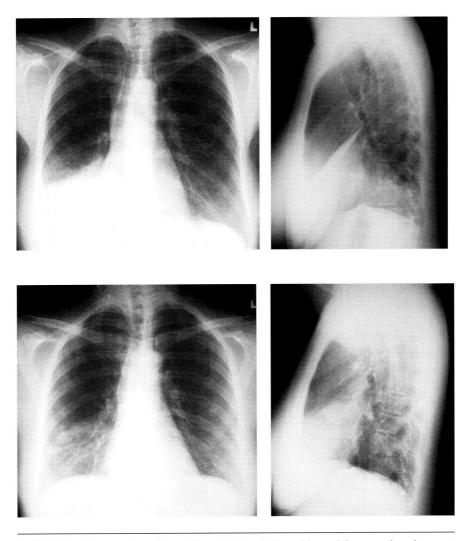

FIGURE 11 Reexpansion of the collapsed right middle and lower lobes over the subsequent 4 days after expectoration of the mucus plug and manual chest percussion by a respiratory therapist.

THE DISAPPEARING DIAPHRAGM

Patient 14B

The same differential diagnosis pertains to Patient 14B, although, the radiographic findings and ultimate diagnosis are different.

On the **PA view,** the superior margin of the opacity makes a concave acute angle with the pleural margin (Figure 12, *arrowheads*). This implies that the opacity is either a pleural effusion or a pleural-based mass, rather than being intrapulmonary. An intraparenchymal infiltrate or mass would make an angle of ≥ 90° with the pleural margin, as seen in Patient 14A (Figure 7). However, the superior margin of the opacity is not horizontal as would be expected with a pleural effusion (Figure 12). In addition, a left lateral decubitus view was obtained to detect a free-flowing pleural effusion, but there was no layering (Figure 13).

When a pleural effusion is loculated, i.e., held in place by a fibrous capsule, it does not layer or move when the patient changes position. A plaster cast simulating the shape of a pleural effusion has a similar radiographic appearance to that seen on this patient's PA view (Figure 14). (In this patient, because the effusion is loculated, its medial extent curves inferiorly giving it the rounded appearance seen on the PA view.)

On the **lateral view,** the opacity (loculated effusion) is, paradoxically, invisible (Figures 2B and 15). The radiographic appearance of an object depends not only on its radiopacity, but also its shape and whether its margins are sharp and parallel to the direction of the x-ray beam. When an object fades gradually into its surroundings, it may be invisible. This is the case in this patient. When viewed from the side, the margins of the loculated effusion become gradually thinner and are therefore invisible on the lateral view (Figures 15 and 16).

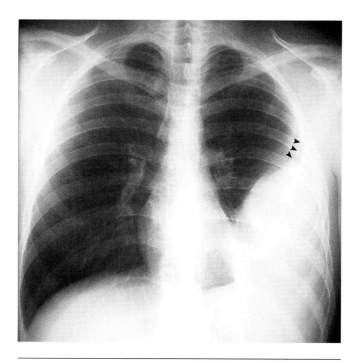

FIGURE 12   PA view showing a curved concave junction between the opacity and the pleural margin (*arrowheads*).

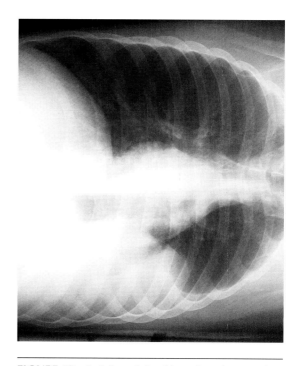

FIGURE 13   Left lateral decubitus view shows no layering as would be expected with a pleural effusion.

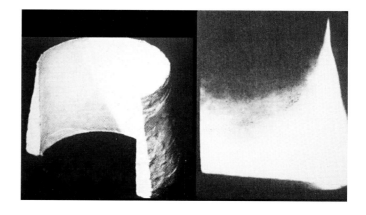

FIGURE 14   Plaster cast of a pleural effusion and a radiograph depicting its appearance on a PA radiograph.
[From: Heitzman ER: *The Lung: Radiologic-Pathologic Correlations*, 2nd ed., Mosby-Year Book, 1984, with permission.]

There is, however, indirect evidence on the lateral view that an effusion is present. Because the effusion merges gradually with the dome of the left hemidiaphragm, the diaphragm looses its well-defined margin with the lung and becomes invisible. On this patient's lateral view, only one side of the diaphragm is visible, the right side. The left hemidiaphragm is obscured by the loculated pleural effusion. This is known as the *single diaphragm sign* (Figure 15).

Patient 14B Outcome

When the patient was questioned further about his medical history, he stated that he had been stabbed to the chest two months earlier. He was hospitalized elsewhere and treated with a chest tube for several days. He had not returned for follow-up visits. He had persistent pain at the thoracostomy site, but no recent change or worsening. The radiographic finding was therefore likely a loculated, incompletely drained hemothorax.

A thoracic surgery consultant reviewed this patient's case with regard to performing a thoracotomy or thorascopic surgery to remove the loculated hemothorax. He decided instead to follow the patient in the clinic for evidence of resorption over time, as occurs in most patients. If considerable fibrosis were to develop (fibrothorax), there could be long-term restrictive lung disease. This is treated surgically by pleural decortication. Fibrothorax develops in less than 1% of patients with hemothorax, even when small to moderate amounts of blood remain in the pleural space. Fibrothorax is more common following hemopneumothorax or when a pleural space infection occurs.

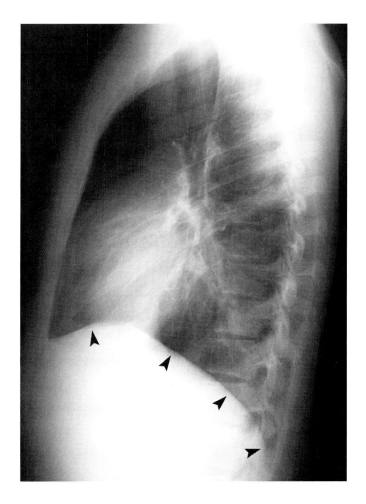

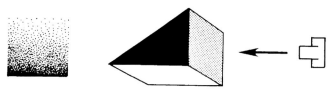

FIGURE 16   Without a sharp margin in the plane of the x-ray beam, a radiopaque mass may be completely invisible.

FIGURE 15   The lateral view shows only the right side of the diaphragm (*arrowheads*). The left hemothorax is not visible—the *single diaphragm sign*. The left side is obscured on the lateral view by the loculated hemothorax.

The hemothorax itself is not visible because its superior surface tapers gradually with respect to the x-ray beam.

SUGGESTED READING

Felson B: *Chest Roentgenology*. Saunders, 1973.

Huggins JT, Sahn SA: Causes and management of pleural fibrosis. *Respirology* 2004;9:441–447.

Light RW, Lee YCG: Pneumothorax, chylothorax, hemothorax, and fibrothorax. In Mason RJ, Murray JF, Broaddus VC, Nadel JA, eds. *Murray and Nadel's Textbook of Respiratory Medicine*, 4th ed. Elsevier, 2005:1979–1980.

ABDOMINAL RADIOGRAPHY

Diagnostic imaging plays a key role in the management of patients with acute abdominal pain. A precise diagnosis based on clinical findings alone is usually not possible, and diagnostic imaging should therefore be used liberally, especially if surgical treatment might be necessary. In elderly or debilitated patients, the clinical presentations of serious abdominal conditions can be muted, so a low threshold for ordering radiography and especially CT should be maintained (Esses et al. 2004). However, when a patient is unstable or an imaging study would delay emergency surgery, diagnostic imaging should be omitted.

In the past, abdominal radiography was the primary imaging modality even though its diagnostic accuracy for most disorders is limited. With the introduction of CT and ultrasonography, the scope of imaging diagnosis has expanded greatly. Other imaging modalities include nuclear scintigraphy, enteric contrast studies, and angiography. The choice of imaging study is based on the diagnoses suspected (Table 1).

CT has the greatest diagnostic capabilities and is the test of choice in most patients presenting with significant abdominal pain. CT has high sensitivity for many abdominal disorders and can often detect alternative diagnoses when the primary disorder is not present.

Radiography is indicated in patients with suspected peptic ulcer perforation and small or large bowel obstruction. Because emergency clinicians are often called upon to interpret radiographs, conventional radiography is the focus of the cases in this section. In addition, knowledge about the radiographic manifestations of these disorders is important in understanding the radiologist's report.

TABLE 1

Diagnostic Imaging Based on Suspected Diagnosis

Perforated peptic ulcer (pneumoperitoneum)	Radiography—upright chest or left lateral decubitus abdominal view CT
Small bowel obstruction	Radiography—abdomen (supine and upright) CT (IV contrast, oral contrast not essential) Upper GI contrast study (enteroclysis)—not in ED
Large bowel obstruction (tumor or volvulus)	Radiography CT; Contrast enema
Intussusception (children)	Radiography; ultrasonography Contrast or air enema—therapeutic (reduces the intussusception)
Appendicitis	CT, MRI (pregnancy) Ultrasonography (graded-compression technique)
Diverticulitis	CT
Ovarian cyst (bleed or torsion), pelvic abscess	Ultrasonography (transvaginal, including Doppler) CT (if enteric disorders are also being considered)
Early pregnancy (ectopic)	Ultrasonography (transvaginal)
Colitis, enteritis	No imaging needed for infectious diarrhea CT for Crohn's disease or ischemic colitis
Mesenteric ischemia	CT; angiography for acute arterial occlusion Emergency surgery, if bowel infarction and peritonitis Radiography—intramural gas and hepatic portal venous gas (rare)
Abdominal aortic aneurysm or dissection	Ultrasonography—detects aneurysm, not leakage CT—noncontrast to detect aneurysm leakage, IV contrast for dissection
Renal colic	Helical CT (noncontrast); radiography (to follow a known stone) Ultrasonography—hydronephrosis, Contrast urography (if no CT)
Cholecystitis	Ultrasonography; CT; radiography (gallstones, gallbladder gas) Hepatobiliary scintigraphy (HIDA)
Pancreatitis	CT—prognostic assessment in severe pancreatitis, complications (pseudocyst), negative in mild pancreatitis

ABDOMINAL RADIOGRAPHY

Radiographic Views

Three radiographic views should be obtained in an abdominal series: supine and upright abdominal views and an upright chest radiograph (Table 2). If possible, a lateral chest radiograph should also be obtained. The *supine abdominal view* shows bowel, soft tissues, and bones. The *upright view* is used to demonstrate air/fluid levels within the bowel that aid in the diagnosis of mechanical small bowel obstruction.

The upright view of the *chest* is obtained to look for free air under the diaphragm (pneumoperitoneum). The chest radiograph can also reveal intrathoracic disorders that may be responsible for abdominal pain such as a lower lobe pneumonia or pleural effusion.

When the patient is too ill or frail to be positioned for upright radiographs (abdomen and chest), a *left lateral decubitus abdominal radiograph* should be obtained. The left lateral decubitus view is an AP view of the abdomen that is obtained with the patient lying with the left side down; the x-ray beam is directed horizontally. This view is obtained to detect air/fluid levels and pneumoperitoneum.

Radiographic Anatomy

Five tissue densities can be distinguished on abdominal radiographs: air, fat, fluid (solid organs), bone (calcifications), and metal. Fat is slightly less radiopaque than fluid. Solid organs are visible when they are surrounded by fat tissue, e.g., perinephric fat (Figure 1).

BOWEL GAS   Bowel gas provides the most clinically useful information on an abdominal radiograph. Most gas in the bowel is *swallowed air.* Only a small portion of bowel gas (less than 5%) originates from digestion of bowel contents. Gas is normally seen within the stomach and colon. Small bowel normally contains little or no gas. When intestinal motility is disturbed either by mechanical obstruction or nonobstructive adynamic ileus, gas accumulates within small bowel. Gas within the different segment of the alimentary tract can be differentiated by its location and appearance (Figures 1, 2, and 3A).

The **stomach** occupies the mid upper abdomen and left upper quadrant on the supine view. Thick irregular rugal folds may be visible (Figures 1 and 2). On the upright view, a distinctive air/fluid level is seen below the left hemidiaphragm (Figure 3B).

Small and large bowel have distinctive radiographic features (Table 3). **Small bowel** has a central location in the abdomen. When small bowel (jejunum) is distended, mucosal folds known as **valvulae conniventes** (*plicae circularis*) make thin transverse indentations on the bowel gas. The valvulae are numerous and extend completely across the bowel lumen. The valvulae conniventes are best seen when the bowel is distended (Figures 3A and 4A). The *distal ileum* does not have valvulae conniventes and, when distended, has a smooth tubular appearance. Small bowel can fold back on itself, and when distended, has a *"bent finger"* appearance (Figure 3A).

Large bowel is generally *peripheral* in location, although the transverse colon spans the mid-abdomen, and an elongated sigmoid colon may migrate up from the lower abdomen (Figure 2). The transverse colon tends to fill with air on a supine radiograph because it is anteriorly located. The colon has characteristic mucosal indentations called **haustra**, which are thick, few in number, and do not extend completely across the bowel lumen (Figure 2). Finally, the colon contains *fecal matter,* which has a stippled appearance owing to embedded air (Figure 1).

Radiograph Interpretation

A **systematic approach** to radiograph interpretation entails examination of each tissue density in all regions of the radiograph: air, soft tissue, and bones and calcification. Air may be located within the bowel lumen, free within the peritoneal cavity, or in other abnormal locations.

A **targeted approach** focuses on the radiographic manifestations of the diseases under consideration, mainly **bowel obstruction** and **perforation,** although other disorders can occasionally be detected.

TABLE 2

Radiographic Views

Supine abdomen

Upright abdomen

Chest (upright preferred)

Left lateral decubitus abdominal view
   (if upright views of abdomen and chest not obtained)

TABLE 3

Intestinal Gas

Small bowel	Colon
Central	Peripheral
Valvulae conniventes	Haustra
Pliable—bent finger	Contains feces

The evaluation begins by examining the **bowel gas pattern** for evidence of bowel obstruction or adynamic ileus. Next, **free intraperitoneal air** is sought primarily on the upright chest radiograph (or the left lateral decubitus view if upright radiographs were not obtained). **Other abnormal gas collections** are then identified, such as gas in the biliary tract or gall bladder, hepatic portal veins, within the bowel wall (intramural gas), within abscesses, and in retroperitoneal tissues (Table 4).

Soft tissue organs are examined, including the liver, spleen, and kidneys. Soft tissue masses are identified by the displacement of other intra-abdominal structures.

Calcifications may be incidental findings (phleboliths) or may have potential pathological significance (gallstones, renal calculi, vascular calcifications or calcified tumors). The **bones** are then examined, including the pelvis, spine, and lower ribs. Finally, **metallic foreign bodies** may be found, depending on the clinical circumstances (ingestion or rectal insertion, or surgical clips).

Bowel Gas Patterns

There are five different bowel gas patterns (Table 5). The **primary goal** is identifying bowel obstruction. Obstructive patterns must be differentiated from adynamic ileus, since both are characterized by bowel distention.

NORMAL   Normally, in an asymptomatic individual, bowel gas is found only in the stomach and large intestine (mainly in feces). Small bowel normally contains minimal or no gas (Figure 1).

NON-SPECIFIC   As intestinal motility diminishes in response to a wide variety of disorders (including the minor painful stimulus of a venipuncture), air begins to accumulate within small bowel, although the small bowel is not distended (diameter <3 cm) (Figure 2). The *nonspecific bowel gas pattern* has little clinical significance. Some authors consider this pattern normal and others use the term "nonspecific" to denote mild ileus (an abnormal pattern with less than three distended loops of small bowel). Because of this inconsistency, some authors recommend that the term "nonspecific bowel gas pattern" be abandoned, even though its use is widespread (Maglinte 1996, Patel 1995). Some authors use nonspecific to mean nonobstructive, although this is not valid because obstruction can be present with a normal or nonspecific bowel gas pattern.

ADYNAMIC ILEUS   As intestinal motility is further diminished, air continues to accumulate and the bowel becomes distended (diameter >3 cm for small bowel, >8 cm for large bowel). Fluid also accumulates within the bowel lumen, and air/fluid levels (usually small) may be seen on an upright radiograph (Figure 3).

The key feature distinguishing adynamic ileus from mechanical obstruction is that with adynamic ileus, distention is uniform throughout the intestinal tract, whereas with obstruction, distention only occurs proximal to the site of obstruction.

Ileus occurs with pathologic processes of practically any sort, including intra-abdominal disorders (appendicitis and cholecystitis), and extra-abdominal and systemic disorders (pneumonia, electrolyte disturbances, etc). Bowel distention also occurs in diarrheal illnesses such as infectious enteritis (Table 6). Adynamic ileus may be acute, chronic, or intermittent.

In **mild ileus,** bowel distention and gas accumulation is limited. When a single dilated air-filled loop of bowel is located near an intra-abdominal inflammatory process, it is called a *localized ileus* or *"sentinel loop."* This is associated with finding in appendicitis, pancreatitis, or cholecystitis. It is difficult to identify with any certainty and is of limited diagnostic value.

With **severe adynamic ileus,** there is marked distention of both small and large bowel. This is sometimes referred to as *colonic pseudo-obstruction* because when the colon is markedly distended it has a similar radiographic pattern to distal large bowel obstruction (Figure 5). Contrast enema or CT may be needed to distinguish the two. When there is no underlying cause such as an electrolyte disturbance or neurological disorder, colonic ileus is idiopathic and is termed *Ogilvie's syndrome.*

SMALL BOWEL OBSTRUCTION   A mechanical small bowel obstruction (SBO) is characterized by loops of small bowel that are dilated proximal to the point of obstruction, and collapsed or nondistended distal to the obstruction. On abdominal radiography, the colon is assessed to determine whether distal bowel is collapsed or dilated. With SBO, there need not be complete absence of colonic gas (Figure 4A). When there is gas in the colon, it is often referred to as a "partial obstruction", although this term is misleading because distal gas may be present with a physiologically complete obstruction when the colon has not yet emptied all its contents. In addition, a partial SBO can be difficult to distinguish from an adynamic ileus.

(continued on page 144)

TABLE 4

Systematic Approach to Abdominal Radiographs

Gas
  Intraluminal gas—bowel gas pattern
  Free intraperitoneal air—pneumoperitoneum
  Other gas collections—biliary, intramural, etc.

Soft tissues—solid organs, masses

Calcifications and bones

Foreign bodies—radiopaque

TABLE 5

Bowel Gas Patterns

Normal
Nonspecific
Adynamic ileus
  Mild—localized ileus or "sentinel loop"
  Severe—"colonic pseudo-obstruction"
Small bowel obstruction
Large bowel obstruction

BOWEL GAS PATTERNS

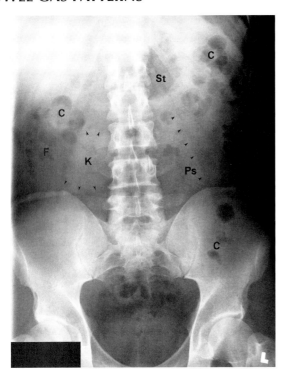

FIGURE 1   Normal bowel gas pattern.

Gas is in the stomach (St) and colon (C). There is practically no gas in small bowel. Feces (F) in the colon has a stippled gas appearance. The kidney (K) and psoas margins (Ps) are visible because they are outlined by fat (*arrowheads*).

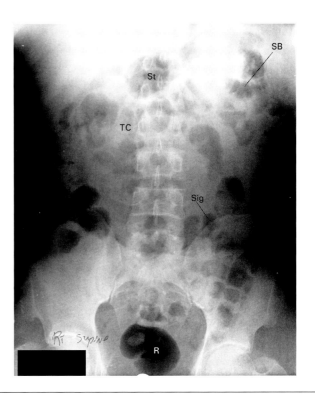

FIGURE 2   Nonspecific bowel gas pattern.

Gas is in the stomach (St), transverse colon (TC), sigmoid colon (Sig) with haustra, small bowel (SB) with valvulae conniventes, and rectum (R).

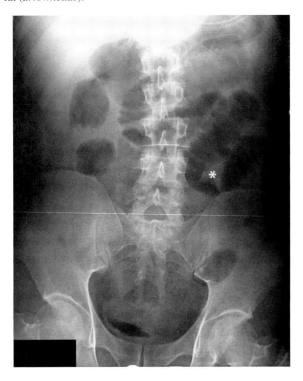

FIGURE 3A   Adynamic ileus.

There is increased gas in the small bowel and colon. Dilated small bowel is central in location, has valvulae conniventes extending across the lumen, and a "bent finger" appearance (*).

This patient had an adynamic ileus due to appendicitis.

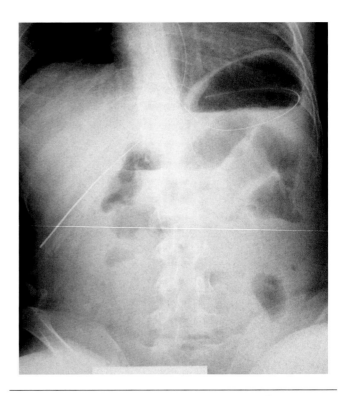

FIGURE 3B   Adynamic ileus—Upright radiograph.

There are a few scattered intestinal air/fluid levels and a large air/fluid level in the stomach. A nasogastric tube is coiled in the stomach.

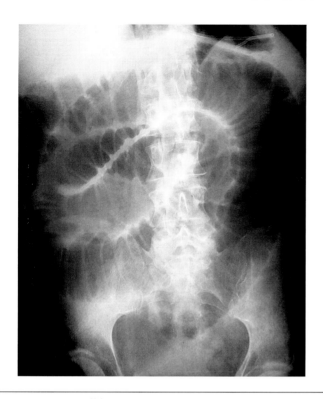

FIGURE 4A   Small bowel obstruction.
Marked dilation of small bowel with numerous valvulae conniventes (mucosal indentations that extend entirely across the small bowel lumen). No gas is in the colon.

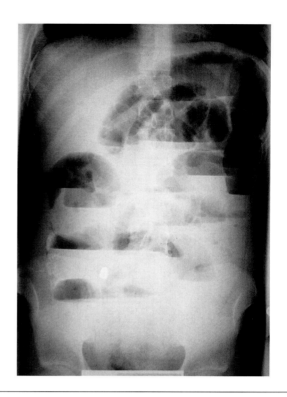

FIGURE 4B   Small bowel obstruction—Upright view.
Multiple broad air/fluid levels. No gas is in the colon.

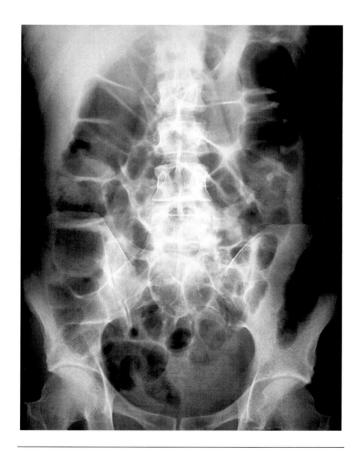

FIGURE 5   Severe adynamic ileus.
Marked dilation of small and large bowel. This patient had appendicitis.

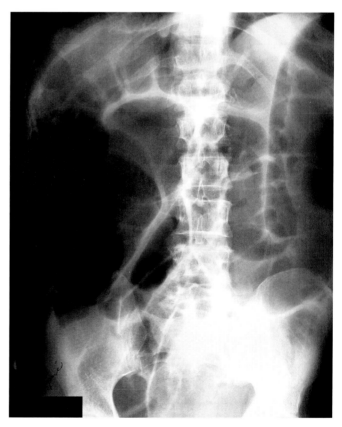

FIGURE 6   Large bowel obstruction.
Marked dilation of large and small bowel. Contrast enema revealed an obstructing tumor in the sigmoid colon.

On the **upright abdominal radiograph** in patients with small bowel obstruction, **air/fluid levels** have distinctive characteristics. *Differential (dynamic) air/fluid levels* occur at different heights within an inverted U-shaped loop of bowel. Multiple differential air/fluid levels create a "stepladder" appearance (Figure 4B). *Broad air/fluid levels* have a "tortoise-shell" appearance. The *"string-of-pearls"* sign is due to small pockets of air trapped under valvulae conniventes.

LARGE BOWEL OBSTRUCTION   In mechanical large bowel obstruction, there is distention of large bowel and often small bowel (Figure 6). Large bowel obstruction may be caused by a colonic tumor, volvulus of the sigmoid colon or cecum, an intraluminal mass (fecal impaction), or extraluminal mass (diverticular abscess). When the cecum is markedly distended (diameter >11–13 cm), there is risk of perforation.

Distal large bowel obstruction can be difficult to distinguish from a severe adynamic ileus. **Contrast enema** or **CT** may be needed to differentiate a colonic tumor or volvulus, from severe adynamic ileus.

TABLE 6

Causes of Adynamic Ileus

Intra-abdominal disorders–Appendicitis, pancreatitis, peritonitis, immediate postsurgical period, etc.

Nonabdominal disorders–Pneumonia, MI, head trauma

Systemic disorders–Electrolyte disorders (hypokalemia), sepsis

Medications–Opiates, anticholinergics

Bed-bound debilitation

ABDOMINAL CT

Emergency physicians should be knowledgeable about the key CT findings of the various diseases that cause acute abdominal pain. This will help in reviewing the CT images, in understanding the radiologist's report, and in facilitating communication with the radiologist, surgeon, or internist.

Various CT protocols are used to improve visualization of particular anatomical structures. **Intravenous contrast** opacifies solid organs, the bowel wall, and vascular structures, and is essential in visualizing lesions in these organs. A rapid bolus of IV contrast is administered for CT angiographic studies, e.g., for aortic dissection.

Enteric contrast is administered to opacify the bowel lumen. Without enteric contrast, it can be difficult to distinguish collapsed small bowel from other soft tissue structures in the peritoneal cavity.

Certain disorders do not require contrast material. In high-grade small bowel obstruction, enteric contrast is not necessary (and it is usually not tolerated by a patient who is vomiting) because distended bowel is readily visualized. A noncontrast CT

scan is used in patients with renal colic since contrast is not necessary to visualize calculi in the ureters. Finally, intra-abdominal fat provides "intrinsic contrast" when it surrounds intra-abdominal organs.

CT Interpretation

CT interpretation depends on knowledge of cross-sectional anatomy as well as the CT findings associated with various disorders (Figure 7). In a systematic approach to interpretation, every organ is examined in every slice (Table 7). Structures that traverse multiple slices should be followed for their full extent. In a targeted approach, the images are reviewed with attention to findings associated with the diseases suspected. For example, if the patient has right lower quadrant pain, the appendix is first examined. Abnormalities in other organs that could be responsible for the patient's symptoms are then sought, particularly if the primary disorder is not found.

TABLE 7

Systematic Approach to CT Interpretation
"Every Organ in Every Slice"

Solid organs	Liver, spleen, pancreas, kidneys, pelvic organs
Blood vessels	Aorta and branches, IVC, portal vein
Bowel	Stomach, duodenum, small bowel, colon, appendix
Mesentery and peritoneum	Abnormal fluid. Free air (use "lung windows")
Muscles	Abdominal wall, diaphragm, psoas, and iliac muscles
Bones	Spine, pelvis (use bone windows)
Thorax	Diaphragm, lungs, heart

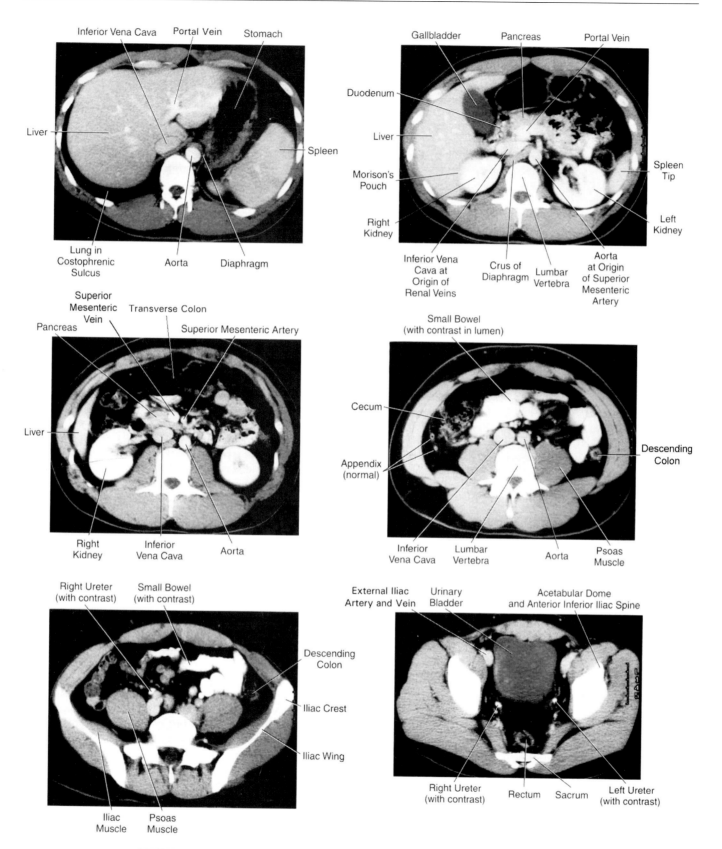

FIGURE 7   Cross-sectional anatomy: Normal abdominal CT in a 26-year-old man.

Both oral and intravenous contrast have been administered.

Contrast is in the ureters but has just begun to be excreted into the bladder (image 6).

Intra-abdominal fat provides "intrinsic contrast" for intraperitoneal and retroperitoneal organs.

[From Schwartz DT, Reisdorff EJ: Emergency Radiology, McGraw-Hill, 2000.]

SUGGESTED READING

Abdominal Radiology

Baker SR, Cho KC: *The Abdominal Plain Film,* 2nd ed. McGraw-Hill, 1999.

Balthazar EJ, ed.: Imaging the acute abdomen. *Radiol Clin North Am* 1994;32:829–1044.

McCort JJ: *Abdominal Radiology.* Williams and Wilkins, 1981.

Mori PA, Mori KW: Abdomen. In Keats TE, ed. *Emergency Radiology,* 2nd ed. Year Book Medical Publishers, 1989.

RS Jones, Claridge JA: Acute abdomen. In Townsend CM, Beauchamp RD, Evers BM, Mattox KL, eds. *Sabiston's Textbook of Surgery,* 17th ed. Saunders, 2004:1219–1240.

Silen W: *Cope's Early Diagnosis of the Acute Abdomen,* 20th ed. Oxford Univ. Press, 2000.

Spates MJ, Schwartz, DT, Savitt D: Abdominal radiography. In Schwartz DT, Reisdorff EJ, eds. *Emergency Radiology.* McGraw-Hill, 2000.

West OC, Tamm EP, Kawshima A, Jarolimek AM: Abdomen: Non-traumatic emergencies. In Harris JH, Harris WH, eds. *The Radiology of Emergency Medicine,* 4th ed. Lippincott Williams and Wilkins, 2000.

Abdominal Radiography—Indications

Ahn SH, Mayo-Smith WW, Murphy BL, et al. Acute nontraumatic abdominal pain in adult patients: Abdominal radiography compared with CT evaluation. *Radiology* 2002;225:159–164.

Bohner H, Yang Q, Franke C, et al.: Simple data from history and physical examination help to exclude bowel obstruction and to avoid radiographic studies in patients with acute abdominal pain. *Eur J Surg* 1998;164:777–784. (A clinical decision rule for SBO.)

Eisenberg RL, Heineken P, Hedgcock MW, et al.: Evaluation of plain abdominal radiographs in the diagnosis of abdominal pain. *Ann Surg* 1983;197:464–469.

Flak B, Rowley VA: Acute abdomen: Plan film utilization and analysis. *Can Assoc Radiol J* 1993;44:423–428.

Mindelzun RE, Jeffrey RB: Unenhanced helical CT for evaluating acute abdominal pain: A little more cost, a lot more information. *Radiology* 1997;205:43–45. (Comment pp. 45–47.)

Abdominal Radiograph Interpretation

Cho KC, Baker SR: Extraluminal air: Diagnosis and significance. *Radiol Clin North Am* 1994;32:829–845.

Maglinte DDT: Nonspecific abdominal gas pattern: An interpretation whose time is gone. *Emerg Radiol* 1996;3:93–95.

Markus JB, Sommers S, Franic SE, et al.: Interobserver variation in the interpretation of abdominal radiographs. *Radiology* 1989;171:69–71. (Comment: *Radiology* 1989;173:283.)

Patel NH, Lauber PR: The meaning of a nonspecific abdominal gas pattern. *Acad Radiol* 1995;2:667–669.

Plewa MC: Emergency abdominal radiology. *Emerg Med Clin North Am* 1991;9:827–852.

Shaffer HA: Perforation and obstruction of the gastrointestinal tract: Assessment by conventional radiology. *Radiol Clin North Am* 1992;30:405–426.

Computed Tomography

Esses D, Birnbaum A, Bijur P, et al.: Ability of CT to alter decision making in elderly patients with acute abdominal pain. *Am J Emerg Med* 2004;22:270–272.

Gore RM, Miller FH, Pereles FS, et al.: Helical CT in the evaluation of the acute abdomen. *AJR* 2000;174:1041–1048.

Jacobs JE, ed. Acute conditions of the abdomen and pelvis. *Semin Roentgenol* 2001;36 (2)

Mindelzun RE, Jeffrey RB: Unenhanced helical CT for evaluating acute abdominal pain: A little more cost, a lot more information. *Radiology* 1997;205:43–45. (Comment pp. 45–47.)

Nagurney JT, Brown DFM, Chang Y, et al.: Use of diagnostic testing in the emergency department for patients presenting with non-traumatic abdominal pain. *J Emerg Med* 2003;25:363–371.

Novelline RA, Rhea JT, Rao PM, Stuk JL: Helical CT in emergency radiology. *Radiology* 1999;213:321–339.

Rosen MP, Sands DZ, Longmaid HE, et al.: Impact of abdominal CT on the management of patients presenting to the emergency department with acute abdominal pain. *AJR* 2000;174:1391–1396.

Rosen MP, Siewert B, Sands DZ, et al.: Value of abdominal CT in the emergency department for patients with abdominal pain. *Eur Radiol* 2003;13:418–424.

Urban BA, Fishman EK: Tailored helical CT evaluation of acute abdomen. *Radiographics* 2000;20:725–749.

Abdominal Radiology: Patient 1

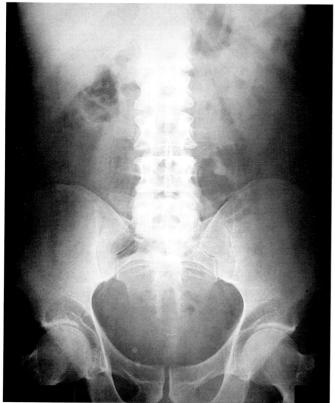

Supine view.

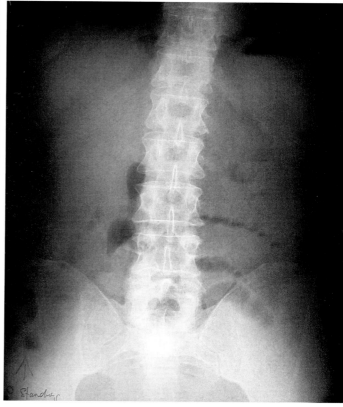

Upright view.

FIGURE 1

Periumbilical and left lower quadrant abdominal pain in a middle-aged man

A 50-year-old man complained of periumbilical and left lower quadrant abdominal pain that began earlier in the day. The pain was intermittent, "crampy" in character, and accompanied by anorexia and vomiting. He had a normal bowel movement the previous day. He had not experienced similar pain in the past. There was no history of prior abdominal surgery.

On examination, the patient was afebrile and in moderate distress due to his abdominal pain. Bowel sounds were present,

and the abdomen was mildly distended with periumbilical tenderness, but no rebound tenderness.

Abdominal radiographs (Figure 1) and chest radiographs were obtained.

The abdominal radiographs were interpreted as showing a "nonspecific bowel gas pattern."

- Do you agree with this interpretation?

STRING OF PEARLS

Although not immediately obvious, this patient's radiographs have findings suggestive of mechanical small bowel obstruction (SBO). Detection of SBO is the primary role for abdominal radiography in patients presenting to the ED with abdominal pain. However, radiographs are diagnostic of obstruction in only 50% of cases; in 30% of cases, they are suggestive, but not diagnostic; and in 20%, they are negative (Mucha 1987). Interpretation of bowel gas patterns can be difficult, and there is considerable interobserver variability, even among radiologists (Suh et al. 1995, Markus et al. 1989).

Clinical Features of Small Bowel Obstruction

There is a wide range of clinicial presentations of mechanical SBO. The **classical clinical presentation** includes intermittent, crampy, periumbilical abdominal pain accompanied by vomiting, and nonpassage of feces or flatus. On examination, the patient's abdomen is distended and tympanitic, and the bowel sounds are typically high-pitched and hyperactive. The abdomen may be mildly tender, but there should be no rigidity or rebound tenderness, unless the obstructed bowel is ischemic. Most patients have had prior abdominal surgery causing postoperative adhesions.

In patients with classical clinical presentations, the diagnosis is usually obvious on clinical examination. Radiographic studies serve mainly to confirm the clinical impression.

Many patients with SBO have **atypical clinical presentations.** Pain may be constant, mild, and even localized. Abdominal distention and vomiting may be minimal, and passage of feces and flatus may continue until bowel distal to the obstruction has evacuated its contents which can take 1–3 days or more. Muted clinical presentations are common in elderly and debilitated patients.

SBO should be considered as a cause of abdominal pain in all patients with prior abdominal surgery. However, obstruction can have etiologies other than postoperative adhesions (Table 1).

Management of Patients with SBO

Initial management of patients with SBO includes nasogastric suction to decompress the stomach, prevent further intestinal distention, and reduce the risk of aspiration. Intravenous fluids are administered to restore intravascular volume and electrolytes.

When **bowel ischemia** is suspected, **emergency surgery** is indicated. Some surgeons will operate when radiography shows complete/high-grade obstruction because of the increased risk for ischemia.

The rationale for the traditional aggressive surgical approach ("never let the sun rise or set on a bowel obstruction") is that clinical parameters are unreliable in excluding ischemia, and delay in operative intervention results in increased morbidity and mortality. However, current selective surgical management allows many patients with SBO to be managed without surgery. Nonetheless, morbidity and mortality are still substantially increased if there is delay in operating on patients with ischemic bowel obstruction (Fevang et al. 2003).

When there are no clinical signs of bowel ischemia, and no high risk factors such as an incarcerated hernia or closed-loop obstruction, most surgeons will attempt a **trial of nonoperative (conservative) care**. Surgery is performed if signs of ischemia develop or if the obstruction does not resolve over a period of time—usually 24–48 hours. If successful, a conservative approach avoids the short-term morbidity associated with laparotomy and the potential creation of additional adhesions (Cox et al. 1993, Serror et al. 1993, Fevang et al. 2002, Shih et al. 2003).

TABLE 1

Causes of SBO

Adhesions (postoperative):	50–80%
Hernias (external):	5–15%
Malignancy (peritoneal):	5–15%
Crohn disease:	up to 7%
Other:	10–20%
Bowel wall lesions (causing intussusception)	
Intraluminal mass: foreign body, gallstone ileus	
Extrinsic inflammatory lesions (appendiceal)	
Internal hernia	

Range of frequencies as found in several series (Miller et al. 2000, Evers 2001, Turnage and Berger 2002).

Ischemic Obstruction and Closed-Loop Obstruction

Bowel wall ischemia is the most dangerous complication of bowel obstruction, and is the principal indication for emergency surgery. There are **two mechanisms**: (1) marked bowel distention that impedes bowel wall perfusion and (2) mesenteric vascular compression that occurs with an incarcerated hernia or small bowel volvulus. Volvulus occurs when a loop of bowel twists around its mesentery. Small bowel **volvulus** is also called a "**closed-loop obstruction**" because a single loop of bowel is occluded at both ends (Figure 2).

The **spectrum** of bowel wall ischemia ranges from reversible ischemia that resolves when the obstruction is relieved, to irreversible ischemia and infarction that requires resection of the involved bowel segment. The **incidence** of ischemia in patients with SBO ranges from 8% to 38% (Miller et al. 2000, Shih et al. 2003, Fevag 2002).

Clinical signs of ischemia include pain that is *constant* (rather than intermittent), marked abdominal tenderness, rigidity or rebound tenderness, fever or leukocytosis, tachycardia, and signs of sepsis (Table 2). Small bowel **volvulus** typically causes an abrupt onset of abdominal pain.

The absence of these clinical signs, however, does not reliably exclude ischemia. Therefore, patients being managed nonsurgically must be observed closely. Patients at higher risk of ischemia are those with advanced high-grade obstruction (marked bowel distention on the abdominal radiograph), an incarcerated hernia, or a closed-loop obstruction.

Computed tomography (CT) can detect signs of bowel wall ischemia or closed-loop obstruction (Donecker 1998).

However, CT has only moderate sensitivity (70–96%) and specificity (60–95%) for bowel ischemia (Sheedy et al. 2006, Zalcman et al. 2000, Frager et al. 1996). Therefore, although helpful, CT should not be used alone to diagnose ischemic bowel obstruction; the decision to operate or to continue nonoperative care is based on the entire clinical scenario.

Diagnostic Imaging Principles of SBO

With SBO, both gas and fluid accumulate within bowel proximal to the obstruction, and bowel distal to the obstruction empties its contents. Distal small bowel becomes collapsed soon after the onset of obstruction, whereas the colon does not empty for 1–2 days or longer. The **principal diagnostic imaging finding** of SBO is, therefore, distention of small bowel proximal to the obstruction and collapse or a relative paucity of gas and fluid in bowel distal to the obstruction.

Bowel distention also occurs in **adynamic ileus**; however, with adynamic ileus, there is no disparity in distension between proximal and distal bowel. Adynamic ileus is caused by diminished gut motility due to a wide variety of abdominal and systemic disorders (see "Introduction to Abdominal Radiology," Table 6, page 144). With mild or localized ileus, only a portion of bowel is distended, whereas with severe adynamic ileus, the entire large and small bowel is distended. Diffuse bowel dilation also occurs with distal large bowel obstruction.

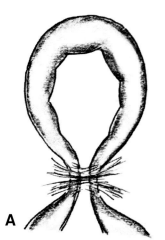
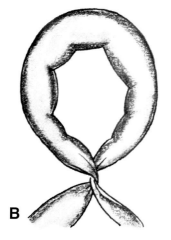

FIGURE 2   **Closed-loop SBO and volvulus.**
(*A*) Adhesive band causes obstruction.
(*B*) Small bowel volvulus closed-loop.
[From Balthazar et al. Closed-loop and strangulating intestinal obstruction: CT signs. *Radiology* 1992;185:769, with permission.]

TABLE 2

Ischemic Bowel Obstruction

Suspect when:

Pain is constant, not intermittent

Marked abdominal tenderness, rigidity, rebound tenderness

Fever or leukocytosis

Signs of sepsis

Small bowel markedly distended (on abdominal radiography)

Incarcerated hernia

Closed-loop obstruction (on CT)

CT signs of bowel wall ischemia

Abdominal radiography readily demonstrates bowel gas and is therefore useful for the diagnosis of bowel obstruction, when there is a considerable quantity of air within bowel proximal to the obstruction. Collapsed distal small bowel cannot be seen on abdominal radiography and the colon is therefore the portion of distal bowel that is observed to ascertain whether distal bowel is collapsed. However, the colon is often not totally devoid of gas and feces in patients with SBO because it can take two days or longer for large bowel to evacuate its contents.

When there is less disparity in caliber between small and large bowel, SBO has an appearance similar to adynamic ileus. In addition, when the obstructed small bowel is entirely fluid-filled, it is not visible on abdominal radiography. Abdominal radiography should therefore not be used to exclude the diagnosis of SBO.

Computed tomography can diagnose SBO when conventional radiography is not conclusive (50% of patients). On CT, collapsed distal small bowel can be directly visualized. In addition, CT can visualize dilated loops of bowel that are completely fluid-filled and are therefore not visible on conventional radiography. The sensitivity of CT for SBO is as high as 95% (Megibow et al. 1991).

CT can also determine the cause of obstruction (adhesions, tumors, hernias, etc.) and detect signs of bowel ischemia and closed-loop obstruction.

Diagnostic Imaging Strategy in Patients with Suspected SBO

Abdominal radiography is the traditional diagnostic test in patients with suspected SBO. However, abdominal radiography is diagnostic in only 50% of patients with SBO. Abdominal radiography is most likely to be diagnostic in patients with abdominal distention due to gas-filled bowel.

CT is indicated when abdominal radiography is nondiagnostic. In many hospitals, CT is also used whenever SBO is being managed nonoperatively to detect signs of bowel ischemia or a closed-loop obstruction that might not be evident clinically. CT is also indicated when the cause of obstruction is uncertain such as in patients who have not had prior abdominal surgery or in patients who have had both an intra-abdominal malignancy and prior abdominal surgery.

In EDs where CT is readily available, CT can be used as the initial imaging test. CT is more often diagnostic and can provide information about other disorders responsible for the patient's abdominal pain.

Abdominal radiography still has a role in the diagnosis of SBO, although its use should be limited to patients in whom the clinical presentation is classic—crampy abdominal pain and vomiting with gaseous distention of the abdomen, particularly in a patient who has had prior abdominal surgery. Abdominal radiography can be performed more quickly than CT and, when the diagnosis of SBO is confirmed, an earlier surgical consultation can be made. If CT will be ordered irrespective of the abdominal radiograph results or the clinical presentation is not classic for SBO, it is reasonable to omit abdominal radiography and proceed directly to CT, because abdominal radiography is unlikely to be diagnostic.

One precaution in the use of CT is that patients with SBO often cannot tolerate oral contrast due to vomiting, which could lead to substantial delays in obtaining CT. In these cases, oral contrast should be omitted because it is not essential to making the diagnosis of SBO on CT.

Radiographic Signs of Mechanical SBO

SUPINE ABDOMINAL RADIOGRAPH   On the supine abdominal radiographs, the principal diagnostic finding is dilated gas-filled, small bowel proximal to the obstruction and a relative paucity of air and feces in large bowel (Table 3). The presence of gas in the distal bowel (colon or rectum) does not negate the diagnosis of obstruction; it means simply that the distal bowel has not yet evacuated all of its contents.

Distended small bowel has a diameter greater than 3 cm. The valvulae conniventes make distinctive thin transverse bands extending completely across the bowel lumen (Figures 3 and 4). Numerous valvulae conniventes in distended small bowel can have a *"stack-of-coins"* appearance (Figure 5A). Valvulae conniventes are not present in the distal ileum, which, when distended, has a smooth tubular appearance.

UPRIGHT ABDOMINAL RADIOGRAPH   The upright radiograph can be helpful in confirming the diagnosis of SBO. Occasionally, SBO is more evident on the upright than the supine radiograph.

Fluid and gas within the bowel lumen create distinctive **air/fluid levels.** The upright radiograph is especially helpful when the obstructed bowel is mostly fluid-filled and signs of SBO are less evident on the supine view.

Air/fluid levels occur in both obstruction and adynamic ileus. However, the air/fluid levels associated with SBO have several distinguishing features. With SBO, the air/fluid levels at opposite ends of an inverted U-shaped loop of bowel are often at different heights. These are known as **differential (dynamic) air/fluid levels** (Figure 4B). This effect is presumably due to the action of peristalsis. Air/fluid levels are more specific for SBO when there is greater height differential (>15 mm) (Harlow et al. 1993, Lappas et al. 2001).

Multiple differential air/fluid levels have a **"step-ladder"** appearance. Broad air/fluid levels (**"tortoise-shell"** sign) are also characteristic of mechanical obstruction (Figure 3B). With **adynamic ileus;** air/fluid levels tend to be less prominent and, when present, are usually small and isolated.

One type of air/fluid level that is highly suggestive of obstruction is the **string-of-pearls** sign. Small pockets of air are trapped under the valvulae conniventes when the patient assumes an upright position. This appears as a row of small air bubbles on the radiograph (Figures 3B, 5B, 6, and 7). The string of pearls sign is especially helpful when the small bowel is nearly entirely fluid-filled, which makes bowel distention impossible to detect on the supine radiograph.

When the patient is too ill to stand upright, a left lateral decubitus view should be obtained to detect air/fluid levels (a cross-table AP view of the abdomen with the patient lying left-side down) (see Figure 9B on page 157). This view is also used to detect free intraperitoneal air (see Patient 3, Figure 8 on page 195).

Complete Versus Partial SBO

In traditional radiographic nomenclature, when there is a total absence of gas in large bowel and marked proximal bowel distention, obstruction is termed **"complete"** (Figure 3). When there is any gas in the colon or rectum, the obstruction is termed **"partial"** or **"early"** (Figure 4).

This terminology can be problematic because it does not distinguish between a "partial" obstruction, in which there is a great disparity in caliber between proximal small bowel and colon, i.e., the radiographs are definitely diagnostic of SBO (Figure 4), and a "partial" obstruction in which there is little

---

TABLE 3

Radiographic Signs of SBO

Supine view

    Distended small bowel (>3 cm)
      ("stack-of-coins")

    Relative paucity of air and feces in colon

Upright view

    Differential air/fluid levels ("step-ladder")

    Broad air/fluid levels ("tortoise-shell")

    "String-of-pearls" sign

disparity in bowel distention, i.e., the radiographs are merely "suggestive" of or "equivocal" for SBO (Figure 8). In addition, the terminology is potentially confusing because a radiographically "partial obstruction" can be physiologically complete (i.e., no bowel contents can pass the point of obstruction) or advanced (if proximal bowel is markedly distended), when the distal bowel has simply not emptied all of its contents, i.e., an "early" SBO. The term "partial" or "early" SBO could create an erroneous impression that the obstruction is mild or the diagnosis is questionable.

Rather than categorize the radiographic findings of SBO as "partial (early)" or "complete," an interpretation can be based on diagnostic certainty (Harlow et al. 1993). "**Definite SBO**" or "**probable SBO**" is reported when there is marked distention in proximal small bowel and little or no gas or feces in the colon (Figures 3–5). "**Possible SBO**" is reported when there is more gas in the colon and less distention in proximal small bowel such that SBO is questionable and further testing with CT is needed (Figure 8). Finally, radiographs can be negative for signs of SBO even though obstruction is present (Figure 9).

Limitations of Abdominal Radiography for SBO

There are several reasons that abdominal radiographs may be nondiagnostic in patients with small bowel obstruction (Table 4). These are: (1) partial or early obstruction with less disparity in distention between small and large bowel makes differentiation from adynamic ileus difficult (Figure 8); (2) obstructed bowel is filled with fluid and therefore not visible on the radiographs (Figure 9); and (3) proximal small bowel obstruction such that only a short segment of bowel becomes dilated. When obstructed bowel is entirely filled with fluid, the abdomen may appear relatively *gasless*, i.e., radiographs are normal or negative for signs of SBO. Therefore, negative, nonspecific, and mild ileus patterns do not exclude bowel obstruction.

The **specificity of abdominal radiography** is limited, particularly when there is a partial or "early" obstruction—because adynamic ileus has a similar radiographic picture (Figure 10). In addition, acute mesenteric ischemia can produce a "pseudo SBO" pattern in which a segment of small bowel is ischemic and therefore dilated and there is a disparity in distention between small bowel (the ischemic segment) and large bowel.

Finally, undue **equivocation in the radiologist's report** can also be a source of misdiagnosis. When gas is present in large bowel, the obstruction may be termed "partial" or "early." However, this does not adequately differentiate high-grade partial obstruction that has relatively definitive radiographic findings from partial obstruction in which the radiographs are equivocal. Even when there is great disparity in caliber between proximal and distal bowel, the radiograph might still be reported as "possible partial or early obstruction versus ileus," even though the diagnosis of obstruction is likely and the obstruction is more advanced. Because radiologist's reports of bowel gas patterns often are equivocal, the clinician should review the radiographic images themselves rather than rely solely on the radiologist's report (Figure 11).

TABLE 4

**Reasons for Nondiagnostic Radiographs
      in Patients with SBO**

Partial or early SBO

Fluid-filled bowel

Proximal obstruction

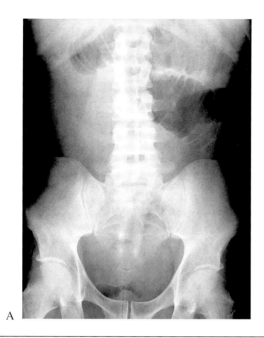
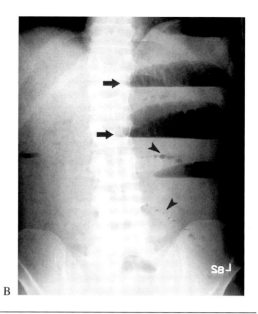

FIGURE 3   Complete small bowel obstruction.

(*A*) There is marked distention of small bowel and nearly complete absence of air in distal bowel (a small amount of air remains in the rectum).

(*B*) The upright radiograph shows characteristic broad air/fluid levels ("tortoise-shell" sign) (*arrows*) and a "string-of-pearls" (*arrowheads*).

  The patient had adhesions due to a prior laparotomy for a stab wound to the abdomen. Because of the marked bowel distention, surgery was performed shortly after admission for lysis of adhesions.

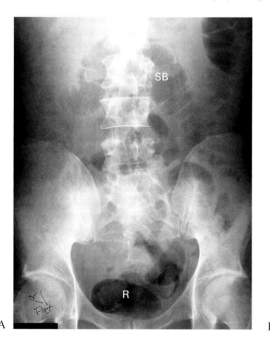
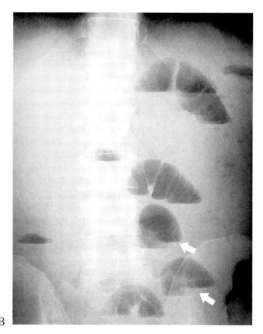
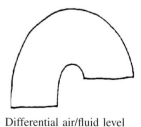

Differential air/fluid level

FIGURE 4   "Partial," although definite, SBO and differential air/fluid levels.

(*A*) On the supine radiograph, there are dilated loops of small bowel (SB) and a relative paucity of air in the colon. Air in the rectum (R) does not negate the diagnosis of bowel obstruction, but indicates only that the distal colon has not yet expelled all of its contents. This radiographic pattern may be referred to as a "partial" small bowel obstruction even though it is advanced and is "definite" for the diagnosis of SBO.

(*B*) The upright radiograph shows *differential (dynamic) air/ fluid levels*— air/fluid levels that are at different heights in a single

loop of bowel (*arrows*). Differential air/fluid levels are suggestive of mechanical obstruction. Simple (nondifferential) air/fluid levels are seen in both mechanical obstruction and adynamic ileus (see "Introduction to Abdominal Radiography," Figure 3B on page 142).

This patient developed SBO two weeks after a laparotomy performed for lysis of adhesions due to a prior stab wound to the abdomen. This early postoperative bowel obstruction was successfully managed using nasogastric decompression.

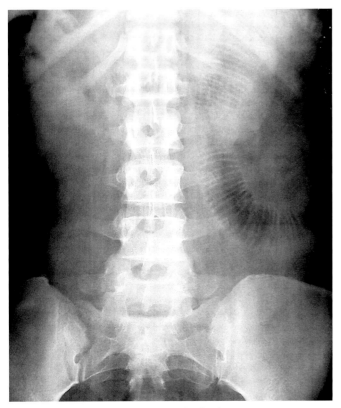

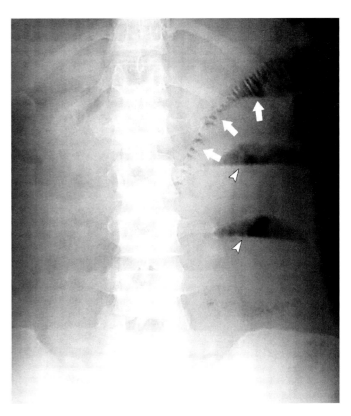

A. Dilated loop of small bowel–Stack of coin

B. Upright view—Genesis of the "string of pearls" sign

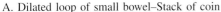

FIGURE 5   "Stack-of-coins" and "string of pearls" signs.

(*A*) On the supine radiograph, a single distended loop of dilated small bowel has numerous valvulae conniventes extending across the bowel lumen, giving it a "stack-of-coins" appearance.

(*B*) The upright radiograph illustrates the genesis of the "string-of-pearls" sign". There is a row of small air pockets representing gas that had become trapped under valvulae conniventes when the patient assumed an upright position (*arrows*). In addition, there are two broad air/fluid levels, which are also characteristic of mechanical small bowel obstruction (*arrowheads*).

This patient presented with periumbilical abdominal pain and vomiting and had not had prior abdominal surgery. After abdominal radiography, she was reexamined and a small incarcerated umbilical hernia was found (*C*). The hernia was reduced in the ED and the patient was hospitalized for urgent, rather than emergent, hernia repair.

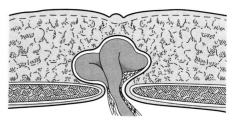

C   Incarcerated umbilical hernia.

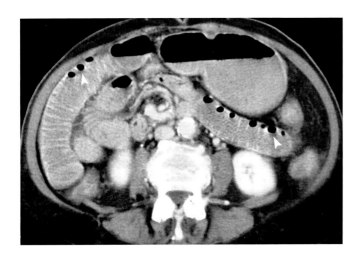

FIGURE 6   "String-of-pearls" sign depicted on CT.

In another patient with SBO, the abdominal radiographs were negative because the bowel was nearly entirely filled with fluid. On CT, obstructed small bowel is markedly dilated and fluid-filled. There are several small pockets of air trapped under valvulae conniventes producing a CT "string-of-pearls" sign (*arrowheads*).

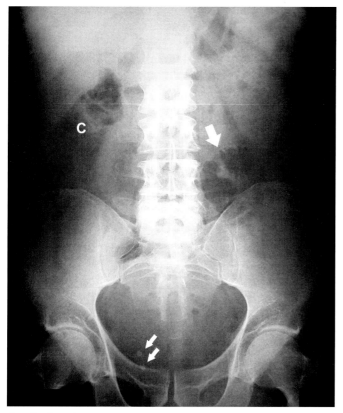

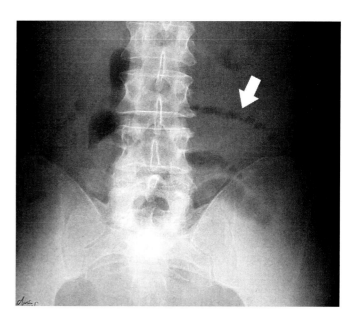

A.   Supine view   B.   Upright view

FIGURE 7   Patient 1

(A) This patient's supine radiograph showed a single loop of dilated small bowel in the mid-abdomen (*large arrow*) and air in the colon (C). Although this dilated small bowel loop is abnormal, SBO cannot be diagnosed on the supine view because there is no clear disparity in distention between proximal and distal bowel. The single dilated loop of small bowel could be interpreted as a localized or mild ileus.

Most of the obstructed small bowel was not visible on the radiograph because it wasfilled with fluid. Gas in large bowel was *not* relatively diminished compared to small bowel because the obstruction developed rapidly and the colon did not have time to empty its contents.

Incidentally, two small pheleboliths are seen in the pelvis (*small arrows*).

(B) The upright radiograph is suggestive of obstruction. Most of the bowel is fluid-filled, so there are few air/fluid levels. However, there is a **string-of-pearls sign,** which is indicative of mechanical small bowel obstruction (*arrow*).

Patient Outcome

After the abdominal radiographs were reviewed, the patient was carefully reexamined and a small left inguinal hernia was found. The hernia could not be reduced in the ED. An incarcerated (irreducible) hernia requires emergency surgery when it is causing bowel obstruction or ischemia (strangulation).

The patient was taken to the operating room for reduction and repair of the incarcerated hernia.

In all patients with abdominal pain, a careful search should be made for hernias, even if the patient is not complaining of localized pain or swelling.

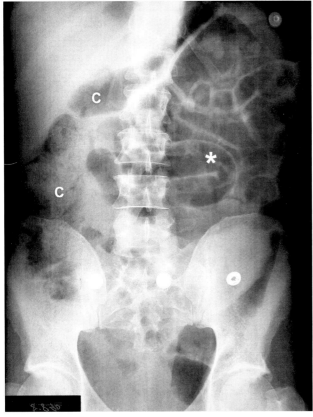

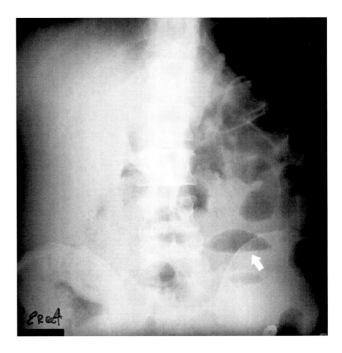

A. Supine radiograph. There is gaseous distention of small bowel and considerable gas and feces in large bowel. Small bowel is centrally located. One distended loop of ileum has a "bent finger" appearance (*). The colon (C) is peripheral and contains feces .

B. Upright radiograph. A few nondifferential air/fluid levels are present. One broad air/fluid level is seen in the left lower quadrant—the "tortoise-shell" sign (*arrow*).

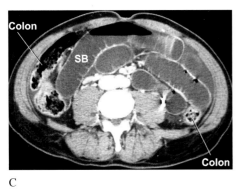

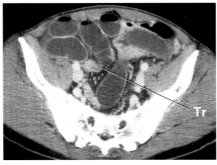

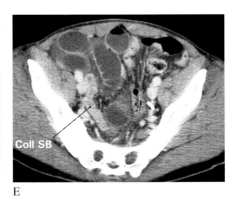

C   D   E

(C) Small bowel is markedly distended and mostly fluid-filled **(SB).** The small bowel wall is normal — thin and uniformly enhancing with visible valvulae conniventes. Large bowel is not distended but contains air and feces **(Colon),** which is why the abdominal radiographs were not diagnostic of obstruction.

The obstruction could be termed "partial" even though it is a "high-grade" obstruction with markedly distended small bowel proximal to

the obstruction. Oral contrast was administered, but it did not reach the obstructed small bowel. Enteric contrast is not necessary to visualize distended bowel containing fluid or air.

(D) The distended bowel tapers to the transition point **(Tr).** There is no lesion at the transition point, implying that postoperative adhesions are the cause of obstruction.

(E) Distal small bowel is collapsed (Coll SB).

FIGURE 8   Small bowel obstruction with suggestive but not diagnostic radiographs.

A 45-year-old man presented with abdominal pain, vomiting, and abdominal distention. Two years earlier, he had undergone laparotomy following a stab wound to the abdomen.

The initial radiographs were suggestive but not diagnostic of obstruction. Adynamic ileus can have a similar radiographic appearance. An abdominal CT obtained several hours later revealed a high-grade mechanical SBO. The patient was treated with laparotomy for lysis of adhesions.

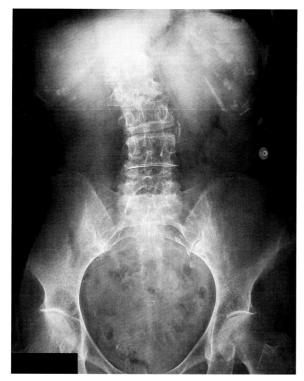

(A) Supine radiograph is "negative," i.e., no signs of obstruction. The abdomen is nearly entirely gasless.

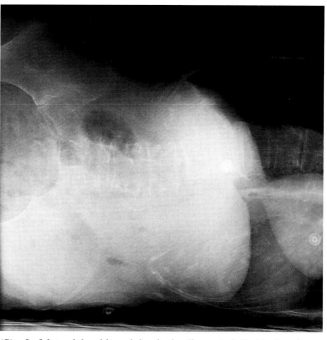

(B) Left lateral decubitus abdominal radiograph (left-side down) was obtained because the patient was too weak to stand upright.
There is a single dilated loop of bowel with an isolated air/fluid level.

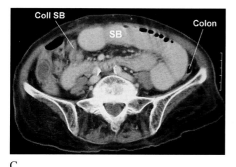

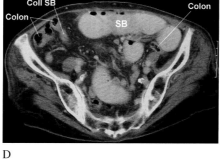

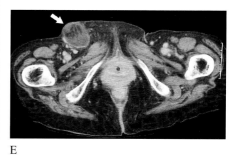

C   D   E

(C and D) CT slices through the lower abdomen at the level of the iliac crests. There is markedly dilated small bowel (SB). The obstructed small bowel is nearly entirely fluid-filled, which accounts for the negative (gasless) abdominal radiograph. Oral contrast is present in the obstructed small bowel. There is collapsed small bowel (Coll SB) in the right lower quadrant. The colon is also collapsed (Colon).

(E) CT slice of the lower pelvis reveals a large femoral hernia (arrow), which was the cause of the patient's obstruction.

(F) A femoral hernia follows the course of the femoral artery and vein into the anterior thigh inferior to the inguinal ligament.

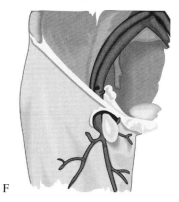

F

FIGURE 9   Small bowel obstruction with negative radiographs.

An 84-year-old woman presented with abdominal pain. Abdominal radiographs were "negative." A CT of the abdomen revealed distal SBO.

CT slices through the lower pelvis demonstrated that the cause of obstruction was an incarcerated femoral hernia (E). The large incarcerated femoral hernia was not noted initially due to an incomplete physical examination.

A nearly gasless abdomen can be seen in patients with high-grade obstruction when the obstructed bowel is entirely fluid-filled.

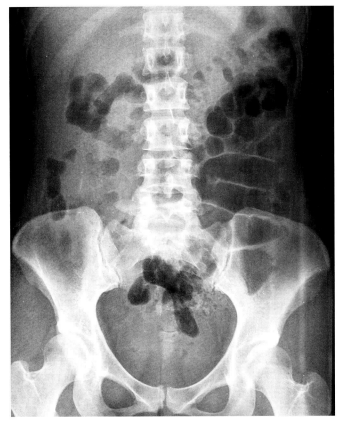

A

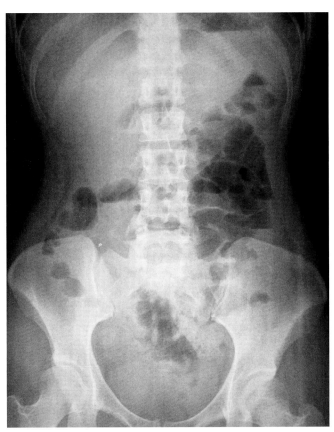

B

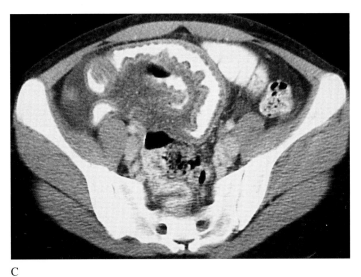

C

FIGURE 10   Radiographs suggestive of obstruction but not due to obstruction.

A 25-year-old woman presented with lower abdominal pain and nausea.

The abdominal radiographs were "suggestive" of partial SBO. The supine radiograph shows moderately dilated small bowel and a relative paucity of air in the colon. The upright radiograph shows several non-differential air/fluid levels.

An abdominal CT revealed markedly thickened bowel wall of the distal small bowel, including the terminal ileum, consistent with Crohn disease. There was no bowel obstruction; bowel dilation was due to adynamic ileus.

Radiographs that are "suggestive" of obstruction (especially partial SBO) should not be considered diagnostic of obstruction. Clinical correlation and further diagnostic testing, i.e., CT, is necessary. (See Introduction to Abdominal Radiology, Figure 3 on page 142 —radiographs in a patient with appendicitis showing "early SBO versus localized ileus.")

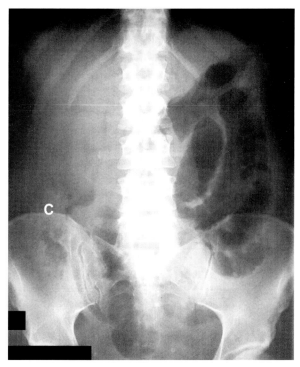

A. Supine view

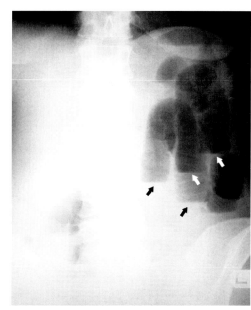

B. Upright view

Radiologist's Report

LOCALIZED SEGMENT OF SMALL BOWEL FILLED WITH AIR WITH DIFFERENTIAL
AIR FLUID LEVELS. AIR IS ALSO SEEN IN THE DISTAL LARGE BOWEL.
FINDINGS CONSISTENT WITH LOCALIZED ILEUS VERSUS EARLY SBO. NO FREE
AIR. MULTIPLE PELVIC CALCIFICATIONS SEEN.

IMPRESSION: LOCALIZED SMALL BOWEL ILEUS VERSUS EARLY SBO. F/U AXR
ADVISED FOR CORRELATION AS INDICATED.

FIGURE 11   Delayed diagnosis of bowel obstruction due to an unduly equivocal radiologist's report.

A 42-year-old woman presented to the ED with upper abdominal pain and vomiting. She had a uterine myomectomy four months earlier.

The radiographic findings were correctly noted in the **radiologist's report**, although the "impression" understates their significance. With gas in the colon, obstruction is traditionally called "partial" or "early." These terms do not, however, distinguish between "definite" obstruction (present in this patient, despite the gas in the colon) and "possible" obstruction, which cannot be differentiated from adynamic ileus. This ambiguity contributed to the delay in diagnosis.

After the radiologist's interpretation was reviewed, an ultrasound of the right upper quadrant was ordered because the patient had tenderness in that location. The sonogram revealed gallstones without definite signs of cholecystitis. On the advice of a surgical consultant, a HIDA (hepatobiliary) scan was obtained to determine whether the gallstones were responsible for the patient's abdominal pain. The scan was normal.

After that, the patient had an **abdominal CT** scan which revealed SBO (*C*). Twenty hours after her arrival, the patient was taken to surgery. Bowel obstruction with mural ischemia was found and treated with lysis of adhesions. Bowel resection was not necessary.

Review of the **initial radiographs** (*A* and *B*) reveals that they were, in fact, diagnostic of obstruction. Small bowel was markedly dilated and only a small amount of air and feces were in the cecum

(C in Figure 11A). There were several *differential* air/fluid levels on the upright radiograph (*arrows* in Figure 11B).

Because written reports of bowel gas patterns are often vague, it is important for the clinician to examine the radiographs, rather than rely solely on the radiologist's report.

Had cholecystitis been a plausible concern, CT would have been a better test than HIDA scan because CT has good sensitivity for cholecystitis (>90%), can detect other abdominal disorders, and can be performed more quickly. However, had the radiologist's report been less equivocal, the diagnosis of SBO would have been made earlier.

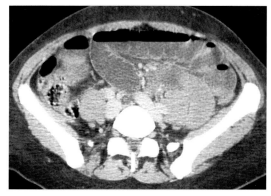

C. CT showed mechanical bowel obstruction with markedly dilated small bowel.

CT Diagnosis of SBO

CT scanning is a major advance in diagnostic imaging for bowel obstruction. In addition to being more sensitive and specific than radiography, CT can determine the cause of obstruction in 75–90% of cases, and can detect signs of bowel ischemia and closed-loop obstruction (Table 5) (Megebow 1991, Balthazar 1994, Maglinte 1997, Macari 2001).

The **CT diagnosis of SBO** is based upon seeing: (1) dilated small bowel proximal to the obstruction, (2) collapsed *small bowel* distal to the obstruction, and (3) a transition zone (Table 6, Figures 8 and 9). A transition zone without a lesion or mass implies that the obstruction is due to an adhesion (Figure 8). With an adhesion, the obstructed small bowel may taper at the transition zone and have a "bird's beak" appearance. Large bowel is usually not totally collapsed and devoid of gas and feces (Figure 8).

The principal **advantages of CT** over abdominal radiography are (1) that the diagnosis of SBO does not depend on collapse of the colon (collapsed distal small bowel is directly visualized), and (2) CT can detect dilated fluid-filled small bowel that is not visible on radiography (Figure 9).

A secondary sign of SBO is the **small bowel feces sign** (Figure 12). Enteric contents within obstructed bowel undergo digestion and develop feces-like air stippling. This sign is suggestive, although not entirely specific, for obstruction. In addition, it can help locate the transition zone because it usually occurs in the distal portion of obstructed small bowel (Mayo-Smith et al. 1995).

Intravenous contrast causing bowel wall enhancement is needed to detect bowel wall thickening, which is a sign of ischemia, as well as other bowel wall and solid organ lesions. **Oral contrast** is not essential to diagnose SBO because distended bowel containing fluid and air can be visualized without intraluminal contrast (Figure 8) (Macari and Megibow 2001). Oral contrast is often not tolerated by patients who are vomiting due to SBO, and the oral contrast may not reach the lumen of the obstructed bowel. However, when the obstruction is less severe and the patient is able to tolerate oral contrast, enteric contrast provides a more comprehensive CT examination and better evaluation of other abdominal conditions that could be responsible for the patient's pain. Some authors recommend administration of oral contrast whenever possible because passage of contrast into the colon is a sign that obstruction is not complete and that nonoperative care is more likely to be successful (Frager 2002).

CT is indicated in patients with suspected SBO whenever abdominal radiography is nondiagnostic (50% of cases). CT can confirm the diagnosis of SBO more reliably than abdominal radiography and, when obstruction is not found, it can often detect other disorders responsible for the patient's symptoms (Figure 10). CT is also useful when nonoperative management of SBO is being considered because it can detect signs of ischemia and closed-loop obstruction that mandate surgery (Donecker 1998).

CT can frequently **identify the lesion causing obstruction.** This is particularly important when a lesion other than an adhesion is found, which may require specific treatment, such as a tumor, abscess, or hernia (Figures 9 and 13). CT is therefore especially useful in patients with SBO who have not had prior abdominal surgery because etiologies other than adhesions are likely. Even when urgent surgery is planned, many surgeons obtain a preoperative CT if it does not delay operative intervention in order to delineate intra-abdominal pathology prior to laparotomy.

TABLE 5

Role of CT in SBO Diagnosis

Confirm obstruction—sensitivity up to 95%

Cause of obstruction—adhesions, hernia, tumor

Closed-loop obstruction

Bowel ischemia—sensitivity 70–96%

TABLE 6

CT Signs of SBO

Dilated proximal small bowel (> 2.5 cm diameter)

Collapsed distal small bowel

Transition zone

Obstructing lesion (adhesions presumed if no lesion seen)

Small bowel feces sign

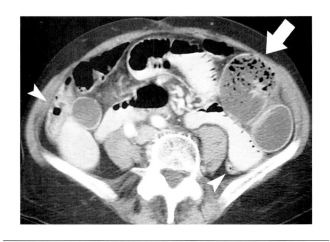

FIGURE 12   Small bowel feces sign.
Feculent enteric contents in obstructed small bowel (*arrow*).
Arrowheads—collapsed ascending and descending colon.

The reported **sensitivity of CT** for SBO varies among published studies, although differences in patient selection account for much of this variation. CT is most useful in patients with acute onset of symptoms, i.e., those most likely to be seen in the ED. Sensitivity and specificity in such patients is as high as 90–100% (Megibow et al. 1991, Fukuya et al. 1992, Frager et al. 1994, 1995, Gazelle et al. 1994). Other investigators found considerably lower sensitivity (64%) and specificity (80%) (Maglinte et al. 1993 and 1996). However, all of their patients had been referred for *enteroclysis* and are therefore not representative of patients with SBO seen in the ED. Sensitivity was especially low (50%) in patients with low-grade partial obstruction (as defined by enteroclysis). (CT sensitivity was 83% in patients with high-grade obstruction). Despite its limitations, this study does demonstrate that CT can miss the diagnosis of low-grade partial SBO.

CT's accuracy has likely been improved with the advent of helical CT and particularly, **multidetector CT** (Caoili and Paulson 2000, Furukawa et al. 2001, Boudiaf et al. 2001, Khurana et al. 2002, Taourel et al. 2002). Reformatted images in the coronal or sagittal planes further improve CT's capabilities by, for example, helping to identify a transition zone that does not lie in the axial plane (Jaffe et al. 2006).

Macari and Megibow (2001) proposed an approach for examining CT scans in patients with suspected SBO. First, the colon is followed on sequential images from the rectum and sigmoid colon proximally to the cecum looking for lesions that could be causing obstruction. Identification of the entire colon also allows the reader to confidently distinguish small bowel from colon on the CT images. Next, the terminal ileum is identified near the ileocecal valve. If the terminal ileum is dilated, SBO is excluded. If the terminal ileum is collapsed, the remaining small bowel is examined to identify dilated and collapsed segments of bowel and a transition zone.

CT Signs of Ischemic Obstruction and Closed-Loop Obstruction

CT signs of **bowel ischemia** include bowel wall thickening, bowel wall edema (target sign), congestion of mesenteric fat due to edema and hemorrhage (increased attenuation), and hemorrhagic ascites (Table 7 Figure 14). Absence of bowel wall enhancement and intramural gas are signs of **infarction.**

Detecting ischemia is one of CT's most important roles in patients with SBO because ischemic bowel mandates surgical treatment and clinical signs of ischemia are not always present (Table 2) (Donecker 1998). However, CT has limited sensitivity for detecting bowel ischemia, ranging from 70% to 96% (the latter using helical CT) (Balthazar et al. 1997, Zalcman et al. 2000). Therefore, despite a negative CT, when there is clinical suspicion of ischemia, the patient should undergo laparotomy.

A **closed-loop obstruction** is at high risk of ischemia due to the potential for mesenteric vascular occlusion at the neck of the obstruction (Figure 15) (Balthazar et al. 1992, Batlhazar 1994). **CT signs** of closed-loop obstruction include: (1) a cluster of dilated fluid-filled loops of bowel arranged in a radial distribution; (2) mesenteric vessels converging to a central point, ("*spoke wheel sign*"); (3) a C-shaped loop of dilated bowel; (4) two adjacent collapsed, triangular-shaped loops of bowel; and (5) the "whirl sign"—twisted mesenteric vessels at point of volvulus (Table 7, Figures 15 to 18). Because of the increased risk of ischemia, surgery is indicated even when there are no CT signs of bowel wall ischemia.

An **internal hernia** (herniation of bowel through a defect in the mesentery) has a similar CT appearance and risk of ischemia as a closed-loop obstruction. Defects in the mesentery are either congenital (paraduodenal is most common) or postsurgical in origin (Takeyama et al. 2005, Blanchar 2001).

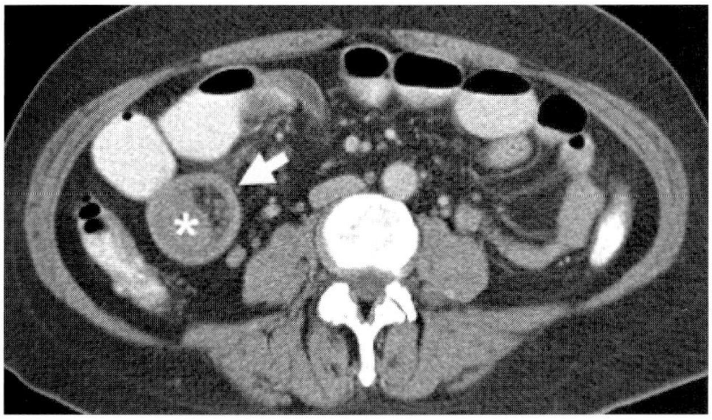

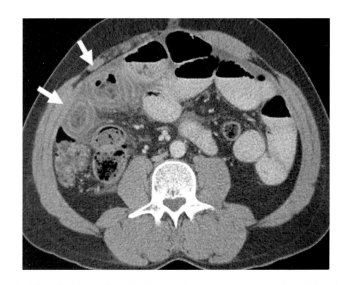

FIGURE 13   Ileoileal intussusception causing SBO.
A pedunculated ileal polyp was the lead point for intussusception causing SBO. A segment of ileum, the intussusceptum (*asterisk*), along with mesenteric fat and vessels were pulled into an outer segment of bowel, the intussuscipiens (*arrow*).

FIGURE 14   Ischemic SBO—Target sign.
Adhesive SBO with bowel wall thickening. At laparotomy, the bowel was ischemic but salvageable following relief of obstruction. Other disorders that can cause a target sign include infectious enteritis, inflammatory bowel disease and acute mesenteric ischemia.

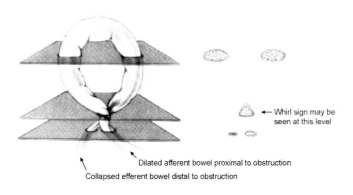

FIGURE 15   CT signs of closed-loop obstruction.

Upper slice shows two or more adjacent dilated loops of bowel. At the level of twisting, compressed triangular-shaped bowel is seen. A "whirl" sign may be present at this level.

When the closed-loop is in the same plane as the CT slice, a C-shaped loop of bowel is seen (Figure 16).

[From: Balthazar, et al: Closed-loop and strangulating intestinal obstruction: CT signs. *Radiology* 1992;185:770.]

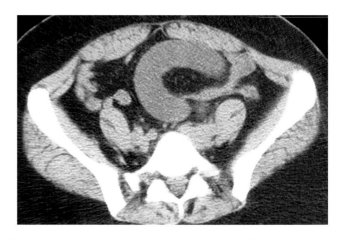

FIGURE 16   Closed-loop obstruction.

A C-shaped loop of obstructed bowel lies in the plane of the CT slice. (Non-contrast CT was done in a patient with abrupt onset lower abdominal pain for suspected renal colic).

TABLE 7

CT Signs of Ischemic and Closed-Loop Obstruction

Ischemic Obstruction

  Bowel wall thickening, "target sign," increased enhancement

  Mesenteric congestion—edema, hemorrhage

  Ascites—bloody

  Infarcted bowel—poorly enhancing, paper-thin bowel wall; intramural gas

Closed-loop obstruction

  Dilated loops of bowel in a cluster or radial distribution

  Mesenteric vessels converging to a central point—"Spoke-wheel" sign

  C-shaped or U-shaped loop of dilated bowel

  Two adjacent collapsed, triangular-shaped loops of bowel

  Whirl sign—twisted mesenteric vessels at point of volvulus

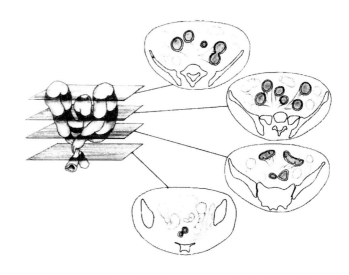

FIGURE 17   CT depiction of closed-loop obstruction.

A cluster of distended loops of bowel arranged in a radial distribution. The mesentery radiates from the central point of the volvulus. This forms the "spoke-wheel" sign.

[From: Balthazar EJ: CT of small bowel obstruction. *AJR* 1994;162: 258 with permission.]

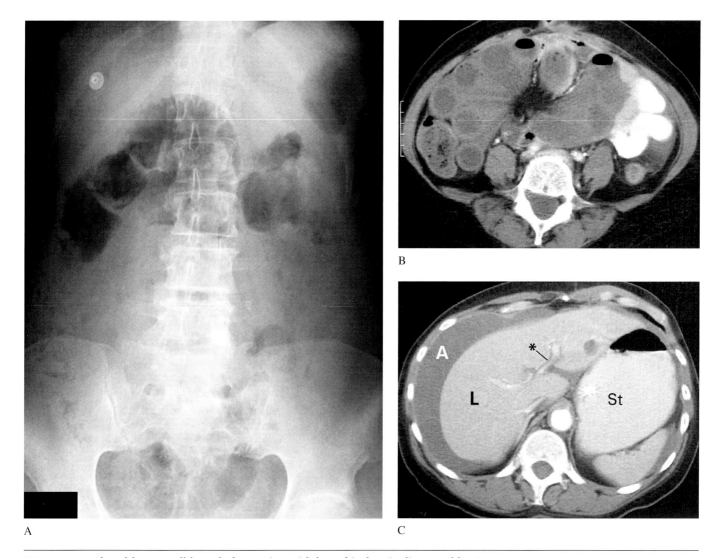

A

B

C

FIGURE 18   Closed-loop small bowel obstruction with bowel ischemia diagnosed by CT.

A 64-year-old woman presented with abrupt onset of mid-abdominal pain. Initially, her abdomen was soft and mildly tender, and her pain seemed out of proportion to the abdominal tenderness. The abdominal radiographs and blood tests were "negative" (WBC count 8,400 cells/mm^3)

(*A*) Abdominal radiography showed a considerable amount of air in the transverse colon and practically no gas in small bowel. This finding would seem to go against SBO because it is opposite the expected pattern of small bowel dilation and large bowel collapse.

After two hours of observation in the emergency department, the patient's abdomen was distended and increasingly tender.

(*B*) A CT of the abdomen revealed a closed-loop small bowel obstruction. A cluster of dilated fluid-filled small bowel loops was arranged in a radial distribution, the "**spoke wheel sign**." The congested edematous mesentery radiated from the point of volvulus. The bowel wall was thickened, indicative of ischemia.

(*C*) A second CT slice showed ascites (**A**) surrounding the liver (**L**), also a sign of bowel ischemia. The ascites extended along the portal vein (*). A radiopaque nasogastric tube was in the dilated fluid and contrast-filled stomach (**St**).

At surgery, an **internal hernia** was found and was reduced. Blood flow to the bowel returned, and there was no need for bowel resection. Bloody ascites was present.

An **abdominal radiographic finding** associated with closed-loop obstruction is the *"pseudo-tumor sign."* The fluid-filled obstructed bowel appears like a soft-tissue mass displacing adjacent abdominal organs (Balthazar et al. 1992). This is rarely seen.

The gasless mid abdomen on this radiograph (A) may represent a pseudo-tumor sign (fluid-filled loops of dilated bowel), although this finding would be impossible to identify without knowing the CT results. Gas in the colon is often seen in closed-loop obstruction because the onset of obstruction is rapid and gut motility is diminished due to the severity of pain.

SUGGESTED READING

SBO

Baker SR, Cho KC: *The Abdominal Plain Film,* 2nd ed. McGraw-Hill, 1999.

Evers BM: Small bowel. In Townsend et al., eds. *Sabiston's Textbook of Surgery,* 16th ed. Saunders, 2001 : 882–887.

Frimann-Dahl J: *Roentgen Examination in Acute Abdominal Diseases,* 3rd ed. CC Thomas, 1974.

McCort JJ, Mindelzun RE, Filpi RG, Rennell C: *Abdominal Radiology.* Williams & Wilkins, 1981.

Spates MJ, Schwartz, DT, Savitt D: Abdominal imaging. In Schwartz DT, Reisdorff EJ, eds. *Emergency Radiology.* McGraw-Hill, 2000.

Torrey SP, Henneman PL: Small intestine. In Marx J et al., eds. *Rosen's Emergency Medicine: Concepts and Clinical Practice,* 5th ed. Mosby 2002 :1284–1287.

Turnage RH, Bergen PC: Intestinal obstruction and ileus. In Feldman et al., eds. *Sleisenger & Fordtran's Gastrointestinal and Liver Disease,* 7th ed. Elsevier, 2002 : 2113– 2127.

Clinical Series and Management

Bohner H, Yang Q, Franke C, et al.: Simple data from history and physical examination help to exclude bowel obstruction and to avoid radiographic studies in patients with acute abdominal pain. *Eur J Surg* 1998;164:777–784. (A clinical decision rule for SBO.)

Brolin RE, Krasna MJ, Mast BA: Use of tubes and radiographs in the management of small bowel obstruction. *Ann Surg* 1987;206: 126–133.

Cox MR, Gunn IF, Eastman MC, et al.: The operative aetiology and types of adhesions causing small bowel obstruction. *Aust N Z J Surg* 1993;63:848–852.

Cox MR, Gunn IF, Eastman MC, et al.: The safety and duration of non-operative treatment for adhesive small bowel obstruction. *Aust N Z J Surg* 1993;63:367–371.

Fevang BT, Fevang JM, Soreide O, et al.: Delay in operative treatment among patients with small bowel obstruction. *Scand J Surg* 2003;92:131–137.

Fevang BT, Jensen D, Svanes K, Viste A: Early operation or conservative management of patients with small bowel obstruction? *Eur J Surg* 2002;168:475–481.

Kingsnorth A, LeBlanc K: Hernias: Inguinal and incisional. *Lancet* 2003;362:1561–1571.

Miller G, Boman J, Shrier I, et al.: Etiology of small bowel obstruction. *Am J Surg* 2000;180:33–36.

Miller G, Boman J, Shrier I, et al.: Natural history of patients with adhesive small bowel obstruction. *Br J Surg* 2000;87:1240–1247.

Mucha P: Small intestinal obstruction. *Surg Clin North Am* 1987;67:597–620.

Perrott CA: Inguinal hernias: Room for a better understanding. *Am J Emerg Med* 2004; 22: 48–50.

Serror D, Feigin E, Szold A, et al.: How conservatively can postoperative small bowel obstruction be treated? *Am J Surg* 1993;165: 121–126.

Shih SC, Jeng KS, Lin SC, et al.: Adhesive small bowel obstruction: How long can patients tolerate conservative treatment? *World J Gastroenterol* 2003;9:603–605.

Diagnostic Imaging Strategy

Frager D: Intestinal obstruction: Role of CT. *Gastroenterol Clin North Am* 2002;31:777–799.

Kahi CJ, Rex DK: Bowel obstruction and pseudo-obstruction. *Gastroenterol Clin North Am* 2003;32:1229–1247.

Macari M, Megibow A: Imaging of suspected acute small bowel obstruction. *Semin Roentgenol* 2001;36:108–117.

Maglinte DD, Heitkamp DE, Howard TJ, et al.: Current concepts in imaging of small bowel obstruction. *Radiol Clin North Am* 2003;41:263–283.

Maglinte DDT, Balthazar EJ, Kelvin FM, Megibow AJ: The role of radiology in the diagnosis of small-bowel obstruction. *AJR* 1997;168:1171–1180.

Taourel P, Kessler N, Lesnik A, et al.: Imaging of acute intestinal obstruction. *Eur Radiol* 2002;12:2151–2160.

Abdominal Radiography

Flak B, Rowley VA: Acute abdomen: Plain film utilization and analysis. *Can Assoc Radiol J* 1993;44:423–428.

Green J. Ryan J, Baro O: Characteristics of ED patients with CT-proven small bowel obstruction and discordant negative plain abdominal radiography. Acad Emerg Med 2007 14 (5 Supplement 1): S38.

Harlow CL, Stears RLG, Zeligman BE, Archer PG: Diagnosis of bowel obstruction on plain abdominal radiographs: Significance of air-fluid levels at different heights in the same loop of bowel. *AJR* 1993;161:291–295.

Lappas JC, Reyes BL, Maglinte DDT: Abdominal radiography findings in small-bowel obstruction: Relevance to triage for additional diagnostic imaging. *AJR* 2001;176:167–174.

Maglinte DDT, Reyes BL, Harmon BH, et al.: Reliability and role of plain film radiography and CT in the diagnosis of small-bowel obstruction. *AJR* 1996;167:1451–1455.

Markus JB, Sommers S, Franic SE, et al.: Interobserver variation in the interpretation of abdominal radiographs. *Radiology* 1989;171:69–71.

Mucha P: Small intestinal obstruction. *Surg Clin North Am* 1987;67:597–620.

Nevitt PC: The string of pearls sign. *Radiology* 2000;214:157–158.

Shaffer HA: Perforation and obstruction of the gastrointestinal tract: Assessment by conventional radiology. *Radiol Clin North Am* 1992;30:405–426.

Shrake PD, Rex DK, Lappas JC, Maglinte DDT: Radiographic evaluation of suspected small bowel obstruction. *Am J Gastroenterol* 1991;86:175–178.

Suh RS, Maglinte DDT, Lavonas EJ, Kelvin FM: Emergency abdominal radiography: Discrepancies of preliminary and final interpretation and management relevance. *Emerg Radiol* 1995;2:315–318.

Thompson WM, Kilani, RK: Smith BB, et al: Accuracy of abdomial radiography in acute small-bowel obstruction: Does experience matter? AJR 2003: 188: W233-W238.

Ogata M, Mateer JR, Condon RE: Prospective evaluation of abdominal sonography for the diagnosis of bowel obstruction. *Ann Surg* 1996;223:237–241.

CT — Small Bowel Obstruction

Balthazar EJ: CT of small bowel obstruction. *AJR* 1994;162:255–261.

Blachar A, Federle MP, Brancatelli G, et al.: Radiologist performance in the diagnosis of internal hernia by using specific CT findings with emphasis on transmesenteric hernia. *Radiology* 2001;221: 422–428.

Boudiaf M, Soyer P, Terem C, et al.: CT evaluation of small bowel obstruction. *Radiographics* 2001;21:613–624.

Caoili EM, Paulson EK: CT of small-bowel obstruction: Another perspective using multiplanar reformations: Pictorial essay. *AJR* 2000;174:993–998.

Choi SH, Han JK, Kim SH, et al.: Intussusception in adults: From stomach to rectum. *AJR* 2004;183:691–698.

Daneshmand S, Hedley CG, Stain SC: The utility and reliability of computed tomography scan in the diagnosis of small bowel obstruction. *Am Surg* 1999;65(10): 922–927.

Delabrousse E, Destrumelle N, Brunelle S, et al.: CT of small bowel obstruction in adults: Pictorial review. *Abdom Imaging* 2003;28:257–266.

Donckier V, Closset J, Van Gansbeke D, et al.: Contribution of computed tomography to decision making in the management of adhesive small bowel obstruction. *Br J Surg* 1998;85:1071–1074.

Frager D, Medwid SW, Baer JW, et al.: CT of small-bowel obstruction: Value in establishing the diagnosis and determining the degree and cause. *AJR* 1994;162:37–41.

Frager DH, Baer JW, Rothpearl A, Bossart PA: Distinction between postoperative ileus and mechanical small bowel obstruction: Value of CT compared with clinical and other radiographic findings. *AJR* 1995;64:891–894.

Fuchsjager MH: The small bowel feces sign. *Radiology* 2002;225: 378–379.

Fukuya T, Hawes DR, Lu CC, et al.: CT diagnosis of small bowel obstruction: Efficacy in 60 patients. *AJR* 1992;158:765–769. (90% accuracy for CT.)

Furukawa A, Yamasaki M, Furuichi K, et al.: Helical CT in the diagnosis of small bowel obstruction. *Radiographics* 2001;21:341–355.

Gazelle GS, Goldberg MA, Wittenberg J, et al.: Efficacy of CT in distinguishing small-bowel obstruction from other causes of small-bowel dilatation. *AJR* 1994;162:43–47.

Ha HK, Shin BS, Lee SI, Yoon KH: Usefulness of CT in patients with intestinal obstruction who have undergone abdominal surgery for malignancy. *AJR* 1998;171:1587–1593.

Jabra AA, Eng J, Zaleski CG, et al.: CT of small-bowel obstruction in children: Sensitivity and specificity. *AJR* 2001;177:431–436.

Jaffe TA, Martin LC, Thomas J, et al.: Small-bowel obstruction: Coronal reformations from isotropic voxels at 16-section multi-detector row CT. *Radiology* 2006;238:135–142.

Khurana B, Ledbetter S, McTavish J, et al.: Bowel obstruction revealed by multidetector CT: Pictorial essay. *AJR* 2002;178:1139–1144.

Kim AY, Bennett GL, Bashist B, et al.: Small-bowel obstruction associated with sigmoid diverticulitis: CT evaluation in 16 patients. *AJR* 1998;170:1311–1313.

Maglinte DDT, Gage SN, Harmon BH, et al.: Obstruction of the small intestine: Accuracy and role of CT in diagnosis. *Radiology* 1993;188:61–64.

Maglinte DDT, Reyes BL, Harmon BH, et al.: Reliability and role of plain film radiography and CT in the diagnosis of small-bowel obstruction. *AJR* 1996;167:1451–1455.

Makanjuola D: Computed tomography compared with small bowel enema in clinically equivocal intestinal obstruction. *Clin Radiol* 1998;53:203–208.

Martin LC, Merkle EM, Thompson WM: Review of internal hernias. *AJR* 2006;186:703–717.

Mayo-Smith WW, Wittenberg J, Bennett GL, et al.: The CT small bowel faeces sign: Description and clinical relevance. *Clin Radiol* 1995;50:765–767.

Megibow AJ, Balthazar EJ, Cho KC, et al.: Bowel obstruction: Evaluation with CT. *Radiology* 1991;180:313–318. (The seminal paper describing use of CT. 95% accuracy.)

Obuz F, Terzi C, Sokmen S, et al.: The efficacy of helical CT in the diagnosis of small bowel obstruction. *Eur J Radiol* 2003;48:299–304.

Peck JJ, Milleson T, Phelan J: The role of computed tomography with contrast and small bowel follow-through in management of small bowel obstruction. *Am J Surg* 1999;177:375–378.

Rubesin SE, Herlinger H: CT evaluation of bowel obstruction: A landmark article—implications for the future (editorial). *Radiology* 1991;180:307–308.

Stewart ET: CT diagnosis of small bowel obstruction (editorial). *AJR* 1992;158:771–772.

Suri S, Gupta S, Sudhakar PJ, et al.: Comparative evaluation of plain films, ultrasound and CT in the diagnosis of intestinal obstruction. *Acta Radiol* 1999;40:422–428.

Taourel PO, Fabre JM, Pradel JA, et al.: Value of CT in the diagnosis and management of patients with suspected acute small-bowel obstruction. *AJR* 1995;165:1187–1192.

Warshauer DM, Lee JKT: Adult intussusception detected at CT or MR imaging: Clinical-imaging correlation. *Radiology* 1999;212:853-860.

CT—Closed-Loop and Ischemic Small Bowel Obstruction

Ahualli J: The target sign. *Radiology* 2005;234:549–550.

Balthazar EJ et al.: Closed-loop and strangulating obstruction: CT signs. *Radiology* 1992;185:769–775.

Balthazar EJ, Liebeskind ME, Macari M: Intestinal ischemia in patients in whom small bowel obstruction is suspected: Evaluation of accuracy, limitations, and clinical implications of CT in diagnosis. *Radiology* 1997;205:519–522.

Frager D, Baer JW, Medwid SW, et al.: Detection of intestinal ischemia in patients with acute small-bowel obstruction due to adhesions or hernia: Efficacy of CT. *AJR* 1996;166:67–71.

Ha HK, Kim JS, Lee MS: Differentiation of simple and strangulated small-bowel obstructions: Usefulness of known CT criteria. *Radiology* 1997;204:507–512.

Khurana B: The whirl sign. *Radiology* 2003;226:69–70.

Makita O, Ikushima I, Matsumoto N, et al.: CT differentiation between necrotic and nonnecrotic small bowel in closed loop and strangulating obstruction. *Abdom Imaging* 1999;24:120–124.

Rudloff U: The spoke wheel sign. *Radiology* 2005;237:1046–1047.

Sheedy SP, Earnest F, Fletcher JG, et al.: CT of small-bowel ischemia associated with obstruction in emergency department patients: Diagnostic performance evaluation. *Radiology* 2006;241:729–736.

Singer A, Handler BJ, Simmons MZ, Baker SR: Acute small bowel ischemia: Spectrum of computed tomographic findings. *Emerg Radiol* 2000;7:302–307.

Zalcman M, SY M, Donckier V, et al.: Helical CT signs in the diagnosis of intestinal ischemia in small-bowel obstruction. *AJR* 2000;175:1601–1607.

CT—Internal Hernias and Intussusception

Blachar A, Federle MP, Brancatelli G, et al.: Radiologist performance in the diagnosis of internal hernia by using specific CT finding with emphasis on transmesentric hernia. *Radiology* 2001;221:422–428.

Choi SH, Han JK, Kim SH, et al.: Intussusception in adults: From stomach to rectum. *AJR* 2004;183:691–698.

Martin LC, Merkle EM, Thompson WM: Review of internal hernias *AJR* 2006;186:703–717.

Mathieu D, Luciani A for the GERMAD Group: Internal abdominal herniations. *AJR* 2004;183:397–404.

Takeyama N, Gokan T, Ohgiya Y, et al.: CT of internal hernias. *Radiographics* 2005;25:997–1015.

Warshauer DM, Lee JKT: Adult intussusception detected at CT or MR imaging: Clinical-imaging correlation. *Radiology* 1999;212:853–860.

Abdominal Radiology: Patient 2

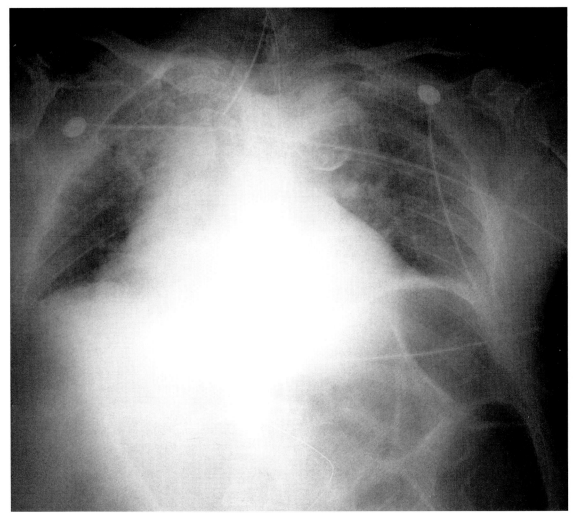

FIGURE 1A

Severe respiratory distress in an elderly man

An 83-year-old man was brought to the ED by ambulance for progressive shortness of breath of one day duration. On arrival, he was in severe respiratory distress and was unable to provide a detailed medical history.

Vital signs: blood pressure: 150/80 mm Hg; pulse: 120 irregular beats/min; respirations: 36 breaths/min; pulse oximetry SO_2 78% on room air.

On examination, there was poor air movement bilaterally. His abdomen was distended, tympanitic to percussion, and non-tender. Bowel sounds were quiet, but present. The patient stated that he had been constipated for six days, but had a bowel movement the previous day.

On 100% oxygen by face mask, the pulse oximetry SO_2 was 92%.

ABG: pH 7.20, P_{CO_2} 59 mm Hg, 79 mm Hg, P_{O_2} 79 mm Hg
The patient was intubated.

His chest and abdominal radiographs are shown in Figure 1.

- What is this patient's diagnosis?

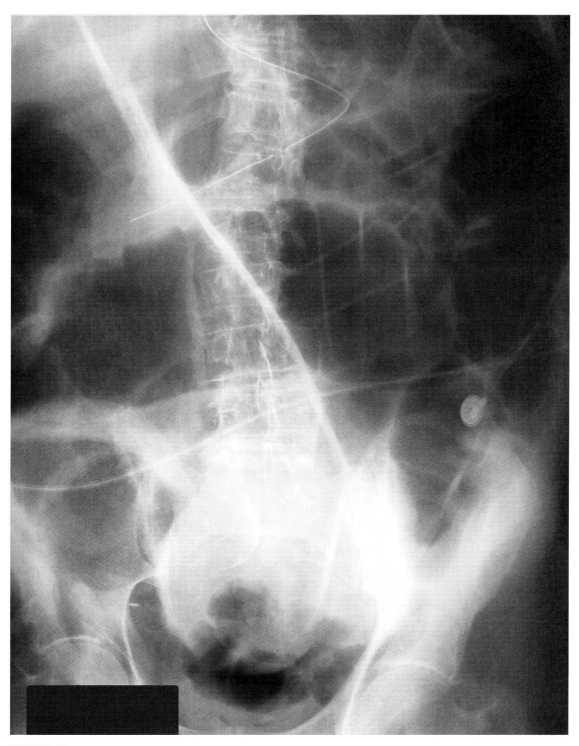

FIGURE 1B

COFFEE BEAN

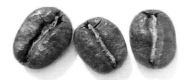

Chest radiography often provides useful information about the cause of a patient's respiratory failure, for example pulmonary edema or pneumonia. In this patient, although the lungs are clear, the chest radiograph does provide a clue to the cause of respiratory failure—a very shallow level of inspiration (Figure 1A). Although shallow inspiration is common in technically suboptimal, supine portable radiographs in critically ill patients, in this case, the shallow inspiration was due to massive abdominal distention—the cause of the patient's respiratory failure.

The **abdominal radiograph** shows markedly distended, air-filled bowel (Figure 2). The **first issue** is whether this is distended small or large bowel. One bowel segment extends horizontally across the midabdomen (T). Small bowel tends to have a central location, although the transverse colon is also centrally located. The mucosal indentations of small bowel are numerous, closely spaced, and extend entirely across the bowel lumen, in contrast to large bowel haustra. However, markedly distended small bowel can have an appearance similar to large bowel (Figure 3). Nonetheless, it is unusual for small bowel to dilate to this extent (10 cm). In addition, although the mucosal indentations are long and thin, like in small bowel, they do not extend entirely across the bowel lumen, which is characteristic of haustra (Figure 2). This segment of bowel is therefore the transverse colon.

The **second issue** is whether the colonic distention is due to a distal large bowel obstruction (LBO) or severe adynamic ileus. Gas is seen in the rectosigmoid colon (Figure 2, R). However, the mere presence of gas in distal bowel does not exclude a mechanical obstruction because distal gas may be present when the colon has not yet completely evacuated its contents. The principal radiographic feature of obstruction, namely the presence of less gas and distention of bowel distal to the obstruction, is often difficult to discern in patients suspected of having LBO. Instead the diagnosis of LBO depends on identifying one segment of large bowel that is especially dilated such as the sigmoid colon or cecum.

In this patient, the key radiographic finding is a distinctive **soft tissue stripe** that extends diagonally across the abdomen (Figure 2, *arrows*). However, because the abdominal radiograph did not encompass the entire abdomen, the nature of this finding was enigmatic.

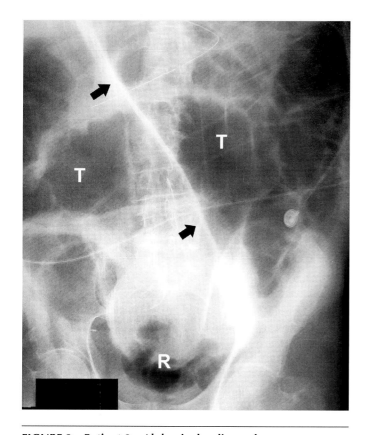

FIGURE 2 Patient 2—Abdominal radiograph
There is a markedly distended loop of bowel extending across the midabdomen (T) and air in the rectosigmoid colon (R). A thin soft tissue stripe extends diagonally across the abdomen (*arrows*).

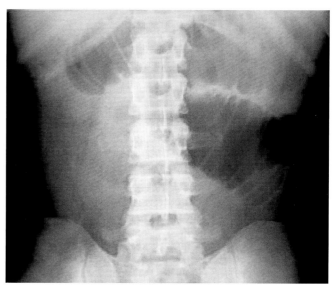

FIGURE 3 Another patient—Small bowel obstruction
Markedly dilated small bowel in a mechanical small bowel obstruction can have a similar appearance to dilated large bowel, particularly the transverse colon.

Because the patient's diagnosis was uncertain based on his abdominal radiograph, an **abdominal CT** was obtained. The CT revealed diffuse dilation of the large bowel as well as fecal matter and air in the rectum (Figure 5). The scan was interpreted as showing an *adynamic ileus* and the patient was admitted to the Medical Intensive Care Unit.

When the CT was re-read the next day, the diagnosis of **sigmoid volvulus** was made. The CT scout digital radiograph is easier to interpret than the abdominal radiograph and the axial CT axial images because it encompasses the entire abdomen (Figure 4). The perplexing diagonal soft tissue stripe (Figure 2, *arrows*) can now be recognized as the apposed walls of an elongated, distended sigmoid colon that has twisted on itself—the central stripe of the **coffee bean sign,** which is diagnostic of sigmoid volvulus (Figure 4, *arrowheads*). The initial abdominal radiograph was, in fact, also diagnostic of sigmoid volvulus, although only the central stripe was visible. Large bowel proximal to the sigmoid volvulus was markedly dilated. The dilated bowel extending horizontally across the mid-abdomen can be more easily identified as the transverse colon on the CT scout image (Figure 4).

The **CT axial images** are more difficult to interpret. The entire colon is markedly dilated (Figure 5). The rectum is neither distended or collapsed making it difficult to distinguish obstruction from ileus. However on one of the images, the point of obstruction is seen where the sigmoid colon is twisted upon itself—the *"whirl sign,"* which is diagnostic of volvulus (Figure 5B, *arrow*).

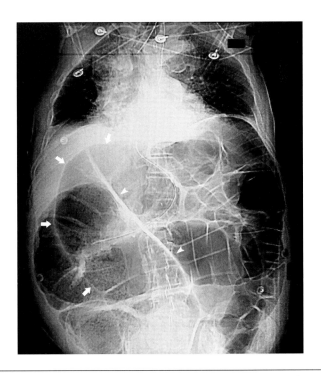

FIGURE 4 CT abdominal scout view showing the outer margins of the "coffee bean" (*arrows*) and the central stripe formed by the apposed walls of the volvulus (*arrowheads*).

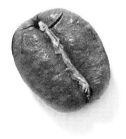

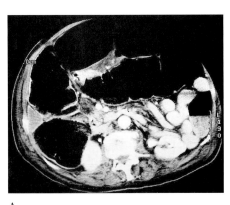

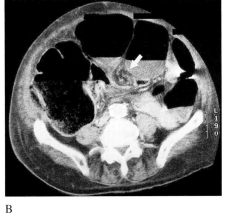

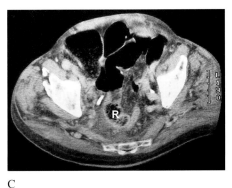

A B C

FIGURE 5 CT axial images.

(*A*) The entire colon is markedly dilated.

(*B*) Two segments of dilated colon twist upon each other forming the *"whirl sign"* at the point of volvulus (*arrow*). This finding is diagnostic of volvulus.

(*C*) Gas and feces is seen in the rectum (R). The rectum is neither distended nor collapsed. A diagnosis of ileus or obstruction cannot be clearly made by assessing rectal filling.

(The CT scout abdominal image is more easily interpreted than the CT axial slices.)

Patient Outcome

After the patient's CT scan was re-read as showing sigmoid volvulus, a contrast enema was performed to confirm the diagnosis (Figure 6). The contrast enema revealed blockage to retrograde flow of contrast at the sigmoid colon that had a tapering "bird's beak" appearance characteristic of sigmoid volvulus.

The patient underwent flexible sigmoidoscopy and placement of a rectal tube. This successfully decompressed the volvulus. Dark, hemorrhagic ischemic mucosa was noted at sigmoidoscopy. The patient was taken to the operating room later that evening. The involved segment of sigmoid colon was necrotic, but not perforated. It was resected and a colostomy was fashioned. The patient made a good recovery.

LARGE BOWEL OBSTRUCTION

Large bowel obstruction represents 15% of cases of bowel obstruction; the remaining cases are small bowel obstruction. In most patients, the obstruction involves the distal colon. Common causes of LBO include colonic tumors, volvulus of the sigmoid colon or cecum, fecal impaction, and benign strictures or abscesses due to diverticulitis, inflammatory bowel disease, or ischemic colitis (Table 1). Tumors constitute 60% of cases of LBO, of which 75% involve the sigmoid or descending colon.

Clinically, LBO usually causes marked abdominal distention that progresses over days to weeks, although with sigmoid or cecal volvulus, the onset is more rapid (Figure 7). Pain may or may not be present and vomiting is often not a prominent symptom. Respiratory failure due to massive abdominal distention occasionally occurs, as in the patient presented here.

The most feared complication of LBO is mural ischemia and **perforation** due to marked bowel distention. A bowel diameter of greater than 11–13 cm on abdominal radiography is at high risk for perforation. The risk of perforation depends also on the rapidity of distention; bowel that is chronically dilated can tol-

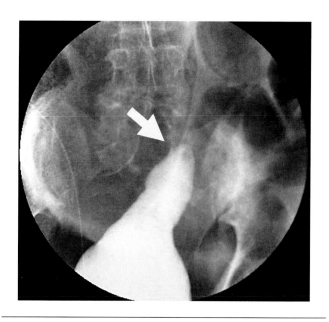

FIGURE 6   Contrast enema of sigmoid volvulus showing the contrast column tapering to a "bird's beak" (*arrow*).

TABLE 1

Causes of Large Bowel Obstruction

Tumor (usually sigmoid carcinoma)

Volvulus (sigmoid, cecal)

Fecal impaction

Benign stricture or abscess

erate greater distention without perforating. Distention greater than 11–13 cm is an indication for emergency surgical decompression using diverting colostomy (for tumors) or sigmoidoscopy (for sigmoid volvulus). Perforation (free intraperitoneal air) requires emergency laparotomy.

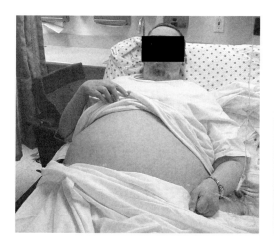
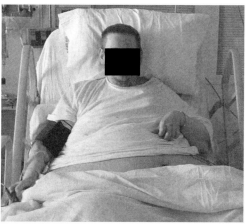

FIGURE 7   Clinical presentation of sigmoid volvulus.

A patient who was chronically bed-bound due to a neurodegenerative disease presented with marked abdominal distention (*A*). The diagnosis of sigmoid volvulus was confirmed by contrast enema. The patient's abdomen rapidly deflated after decompression using sigmoidoscopy and rectal tube insertion (*B*). The patient then underwent elective resection of the sigmoid colon.

IMAGING MODALITIES FOR LARGE BOWEL OBSTRUCTION

The diagnostic evaluation of patients suspected of having LBO begins with abdominal radiography. However, the radiographic findings are often not definitive and confirmatory testing with contrast enema or CT is usually necessary.

Abdominal Radiography

The key radiographic feature of LBO is *distention of large bowel* (> 5 cm). Colonic distention also occurs with *adynamic ileus*. It is often difficult to distinguish severe ileus from distal LBO. Severe adynamic ileus is therefore sometimes referred to as *(colonic) pseudo-obstruction.*

The radiographic principle of small bowel obstruction—dilation of bowel proximal to the obstruction and collapse of distal bowel—often does not pertain to LBO. There are three reasons.

First, large bowel that is distal to an obstruction often does not collapse due to retention of fecal matter. Second, the distribution of air in the segments of the colon is determined more by anatomical location than by whether it is proximal or distal to an obstruction. For example, the transverse colon has an anterior location and tends to fill with air on a supine radiograph, whereas the descending colon is posterior and therefore fills with fluid, which makes the assessment of distention difficult. Third, the rectum is the most dependent portion of the bowel and is usually fluid-filled and not radiographically visible irrespective of whether it is distended or collapsed.

Rather than looking for differences in colonic distention proximal and distal to the obstruction to distinguish LBO from adynamic ileus, the examiner should look for disproportionate distension of a segment of colon (Table 2). For instance, a massively dilated ahaustral loop of colon is seen in patients with volvulus (sigmoid or cecal). In patients with distal LBO, disproportionate distention of the cecum occurs in up to 75% of patients.

Nonetheless, differentiating LBO from adynamic ileus is often difficult based on abdominal radiography alone. Contrast enema or CT is usually needed to confirm the diagnosis of LBO.

TABLE 2

Radiographic Signs of Volvulus, LBO, and Ileus*

Sigmoid volvulus

   Coffee bean—a doubled-back and dilated bowel segment

   Extends from left lower quadrant to right upper quadrant

   Proximal large bowel dilated

Cecal volvulus

   Single dilated segment (kidney-shaped) in mid or upper abdomen

   Distal large bowel collapsed, unless concomitant colonic ileus

   Small bowel often dilated (effectively obstructed at terminal ileum)

Large bowel obstruction—distal

   Diffuse distention of large bowel and often small bowel

   Cecum disproportionately distended (75% of cases)

   Rectum not distended

Ileus—pseudo-obstruction

   Diffuse distention of colon and often small bowel

   Rectum distended on CT or prone rectal view (air filled)

Toxic megacolon

   Distended colon with focal bowel wall edema (nodularity)

*Illustrative cases are given below.

Contrast Enema

Contrast enema may be performed either following abdominal radiography or after a suspicious but nondiagnostic CT. A contrast enema directly demonstrates LBO by retrograde filling of the colon to the point of obstruction. A contrast enema can also characterize the nature of the obstructing lesion. With **volvulus,** the contrast column tapers abruptly at the point of obstruction, having a *"bird's beak"* appearance (Figure 6). With an obstructing **carcinoma,** the contrast is blocked by a mass-like luminal filling defect, or, if the tumor is circumferential, an "apple core" lesion (see Figures 16 and 17 on p.181). With **adynamic ileus,** the contrast column fills the entire colon to the terminalileum (see Figure 21 on p.184). (Although contrast enema is used to reduce intussusception in children, it is not used to reduce a colonic volvulus.)

Evaluation of suspected LBO is the remaining role for contrast enema in adult ED patients. Water-soluble contrast is preferred to barium because it can fill an unprepared colon adequately to diagnose an obstructing lesion. The mucosal detail provided by a standard barium enema is not needed and is usually not feasible. Emergency contrast enema studies may be technically suboptimal if the patient is unable to retain the rectal tube and contrast. In addition, a partially obstructing colonic mass may not be adequately demonstrated or may be missed entirely. Elective colonoscopy or double-contrast barium enema is needed.

Computed Tomography

CT is the most widely used imaging test in emergency patients with abdominal pain. CT is diagnostic of **LBO** when an obstructing lesion is identified, such as a stricture, carcinoma or diverticular abscess (see Figure 18 on p.182). CT is diagnostic of **volvulus** when a *whirl sign* is seen (Figure 5B). The whirl is due to torsion of the bowel and its mesentery at the point of volvulus (Khurana 2003). When there is diffuse large bowel dilation and marked rectal distention, non-obstructive *adynamic ileus* is confirmed on CT (see Figure 20 on p.183).

However, differentiating large bowel obstruction from severe adynamic ileus by CT can be difficult. Because it is difficult to distinguish the various segments of distended large bowel on CT, the defining characteristic of bowel obstruction—distention of bowel proximal to the obstruction and distal collapse—is sometimes impossible to determine on CT (Figure 5). Furthermore, in some patients with LBO, the distal colon and rectum is not collapsed due to retained fecal material, whereas in some patients with ileus, the rectum is not markedly distended.

When a segment of the colon is in an abnormal position, such as finding the cecum in the mid abdomen, volvulus should be suspected. Nonetheless, if an obstructing lesion or whirl sign is not seen, the diagnosis of obstruction often is uncertain and a contrast enema should be performed.

Another option would be to perform CT with rectal contrast when the abdominal radiographs suggest volvulus or LBO. Oral contrast might not reach the point of obstruction in large bowel, whereas rectal contrast may detect the site of obstruction by retrograde filling of the colon and directly confirm the diagnosis (see Figure 13 on p.178).

Accuracy of CT and Contrast Enema for the Diagnosis of LBO

The accuracy of CT in the diagnosis of LBO was evaluated in one prospective series involving 75 patients (Frager 1998). CT sensitivity was 96% and specificity 93%. There have only been individual case reports and small case series on the use of CT for the diagnosis of **volvulus.** The sensitivity and specificity of CT has therefore not been determined. CT can occasionally miss the diagnosis of colonic volvulus and when there is uncertainty, a contrast enema should be performed. In one series of 140 patients, **contrast enema** had a sensitivity of 96% and specificity of 98% for LBO (Chapman 1992).

Prone Abdominal Radiography

In patients in whom the most likely diagnosis is adynamic ileus ("pseudo-obstruction"), prone abdominal radiography can be employed. The patient assumes a prone position in order to fill the rectum with air. A *cross-table lateral radiograph* of the rectal area is then obtained. If the rectum is air-filled and distended, the patient has an ileus and the diagnosis of LBO is excluded. When the rectum does not fill with air, the diagnosis of obstruction remains a possibility (Low 1995). The underlying cause of ileus must then be determined. This technique is most useful is chronically bed-bound patients with colonic stasis (see Figure 22 on p.184).

SIGMOID VOLVULUS

Sigmoid volvulus accounts for 60–75% of cases of large bowel volvulus. Sigmoid volvulus typically occurs in older individuals who have developed an elongated redundant sigmoid colon with a narrow mesenteric base. The sigmoid colon then twists upon itself forming a closed-loop obstruction (Figure 8). The volvulus rapidly becomes distended. There is a high risk of ischemia and perforation due to compression of mesenteric blood vessels and extreme bowel distention.

Treatment entails emergency decompression using sigmoidoscopy and rectal tube insertion. After reduction, the redundant sigmoid colon should be resected because sigmoid volvulus recurs in up to 90% of unresected cases (Figure 9).

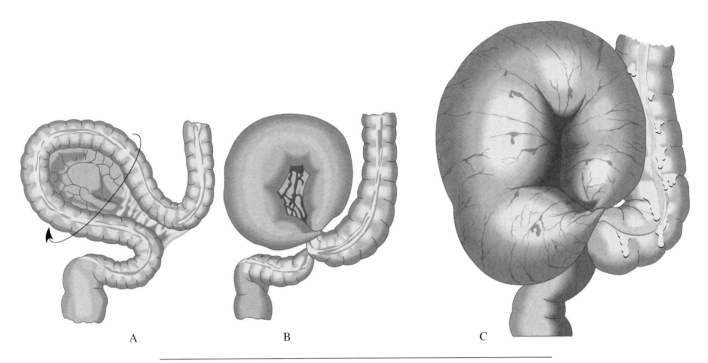

A   B   C

FIGURE 8   Pathogenesis of sigmoid volvulus.

(*A*) Elongated redundant sigmoid loop twists on a contracted base of mesentery.

(*B*) Torsion and closed-loop obstruction.

(*C*) Bowel distention, forming the "coffee bean," and compression of the mesenteric vascular pedicle can cause mural ischemia and perforation.

Abdominal radiography is diagnostic in up to 80% of cases of sigmoid volvulus. The principal finding is the **coffee bean sign**—the redundant sigmoid colon twisted on itself like a "bent inner tube" (Figure 4). The sigmoid colon is massively distended and looses its haustral indentations. The volvulus arises from the left lower quadrant and extends toward the right upper quadrant (Figure 9). The superior margin typically lies under the right hemidiaphragm, although it may extend to the left upper quadrant or midepigastrium. On an upright radiograph, there may be two air/fluid levels, one for each limb of the volvulus. The proximal colon is usually dilated because it is effectively obstructed by the volvulus (Table 2).

When the entire sigmoid volvulus is seen on the radiograph, the diagnosis is usually straightforward. Difficulties arise when the entire volvulus is not seen because it extends beyond the margins of the radiograph. In these situations, only **individual segments of the sigmoid volvulus** are visible. The uppermost extent of the volvulus may appear as a curved line superior to the transverse colon, most often in the right upper quadrant overlying the liver. The ahaustral curved lateral walls of the volvulus may overlap the ascending colon on the right side of the abdomen or the descending colon on the left. The *central stripe* formed by the opposed walls of the volvulus may be seen extending from the left lower quadrant to the right upper quadrant (Figure 1B). In the right lower quadrant, the volvulus may appear as a convergence of three lines: the central stripe and the two lateral walls of the volvulus.

When the proximal colon is markedly distended, the radiographic findings of sigmoid volvulus can be similar to those of adynamic ileus. On the other hand, in patients with an elongated redundant sigmoid colon, adynamic ileus can have a similar radiographic appearance to sigmoid volvulus (see Figure 22 on p.184). When the diagnosis of sigmoid volvulus is clear based on clinical presentation and abdominal radiography, the clinician can proceed directly to sigmoidoscopy and rectal tube insertion to decompress the volvulus. Rapid decompression confirms the diagnosis (Figure 7).

When the diagnosis of sigmoid volvulus remains uncertain, further testing is necessary (Figures 9 and 10). This can be either contrast enema or CT, although contrast enema is usually the more direct and easily interpreted. **Contrast enema** reveals a typical *bird's beak* at the sigmoid colon (Figures 6 and 9B). On **CT,** the entire colon is markedly distended, especially the sigmoid colon and a *whirl sign* is seen at the region of torsion (Figure 10).

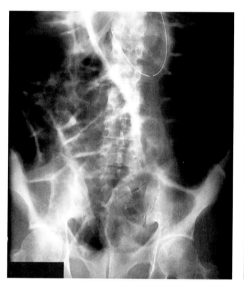

A. **First admission**—Sigmoid volvulus. Interpretation of abdominal radiograph is difficult because entire colon is distended

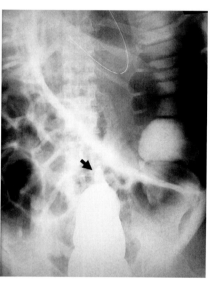

B. Contrast enema showing "bird's beak" at the sigmoid volvulus (*arrow*)

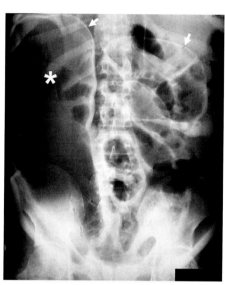

C. **Second admission**—3 weeks later Recurrent volvulus and perforation

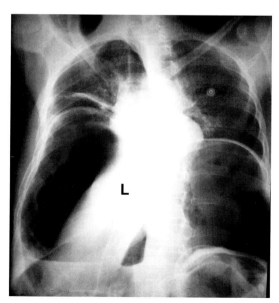

D. Second admission—Chest radiograph. Massive free air. L–liver

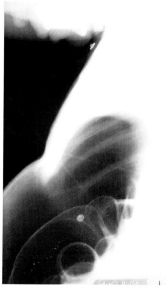

E. Lateral chest view

FIGURE 9   Sigmoid volvulus with perforation.

A 40-year-old man presented with abdominal distention and pain. Three weeks earlier, he had been hospitalized for sigmoid volvulus (*A* and *B*). The volvulus was reduced with a rectal tube, but the patient refused surgery for sigmoid resection.

(*C*) On this second admission, the abdominal radiograph revealed sigmoid volvulus (*asterisk*). However, air outlines both sides of the bowel wall in several locations (*arrows*), a sign of extensive extraluminal air due to perforation of the sigmoid volvulus (*Rigler sign*).

(*D* and *E*) The chest radiographs confirmed massive pneumoperitoneum.

The patient underwent emergency surgery to resect the perforated sigmoid colon.

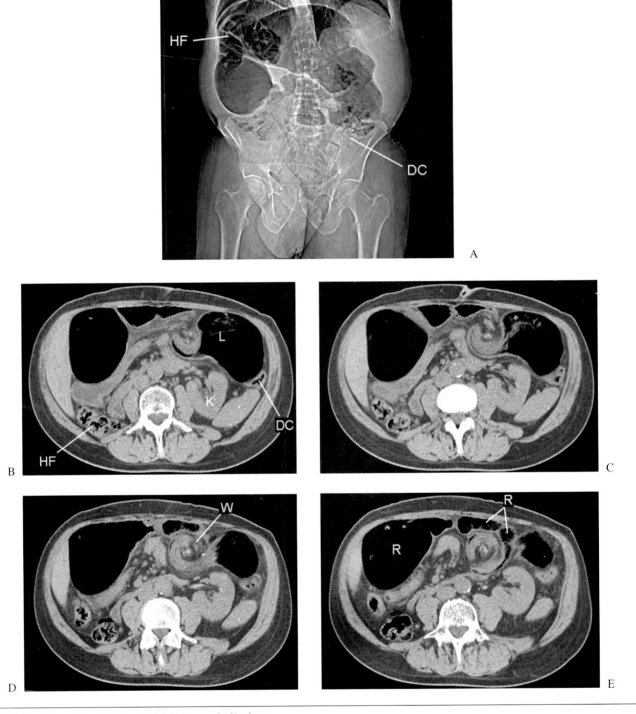

FIGURE 10   Sigmoid volvulus—Whirl sign on helical CT.

A 68-year-old man presented with an abrupt onset of abdominal pain. He appeared restless and vomited once. A CT was performed without oral or intravenous contrast for suspected renal colic, even though the pain was not localized to one side of the abdomen or flank.

(*A.*) The abdominal radiograph shows a markedly distended loop of large bowel in the right upper quadrant under the right hemidiaphragm representing the sigmoid volvulus.

(*B–D.*) Successive CT slices show a progressive *whirl sign* (W) where there is torsion of the volvulus.

The left side of the volvulus (L) is pulled into the whirl and has a "bird's beak" appearance (*B* and *C*). The right side of the volvulus is pulled horizontally across the mid-abdomen (R in *E*). A *coffee bean sign* is therefore not seen on the abdominal radiograph (*A*).

Despite the fact that the proximal colon is effectively obstructed by the volvulus, it is not dilated. Gas and feces are present in the hepatic flexure (HF in *A* and *B*) and descending colon (DC in *B*).

This patient had had a right nephrectomy (K—left kidney), so the hepatic flexure (HF) of the colon is located posterior to the sigmoid volvulus in the right renal fossa.

CECAL VOLVULUS

Cecal volvulus represents 25–40% of cases of large bowel volvulus. The predisposing condition is congenital incomplete fixation of the cecum to the posterior peritoneum. Cecal volvu-lus tends to occur in younger patients (40–60 years old) than does sigmoid volvulus. The mobile cecum twists around the ter-minal ileum and proximal ascending colon (Figure 11).

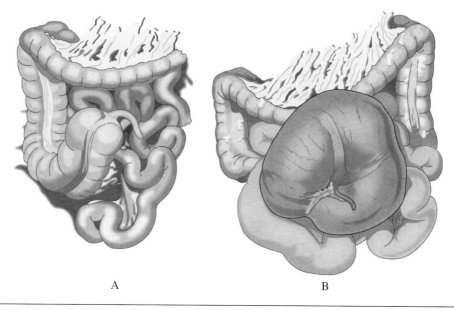

A   B

FIGURE 11 Pathogenesis of cecal volvulus.
(*A*) Congenital incomplete fixation of the cecum to the posterior peritoneum allows the cecum to rotate freely.
(*B*) Torsion of the cecum around the terminal ileum and proximal ascending colon causes cecal volvulus.

The key **radiographic feature** of cecal volvulus is a single, large gas-filled segment of bowel representing the massively distended cecum (Figures 12 and 13). It is kidney-shaped due to indentation of its inferior surface by often the ileocecal valve. The cecal volvulus is most often located in the midabdomen or left upper quadrant, but may be in the right upper quadrant and right or left lower quadrants. The upright radiograph may show a single large air/fluid level. When markedly distended, cecal volvulus can be complicated by perforation (see Patient 3, Fig-ure 11 on page 198).

Large bowel distal to the cecal volvulus is usually collapsed unless there is a concomitant colonic ileus. When there is con-comitant colonic ileus, the radiographic diagnosis of cecal volvu-lus can be difficult because of the diffuse colonic distention.

The small bowel is often distended due to the obstruction at the terminal ileum, in which case, cecal volvulus can have a radiographic appearance similar to distal small bowel obstruction. Cecal volvulus can be mimicked by other disorders associated with a single large gas-filled structure in the ab-domen (Figure 14).

Contrast enema can be used to diagnose cecal volvulus. The contrast column fills the entire colon to the volvulus where it tapers to a "bird's beak" (Figure 12C).

Computed tomography shows a massively dilated cecum in an abnormal location. At the neck of the volvulus, a tapering *bird's beak* or *whirl sign*, representing twisted bowel and mesentery, may be seen (Moore et al. 2001). As with sigmoid volvulus, CT is not always definitive and contrast enema may be necessary to confirm the diagnosis. Alternatively, CT can be performed after the admin-istration of rectal contrast to increase its yield (Figure 13).

Cecal volvulus is not amenable to endoscopic decompres-sion and emergency laparotomy is needed. If the bowel is not ischemic, the cecum can be surgically fixed to the posterior peritoneum (cecopexy) to prevent recurrence.

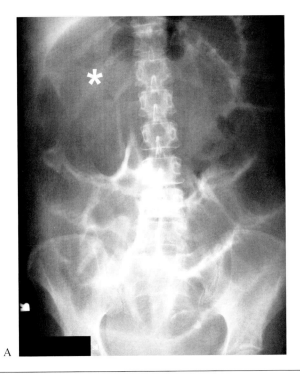
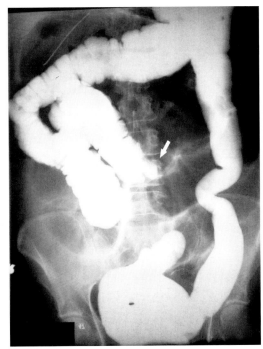

A

B

FIGURE 12   Cecal volvulus.

(*A*) The classic radiographic findings of cecal volvulus include massively dilated cecum displaced superiorly to occupy the upper abdomen (*asterisk*). Dilated small bowel in the lower abdomen is due to the concomitant small bowel obstruction at the distal ileum.

(*B*) Contrast enema confirms cecal volvulus. Contrast fills the colon from the sigmoid, descending, transverse and ascending colon until reaching the obstruction at the point of volvulus (*arrow*).

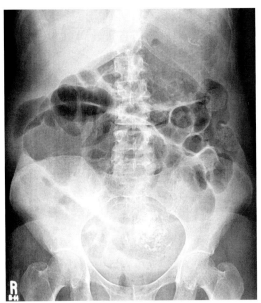
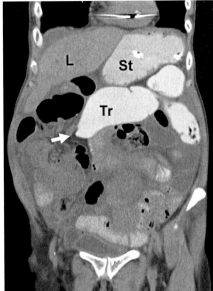
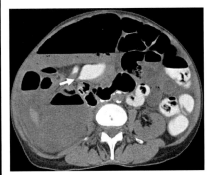

FIGURE 13   Ascending colonic volvulus—Rectal contrast CT.

A 75-year-old woman presented with abdominal pain and distention. Abdominal radiography showed a markedly distended colonic segment in mid-abdomen suggestive of volvulus, although it was uncertain whether this was sigmoid or cecal volvulus.

A CT was performed after the administration of oral and rectal contrast. Intravenous contrast was not given due to renal insufficiency.

Rectal contrast filled the distal colon to a point near the hepatic flexure. The contrast column tapers to a bird's beak (*arrows*). The use of rectal

contrast assisted in making the diagnosis of cecal volvulus by retrograde filling of the colon to the point of volvulus.

The patient underwent surgery, where an ischemic cecal and ascending colonic volvulus was found that required a right hemicolectomy.

Tr—transverse colon, St—stomach, L—liver

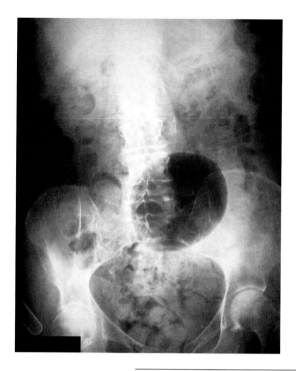
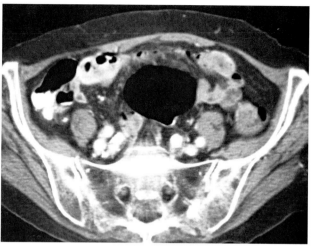

14 A and B   Giant sigmoid diverticulum.

A massively distended air-filled sigmoid diverticulum was causing extrinsic compression on the small bowel and a partial small bowel obstruction. The sigmoid diverticulum was resected.

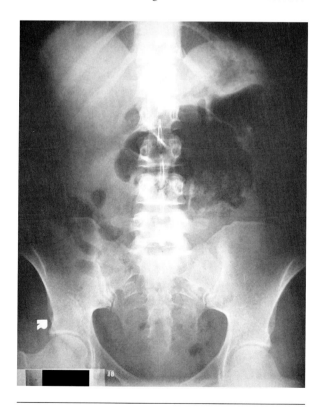
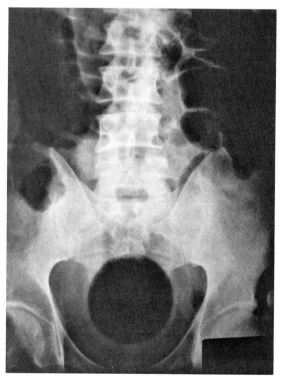

14C   Cecum-in-bascule.

The nonfixed cecum has migrated up to the mid-abdomen. There was no evidence of volvulus on contrast enema.

14D   Tennis ball inserted in rectum.

The radiolucent object is a perfect sphere.

Emphysematous cystitis also causes a round pelvic gas collection, although the clinical presentation is considerably different.

FIGURE 14   Radiographic findings that can mimic cecal volvulus.
Gas-filled structure in mid-abdomen.

DISTAL LARGE BOWEL OBSTRUCTION

Distal large bowel obstruction may be caused by a sigmoid carcinoma, stricture, extrinsic compression (e.g., diverticular abscess), or fecal impaction.

Abdominal radiography is the initial test in evaluating patients with abdominal distention, particularly when a small or large bowel obstruction might be present. Abdominal radiographs often have findings useful in distinguishing large and small bowel obstruction and adynamic ileus. Nonetheless, further testing with CT or contrast enema is often needed.

With distal LBO, there is dilation of large bowel (>5 cm) up to the point of obstruction. Obstruction usually occurs in the rectosigmoid colon. Distal LBO must be differentiated from adynamic ileus in which there is also diffuse colonic distention. Although it would seem logical that identifying collapse of the colon distal to the obstruction (i.e., the rectum) would be a useful sign of LBO, this is often difficult to detect on abdominal radiography. Even with obstruction, the rectosigmoid usually contains some air and feces (Figures 2 and 17). In addition, in a supine or standing position, the rectum fills with fluid and is therefore not often visible radiographically (Chapman et al. 1992).

The key radiographic finding that distinguishes a distal large bowel obstruction from adynamic ileus is disproportionate **distention of the cecum** (Wittenberg 1993). The cecum tends to become especially dilated in mechanical LBO because it is the segment of the colon with the greatest diameter. In accordance with Laplace's law regarding distensible tubular structures, the bowel segment with the greatest diameter has the greatest wall tension and therefore tends to become most distended (Figures 16 and 17).

There are **three radiographic patterns** of distal LBO (Figure 15). In 75% of cases, the ileocecal valve is competent, and the cecum is markedly dilated. In type A, only the colon is dilated, whereas in type B, both small and large bowel are dilated. In 25% of cases (type C), the ileocecal valve is incompetent, the cecum decompresses into the terminal ileum and is therefore not disproportionately dilated. The diagnosis of LBO is especially difficult in these cases. Further testing with contrast enema or CT is usually needed.

Computed tomography   CT is effective at detecting an obstructing cancerous lesion. CT can assess extension into adjacent tissues and lymph nodes as well as more distant metastasis, particularly to the liver (Horton 2000). However, in 10% of cases, CT is unable to distinguish neoplastic lesions from benign strictures that are caused by diverticulitis, inflammatory bowel disease, or ischemic colitis. Double-contrast barium enema or colonoscopy with biopsy is necessary to make the diagnosis (Figure 18).

Supplementary CT maneuvers are occasionally needed to detect short annular lesions and to distinguish apparent wall thickening due to incomplete distention. There maneuvers include rectal insufflation of air, instillation of rectal contrast, decubitus positioning, or delayed CT imaging (Frager 1998, 2002). Consultation with the radiologist or close clinical follow-up should be arranged in such cases.

Contrast enema   A contrast enema is traditionally the test of choice for the diagnosis of LBO and, depending on local resources and expertise, can still be used in the ED (Chapman 1992). Water-soluble contrast is used in these situations. An occluding mass or circumferential narrowing ("apple core") is seen in the region of obstruction (Figures 16 and 17).

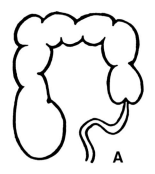 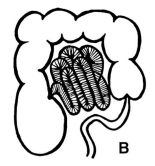 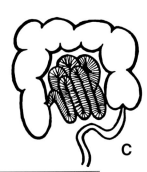

FIGURE 15   LBO due to an obstructing sigmoid lesion.

(A) Competent ileocecal valve—large bowel is dilated and the cecum is especially dilated

(B) Competent ileocecal valve—both large and small bowel are dilated and the cecum is especially dilated

(C) Incompetent ileocecal valve—the cecum decompresses into the terminal ileum

[From: Plewa: Emerg Med Clin North Am 1991, with permission]

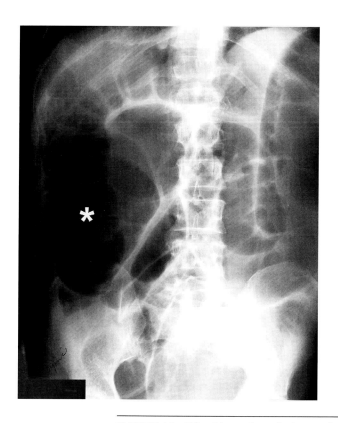

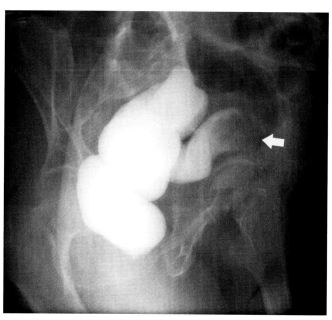

FIGURE 16   Distal large bowel obstruction due to sigmoid carcinoma

A 60-year-old man presented to the ED with progressive abdominal distention that developed over two weeks. His abdomen was tympanitic and firm, but not tender.

The abdominal radiograph shows marked dilation of large and small bowel with disproportionate distention of the cecum characteristic of distal large bowel obstruction (*asterisk*). The contrast enema revealed occlusion at the sigmoid colon by the tumor mass (*arrow*).

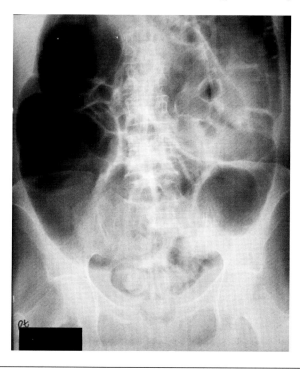

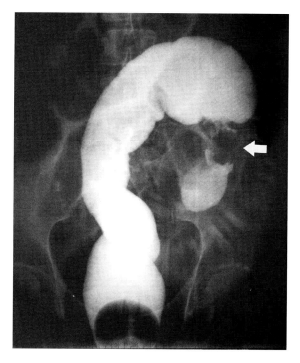

FIGURE 17   Another patient with abdominal distention due to LBO.

The abdominal radiograph shows diffuse dilation of large and small bowel. There is disproportionate distention of the cecum suggestive of mechanical LBO rather than ileus. Air in a low-lying sigmoid colon should not be mistakenly identified as being in the rectum, thereby incorrectly excluding LBO.

Contrast enema revealed an "apple core" lesion with nearly complete occlusion of the sigmoid colon by a circumferential tumor (*arrow*).

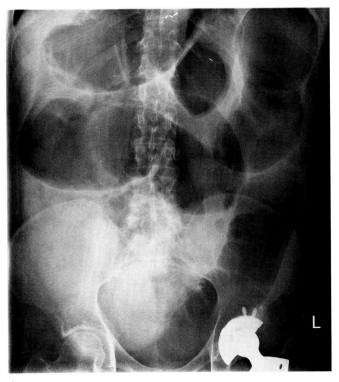

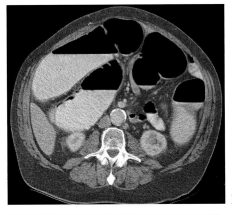

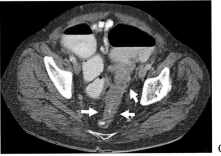

A

FIGURE 18   Distal LBO due to a sigmoid stricture suspicious for carcinoma

A 57-year-old man presented with one week of abdominal distention and constipation.

(*A*) The abdominal radiograph showed markedly dilated large bowel. The cecum and ascending colon are fluid-filled and cannot be assessed for distention.

(*B* and *C*) An abdominal CT showed colonic distention due to obstruction at the sigmoid colon. There was a long (10 cm) segment of colonic wall thickening and luminal stenosis (*arrows*). This was suspicious for an infiltrating adenocarcinoma.

The patient underwent sigmoid resection with colostomy. Pathology revealed diverticulosis with muscular hypertrophy, focal fibrosis and chronic inflammation. There was no evidence of malignancy.

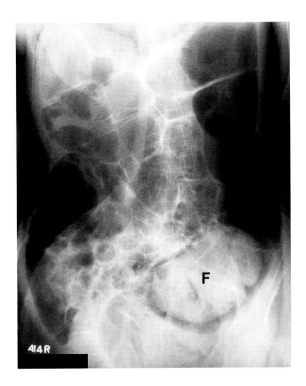

FIGURE 19   LBO due to fecal impaction.

A large fecal mass is seen in the distal descending colon (F). The proximal large bowel is markedly dilated.

Despite the benign nature of the obstructing lesion, there is a risk of colonic ischemia and perforation due to pressure necrosis and marked distention—stercoral colitis (Heffernan, et al 2005). The patient was manually disimpacted and admitted to the hospital for observation.

ADYNAMIC ILEUS (PSEUDO-OBSTRUCTION)

In adynamic ileus, there is diffuse dilation of both small and large bowel. In some instances, colonic distention predominates, which is referred to as *colonic ileus*. Because of similarities in the radiographic appearance of ileus and distal LBO, severe adynamic ileus is sometimes referred to as colonic *"pseudo-obstruction."*

A dynamic ileus may be acute or chronic, and is caused by a variety of intra-abdominal and systemic disorders (see Introduction to Abdominal Radiology, Table 6 on page 144). When there is no evident underlying cause, it is given the eponym *Ogilvie syndrome*. Although colonic ileus does not require surgical treatment, bowel distention should be relieved by rectal tube decompression, and occasionally colonoscopy (Kahi and Rex 2003, Heffernan 2005).

When the distinction between obstruction and ileus is uncertain, further diagnostic testing is needed—CT or contrast enema. In many patients with diffuse bowel dilation due to adynamic ileus, disorders other than obstruction are diagnostic considerations and appropriate testing should be undertaken (e.g., CT for appendicitis—see Introduction to Abdominal Radiology, Figure 5 on page 143). With adynamic ileus, the critical finding on CT is dilated large bowel extending to the rectum. **Contrast enema** shows contrast filling the entire colon (Figure 21).

In chronically bed-bound patients with recurrent adynamic ileus in whom excluding obstruction is the only diagnostic consideration, a simple imaging technique can be employed. The patient is placed in a **prone position** so that the rectum will fill with air if it is not obstructed. A cross-table lateral radiograph of the rectal area is then obtained. If the rectum is distended with air, a distal LBO is excluded (Figure 22) (Low 1995).

Although ileus is a nonspecific radiographic finding, it is not a benign entity. Adynamic ileus is associated with a wide range of serious disorders that may require definitive treatment such as appendicitis, mesenteric ischemia, pneumonia, and electrolyte abnormalities.

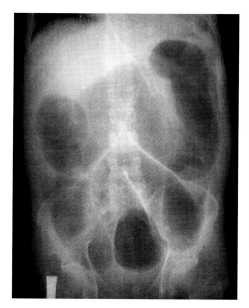 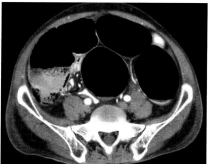 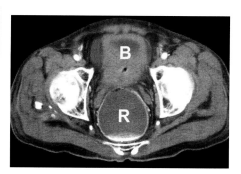

FIGURE 20   Adynamic ileus diagnosed by CT

A bed-bound nursing home resident presented to the ED with abdominal distention. Abdominal radiography showed markedly dilated air-filled colon.

CT confirmed the colonic dilation. A CT slice thorough the lower pelvis shows a dilated fluid-filled rectum (R) posterior to the bladder (B). Colonic dilation extending to the rectum is diagnostic of adynamic ileus.

No underlying medical condition was found as aside from his immobility and the patient was treated with rectal tube decompression.

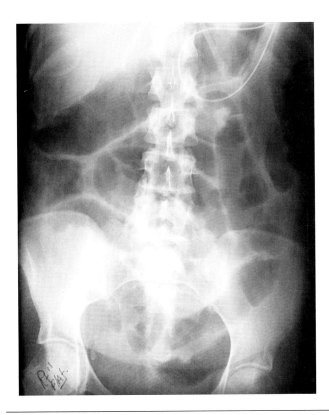

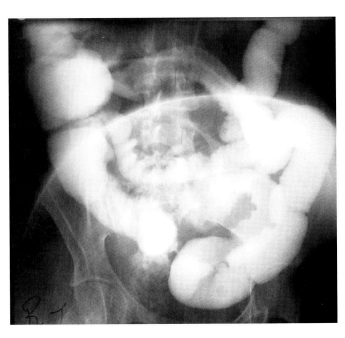

FIGURE 21 A 40-year-old woman with AIDS and pneumonia was noted to have abdominal distention. There was diffuse dilation of small and large bowel. Although this was likely due to an adynamic ileus, there was concern about a distal large bowel obstruction. A contrast enema filled the colon and contrast refluxed into the terminal ileum confirming non-obstructive adynamic ileus.

A clinical diagnosis of adynamic ileus can be made in most cases, and diagnostic imaging is not necessary.

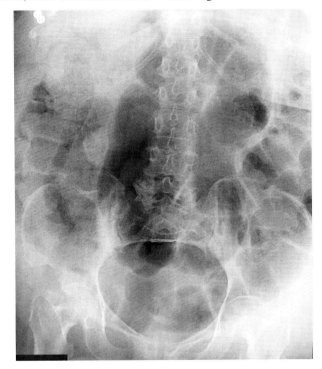

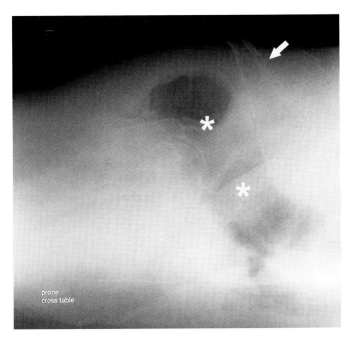

FIGURE 22 A bed-bound 80-year-old woman was transferred from a nursing home because of abdominal distention. Her abdomen was soft and non-tender. She had has several prior ED visits for the same problem.

The abdominal radiograph showed diffuse dilation of large bowel with a dilated redundant sigmoid colon occupying the entire mid-abdomen. The radiographic findings were suspicious for sigmoid volvulus.

The patient was placed in a prone position and a cross-table lateral radiograph of the rectal area revealed gas in a dilated rectum (*asterisks*), excluding mechanical obstruction. This effectively excludes mechanical obstruction. (The sacrum is indicated for orientation (*arrow*)).

No other disorders were under consideration, so additional imaging (i.e., CT) was not needed.

TOXIC MEGACOLON

Toxic megacolon is a disorder characterized by colonic distention ("megacolon") in patients with clinical signs of *systemic toxicity*. Toxic megacolon is most commonly a complication of *ulcerative colitis*. It may also be associated with *infections colitis* such as *Clostridium difficile* colitis, amebic dysentery, or Shigellosis, particularly following the use of antiperistaltic medications (Figure 23).

With toxic megacolon there is bowel wall inflammation and necrosis and a high risk of perforation and sepsis. Contrast enema and colonoscopy should be avoided due to the risk of perforation.

Abdominal radiography shows colonic distention, loss of haustral markings, and *mucosal nodules* due to focal bowel wall edema, hemorrhage, and pseudo-polyps (areas of intact mucosa surrounded by areas of deep ulceration).

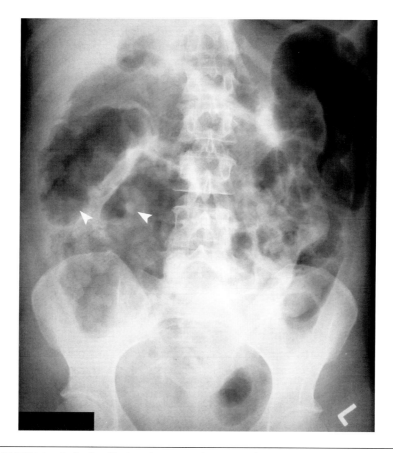

FIGURE 23   Colonic dilation due to toxic megacolon.

A 41-year-old woman with AIDS had been taking diphenoxylate and atropine (Lomotil®) in addition to ganciclovir for CMV colitis. She presented with abdominal pain, distention, fever, and hypotension. The radiograph shows colonic distention and characteristic mucosal nodules (*arrowheads*) consistent with toxic megacolon.

This patient initially improved with supportive care and intravenous antibiotics, but subsequently developed septic shock possibly due to colonic perforation. She died several days later.

SUMMARY—IMAGING FOR SUSPECTED LBO AND VOLVULUS

Abdominal radiography remains to initial diagnostic test in patients suspected of having bowel obstruction, either SBO or LBO. In most cases, additional testing is needed to confirm the diagnosis. The choice of confirmatory imaging test, either CT or contrast enema, depends on the most likely diagnosis (LBO or volvulus), as well as the resources and expertise at the practitioner's institution (Table 3). Consultation should be made with the radiologist regarding which imaging examination to perform. If a definitive result is not obtained with the first test, an alternative study may be needed.

CT is the most comprehensive examination and should be used whenever there is suspicion of other intra-abdominal pathology, such as appendicitis causing adynamic ileus. For colonic malignancy or benign strictures (e.g., diverticulitis), CT provides more information than contrast enema about the extra-luminal component of disease. If, however, the immediate question is simply whether or not there is a distal LBO as opposed to a dynamic ileus, a **contrast enema** is usually sufficient. If pseudo-obstruction is the most likely diagnosis, a **prone rectal radiograph** showing a dilated air-filled rectum will confirm nonobstructive ileus and exclude mechanical LBO. In a chronically bed-bound patient, this approach may provide sufficient information.

Sigmoid volvulus can be diagnosed solely with abdominal radiography. This can be followed by emergency decompression using sigmoidoscopy and/or a rectal tube. Abrupt decompression confirms the diagnosis of sigmoid volvulus. When diagnostic uncertainty exists, a contrast enema can provide confirmation of sigmoid volvulus. CT would probably also be diagnostic, although the published experience is less extensive.

The diagnosis of **cecal volvulus** based on abdominal radiography is usually less certain that of sigmoid volvulus, and either contrast enema or CT may be needed. If, after CT, the diagnosis remains uncertain, contrast enema can be performed. Operative reduction of the volvulus and cecopexy is the definitive treatment.

With the current widespread and ready availability of CT in the ED, it would seem preferable to obtain CT rather than contrast enema. If LBO or volvulus is suspected, the CT technique could be modified to include rectal contrast, which would serve a similar function as in a contrast enema. Retrograde filling of the colon could potentially increase the yield of CT in detecting large bowel obstruction, volvulus or other colonic lesions (Figure 13).

TABLE 3

Diagnostic imaging for suspected LBO, volvulus, or adynamic ileus*

Probable diagnosis based on clinical presentation and abdominal radiography	Confirmatory test for definitive management
Sigmoid volvulus	Sigmoidoscopy or contrast enema (CT—alternative test)[†]
Cecal volvulus	Contrast enema or CT[†]
Distal LBO (possible colonic tumor)	CT or contrast enema[†]
Ileus (pseudo-obstruction)	Prone view of rectum, CT (contrast enema - alternative test)
Toxic megacolon	CT (contrast enema and colonoscopy are contraindicated due to risk of perforation)

*If colon diameter is >11-13 cm, emergency decompression is indicated to prevent perforation
 If free intraperitoneal air is seen (perforation), emergency surgery is indicated
† If after CT, the diagnosis remains uncertain, contrast enema should be performed. To increase the diagnostic yield of
 CT, it could be performed following the administration of rectal contrast.

SUGGESTED READING

Large Bowel Obstruction

Bryk D: Diagnosis of colonic obstruction based on findings on plain radiographs. *AJR* 1994; 163:225.

Chapman AH, McNamara M, Porter G: The acute contrast enema in suspected large bowel obstruction: Value and technique. *Clin Radiol* 1992;46:273–278.

Day JJ, Freeman AH, Coni NK, et al.: Barium enema or computed tomography for the frail elderly patient? *Clin Radiol* 1993;48:48–51.

Frager D: Intestinal obstruction: Role of CT. *Gastroenterol Clin North Am* 2002;31:777–799.

Frager D, Rovno HDS, Baer JW, et al.: Prospective evaluation of colonic obstruction with computed tomography. *Abdom Imaging* 1998;23:141–146.

Hazelwood S, Burton D: Colonic ileus. *N Engl J Med* 2006;354:e6.

Heffernan C, Pachter HL, Megibow AJ, Macari M: Stercoral colitis leading to fatal peritonitis: CT findings. *AJR* 2005;184:1189–1193.

Horton KM, Abrams RA, Fishman EK: Spiral CT of colon cancer: Imaging features and role in management. *Radiographics* 2000;20:419–430.

Kahi CJ, Rex DK: Bowel obstruction and pseudo-obstruction. *Gastroenterol Clin North Am* 2003;32:1229–1247.

Koruth NM, Koruth A, Matheson NA: The place of contrast enema in the management of large bowel obstruction. *J R Coll Surg Edinb* 1985;30:258–260.

Loubières Y, Chereau O: Severe fecal impaction. *New Engl J Med* 2005;352:e12.

Love L: Large bowel obstruction. *Semin Roentgenol* 1971;8:299–322.

Low VH: Colonic pseudo-obstruction: Value of prone lateral view of the rectum. *Abdom Imaging* 1995;20:531–533.

Macari M, Balthazar EJ: CT of bowel wall thickening: Significance and pitfalls of interpretation. *AJR* 2001;176:1105–1116.

Megibow AJ: Bowel obstruction: Evaluation with CT. *Radiol Clin North Am* 1994;32:861–870.

Megibow AJ, Balthazar EJ, Cho KC, et al.: Bowel obstruction: Evaluation with *CT. Radiology* 1991;180:313–318.

Stewart J, Finan PJ, Courtney DF, et al.: Does a water soluble contrast enema assist in the management of acute large bowel obstruction? A prospective study of 117 cases. *Br J Surg* 1984;71:799–801.

Taourel P, Kessler N, Lesnik A, et al.: Helical CT of large bowel obstruction. *Abdom Imaging* 2003;28:267–275.

Taorel P, Kessler N, Lesnik A, et al.: Imaging of acute intestinal obstruction. *Eur Radiol* 2002;12:2151–2160.

Turnage RH, Bergen PC: Intestinal obstruction and ileus. In Feldman et al., eds. *Sleisenger and Fordtran's Gastrointestinal and Liver Disease*, 7th ed. Elsevier, 2002:2113–2127.

Wittenberg J: The diagnosis of colonic obstruction on plain abdominal radiographs: Start with the cecum, leave the rectum to last. *AJR* 1993;161:443–444.

Wittenberg J, Harisinghani MG, Jhaveri K, et al.: Algorithmic approach to CT diagnosis of the abnormal bowel wall. *Radiographics* 2002;22:1093–1107.

Volvulus

Hiltunen KM, Syrja H, Matikainen M: Colonic volvulus. Diagnosis and results of treatment in 82 patients. *Eur J Surg* 1992;158:607–611.

Jones DJ: ABC of colorectal diseases: Large bowel volvulus. *BMJ* 1992;305:358–360.

Kerry RL, Lee F, Ransom HK: Roentgenologic examination in the diagnosis and treatment of colon volvulus. *AJR* 1971;113:343–348.

Khurana B: The whirl sign. *Radiology* 2003;226:69–70.

Pickhardt PJ, Bhalla S: Intestinal malrotation in adolescents and adults: Spectrum of clinical and imaging features. *AJR* 2002;179:1429–1435.

Shaff MI, Himmelfarb E, Sacks GA, et al.: The whirl sign: A CT finding in volvulus of the large bowel. *J Comput Assist Tomogr* 1985;9:410.

Theuer C, Cheadle WG: Volvulus of the colon. *Am Surg* 1991;57:145–150.

Sigmoid Volvulus

Burrell HC, Baker DM, Wardrop P, Evans AJ: Significant plain film findings in sigmoid volvulus. *Clin Radiol* 1994;49:317–319.

Catalano O: Computed tomographic appearance of sigmoid volvulus. *Abdom Imaging* 1996;21:314–317.

Chin LW, Lin MT, Wang HP, et al.: Rapid diagnosis of sigmoid volvulus with water soluble urograffin in emergency service. *Am J Emerg Med* 2001;19:600.

Feldman D: The coffee bean sign. *Radiology* 2000;216:178–179.

Gibney EJ: Volvulus of the sigmoid colon. *Surg Gynecol Obstet* 1991;173:243–255.

Madiba TE, Thomson SR: The management of sigmoid volvulus. *J R Coll Surg Edinb* 2000;45;74–80.

Young WS, Engelbrecht HE, Stoker A: Plain film analysis in sigmoid volvulus. *Clin Radiol* 1978;29:553–560.

Cecal Volvulus

Anderson JR, Lee D: Acute caecal volvulus. *Br J Surg* 1980;67:39–41.

Anderson JR, Mills JOM: Caecal volvulus: A frequently missed diagnosis? *Clin Radiol* 1984;35:65–69.

Frank AJ, Goffner LB, Fruauff AA, Losada RA. Cecal volvulus: The CT whirl sign. *Abdom Imaging* 1993;18:288–289.

Moore CJ, Corl FM, Fishman EK: CT of cecal volvulus: Unraveling the image. *AJR* 2001;177:95–98.

Perrer RS, Kunberger LE: Cecal volvulus. *AJR* 1998;171:860.

Rabinovici R, Simansky DA, Kaplan O, et al.: Cecal volvulus. *Dis Colon Rectum* 1990;33:765–769.

Wright TP, Max MH: Cecal volvulus: Review of 12 cases. *South Med J* 1988;81:1233–1235.

Toxic Megacolon

Beaugerie L, Ngo Y, Goujard F, et al.: Etiology and management of toxic megacolon in patients with human immunodeficiency virus infection. *Gastroenterology* 1994;107:858–863.

(Patients had CMV colitis or pseudomembranous colitis. Mortality was 80%.)

Sheth SG, LaMont JT: Toxic megacolon. *Lancet* 1998;351:509–513.

Abdominal Radiology: Patient 3

Abdominal pain and vomiting in a middle-aged man with history of alcoholism

A 51-year-old man presented to the ED with progressive abdominal pain of one day's duration. He had not eaten all day and had vomited twice. There was no associated diarrhea or melena.

He had a history of alcoholic hepatitis, COPD, and surgical repair of a colonic-bladder fistula 10 years earlier. He had mild constipation and abdominal discomfort for the past few months.

On examination, the patient was in moderate distress due to abdominal pain. Vital signs: blood pressure 130/70 mm Hg; pulse 118 beats/min; respirations 24 breaths/min; temperature 100.8° F (rectal).

His abdomen was distended but soft, with mild diffuse tenderness and no rebound tenderness. His stool was negative for occult blood. He was anicteric.

The initial chest and abdominal radiographs were interpreted as negative (Figure 1A–C). Upon his return from the radiology suite, he vomited dark bilious material that tested positive for blood. A nasogastric tube was inserted. Because of concern that he might have a perforated peptic ulcer, 300 mL of air was insufflated via a nasogastric tube and the upright abdominal radiograph was repeated (Figure 1D). The air noted under the left hemidiaphragm was interpreted as being in the patient's distended stomach.

Two hours later, an abdominal CT was performed that revealed the correct diagnosis.

The diagnosis was evident on the initial radiographs (Figure 1).

- What do they show?

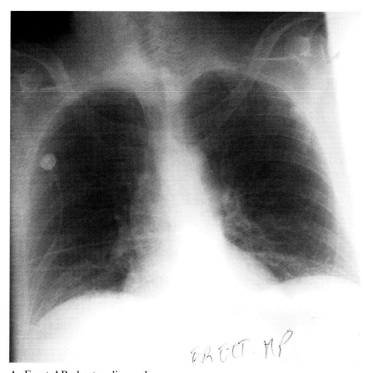

A. Erect AP chest radiograph

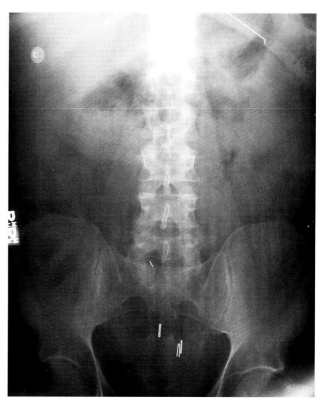

B. Supine abdomen

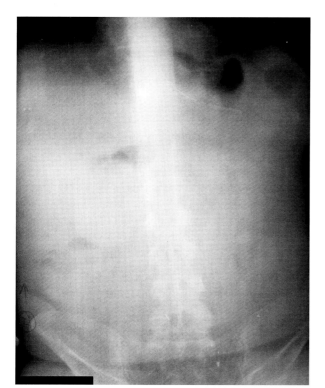

C. Upright abdomen

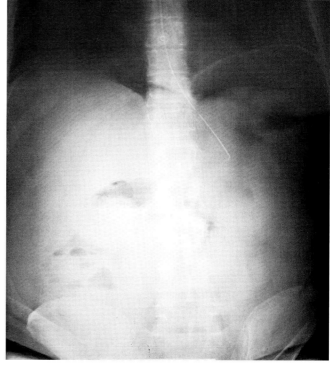

D. Upright abdomen repeated after insufflation of 300 mL air via a nasogastric tube

FIGURE 1

AIR THAT IS FREE ISN'T ALWAYS EASY TO SEE

Detection of free intraperitoneal air (**pneumoperitoneum**) is one of the principal uses of radiography in patients with abdominal pain. Pneumoperitoneum is nearly always due to perforation of the gastrointestinal tract, and virtually all patients require surgery. In 80–90% of cases, free intraperitoneal air is due to a **perforated peptic ulcer.** An upright chest radiograph is the preferred imaging test because it readily detects free air under the diaphragm.

Radiography to detect free intraperitoneal air in indicated in patients suspected of having a perforated peptic ulcar. The patient typically presents with an abrupt onset of severe abdominal pain. The abdomen is diffusely tender with rigidity and rebound tenderness. In many patients, there is no history of prior peptic ulcer disease.

In most cases, the clinical and radiographic findings are obvious, and radiography serves to confirm the diagnosis. Diagnostic difficulty arises when the clinical presentation is muted, particularly in elderly or debilitated patients, or when the radiographic findings are subtle (Cina et al. 1994). Although radiography can detect small amounts of free air, not all cases of peptic ulcer perforation show free air—sensitivity may be as low as 60% (Lee et al. 1993, Maull and Reath 1984).

Other disorders can cause free intraperitoneal air. Cecal perforation in patients with large bowel obstruction is most common (Table 1). Cecal perforation can be distinguished from peptic ulcer perforation both clinically and radiographically by the presence of markedly distended air-filled bowel (see Figure 11 on p.198). Bowel perforation associated with appendicitis or diverticulitis does not usually result in free intraperitoneal air because the extraluminal gas is contained within inflammatory tissue adjacent to the perforation. Nonetheless, in patients with right or left lower quadrant pain, these diagnoses should be considered (see Figure 13 on p.198).

Rare causes of pneumoperitoneum that do not require surgery include rupture of *pneumatosis cystoides intestinalis* (a benign form of bowel wall gas) or air insufflation into the female pelvic organs (Rowe et al. 1998, Freeman 1970, Maltz 2001). In these circumstances, the patient should have minimal abdominal pain and tenderness. Finally, free air is usually present for 3-7 days following an abdominal surgical procedure, and may persist for as long as 2-3 weeks.

Certain radiographic findings can potentially be misinterpreted as pneumoperitoneum and caution must exercised so that unnecessary surgery is not performed (Table 2) (see Figures 14-17 on p.199-200).

Radiography may fail to reveal free air when a perforation is quickly sealed by overlying omentum, when perforation occurs into the lesser sac, when the released air is loculated by peritoneal adhesions, or when small bowel, which normally contains little air, is perforated. CT can often detect these small collections of extraluminal air. Insufflation of air via an NG tube can increase the rate of detection of a perforated peptic ulcer.

Chest Radiography

The best radiographic view for detecting free intraperitoneal air is the **upright chest radiograph.** This was demonstrated by Miller in 1971. Pneumoperitoneum appears as extraluminal air under the diaphragm. In an experiment, Miller had an assistant inject successively smaller quantities of air into his lower abdomen. He determined that by using optimal technique, the chest radiograph can detect as little as 1 ml of free intraperitoneal air (Miller et al. 1971 and 1980).

The chest radiograph is better than an upright abdominal radiograph for detecting subdiaphragmatic air for two reasons. First, on an upright chest radiograph, the x-ray beam is centered near the diaphragm rather than the midabdomen, and is therefore parallel to the intra-abdominal air/fluid level (Figure 2). Second, abdominal radiographs are exposed for soft tissues and subdiaphragmatic air is therefore overpenetrated (too dark) and not visible (Figure 3).

TABLE 1

Causes of Free Intraperitoneal Air

Perforated peptic ulcer (usually duodenal)

Gastric ulcer perforation (benign or malignant)

Large bowel obstruction causing cecal perforation

Cecal or sigmoid volvulus

Perforated appendicitis or diverticulitis (infrequent)

Colonoscopy and biopsy

Residual postoperative gas

Ruptured pneumatosis cystoides intestinalis

Extension from pneumomediastinum

TABLE 2

Radiographic Findings That Mimic Free Air

Hepatodiaphragmantic interposition of the colon

   Idiopathic (Chilaiditi's syndrome)

   Secondary to colonic distention (obstruction or ileus)

Rib margin that parallels diaphragm

Perihepatic fat

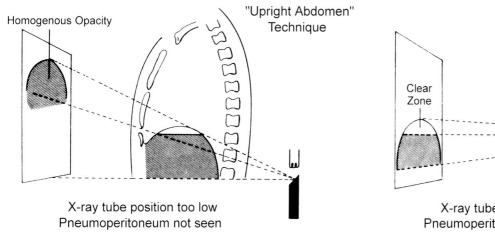
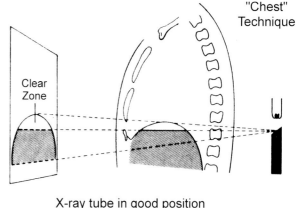

A   B

FIGURE 2   An upright chest radiograph is better than an upright abdominal radiograph to detect free air under the diaphragm.

(A) On an upright abdomen view, the x-ray beam is oblique to the air/fluid interface, which is therefore not well visualized. The radiograph is exposed for soft tissues and so air is overpenetrated (too dark).

(B) Using upright chest technique, the air/fluid level is parallel to the x-ray beam and the air collection is readily distinguished from the abdominal soft tissues. In addition, the radiograph is exposed to show air-filled structures.

[From Miller RE, Nelson SW: *AJR* 1971;112:574–585. Reprinted with permission from the American Journal of Roentgenology.]

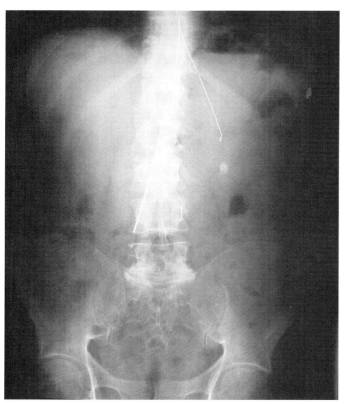
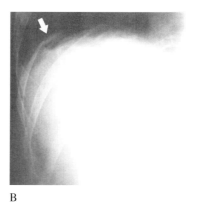

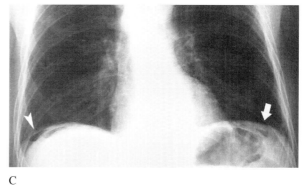

A   C

B

FIGURE 3   Free air under the diaphragm is seen better on an upright chest radiograph than an upright abdominal radiograph.

A 42-year-old man presented with abrupt onset of diffuse abdominal pain. He had no history of peptic ulcer disease.

The upright abdominal radiograph is negative (A). However, when closely inspected using a lightened view (B), free air under the right hemidiaphragm is possibly present (*arrow*). Subdiaphragmatic air is difficult to see because the region is overpenetrated (too dark) and the x-ray beam is obliquely oriented at this level.

The chest radiograph (C) clearly shows free air on the right (*arrowhead*). Free air may be present on the left, although this is difficult to distinguish from air in the stomach (*arrow*).

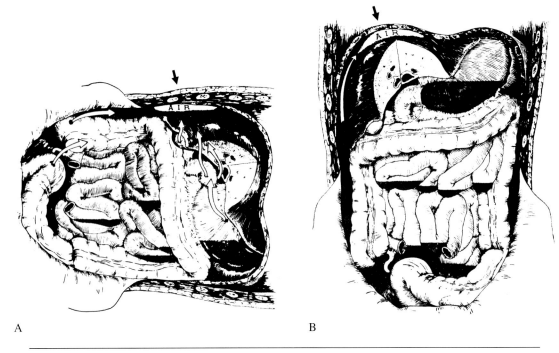

A   B

FIGURE 4   In the left lateral decubitus position (*A*), free air rises to the right side of the abdomen (*arrow*). (This is also the positioning for a left lateral decubitus abdominal radiograph.)

When the patient assumes an upright position (*B*), the free air rises to the space between the liver and right hemidiaphragm (*arrow*), where it is readily detected on an upright chest radiograph.

[From: Miller RE, Nelson SW: *AJR* 1971;112:574–585.]

Free air under the right hemidiaphragm is readily identified because that region is mostly occupied by the uniform soft tissue of the liver. Free air under the *left hemidiaphragm* is often impossible to distinguish from air within the stomach (Figure 3B). If free air is suspected under the left hemidiaphragm, the patient can be placed in the left lateral decubitus position (left side down) for several minutes, which causes the intraperitoneal air to migrate to the right side. The upright chest film is then repeated to visualize the air under the right hemidiaphragm. This was the technique used by Miller to detect small amounts of free intraperitoneal air (Figure 4). If the patient is too ill to assume an upright position, an abdominal radiograph should be obtained while the patient is in the left lateral decubitus position (left side down) (see Figure 8 on p.195).

- **Why was free intraperitoneal air not seen on this patient's chest radiograph?**

Although the upright chest radiograph is the most sensitive view for detecting free air, it must be done with proper technique to be effective. The patient should be standing or sitting *upright* and the x-ray beam should be directed *horizontally.*

This patient was not in a full upright position. The chest radiograph was an AP portable view taken while the patient was sitting "semi-erect" on the stretcher (not supine, but not fully upright), and the x-ray beam was directed downwards (Figure 1A).

Patient Outcome

On this patient's **upright abdominal radiograph,** subdiaphragmatic air can be seen, although the findings are subtle

(Figure 5). One place to look for free air is the "**middle dome of the diaphragm**"—a relatively flat region of the diaphragm that crosses the midline anteriorly. This portion of the diaphragm is not usually visible because both the heart and adjacent abdominal soft tissues have the same radiographic density. Free air under the middle dome of the diaphragm appears as a crescent-shaped air collection crossing the midline at the level of the lower thoracic vertebrae—the **cupola sign** (Grassi et al. 2004, Marshall 2006). It can be seen on an upright abdominal view, or an upright or supine chest radiograph.

Free air under the middle dome of the diaphragm was present in this patient's radiographs both before and after air was insufflated into his stomach (Figures 5A and B). Air under the left hemidiaphragm after NG tube insufflation (Figure 5B) could not be distinguished with certainty from air in a distended stomach (Figure 6). A second chest radiograph would likely have disclosed free air on the right side if it were properly performed in an upright position. Another case of air under the "middle dome" of the diaphragm is shown for comparison (Figure 7).

The **abdominal CT** performed several hours after his arrival revealed a large amount of free air in the upper abdomen, predominantly loculated under the left hemidiaphragm (Figure 5C).

The patient underwent emergency exploratory laparotomy. Copious purulent material was found in the abdomen and a large perforated gastric ulcer was noted in the posterior wall of the stomach. A subtotal gastrectomy with Billroth II gastrojejunostomy was performed. The ulcer was benign.

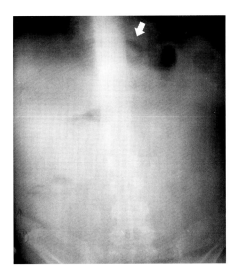

FIGURE 5A   Free air under the "middle dome" of the diaphragm in the Patient 3's first upright abdominal radiograph (*arrow*) – the cupola sign

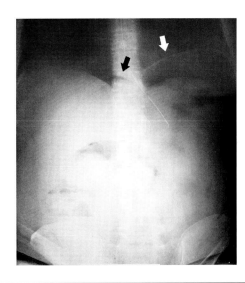

FIGURE 5B   After insufflation of air via the NG tube, free air is again seen under the "middle dome" of the diaphragm (*black arrow*).

Air under the left hemidiaphragm cannot be clearly distinguished from air in a distended stomach (*white arrow*) (see Figure 6).

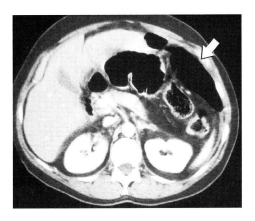

FIGURE 5C   CT in Patient 3 showing free air in the left upper quadrant (*arrow*).

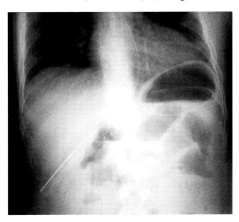

FIGURE 6   In another patient, air in a distended stomach is difficult to distinguish from free air under the left hemidiaphragm (compare with Figure 5B).

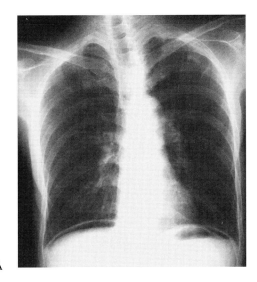

A

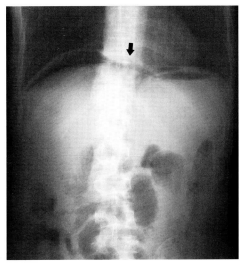

B

FIGURE 7   In another patient with a perforated peptic ulcer, a large amount of free air is seen on the chest radiograph (*A*).

On the upright abdominal radiograph (*B*), free air is visible under the middle dome of the diaphragm—the cupola sign (*arrow*).

Other Radiographic Techniques That Can Detect Free Intraperitoneal Air

When a patient suspected of having a perforated peptic ulcer is unable to be positioned for an upright chest radiograph, a **left lateral decubitus abdominal view** should be obtained. The patient lies with the left side down and an AP abdominal view is obtained (Figure 4A). In this position, free intraperitoneal air collects between the right side of the liver and the ribs. The air may also collect in the region of the right iliac crest.

The radiograph should be exposed using a horizontal x-ray beam and with low penetration ("chest technique"). If the radiograph is taken using "abdominal technique" (greater penetration to visualize abdominal soft tissues), the areas where extraluminal air collects will be over-penetrated (too dark) and the image must be viewed with a "bright light" or lighter monitor setting to detect free intraperitoneal air (Figure 8).

A number of other techniques are useful to detect free intraperitoneal air (Table 3). Occasionally, free air is visible only on the **lateral chest radiograph** (Figure 9). This occurs when the intraperitoneal air has not migrated to the apex of the diaphragm (Markowitz and Ziter 1986, Woodring and Heiser 1995).

A **pneumogastrogram** entails insufflation of 200–400 mL of air into the stomach using an NG tube (Figure 10). This increases the size of the pneumoperitoneum and, in two reports, increased the yield of radiography from 60% to 90% (Lee et al. 1993, Maull and Reath 1984).

The **supine abdominal radiograph** can show signs of a massive pneumoperitoneum (Levine et al. 1991). In the *double bowel wall sign* (*Rigler sign*), both the inner and outer sides of the bowel wall are visible because they are outlined by intra- and extraluminal air, respectively (Figure 11 and Patient 2, Figure 9 on page 175).

Free air underlying the inferior surface of the liver highlights in the falciform ligament or in the space between the left and right hepatic lobes forming a triangular shadow called the **Doge's cap sign.** Air that collects anterior to the liver when the patient is supine appears as a lucent area overlying the liver (Figure 12) (Baker 1998, Baker 2000, Menuck and Siemers 1976).

Finally, free air under the "middle dome" of the diaphragm appears as the **cupola sign** on a supine or upright abdominal radiograph (Figure 5).

Computed tomography is highly sensitive at detecting free intraperitoneal air (Stapakis and Thickman 1992, Jeffrey et al. 1983, Maniatis et al. 2000, Rubesin and Levine 2003). Free air collects anterior to the liver since the patient is supine (Figure 12B) and at the porta hepatis (adjacent to the duodenum) (Figure 9D). Intraperitoneal air is more easily identified when the CT images are displayed using brighter ("lung window") setting in which fat and soft tissues appear light gray and are therefore easier to distinguish from air which appears black (Figure 13). When disorders such as perforated appendicitis or diverticulitis are suspected as causes of pneumoperitoneum, the surgeon may elect to obtain CT before performing surgery.

TABLE 3

Imaging Useful in Detecting Free Intraperitoneal Air

Upright chest radiograph

Left lateral decubitus abdominal radiograph

Lateral chest radiograph

Pneumogastrogram—NG air insufflation

Supine abdominal radiograph (massive free air)

CT

Ultrasonography

Bedside **ultrasonography** can potentially be used to detect pneumoperitoneum. Air between the liver and inner surface of the abdominal wall appears as a bright reverberation or "ring-down" artifact in the midepigastrium (supine position) or right epigastric region (left lateral decubitus position). One investigator found high sensitivity (93%), but only moderate specificity (64%) (Chen et al. 2002). (Ring-down artifact is discussed in Patient 5 on page 213.)

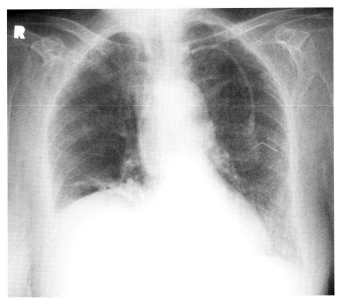

A. AP Chest radiograph.

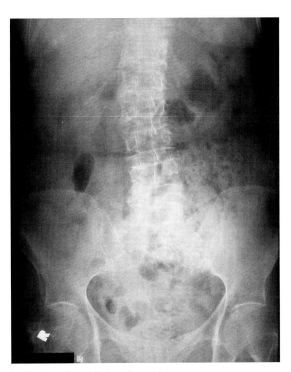

B. Supine abdominal radiograph

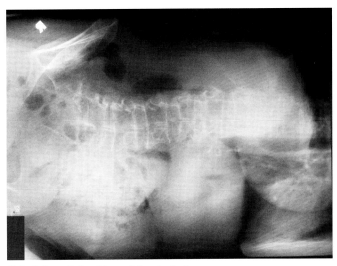

C Left lateral decubitus abdominal view.

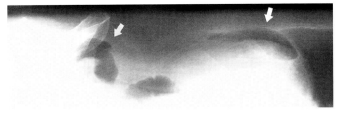

D Detail.

FIGURE 8   Pneumoperitoneum diagnosed on left lateral decubitus radiograph.

(A) A 48-year-old woman with metastatic ovarian cancer presented with abdominal pain of one day's duration. The chest radiograph showed linear atelectasis at the base of the right lung and elevation of the hemidiaphragm. No free air was visible, although this was not an upright radiograph. A MediPort is present on the left.

(B) Supine abdominal radiograph was normal.

(C) The patient was too weak to stand for upright abdominal or chest

radiographs and so a left lateral decubitus abdominal view was obtained instead. It was initially interpreted as negative for free air. However, the radiograph was exposed using "abdominal (soft tissue) technique" rather than "lung technique," resulting in overpenetration along the right lateral abdominal wall.

(D) When the radiograph was re-examined using a lightened image, free air was visible adjacent to the liver and the right iliac crest (*arrows*).

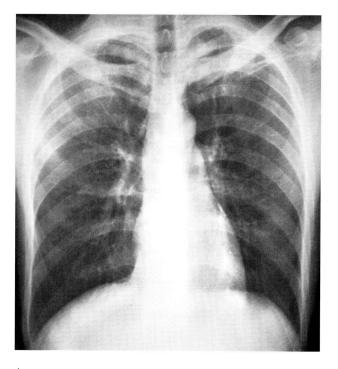

A

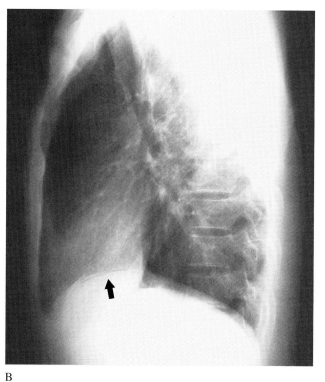

B

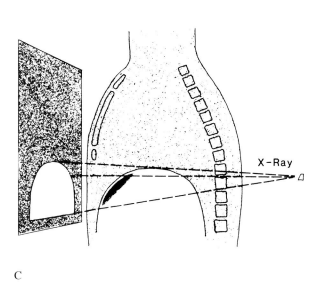

C

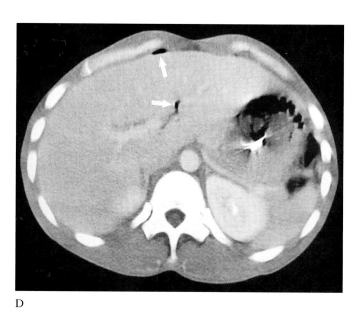

D

FIGURE 9   Pneumoperitoneum seen on a lateral chest radiograph and abdominal CT.

A 30-year-old male complained of abdominal pain after smoking "crack" cocaine.

(A) The upright chest radiograph failed to show free air.

(B) A small amount of free air was visible on the lateral radiograph (*black arrow*).

(C) Free air that has not risen to the apex of the diaphragm may only be visible on a lateral chest radiograph.

(D) A CT scan was performed to confirm the diagnosis prior to laparotomy. Free air is seen anterior to the liver (*upper white arrow*) and at the porta hepatis (*lower white arrow*). The porta hepatis is adjacent to the duodenum and is a common site to see pneumoperitoneum due to a perforated peptic ulcer.

[C from: Markowitz SK, Ziter FHM: The lateral chest film and pneumoperitoneum. *Ann Emerg Med* 1986;15:425–427, with permission.]

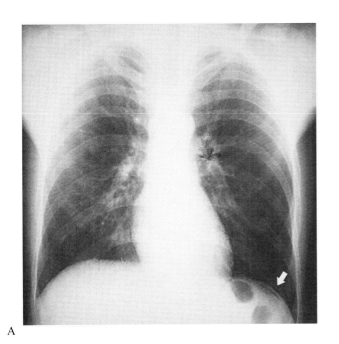
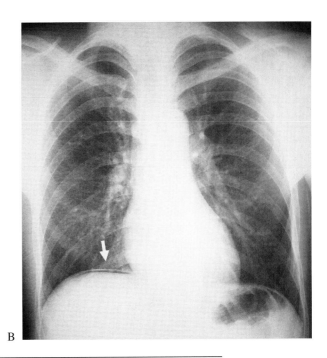

A

B

FIGURE 10   Free air revealed by air insufflation via a nasogastric tube—Pneumogastrogram.

(*A*) The initial chest radiograph did not clearly reveal subdiaphragmatic air. There was a crescent of air under the left hemidiaphragm suspicious for pneumoperitoneum (*arrow*).

(*B*) A second chest radiograph obtained after insufflation of 300 ml of air through a nasogastric tube clearly showed pneumoperitoneum on the right (*arrow*).

Alternatively, the patient could have been placed in a left lateral decubitus position for 10 to 15 minutes so the intraperitoneal air would migrate to the right side of the abdomen, and then repeat an upright chest radiograph (see Figure 4).

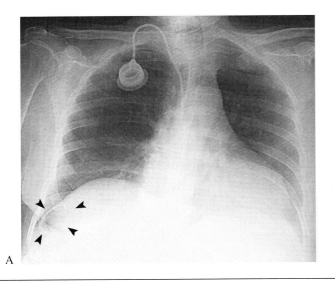
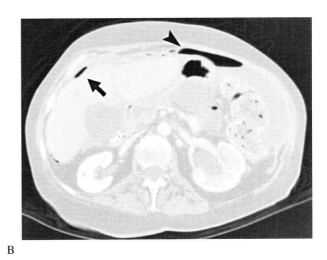

A

B

FIGURE 12   Right upper quadrant gas on a semierect chest radiograph.

(*A*) Gas is present overlying the lateral margin of the liver (*arrowheads*). This was suspicious for pneumoperitoneum, although it was initially misinterpeted as an overlying loop of bowel.

(*B*) CT confirmed that this was pneumoperitoneum (*arrow*). Free air is also present over the stomach (*arrowhead*). (A lung window image is shown.)

The patient was a 50-year-old woman with a history of ovarian cancer who presented with an abrupt onset of severe abdominal pain. At surgery, there was diffuse carcinomatosis and perforation of the rectum at the site of a carcinomatous implant.

A left lateral decubitus abdominal view would have been a less time consuming way to confirm the presence of pneumoperitoneum (see Figure 8).

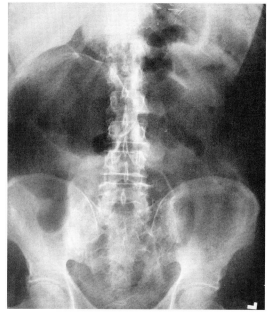

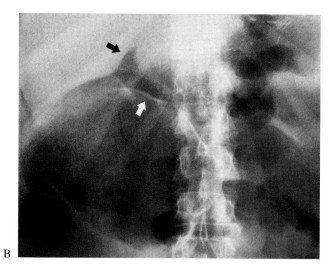

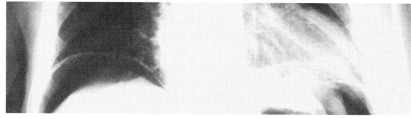

FIGURE 11   Massive free air seen on an abdominal radiograph in a patient with perforated cecal volvulus.

(A) In a patient who presented to the ED with abdominal pain and distention, the supine abdominal radiograph showed a markedly dilated segment of bowel in the right upper abdomen suggestive of cecal volvulus.

(B) A closer view of the right upper quadrant reveals extensive free intraperitoneal air. Both sides of the bowel wall are visible (*white arrow*). The inner surface of the bowel wall is outlined by intraluminal gas and the outer surface by extraluminal gas—the "double bowel wall sign" (Rigler sign).

In addition, free air under the liver outlines in the inferior edge of the liver. A triangular indentation between the left and right hepatic lobes is known as the **Doge's cap sign** because its shape is reminiscent of the hat worn by the rulers of early renaissance Venice (*black arrow*).

These findings on a supine abdominal view are especially useful when a patient is too ill to obtain upright views of the chest or abdomen. In this patient, the upright chest radiograph confirmed the presence of a large amount of free intraperitoneal air (C).

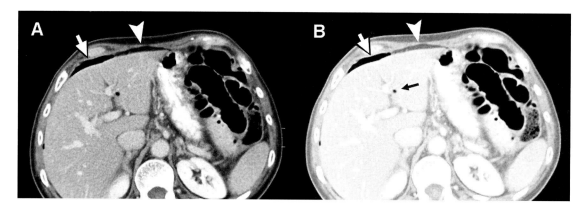

FIGURE 13   CT detection of free intraperitoneal air—Lung windows.

(A) On **soft tissue windows**, free intraperitoneal air (*arrow*) is difficult to distinguish from intraperitoneal fat (*arrowhead*).

(B) On **lung windows,** air (*arrow*) is easily distinguished as being more radiolucent (darker) than fat (*arrowhead*). A small collection of air is also seen in the porta hepatis (*small black arrow*).

The patient was a 70-year-old woman who presented with right lower quadrant pain and fever. CT revealed perforated appendicitis and pneumoperitoneum.

Chest Radiographic Findings That Can Mimic Free Intraperitoneal Air

There are several chest radiograph findings that can mimic free air under the diaphragm. These include a rib margin or discoid atelectasis that parallels the surface of the diaphragm, interposition of bowel between the liver and diaphragm (Chilaiditi syndrome), and abundant subphrenic fat (Figures 14–17). With severe colonic distention (ileus or volvulus), the colon may be seen under the right hemidiaphragm, mimicking pneumoperitoneum.

Caution must be exercised so that abdominal surgery is not performed unnecessarily in such patients (Figure 17).

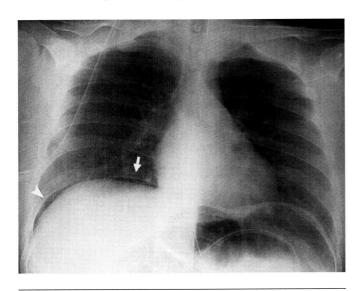

FIGURE 14 Subdiaphragmatic air mimicked by the inferior margin of a rib (arrow). By following the inferior margin of the rib to the lateral chest wall (*arrowhead*), it can be determined that this is not free air.

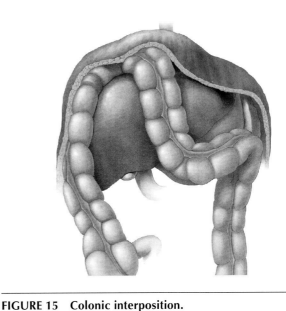

FIGURE 15   Colonic interposition.

The hepatic flexure of the colon has migrated superior to the liver. This can mimic free air under the right hemidiaphragm on a chest radiograph.

[From Horton, et al: CT evaluation of the colon: Inflammatory disease. *RadioGraphics* 2000;20:399–418, with permission.]

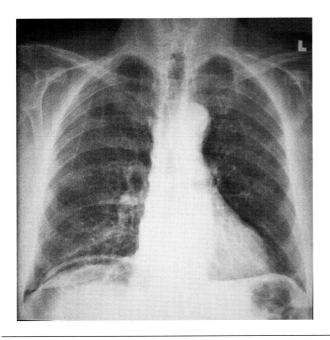

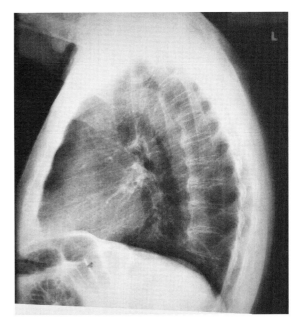

FIGURE 16   Free air mimicked by colonic interposition—Chilaiditi syndrome.

(*A*) A collection of air under the right hemidiaphragm could be mistaken for pneumoperitoneum. However, the air collection has a tubular appearance, the superior margin is thicker than the diaphragm alone, and there are indentations suggestive of intraluminal bowel gas.

(*B*) The lateral view confirms that bowel is interposed between the anterior portion of the liver and the diaphragm.

Colonic interposition is often transient. The clinical scenario usually helps clarify that this is not pneumoperitoneum, i.e., the patient does not have significant abdominal pain. Chilaiditi syndrome is occasionally associated with abdominal pain, and rarely with colonic volvulus.

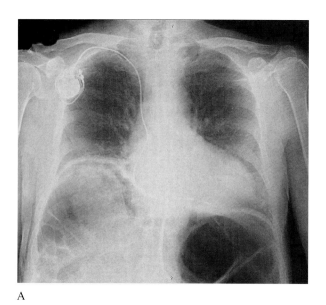

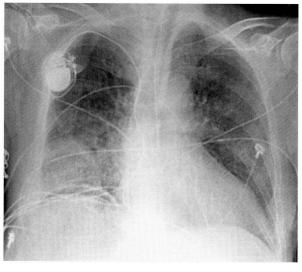

A   B

FIGURE 17   Free air mimicked by colonic distention due to ileus.

A 79-year-old man with dementia presented with abdominal distention but no abdominal tenderness. The initial chest radiograph was suspicious for free air under the right hemidiaphragm, but also showed colonic distention (A). A second chest radiograph obtained a few hours later seemed to show free air under the right hemidiaphragm (B). Colonic distention was not visible on this more limited view and it was interpreted as pneumoperitoneum.

The patient was taken to the operating room. Colonic ileus without perforation was found. Clues to the absence of perforation were the relatively benign clinical presentation and the associated colonic distention. A CT scan would have confirmed the absence of perforation. Post-operative testing did not detect a colonic lesion (malignant or stricture) as a cause of colonic distention.

SUGGESTED READING

Cina SJ, Mims WW, Nichols CA, Conradi SE: From emergency room to morgue: Deaths due to undiagnosed perforated peptic ulcers: Report of four cases and review of the literature. *Am J Forensic Med Pathol* 1994;15:21–27.

Freeman RK: Pneumoperitoneum from oral-genital insufflation. *Obstet Gynecol* 1970;36:162–163.

Gayer G, Hertz M, Zissin R: Postoperative pneumoperitoneum: Prevalence, duration, and possible significance. *Semin Ultrasound CT MRI* 2004;25:286–289.

Kane E, Fried G, McSherry CK: Perforated peptic ulcer in the elderly. *J Am Geriatr Soc* 1981;29:224–227.

Maltz C: Benign pneumoperitoneum and pneumatosis intestinalis. *Am J Emerg Med* 2001;19:242.

Rowe NM, Kahn FB, Acinapura AJ, Cunningham JN: Nonsurgical pneumoperitoneum: A case report and review. *Am Surg* 1998; 64:313–318.

Miller RE, Becker GJ, Slabaugh RD: Detection of pneumoperitoneum: Optimum body position and respiratory phase. *AJR* 1980;135:487–490.

Miller RE, Nelson SW: The roentgenologic demonstration of tiny amounts of free intraperitoneal gas: Experimental and clinical studies. *AJR* 1971;112:574–585.

Shaffer HA: Perforation and obstruction of the gastrointestinal tract: Assessment by conventional radiology. *Radiol Clin North Am* 1992;30:405–426.

Spates MJ, Schwartz, DT, Savitt D: Abdominal imaging. In Schwartz DT, Reisdorff EJ, ed. *Emergency Radiology*. McGraw-Hill, 2000.

Woodring JH, Heiser MJ: Detection of pneumoperitoneum on chest radiographs: Comparison of upright lateral and posteroanterior projections. *AJR* 1995;165:45–47. (In 20% of cases, free air was seen only on the lateral CXR.)

Chest Radiography

Butler J: Detection of pneumoperitoneum on erect chest radiograph. *Emerg Med J* 2002;12:46–47.

Cho KC, Baker SR: Extraluminal air: Diagnosis and significance. *Radiol Clin North Am* 1994;32:829–845.

Grassi R, Romano S, Pinto A, Romano L: Gastro-duodenal perforation: Conventional plain film, US and CT findings in 166 consecutive patients. *Eur J Radiol* 2004;50:30–36.

Markowitz SK, Ziter FMH: The lateral chest film and pneumoperitoneum. *Ann Emerg Med* 1986;15:425–427. (In 14% of cases, free air was seen only on the lateral film.)

Marshall GB: The cupola sign. *Radiology* 2006;241:623–624.

Abdominal Radiography

Baker SR, Cho KC: *The Abdominal Plain Film,* 2nd ed. McGraw-Hill, 1999.

Baker SR: The uppermost abdomen in the recumbent patient: The last neglected area in radiology. *Emerg Radiol* 1998;5:411–415.

Baker SR: Pneumoperitoneum and the plain film: The need to see all of the abdomen. *Emerg Radiol* 2000;7:298–301.

Levine MS, Scheiner JD, Rubesin SE, et at:. Diagnosis of pneumoperitoneum on supine abdominal radiographs. *AJR* 1991;156:731–735.

Abdominal Radiology: Patient 4

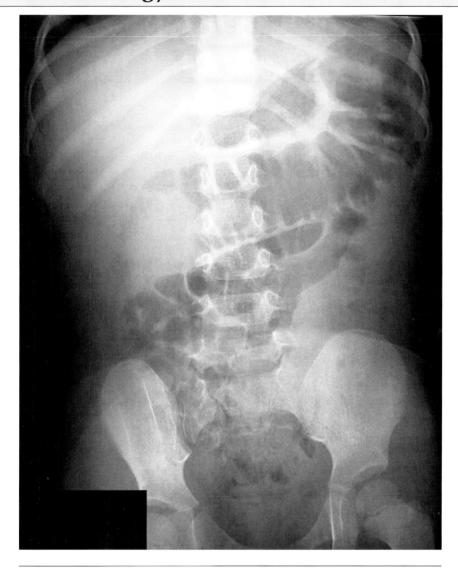

FIGURE 1

A 2-year old girl with intermittent abdominal pain and vomiting

A 2-year-old girl presented to the ED with intermittent abdominal pain that began 18 hours earlier.

The previous evening, she had an episode of abdominal pain accompanied by a large bowel movement. During the night and following day, she had several bouts of abdominal pain. Her oral intake was poor and she vomited after eating. Late that afternoon, her mother brought her to the ED.

The child had been in good health. At age 4 months, she was brought to the ED for abdominal pain, which resolved over several hours. A medical evaluation at that time was normal.

In the ED, her vital signs were: pulse 114 beats/min, respiratory rate 24 breaths/min, and temperature 100.1°F (rectal).

The child appeared well. Her abdomen was soft and nondistended. There was minimal right lower quadrant tenderness with no rebound tenderness or palpable mass. Stool was guiac negative. The child would not eat or drink and was admitted to the hospital for observation. An abdominal radiograph was interpreted as showing a nonspecific bowel gas pattern (Figure 1).

During the night, the child had intermittent episodes of abdominal pain during which she was doubled-over with her legs flexed. In between these episodes, she was comfortable.

- Was an abdominal radiograph indicated in this patient?

- How would you interpret the radiograph?

- Are further diagnostic tests needed?

THE CRESCENT SIGN

In an adult patient with abdominal pain, the principal indication for abdominal radiography is to detect mechanical bowel obstruction. The role of radiography in children with abdominal pain is less certain.

Intussusception is the most common cause of intestinal obstruction in children between the ages of 6 months and 2 years. However, the radiographic findings of intussusception are different from those of mechanical small bowel obstruction.

Diagnostic difficulty with intussusception is due to its variable **clinical presentation**. The classic triad of intussusception consists of intermittent crampy abdominal pain, vomiting, and bloody stools ("currant jelly"). A soft tissue mass may be palpable in the right side of the abdomen, especially during episodes of pain. However, the triad is present in only a minority of cases, and bloody stool, a late sign, is seen in only few cases. The child often appears well between episodes of pain. In some cases, there is no abdominal pain, and the child presents only with listlessness or irritability. Most cases occur between the ages of 6 months and 2 years—60% occur in children younger than 1 year of age and 80% in children younger than 2 years.

Knowledge of the **pathologic anatomy** of intussusception helps in understanding its radiographic features. *Ileocolic intussusception* occurs in about 85% of cases (Figure 2A). The distal ileum invaginates into the cecum and enters the ascending colon. The intussusceptum may extend into the transverse colon or as far as the descending or sigmoid colon.

In most cases, there is no discrete lead point. Intussusception is often associated with an antecedent viral infection causing enlargement of intestinal mucosal lymphoid tissue (Peyer's patches). In neonates, older children, and adults, there is usually an inciting lesion such as a polyp or intramural hematoma.

Ileoileal intussusception occurs in a small number of cases and can be difficult to diagnose. A mass at the lead point is usually present (Figure 2B).

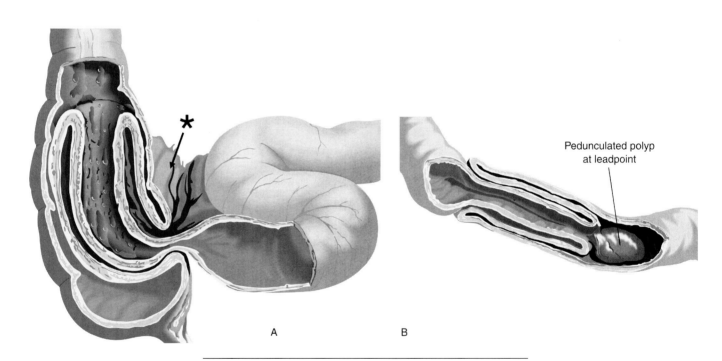

Pedunculated polyp
at leadpoint

A   B

FIGURE 2   Pathologic anatomy of intussusception.

(*A*) Ileocolic intussusception—85% of cases.

  The invaginating mesentery (*asterisk*) is incorporated into the intussusception.

(*B*) Ileoileal intussusception.

Imaging Modalities

The role of **abdominal radiography** in children suspected of having intussusception is controversial. Definitive radiographic signs are seen infrequently and are difficult to identify with certainty. Furthermore, "negative" radiographs do not exclude the diagnosis, although the finding of gas or feces in the cecum argues against intussusception. Nonetheless, radiography is readily available and suggestive findings are present in about 50% of cases.

When intussusception is suspected clinically, a definitive diagnostic test should be ordered irrespective of the radiographic findings. However, in this patient, radiographic signs of intussusception were present and, had they been recognized, a diagnosis might have been made earlier.

The test of choice in suspected intussusception is **contrast enema** because it is both diagnostic and therapeutic. Dilute barium, water-soluble contrast, or air can be used. The contrast enema reliably confirms the diagnosis of intussusception. In addition, reduction of the intussusception can be accomplished in 80–90% of patients using a contrast enema.

Ultrasonography has a more definite role than conventional radiography because it can directly visualize the intussusception (Figures 3 and 4). With experienced operators, sonography has a sensitivity of 98–100% (del Pozo et al. 1999). In addition, sonography has been used to assist reduction of the intussusception using a saline enema technique that avoids exposing the patient to radiation.

Color Doppler sonography can detect lack of blood flow to bowel at the intussusception. In this case, enema reduction should be avoided or attempted with lower pressure because of an increased risk of perforation.

CT can diagnose intussusception, but is generally not used in children due to the relatively high radiation exposure. In adults, CT can detect intussusception as a cause of small bowel obstruction or abdominal mass (see Patient 1, Figure 13 on page 161).

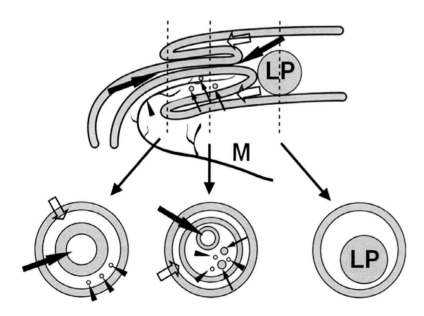

FIGURE 3   **Longitudinal and cross-sectional anatomy of an intussusception.**
The central and everted segments of the **intussusceptum** have invaginated into the outer **intussuscipiens.** Mesenteric fat, vessels (*arrowheads*), and lymph nodes (*small arrows*) have been entrained with the intussusceptum.
A rounded mass lead point is shown in this illustration (LP).
[From: Choi SH, Han JK, Kim SH, et al: Intussusception in adults: From stomach to rectum. *AJR* 2004;183:691–698. Reprinted with permission from the American Journal of Roentgenology.]

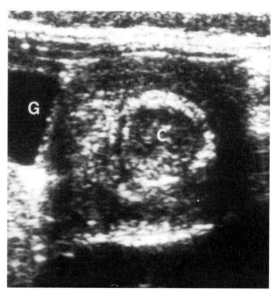

FIGURE 4   **Sonogram of intussusception—The doughnut sign.**
There are concentric sonolucent (smooth muscle) and echogenic layers (mucosa and serosa) formed by the inner intussusceptum (C) and outer intussuscipiens.
G = gallbladder.
[From del-Pozo: RadioGraphics 1999;19:299–319, with permission.]

Radiographic Signs of Intussusception

There are four principal radiographic findings of intussusception: (1) a **soft tissue mass** (absence of gas) on the right side of the abdomen; (2) the **crescent sign** (the visible head of the intussusceptum); (3) the **target sign**; and (4) **small bowel obstruction** with dilated loops of air-filled bowel (Table 1).

A **soft tissue mass** in the right abdomen is the most frequent finding. It is due to filling of the ascending colon with the intussusceptum. The soft tissue mass may obscure the inferior margin of the liver. However, a soft tissue mass can be difficult to identify with certainty and it may be seen in other disorders such as perforated appendicitis with an inflammatory mass.

In the **crescent sign**, the head of the intussusceptum is seen as an intraluminal mass within the ascending or transverse colon. Although not frequently visible, it is a reliable indicator of intussusception (Figure 6A and B).

A mechanical **small bowel obstruction** is seen in some cases, although it is a late finding. In addition, bowel distention may be due to adynamic ileus rather than obstruction, and these bowel gas patterns can be difficult to distinguish.

The **target sign** is a circle of radiolucent fat tissue within a round soft tissue mass that is seen end-on where the intussusception curves anteriorly at the hepatic flexure (Figure 5). In one series, this was identified frequently (68% of cases), although the finding can be subtle (Ratcliffe et al. 1992).

Some radiographic findings **reduce the likelihood of intussusception**. In an ileocolic intussusception, the cecum should not contain gas or feces. Therefore, the presence of gas or feces in the cecum argues against intussusception and may be used to exclude the diagnosis if there is a low clinical suspicion (likelihood ratio 0.11 for cecal feces Sargent—1994). However, this is difficult to identify reliably and, when seen, does not entirely exclude an intussusception when the clinical suspicion is moderate or high.

Patient Outcome

In this patient, the head of the intussusceptum is visible in the right upper quadrant, the **crescent sign** (Figure 6A). If these findings had been recognized, an earlier diagnosis might have been made. The next day, another abdominal radiograph was obtained that again showed a crescent sign, although it was less evident that on the previous day, as well as dilated small bowel (Figure 6B). The child underwent an air enema that confirmed the diagnosis and reduced the intussusception (Figure 6C and D).

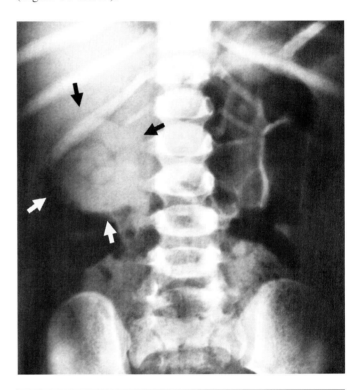

FIGURE 5   Target sign (*arrows*).
[From del-Pozo: *RadioGraphics* 1999;19:299–319, with permission.]

TABLE 1

Radiographic Signs of Intussusception*

Soft tissue mass (gasless) right side of abdomen	Common (74%), not specific
Crescent sign (head of intussusceptum)	Less common (30%) but most specific
Target sign (ring of invaginated mesenteric fat)	Seen in 68%, moderately specific
Small bowel obstruction (distended small bowel)	Seen in 40% but not specific

Signs Arguing Against Intussusception**

Gas in cecum	Likelihood ratio 0.25
Feces in cecum	Likelihood ratio 0.11

*Ratcliffe et al. 1992.
**Sargent et al. 1994 (interobserver agreement was moderate to poor).

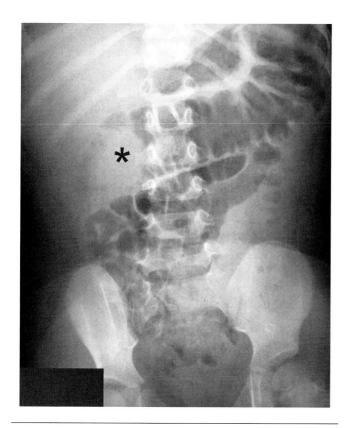

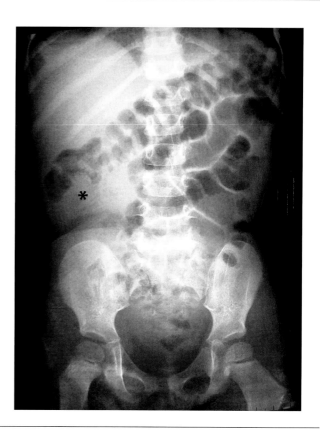

FIGURE 6A   Initial radiograph—Patient 4—The crescent sign.
The crescent-shaped head of the intussusceptum is seen as an intraluminal mass in the gas-filled transverse colon (*asterisk*).

FIGURE 6B   Radiograph the following morning.
The crescent sign is still present but less evident (*asterisk*). There are
dilated loops of small bowel suggestive of mechanical obstruction.

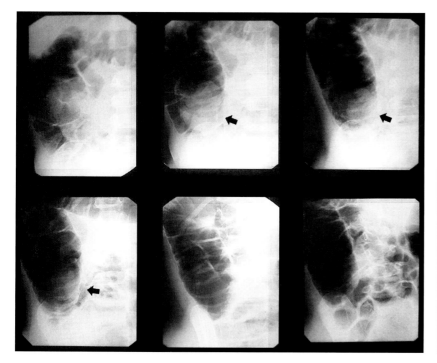

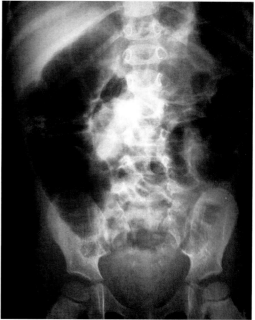

FIGURE 6C   Air enema—Patient 4.
The intussusception is progressively reduced by pressure
from the insufflated rectal air (*arrows*).

FIGURE 6D   A subsequent radiograph shows air
throughout the colon confirming successful reduction
of the intussusception.

Two Additional Patients with Intussusception

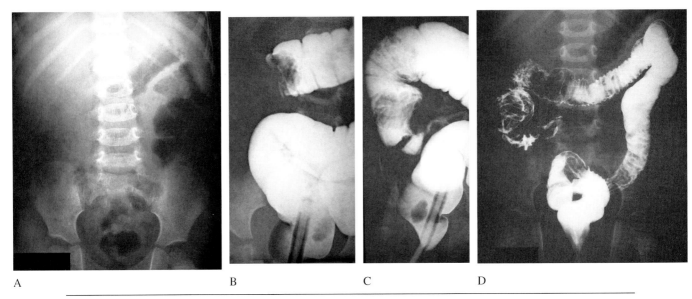

A   B   C   D

FIGURE 7   In a second patient, the initial radiograph is nonspecific (*A*). However, the right side of the abdomen is gasless, a finding suggestive of intussusception. A contrast enema shows progressive reduction of the intussusception (*B–D*).

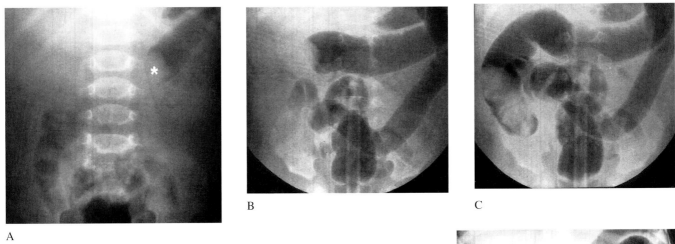

A   B   C

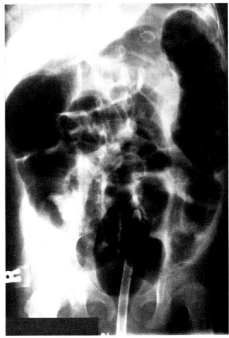

FIGURE 8   In a third patient, the initial radiograph shows a crescent sign in the left side of the transverse colon (*A, asterisk*). An air enema shows progressive reduction of the head of the intussusception (*B* and *C*). The final radiograph shows complete reduction of the intussusception with air in the ileum (*D*).

[From Schwartz DT, Reisdorff EJ. *Emergency Radiology* McGraw-Hill, 2000.]

D

SUGGESTED READING

Diagnosis and Treatment–Reduction by Contrast or Air Enema

Alford BA, McIlhenny J: The child with acute abdominal pain and vomiting. *Radiol Clin North Am* 1992;30:441–454.

del-Pozo G, Albillos JC, Tejedor D, et al.: Intussusception in children: Current concepts in diagnosis and enema reduction. *Radiographics* 1999;19:299–319.

Katz M, Phelan E, Carlin JB, Beasley SW: Gas enema for the reduction of intussusception: Relationship between clinical signs and symptoms and outcome. *AJR* 1993;160:363–366.

Kornecki A, Daneman A, Navarro O, et al.: Spontaneous reduction of intussusception: Clinical spectrum, management and outcome. *Pediatr Radiol* 2000;30:58–63.

McHugh K, Koumanidou C, Mirilas P: Intussusception in children: Observation transformed into irrefutable "fact." *AJR* 2002;179: 1348–1349.

Swischuk LE: *Emergency Radiology of the Acutely Ill or Injured Child*, 4th ed. Williams and Wilkins, 2000.

Abdominal Radiography

Carty HML: Paediatric emergencies: Non-traumatic abdominal emergencies. *Eur Radiol* 2002;12:2835–2848.

Eklof O, Hartelius H: Reliability of the abdominal plain film diagnosis in pediatric patients with suspected intussusception. *Pediatr Radiol* 1980;9:199–206.

Hernandez JA, Swischuk LE, Angel CA: Validity of plain films in intussusception. *Emerg Radiol* 2004;10:323–326.

Lee JM, Kim H, Byun JY, et al.: Intussusception: Characteristic radiolucencies on the abdominal radiograph. *Pediatr Radiol* 1994;24:293–295.

Meradji M, Hussain SM, Robben SG, Hop WC: Plain film diagnosis in intussusception. *Br J Radiol* 1994;67:147–149.

Ratcliffe JF, Fong S, Cheong I, O'Connell PO: The plain abdominal film in intussusception: The accuracy and incidence of radiographic signs. *Pediatr Radiol* 1992;22:110–111.

Ratcliffe JF, Fong S, Cheong I, O'Connell P: Plain film diagnosis of intussusception: Prevalence of the target sign. *AJR* 1992;158:619–621.

Rothrock SG, Green SM, Hummel CB: Plain abdominal radiography in the detection of major disease in children: A prospective analysis. *Ann Emerg Med* 1992;21:1423–1429.

Sargent ME, Babyn P, Alton DJ: Plain abdominal radiography in intussusception: A reassessment. *Pediatr Radiol* 1994;24:17–20.

Smith DS, Bonadio WA, Losek JD, et al.: The role of abdominal x-rays in the diagnosis and management of intussusception. *Pediatr Emerg Care* 1992;8:325–327.

White SJ, Blane CE: Intussusception: Additional observations on the plain radiograph. *AJR* 1982;139:511–513.

Ultrasonography

Munden MM, Bruzzi JF, Coley BD, Munden RF: Sonography of pediatric small-bowel intussusception: Differentiating surgical from nonsurgical cases. *AJR* 2007;188:275–279.

Tiao MM, Wan YL, Ng SH, et al.: Sonographic features of small-bowel intussusception in pediatric patients. *Acad Emerg Med* 2001;8: 368–373.

Vasavada P: Ultrasound evaluation of acute abdominal emergencies in infants and children. *Radiol Clin North Am* 2004;42:445–456.

Yoon CH, Kim HJ, Goo HW: Intussusception in children: US-guided pneumatic reduction. Initial experience. *Radiology* 2001;218: 85–88.

Computed Tomography

Choi SH, Han JK, Kim SH, et al.: Intussusception in adults: From stomach to rectum. *AJR* 2004;183:691–698.

Cox TD, Winters WD, Weinberger E: CT of intussusception in the pediatric patient: Diagnosis and pitfalls. *Pediatr Radiol* 1996;26: 26–32.

Gayer G, Hertz M, Zissin R: CT findings of intussusception in adults. *Semin Ultrasound CT MRI* 2003;24:377–386.

Warshauer DM, Lee JKT: Adult intussusception detected at CT or MR imaging: Clinical-imaging correlation. *Radiology* 1999;212:853–860.

Abdominal Radiology: Patient 5

Right upper quadrant pain in an elderly man with diabetes

A 71-year-old man presented to the ED with right upper quadrant pain of two day's duration.

The pain began as a dull ache in the midepigastrium and then moved to the right upper quadrant and right flank. He vomited several times and was unable to eat. The emesis was a watery brown material. He had a small bowel movement earlier that day.

He had a history of diabetes and hypertension and was taking glyburide and lisinopril.

He had not had prior abdominal surgery.

On examination, he was overweight and in mild distress due to abdominal discomfort. His blood pressure was 148/100 mm Hg, pulse 110 beats/min, respiratory rate 24 breaths/min, temperature 100.4°F (rectal).

He was alert and oriented. His oral mucosa was dry and sclera was anicteric. His lungs were clear and his heart was rapid and regular without a murmur.

Abdominal examination revealed diminished bowel sounds, moderate tenderness in the right upper quadrant, and a Murphy's sign. There was no tenderness on rectal examination and stool was guiac negative.

An intravenous line was started and blood specimens were obtained. Intravenous fluids, insulin, and ampicillin/sulbactam were administered.

Blood test results (units for electrolytes, mEq/L and chemistry values, mg/dL, except where noted):

WBC 19,700/mm^3, hematocrit 49%, platelets 246,000/mm^3.
Na$^+$ 132, K$^+$ 4.1, Cl$^-$ 101, CO$_2^-$ 22, BUN 24, creatinine 1.4, glucose 406.
ALT 100 U/L (normal: 7–37), AST 65 U/L, alkaline phosphatase 61 U/L (normal: 39–117), total bilirubin 1.6 (normal: 0.2–1.2), lipase 110 U/L (normal).

A bedside sonogram was performed and the gallbladder could not be confidently identified. The patient was sent to the radiology department for another abdominal ultrasound study. Selected ultrasound images, including the right upper quadrant, are shown in Figure 1.

- What is this patient's likely diagnosis?

  Hint: Under what circumstances would cholecystitis be difficult to diagnose by ultrasound?

  (What tissue characteristics are disadvantageous for sonographic visualization?)

The correct diagnosis can be confirmed by another simple imaging test.

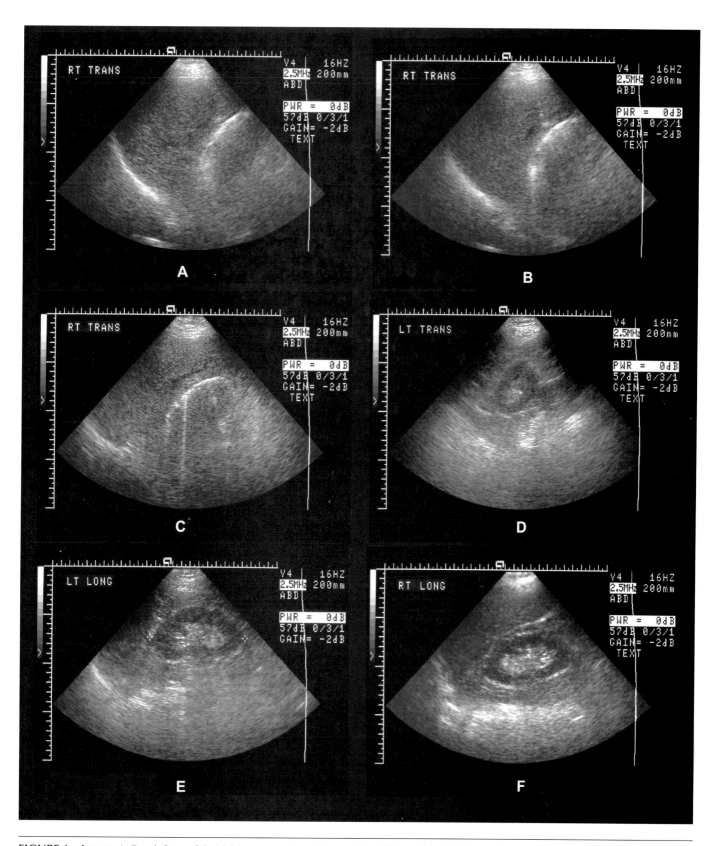

FIGURE 1 Images *A*, *B* and *C* are of the right upper quadrant. Images *D* and *E* are of the left kidney. Image *F* is of the right kidney.

Typical Sonographic Appearance of Gallstones

Gallstones have anatomical characteristics that are advantageous for detection by ultrasonography—a sonolucent fluid-filled sac (the gallbladder) contains an echogenic object (the gallstone). The gallstone is so highly echogenic that the ultrasound beam is entirely reflected and the gallstone casts an *acoustic shadow* (Figures 2 and 3).

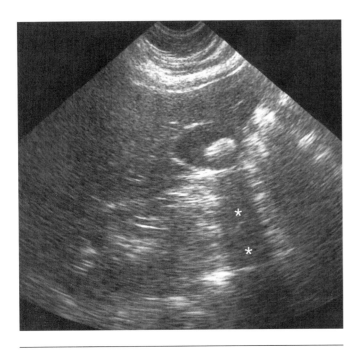

FIGURE 2   A gallstone within the fluid-filled gallbladder casts an acoustic shadow (*asterisks*).

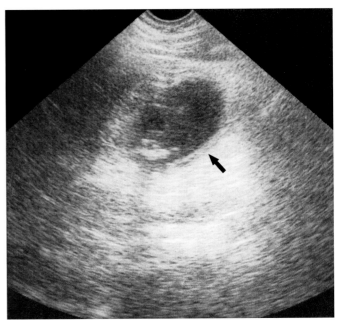

FIGURE 3   An echogenic gallstone within the gallbladder. The gallstone casts an acoustic shadow. There is a thin layer of pericholecystic fluid (*arrow*), a sign of acute cholecystitis.

There are three sonographic criteria for the diagnosis of cholelithiasis:

1. The gallstone is an echogenic focus located within the sonolucent gallbladder.
2. The gallstone casts an acoustic shadow.
3. The gallstone shows gravitational dependency.

Gravitational dependency means that the gallstone is located in the most dependent portion of the gallbladder and that it is mobile, i.e., changes location when the patient moves into another position (lateral decubitus or upright). This third criterion distinguishes a gallstone from a lesion fixed to the gallbladder wall such as a tumor or polyp. In these two images, the gallstones are located in the most dependent portion of the gallbladder.

MODERN DAY ARTIFACTS

Artifact—

1. Something created by humans usually for a practical purpose, especially an object remaining from a particular period (e.g., caves containing prehistoric artifacts).

2. A product of artificial character (as in a scientific test) due usually to an extraneous (as human) agency.*

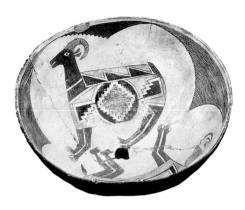

Mimbres Bowl, circa 1100 A.D. Southern New Mexico [Courtesy Millicent Rogers Museum, Taos, New Mexico.]

Although this patient's sonogram does not show typical features of acute cholecystitis, the correct interpretation can be *deduced* by understanding the **principles of ultrasound imaging.**

A sonographic image is formed by the reflection of the ultrasound beam at the interface between two substances of differing acoustic impedance. If the ultrasound beam does not encounter an acoustic interface, no sound is reflected and the object appears black (sonolucent), for example, a fluid-filled gallbladder. If there is a moderate degree of reflection of the ultrasound beam at an acoustic interface, there will be a gray area on the screen and the remaining ultrasound beam continues deeper. If the beam encounters a very echogenic interface, it is entirely reflected, producing a very bright signal and a dark *acoustic shadow* behind it. This is the image produced by a gallstone within the gallbladder (Figure 4).

Air almost entirely obscures an ultrasound image because the ultrasound beam is unable to penetrate air-filled structures such as bowel and lung. Sonography thus differs from conventional abdominal radiography, in which air-filled structures are readily detected because the radiopacity of air is very different from that of adjacent soft tissues. Ultrasonography and abdominal radiography therefore have complementary diagnostic capabilities.

Ultrasonography is subject to a variety of imaging **artifacts.** Artifacts, in general, obscure or distort an imaging study because they produce nonanatomical findings. However, in ultrasonography, artifacts are often helpful for image interpretation. The *acoustic shadow* produced by a gallstone is an example of a sonographic artifact. Although it is nonanatomic, this visually distinctive artifact helps confirm the diagnosis because it is characteristic of a very echogenic object (a gallstone) within the sonolucent gallbladder (Figure 4).

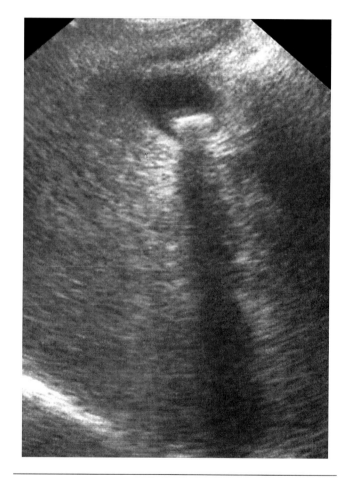

FIGURE 4   An acoustic shadow.

The sonolucent gallbladder contains an echogenic gallstone that casts an acoustic shadow. The acoustic shadow is a *sonographic artifact,* but is often the most conspicuous aspect of a gallstone.

Under what circumstances would the gallbladder not have its typical appearance?

In this patient, a sonolucent gallbladder could not be found. Diffculty in finding the gallbladder occurs most often when a patient has recently eaten. The gallbladder contracts and it is difficult to visualize. When a patient has had multiple prior episodes of cholecystitis, the gallbladder becomes scarred and shrunken and difficult to image by ultrasonography. An antecedent cholecystectomy is, of course, another cause of nonvisualization of the gallbladder, although not in this patient.

In this patient's sonogram, there is a bright crescent next to the inferior surface of the liver in the region of the gallbladder fossa (Figure 1). A similar finding occurs when the gallbladder is filled with stones or is contracted around gallstones. It forms two narrow curvilinear bands and casts an acoustic shadow—the **wall-echo-shadow (WES)** or "double arc" sign (Figure 5).

However in this patient, there is only a single curved echogenic line (Figure 6, *arrow*). This is similar in appearance to the diaphragm/lung interface (D) seen at the posterior surface of the liver. Both of these bright crescents are, in fact, due to air interfaces.

Two sonographic artifacts associated with air interfaces are seen in this patient's sonogram (Figure 7). Deep to the bright crescent, the sonographic image is obscured by shadowing. This is not a black acoustic shadow like that produced by a gallstone, but is instead a grayish shadow that is called **"dirty shadowing."**

A second artifact seen at highly echogenic interfaces is known as **"ring down"** (Figure 7). It is due to reverberation of the ultrasound beam between two reflective interfaces such as a layer of air or a metallic object. This causes repeated reflection

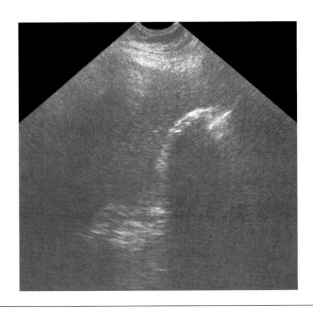

FIGURE 5   The "wall-echo-shadow" (WES) or "double arc" appearance of a gallbladder filled with gallstones that cast an acoustic shadow.

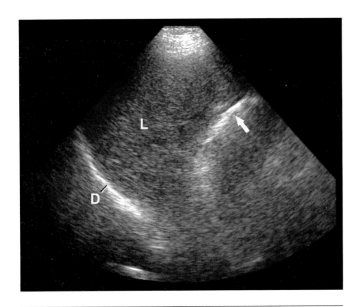

FIGURE 6   Patient 5—Sonogram image A.

There is a bright crescent (*arrow*) along the inferior margin of the liver (L) in the region of the gallbladder fossa. A second bright crescent is seen at the air interface between the lung and diaphragm (D).

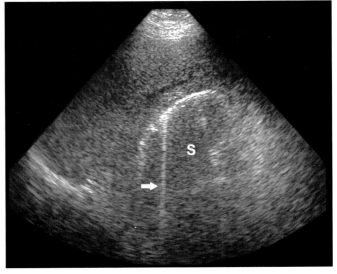

FIGURE 7   Patient 5—Sonogram image C.

There are two artifacts associated with an air interface. **Dirty shadowing** (S) obscures sonographic detail deep to the liver edge. **Ring down** artifact is a bright streak (*arrow*) due to reverberation of the ultrasound beam between two highly reflective interfaces.

of the ultrasound beam back to the transducer (Figure 8) and creates a bright white streak extending down from the white crescent. The bright appearance of the ring-down artifact is the opposite of the black acoustic shadow of a gallstone. When the reverberations are more widely spaced, the bright artifacts appears interrupted rather than continous (Figure 9).

One structure that can create an air interface adjacent to the liver is an air-filled segment of bowel (Figure 9). However in this patient, the gallbladder should still be detectable because he had not had a cholecystectomy.

Another possibility is that the echogenic crescent in the gallbladder's expected location is caused by air within the gallbladder lumen or wall. This is the correct explanation of the patient's sonographic findings. An air-filled gallbladder occurs in *emphysematous cholecystitis*.

Emphysematous cholecystitis occurs in 1% of patients with acute cholecystitis. The patients are typically elderly, usually male, and often have diabetes. The mortality rate is 15% (vs. 1.4% for cholecystitis). Emergency surgery is necessary because of the high risk of perforation. The gas is due to infection by gas-forming bacteria: clostridia (50%), coliform bacilli, or gram-positive cocci (obligate or facultative anaerobes). Emphysematous cholecystitis has a distinctive sonographic appearance, as is seen in this patient.

The diagnostic test of choice for emphysematous cholecystitis is an **abdominal radiograph.** Air within the gallbladder appears as an oval-shaped lucency. An air/fluid level may be seen on an upright abdominal radiograph. Air within the gallbladder wall appears as a curved radioluent line.

Patient Outcome

In this patient, after the sonogram was performed, the radiologist suggested that an abdominal radiograph be performed to confirm the diagnosis. The radiograph showed air in the gallbladder and gallbladder wall (Figure 10). The patient was taken to surgery and a dilated, gangrenous, but nonperforated gallbladder was removed. Numerous stones were found within the gallbladder.

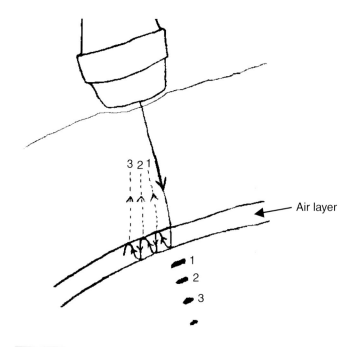

FIGURE 8   Schematic diagram of reverberation artifact.
The sound beam reverberates between two highly reflective surfaces. With each reverberation, an ultrasound signal is returned to the ultrasound probe, which is registered as a signal coming from a deeper structure.

With "ring-down" artifact, the reverberations are very closely spaced, producing a continuous white streak rather than an interrupted series of bright spots.

(NB. The reverberations occur in the same path as the ultrasound beam, not in the sine wave pattern drawn.)

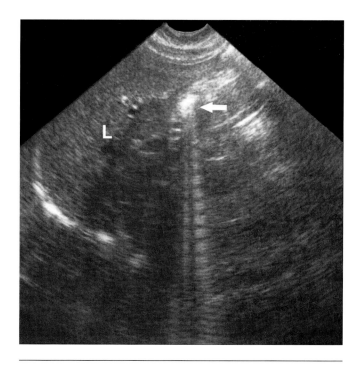

FIGURE 9   Reverberal artifact due to bowel gas.
Bowel gas produces a bright sonographic signal (*arrow*) deep to the liver (L). The highly reflective air collection produces a reverberation artifact (seen here) or ring-down artifact.

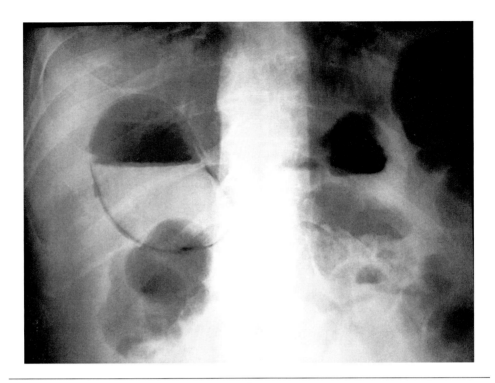

FIGURE 10   Patient 5—Abdominal Radiograph.
The patient's upright abdominal radiograph shows an air/fluid level within the distended gallbladder and gas within the gallbladder wall. This is diagnostic of emphysematous cholecystitis.

Imaging Diagnosis of Emphysematous Cholecystitis

Abdominal radiography is the test of choice to diagnose emphysematous cholecystitis. It shows air within a distended gallbladder or gallbladder wall (Figure 10). Gas in the gallbladder wall is pathognomonic for emphysematous cholecystitis.

Air in the biliary system also occurs with an enteric-biliary fistula (gallstone ileus or surgical anastomosis). However in these cases, the gallbladder is collapsed rather than distended, and a branching air pattern is seen within the biliary ducts.

Suspected emphysematous cholecystitis could be considered a third indication for radiography in patients with abdominal pain (in addition to pneumoperitoneum and bowel obstruction). However, emphysematous cholecystitis is difficult to suspect based on clinical findings alone. Emphysematous cholecystitis occurs predominantly in elderly patients and if radiographs were obtained liberally in elderly patients with abdominal pain, emphysematous cholecystitis could potentially be diagnosed. Nonetheless, detecting emphysematous cholecystitis would be a relatively rare occurrence.

Not all cases of emphysematous cholecystitis have diagnostic radiographs. In one series of eight patients, only one had a diagnostic radiographs (Gill 1997). Reasons for nondiagnostic radiographs include insufficient gas in the gallbladder or gas that cannot be distinguished from bowel gas. In addition, gas collections in the right upper quadrant may also be due to an intrahepatic or subdiaphragmatic abscess infected with gas-forming bacteria (the gas collection usually has a stippled appearance), or a loop of bowel that has migrated anterior to the liver. CT can accurately localize a gas collection when the diagnosis is uncertain (Figure 11).

Because **ultrasonography** is the best initial test for biliary colic/cholecystitis, the sonographer must be able to recognize the sonographic signs of emphysematous cholecystitis—a bright echogenic crescent in the gallbladder fossa with dirty shadowing and ring-down artifacts. Confirmation with abdominal radiography or CT is necessary because other disorders can have similar sonographic appearances. These include a contracted stone-filled gallbladder (WES sign) (Figure 5) or a "porcelain gallbladder" with a calcified wall due to chronic cholecystitis (Figure 12).

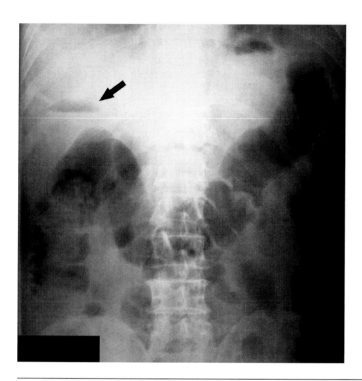

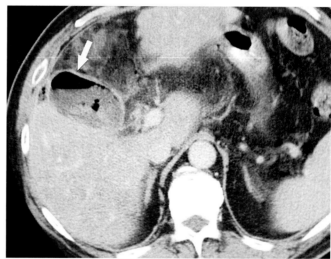

FIGURE 11   Emphysematous Cholecystitis—CT diagnosis.

The upright abdominal radiograph of a 67-year-old man with diabetes shows a gas collection with an air/fluid level in the right upper quadrant superior to the liver edge (*black arrow*). CT confirmed that the gas was within the gallbladder lumen representing emphysematous cholecystitis (*white arrow*).

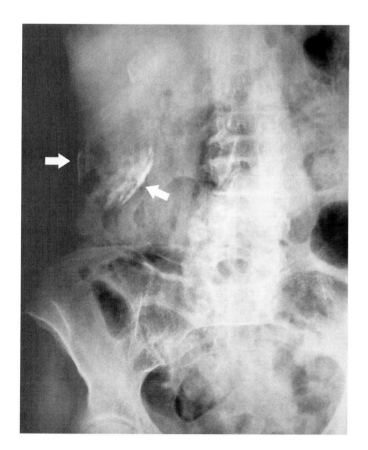

FIGURE 12   Porcelain gallbladder.

Calcification of the gallbladder wall is due to chronic cholecystitis (*arrows*). This may be an incidental finding or be seen in a patient having pain from an exacerbation of cholecystitis.

A porcelain gallbladder has a similar sonographic appearance to emphysematous cholecystitis. There is an increased incidence of gallbladder carcinoma in these patients.

Imaging Diagnosis of Acute Cholecystitis

In the past, **abdominal radiography** was used in patients suspected of having cholecystitis because 15% of gallstones are sufficiently calcified to be detected. However, ultrasonography is a considerably more sensitive test and has supplanted abdominal radiography for suspected biliary colic/cholecystitis.

Ultrasonography can detect nearly all gallstones as well as signs of acute cholecystitis (Figures 2 and 3). However, mere detection of gallstones does not prove that they are responsible for the patient's symptoms. Asymptomatic gallstones are common (up to 80% of patients with gallstones) and gallstones may therefore be an incidental finding unrelated to a patient's pain. Other disorders such as acute coronary syndrome, pneumonia or bowel obstruction, can have clinical presentations similar to biliary colic or cholecystitis—upper abdominal pain, nausea and vomiting. These diagnoses could potentially be missed if incidentally found gallstones are mistakenly considered the cause of a patient's symptoms (Figure 13).

The **diagnosis of acute cholecystitis** is based on the patient's clinical presentation, signs of gallbladder inflammation on sonography or CT, or in some cases, an hepatobiliary scan.

Sonographic signs of acute cholecystitis include gallbladder wall thickening (>3 to 5 mm), pericholecystic fluid, and the sonographic Murphy's sign (Figure 3). With the sonographic Murphy's sign, the site of maximal tenderness is localized with the sonographic transducer overlying the gallbladder. The sensitivity of sonography for acute cholecystitis has been reported to be from 70% to 90%. This depends on the experience of the sonographer and the criteria used. The sonographic Murphy's sign is the most sensitive but least specific sign of acute cholecystitis (specificity as low as 66%) (Ralls 1985, Liang 1992, Shea 1994, Rosen 2001).

Because of the limited sensitivity of ultrasonography for acute cholecystitis, a sonogram that does not show signs of acute cholecystitis does not exclude that diagnosis when a patient has a convincing clinical presentation (persistent pain, focal tenderness or Murphy's sign, leukocytosis or fever). Occasionally additional imaging studies are needed to determine whether a patient's symptoms are due to cholecystitis, biliary colic or another cause, i.e., an hepatobiliary scan or CT.

An **hepatobiliary scan** (also referred to as a "HIDA scan") can directly determine whether gallstones are causing cholecystitis by detecting cystic duct obstruction. An injected radiolabeled tracer (^{99m}technetium-hydroxy-iminodiacetic acid [HIDA] or others) is taken up by the liver and excreted into the bile (Figure 14). In a normal study, (patent cystic duct), tracer fills the gallbladder and common bile duct, and then enters the duodenum and small bowel. In such a patient, gall-stones are either not responsible for the patient's abdominal pain or transient obstruction has caused biliary colic without cholecystitis. With acute cholecystitis, the cystic duct is obstructed and the gallbladder is not visualized. However, other intra-abdominal conditions and systemic illnesses cause delayed uptake of tracer in the gallbladder. When the gallbladder is not seen, additional images at 2–4 hours are necessary to differentiate *nonvisualization* of the gallbladder (cholecystitis) from *delayed visualization* of the gallbladder due to a non biliary condition. Alternatively, if the gallbladder is not visualized after one hour, an injection of low-dose morphine will induce spasm of the sphincter of Oddi, increase intraluminal biliary pressure, and promote filling of the gallbladder if the cystic duct is patent (Grossman and Joyce 1991, Kalimi et al. 2001, Chatziioannou et al. 2000).

Computed tomography is often the initial diagnostic test in patients with abdominal pain when biliary tract disease is not the primary disorder suspected. Although CT is not the usual test of choice for acute cholecystitis, it is able to detect signs of acute cholecystitis (gallbladder wall thickening, pericholecystic fluid and fat stranding). The sensitivity of CT for acute cholecystitis has not been studied in a controlled fashion. One recent study found that CT had a sensitivity of 92% for acute cholecystitis, equivalent to ultrasonography (Bennett et al. 2002). Two earlier studies found a lower sensitivity of 40% to 50%. (Harvey 1999, Fidler 1996). However, gallstones are sufficiently calcified to be detected by CT in only 50% to 75% of cases. Noncalcified gallstones have the same attenuation on CT as bile and are not visible (Figure 15).

Gangrenous cholecystitis is present in 10% (range: 2% to 30%) of patients with acute cholecystitis and can be detected by CT or ultrasonography. Ischemia and necrosis of the gallbladder wall necessitates emergency cholecystectomy. CT signs of gangrenous cholecystitis are: an irregular or absent gallbladder wall (irregular contour or enhancement), intraluminal membranes (also seen on sonography) (Figure 15C), pericholecystic abscess (encapsulated fluid collection adjacent to gallbladder), and gas in gallbladder wall or lumen (emphysematous cholecystitis is only seen in a third of patients with gangrenous cholecystitis). The sensitivity of CT for gangrenous cholecystitis is only 30% and the diagnosis depends largely on clinical findings. However, the specificity of CT for gangrenous cholecystitis is high (96%) and when present, these CT signs should be considered highly suggestive of the diagnosis (Bennett 2002).

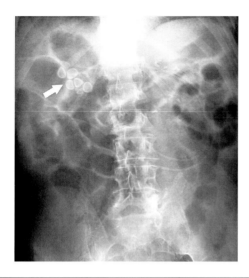
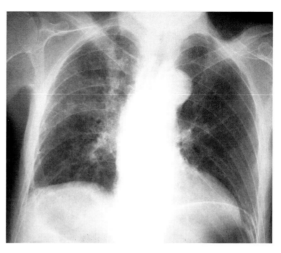

FIGURE 13   Identification of gallstones does not mean they are responsible for a patient's illness

A 75-year-old man presented with fever, altered mental status, and right-sided chest and abdominal pain. The abdominal radiograph showed multiple gallstones (*arrow*) and adynamic ileus. Although the initial impression was that he had acute cholecystitis, the chest radiograph showed pneumonia. A subsequent HIDA scan was normal. The gallstones were asymptomatic and an incidental finding.

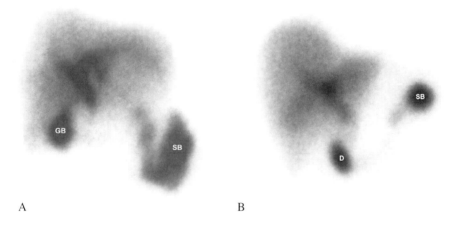

A   B

FIGURE 14   Hepatobiliary scan (HIDA scan).

(*A*) In a normal study (patent cystic duct), the radiolabeled tracer fills the gallbladder (GB) and proximal small bowel (SB). (*B*) With acute cholecystitis, the cystic duct is obstructed and the gallbladder is not visualized (D = duodenum).

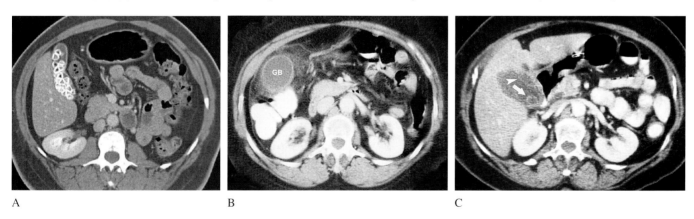

A   B   C

FIGURE 15   CT diagnosis of cholelithiasis and cholecystitis.

(*A*) Multiple calcified gallstones incidentally discovered on CT.

(*B*) In a patient with acute cholecystitis, CT shows stranding of the pericholecystic fat surrounding the gallbladder (GB). Gallstones are not visible because they were not calcified. This should not be misinterpreted as "acalculous cholecystitis." Sonography demonstrated gallstones.

(*C*) A gallstone is visible due to its calcified rim (*arrow*). Gangrenous cholecystitis causes sloughing of the anterior gallbladder wall forming an intraluminal membrane (*arrowhead*).

SUGGESTED READING

Emphysematous Cholecystitis

Andreu J, Perez C, Caceres J, et al.: Computed tomography as the method of choice in the diagnosis of emphysematous cholecystitis. *Gastrointest Radiol* 1987;12:315–318.

Bloom RA, Libson E, Lebensart PD, et al.: The ultrasound spectrum of emphysematous cholecystitis. *J Clin Ultrasound* 1989;17:251–256.

Brandon JC, Glick SN, Teplick SK, et al.: Emphysematous cholecystitis: Pitfalls in its plain film diagnosis. *Gastrointest Radiol* 1988;13: 33–36.

Cho KC, Baker SR: Extraluminal air: Diagnosis and significance. *Radiol Clin North Am* 1994;32:829–845.

Garcia-Sancho TL, Rodriguez-Montes JA, Fernandez de Lis S, Garcia-Sancho ML: Acute emphysematous cholecystitis. Report of twenty cases. *Hepatogastroenterology* 1999;46:2144–2148.

Gill KS, Chapman AH, Weston MJ: The changing face of emphysematous cholecystitis. *Br J Radiol* 1997;70:986–991.

Grayson DE, Abbott RM, Levy AD, Sherman PM: Emphysematous infections of the abdomen and pelvis: A pictorial review. *Radiographics* 2002;22:543–561.

Hawass ND: False-negative sonographic findings in emphysematous cholecystitis. *Acta Radiol* 1987;29:137–138.

Jolly BT, Love JN: Emphysematous cholecystitis in an elderly woman: Case report and review of the literature. *J Emerg Med* 1993;11: 593–597.

Konno K, Ishida H, Naganuma H, et al.: Emphysematous cholecystitis: Sonographic findings. *Abdom Imaging* 2002;27:191–195.

Parulekar SG: Sonographic findings in acute emphysematous cholecystitis. *Radiology* 1982;145:117–119.

Topp SW, Edlund G: Ultrasonic non-visualization of the gallbladder in emphysematous cholecystitis: Case report. *Acta Chir Scand* 1988; 154:153–155.

Sonographic Artifacts

Franquet T, Bescos JM, et al.: Acoustic artifacts and reverberation shadows in gallbladder sonograms: Their cause and clinical implications. *Gastrointest Radiol* 1990;15:223–228.

Kremkau FW, Taylor KJ: Artifacts in ultrasound imaging. *J Ultrasound Med* 1986;5:227–237.

Kremkau FW: *Diagnostic Ultrasound: Principles and Instruments*, 4th ed., Chapter 4, Artifacts. Philadelphia, W.B. Saunders, 1993: 221–251.

Ma OJ, Mateer JR: *Emergency Ultrasound*, pp. 57-63, 353. McGraw-Hill, 2003.

Rubin JM, Adler RS, Bude RO, et al.: Clean and dirty shadowing at US: A reappraisal. *Radiology* 1991;181:231–236.

Scanlan KA: Sonographic artifacts and their origins. *AJR* 1991;156: 1267–1272.

Gallstones, Cholecystitis

Bingener J, Schwesinger WH, Chopra S, et al.: Does the correlation of acute cholecystitis on ultrasound and at surgery reflect a mirror image? *Am J Surg* 2004;188:703–707.

Bortoff GA, Chen MYM, Ott DJ, et al.: Gallbladder stones: Imaging and intervention. *RadioGraphics* 2000; 20:751–766.

Cox GR, Browne BJ: Acute cholecystitis in the emergency department. *J Emerg Med* 1989;7:501–511.

Hanbidge AE, Buckler PM, O'Malley ME, Wilson SR: Imaging evaluation for acute pain in the right upper quadrant. *RadioGraphics* 2004;24:1117–1135.

Indar AA, Beckingham IJ: Acute cholecystitis. *BMJ* 2002;325: 639–643.

Johnson CD: ABC of the upper gastrointestinal tract: Upper abdominal pain: Gallbladder. *BMJ* 2001;323:1170–1173.

Sonography for Cholecystitis

Kendall JL, Shimp RJ: Performance and interpretation of focused right upper quadrant ultrasound by emergency physicians. *J Emerg Med* 2001;21:7–13.

Laing FC: Ultrasonography of the acute abdomen. *Radiol Clin North Am* 1992;30:389–404.

Ralls PW, Colletti PM, Lapin SA, et al.: Real-time sonography in suspected acute cholecystitis. Prospective evaluation of primary and secondary signs. *Radiology* 1985;155:767–771.

Rosen CL, Brown DF, Chang Y, et al.: Ultrasonography by emergency physicians in patients with suspected cholecystitis. *Am J Emerg Med* 2001;19:32–36.

Shea JA, Berlin JA, Escarce JJ, et al.: Revised estimates of diagnostic test sensitivity and specificity in suspected biliary tract disease. *Arch Intern Med* 1994;154:2573–2581.

Hepatobiliary Scintigraphy (HIDA Scan)

Chatziioannou SN, Moore WH, Ford PV, Dhekne RD: Hepatobiliary scintigraphy is superior to abdominal ultrasonography in suspected acute cholecystitis. *Surgery* 2000;127:609–613.

Grossman SJ, Joyce JM: Hepatobiliary imaging. *Emerg Med Clin North Am* 1991;9:853–874.

Kalimi R, Gecelter GR, Caplin D, et al.: Diagnosis of acute cholecystitis: Sensitivity of sonography, cholescintigraphy, and combined sonography-cholescintigraphy. *J Am Coll Surg* 2001;193:609–613.

Kim CK, Tse KK, Juweid M, et al.: Cholescintigraphy in the diagnosis of acute cholecystitis: Morphine augmentation is superior to delayed imaging. *J Nucl Med* 1993;34:1866–1870.

Lorberhoym M, Simon J, Horne T: The role of morphine-augmented cholescintigraphy and real-time ultrasound in detecting gallbladder disease. *J Nucl Med Technol* 1999;27:294–297.

Zeman RK, Garra BS: Gallbladder imaging. *Gastroenterol Clin North Am* 1991;2:127–156.

CT for Cholecystitis

Alterman DD, Hochsztein: Computed tomography in acute cholecystitis. *Emerg Radiol* 1996;3:25–29.

Bennett GL, Rusinek H, Lisi V, et al.: CT findings in acute gangrenous cholecystitis. *AJR* 2002;178:275–281.

Fidler J, Paulson EK, Layfield L: CT evaluation of acute cholecystitis: Findings and usefulness in diagnosis. *AJR* 1996;166:1085–1088.

Grand D, Horton KM, Fishman E: CT of the gallbladder: Spectrum of disease. *AJR* 2004;183:163–170.

Harvey RT, Miller WT: Acute biliary disease: Initial CT and follow-up US versus initial US and follow-up CT. *Radiology* 1999;213: 831–836.

Paulson EK: Acute cholecystitis: CT findings. *Semin Ultrasound CT MR* 2000;21:56–63.

Van Beers BE: Imaging of cholelithiasis: Helical CT. *Abdom Imaging* 2001;26:15–20.

Abdominal Radiology: Patient 6

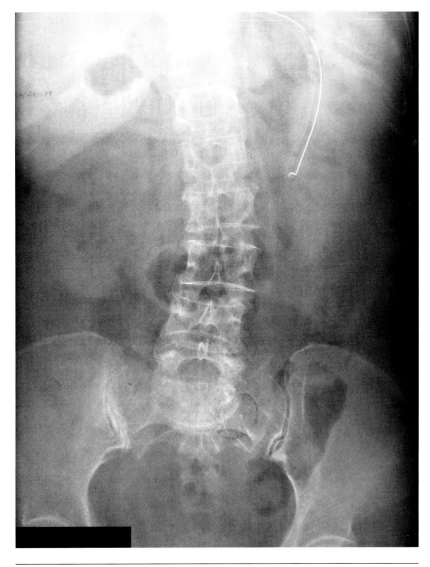

FIGURE 1

Abdominal pain and vomiting in an elderly woman with diabetes

A 71-year-old woman presented to the ED with abdominal pain of one week's duration. The pain was midepigastric in location and radiated upwards. It was associated with nausea, but unrelated to food intake. She had seen another physician two days earlier who prescribed ranitidine. The pain continued and was now associated with vomiting. She also felt "bloated."

The patient had diabetes and was taking glyburide. She had a hysterectomy many years earlier.

On examination, she was an elderly woman in moderate discomfort. Vital signs were: blood pressure 110/72 mm Hg, pulse 80 beats/min, respirations 18 breaths/min, temperature 99.0° F (rectal).

Her abdomen was soft with normal bowel sounds. It appeared slightly distended. There was mild tenderness in the midepigastrium and right upper and lower quadrants, but no rebound tenderness or guarding.

Her blood test results were normal including a complete blood count and chemistries, aside from a blood glucose level of 179 mg/dL.

- The abdominal radiograph provides an exact anatomical diagnosis of the patient's disorder (Figure 1).

219

RIGLER'S TRIAD

Radiography was performed in this patient for suspected bowel obstruction. It shows the classic *Rigler's triad* of gallstone ileus: (1) pneumobilia; (2) small bowel obstruction; and (3) an ectopic gallstone (Rigler et al. 1941) (Figure 2). Rigler's triad is, in fact, seen only in a minority of cases of gallstone ileus (25%).

Gallstone ileus is a disease of the elderly. Despite being called "ileus," it is actually a type of mechanical small bowel obstruction. Cholelithiasis and chronic cholecystitis results in formation of an inflammatory fistula between the gallbladder and the adjacent duodenum (75%) or transverse colon (20%). The gallstone is expelled into the intestine and, if large (3 cm in diameter or greater), the gallstone may lodge in an area of intestinal narrowing, usually at the ileocecal valve, causing bowel obstruction (Figure 3).

In the past, most cases of gallstone ileus were not diagnosed preoperatively because of the lack of specific clinical or radiographic features. With widespread use of CT, preoperative diagnosis is usually possible (Figure 4). It is an uncommon cause of small bowel obstruction (1–2% of cases) but makes up a greater proportion of small bowel obstruction among elderly patients who had not had prior abdominal surgery (historically, up to 25% of such patients). Current widespread use of cholecystectomy for symptomatic gallstones has made gallstone ileus less common. Gallstone ileus has a higher mortality (10–30%) than other causes of small bowel obstruction because of the advanced age of the patients and the more complex surgical procedure required.

(1) **Pneumobilia**—In this patient's radiograph, an oval-shaped air density is located over the liver, too high to be within a loop of bowel. A tubular air collection extends from its medial aspect representing air in the cystic duct. In many cases of gallstone ileus, the gallbladder is collapsed and air is seen only in the biliary tract. By contrast, in emphysematous cholecystitis, the gallbladder is distended and gas may also accumulate within the gallbladder wall. Tubular RUQ gas collections also seen following surgical procedures on the biliary tract (Figure 5) and bowel infarction causing gas in the hepatic portal veins (Figures 6 and 7) (Table 1).

(2) **Small bowel obstruction**—There are several loops of dilated small bowel in the midabdomen. On the upright radiograph, air/fluid levels were seen.

(3) **Ectopic gallstone**—Only 10–15% of gallstones are sufficiently calcified to be visible on conventional radiographs. An intraluminal gallstone can also be visualized by a thin layer of surrounding intestinal air. This is seen on this patient's radiograph overlying the left sacral wing (Figure 2B). The ectopic gallstone is visualized in only 20% of cases of gallstone ileus.

Patient Outcome

The patient was taken to the operating room on the night of admission with a preoperative diagnosis of gallstone ileus. A mechanical small bowel obstruction was present with the point of obstruction in the midjejunum. A luminal mass was palpable and enterotomy revealed two large 3 cm diameter gallstones. The gallbladder was scarred with multiple adhesions to bowel and omentum. Two weeks later, a second operation was performed revealing two intestinal-gallbladder fistulae—cholecystoduodenal and cholecystocolic. The gallbladder was removed and the fistulae were closed.

TABLE 1

Causes of RUQ Gas

Gallstone ileus (biliary-enteric fistula)
Sphincterotomy or surgical anastomosis
Emphysematous cholecystitis (see Patient 4)
Hepatic portal venous gas (bowel infarction)
Hepatic or subdiaphragmatic abscess
Pneumoperitoneum (overlying liver)
  (see Patient 3, Figure 12, page 197)

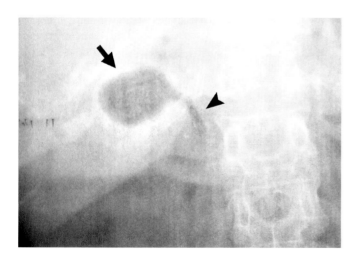

FIGURE 2A   Pneumobilia.
Gas in the gallbladder (*arrow*) and cystic duct (*arrowhead*).

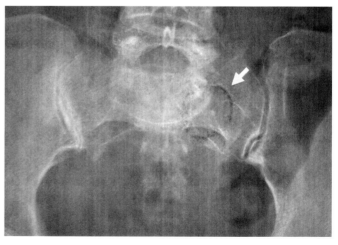

FIGURE 2B   Ectopic gallstone.
A thin layer of gas surrounds the gallstone (*arrow*).

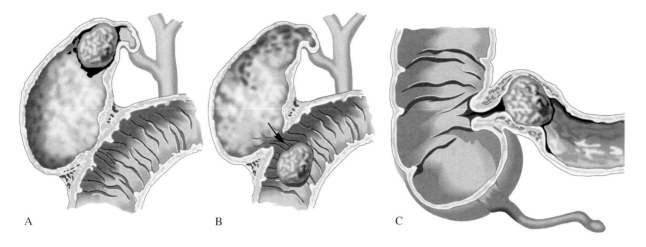

FIGURE 3   Pathogenesis of gallstone ileus.

(*A*) Chronic cholecystitis due to a gallstone causes inflammatory fistula formation to the adjacent bowel (most commonly the duodenum). (*B*) The gallstone is expelled into the intestine across the biliary-enteric fistula.

(*C*) The gallstone migrates through the intestine until it becomes lodged at an area of narrowing (usually the ileocecal valve). This causes a mechanical small bowel obstruction.

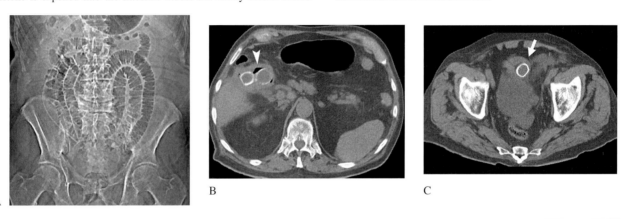

FIGURE 4   Gallstone ileus on CT.

(A) The scout abdominal radiograph showed dilated small bowel indicative of mechanical small bowel obstruction. Air of uncertain orgin was seen overlying the liver. No gallstones were visible.

(*B*) An image of the gallbladder shows two large gallstones and air in the gallbladder (*arrowhead*). (*C*) A large gallstone is lodged in the distal ileum (*arrow*) causing small bowel obstruction.

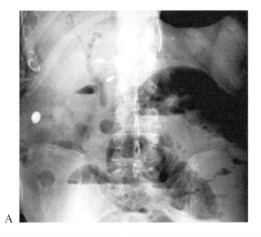
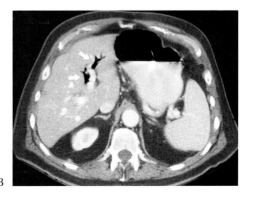

FIGURE 5   Pneumobilia.

The most common cause of air in the biliary tract (*arrows*) is a surgical procedure such as endoscopic sphincterotomy for common bile duct stones, or a surgical anastomosis between the biliary tract and jejunum (choledochojejunostomy) performed to drain an biliary

system obstructed by a tumor or stricture. This patient had had an endoscopic spincterotomy for retained common bile duct stones.

On CT (B), air in the intrahepatic bile ducts (*arrows*) is seen adjacent to a contrast-filled hepatic portal vein.

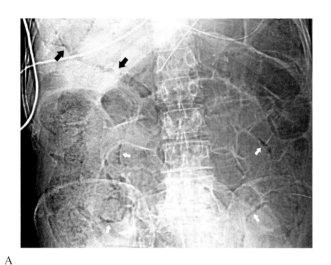

A

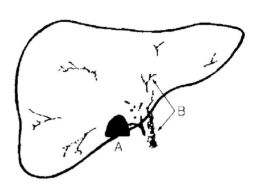

B

FIGURE 6   Hepatic portal venous gas.

Hepatic portal venous gas (HPVG) occurs in the setting of bowel infarction and is generally an ominous sign. HPVG creates a tubular branching gas collection in the right upper quadrant (*black arrows*). It should not be mistaken for pneumobilia. Intramural gas in necrotic bowel wall (*white arrows*) migrates via the mesenteric veins to the portal veins. Hepatic portal venous gas is infrequently seen on abdominal radiography and is more readily detected on CT.

(*B*) Schematically, pneumobilia tends to be central in location and involve the gallbladder (*A*). HPVG extends peripherally in the liver to the small branching hepatic portal veins (*B*).

[From: Plewa MC: Emergency abdominal radiography. *Emerg Med Clin North Am* 1991;9:843, with permission.]

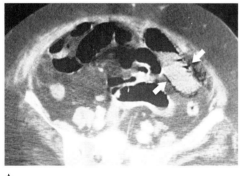

A

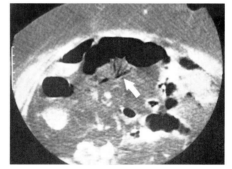

B

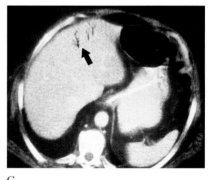

C

FIGURE 7   CT of bowel infarction and HPVG.

A 70-year-old man presented with acute severe abdominal pain, abdominal distention, and hematemesis due to acute mesenteric ischemia.

There is gas within the wall of infarcted bowel (*A*) that extends into the mesenteric veins (*B*) and the hepatic portal veins (*C*).

SUGGESTED READING

Abou-Saif A, Al-Kawas FH: Complications of gallstone disease: Mirizzi syndrome, cholecystocholedochal fistula, and gallstone ileus. *Am J Gastroenterol* 2002;97:249–254.

Balthazar EJ, Schechter LS: Air in gallbladder: A frequent finding in gallstone ileus. *AJR* 1978;131:219–222.

Buljevac M, Busic Z, Cabrijan Z: Sonographic diagnosis of gallstone ileus. *J Ultrasound Med* 2004;23:1395–1398.

Delabrousse E, Bartholomot B, Sohm O, et al.: Gallstone ileus: CT findings. *Eur Radiol* 2000;10:938–940.

Lasson A, Loren I, Nilsson A, et al.: Ultrasonography in gallstone ileus: A diagnostic challenge. *Eur J Surg* 1995;161:259–263.

Lobo DN, Jobling JC, Balfour TW: Gallstone ileus: Diagnostic pitfalls and therapeutic successes. *J Clin Gastroenterol* 2000;30:72–76.

Molmenti EP: Gallstone ileus: Images in clinical medicine. *N Engl J Med* 1996;335:942.

Pannu HK, Fishman EK: Gallstone ileus presenting as small bowel obstruction: Spiral CT evaluation. *Emerg Radiol* 1999;6:170–172.

Reisner RM, Cohen JR: Gallstone ileus: A review of 1001 reported cases. *Am Surg* 1994;60:441–441.

Rigler LG, Borman CN, Noble JF: Gallstone obstruction: Pathogenesis and roentgen manifestations. *JAMA* 1941;117:1753–1759.

Ripolles T, Miguel-Dasit A, Errando J, et al.: Gallstone ileus: Increased diagnostic sensitivity by combining plain film and ultrasound. *Abdom Imaging* 2001;26:401–405.

Swift SE, Spencer JA: Gallstone ileus: CT findings. *Clin Radiol* 1998;53:451–454.

Abdominal Radiology: Patient 7

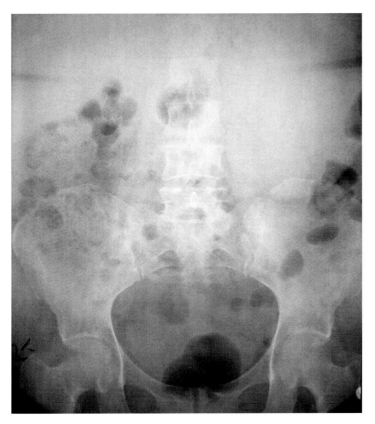 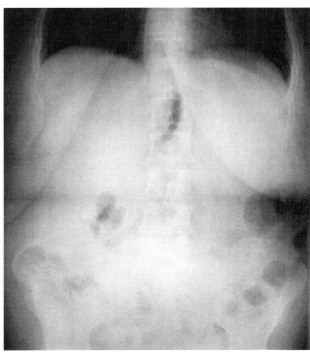

FIGURE 1

Weakness and jaundice in a middle-aged woman

A 60-year-old woman presented to the ED with progressive weakness that developed over two weeks.

Several days earlier, she noted that her eyes were yellow. She also had mild upper abdominal discomfort. She was previously healthy and took no medications. She had had a hysterectomy many years earlier.

On examination, she was an overweight woman in no apparent distress. She was afebrile and her vital signs were normal. There was scleral icterus. Her abdomen was nontender.

The urine dipstick was negative for bilirubin, and the urobilinogen was normal.

Her abdominal radiographs are shown in Figure 1.

- What was the cause of this patient's jaundice?

THE DIFFERENTIAL DIAGNOSIS OF JAUNDICE

An abdominal radiograph is not often helpful in the diagnostic evaluation of a patient with jaundice. In this patient, the radiograph provided worthwhile information before other laboratory results were available.

The most frequent cause of jaundice is **decreased elimination of bilirubin** due to either hepatocellular dysfunction or mechanical obstruction of the extrahepatic biliary tracts. Less frequently, jaundice is due to increased production of bilirubin, as occurs with destruction of red blood cells in hemolytic anemia.

Liver enzyme blood levels can distinguish hepatocellular from obstructive jaundice. In **hepatocellular dysfunction,** elevation of the hepatocellular enzyme aminotransferases predominates. In **obstructive jaundice,** elevation of the biliary canalicular enzyme, alkaline phosphatase, is greater. The serum bilirubin profile—direct (conjugated) versus indirect (unconjugated)—is not helpful in distinguishing obstructive from nonobstructive jaundice. In both, there is elevation of direct and indirect bilirubin.

When jaundice is due to **increased bilirubin production,** as occurs in hemolytic anemia, only unconjugated (indirect) bilirubin levels are elevated (Figure 2). Conjugated bilirubin is excreted into the bile and the serum direct bilirubin is therefore not elevated. Liver enzyme tests are normal and LDH of red blood cell origin is elevated.

In Patient 7, the absence of urinary bilirubin on the bedside dipstick urinalysis suggested that the jaundice was due to hemolysis because the bilirubin was all unconjugated (indirect) and not excreted into the urine.

The abdominal radiographs provide support for the diagnosis of hemolytic anemia by showing a massively enlarged spleen (Figure 3). There is a large round soft tissue mass in the left upper quadrant, which compresses the stomach and displaces the stomach air-bubble to the midline (Figure 3). Splenomegaly was difficult to detect on physical examination because of the patient's obesity.

Splenomegaly is present patients with hemolytic anemia because it is the site where abnormal erythrocytes are removed from the circulation. Alternatively, there could have been a primary splenic disorder causing splenomegaly such as an infiltrative disease (neoplastic or metabolic), infectious disease, or congestive splenomegaly due to portal hypertension. Primary splenomegaly causes *hypersplenism*—pancytopenia due to sequestration and destruction of all blood elements by the enlarged spleen.

The patient's blood test results were:

WBC 7,000 /mm^3, hematocrit 20.9%, reticulocytes 4.7%, platelets 124,000 /mm^3, bilirubin, 4.82 mg/dL (total) and 0.50 mg/dL (direct), ALT 30 U/L, AST 14 U/L, alkaline phosphatase 122 U/L, and LDH 477 U/L.

Coombs Test: Positive (direct) for anti-erythrocyte antibody on RBC surface.

The patient was not taking medications associated with an autoimmune hemolytic anemia such as alpha-methyl dopa, penicillin, quinidine, or isoniazid. Subsequent work-up was negative for lymphoproliferative or infectious diseases involving the spleen. The patient's diagnosis was therefore *idiopathic immunohemolytic anemia.* She was treated with prednisone (1 mg/kg/d) and her hematocrit increased to 30% during the next week.

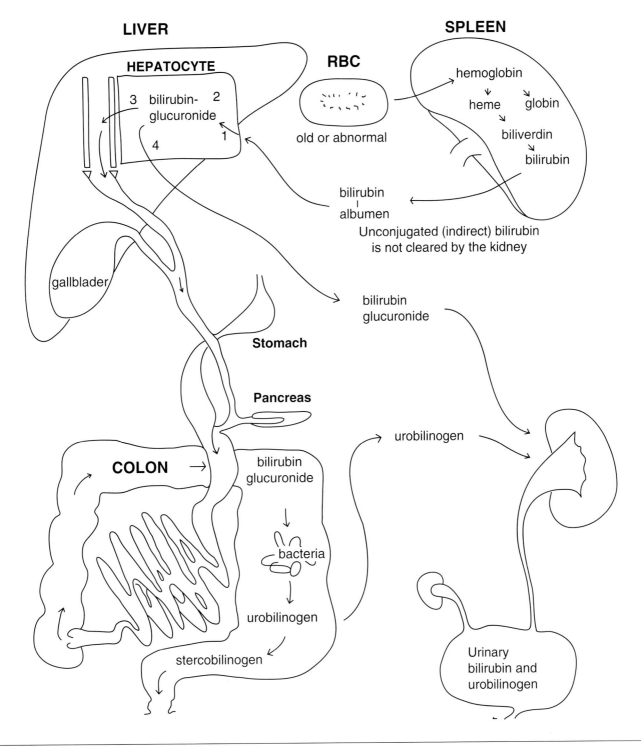

FIGURE 2 Bilirubin metabolism.

Hepatocyte Function:

1. Uptake of unconjugated bilirubin from the systemic circulation.
2. Conjugation by glucuronyl transferase.
3. Excretion of conjugated bilirubin into the bile. (This is the rate limiting step.)
4. When there is hepatocellular dysfunction or bile flow is totally obstructed, conjugated bilirubin "leaks" into the systemic circulation.

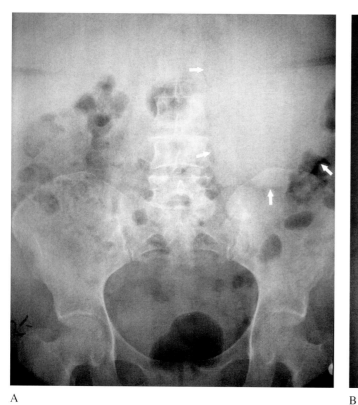

A

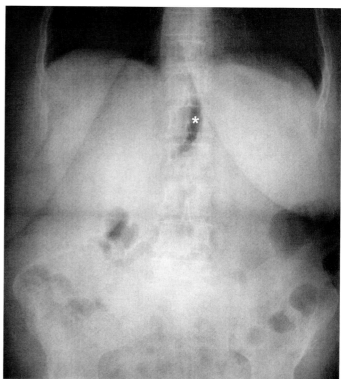

B

FIGURE 3   Patient 7

(*A*) **Supine radiograph**—Massively enlarged spleen is seen in the left upper quadrant, extending both inferiorly and medially (*arrows*).

(*B*) **Upright radiograph**—The stomach bubble is displaced medially and appears as crescent shaped lucency located over the vertebral column (*asterisk*).

The abdominal radiograph is an insensitive test for the detection of splenic enlargement. In approximately half of patients with a normal-sized spleen, the inferior pole of the spleen (the spleen tip) is visible at or above the left costal margin. Numerical measurements of splenic size are unreliable.

Moderate to marked splenomegaly is evident when the spleen tip is displaced significantly below the costal margin. Massive splenomegaly may displace the gastric bubble medially. Both of these finding are present in this patient's radiographs (Figure 3).

Abdominal Radiology: Patient 8

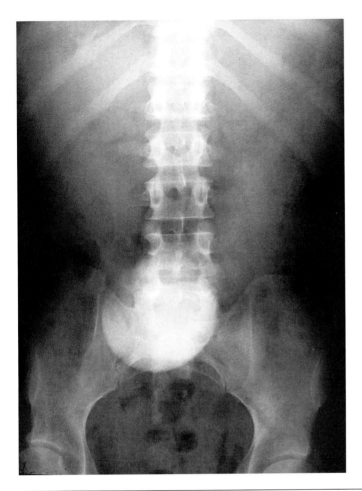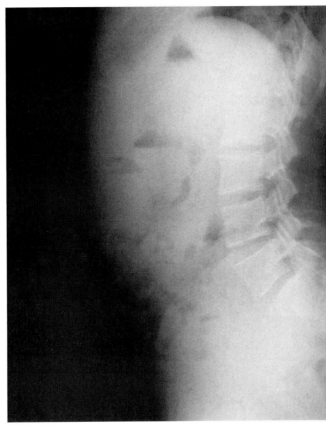

FIGURE 1

Abdominal discomfort in a middle-aged man with renal failure

A 50-year-old man presented to the ED with abdominal pain. He had end-stage renal disease that was being managed with peritoneal dialysis.

His abdominal radiograph is shown in Figure 1.

To better localize the radiopaque object, a lateral view of the abdomen was added by the radiologist.

- What is the radiopaque object seen in the mid-abdomen?

WHAT MAKES SOMETHING RADIOPAQUE?

There are several factors that contribute to the radiopacity of an object. We usually think that the **intrinsic radiopacity** of the material that makes up an object is the major determinant of its radiographic appearance. However, the **shape** of the object can play a major role in determining its radiographic appearance. In this case, the apparently radiopaque object is actually composed of relatively radiolucent material.

The intrinsic radiopacity of a substance depends, in part, on the **atomic numbers** of its constituent atoms. A substance is more radiopaque if it contains atoms of high atomic number such as calcium, iodine, barium, or lead.

X-ray radiation is absorbed when it ejects an electron from one of the inner orbitals of the atom—**the photoelectric effect** (Figure 2). More x-ray energy is absorbed when the electron is tightly bound to its orbital. The force binding an electron to the orbital is determined by the electrical charge of the nucleus, i.e., the number of protons in the nucleus, which is equivalent to the atomic number of the element. This is why bone, which contains calcium (atomic number 20), is more radiopaque than soft tissue, which is made up mostly of carbon (atomic number 6), hydrogen (atomic number 1), and oxygen (atomic number 8). Iodine (atomic number 53) is the key constituent of radiocontrast material and lead (atomic number 82) is an effective barrier to x-rays.

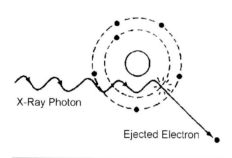

FIGURE 2   The photoelectric effect.

In this patient, however, the **object's shape** (i.e., the patients abdomen) rather than its intrinsic radiopacity is more important in determining its radiographic appearance. The round radiopaque mass seen in the middle of the abdomen on the AP view cannot represent an object within the abdominal cavity, e.g., a solid ball that was swallowed or an intra-abdominal tumor, because such an object would be visible within the abdomen on the lateral view (Figure 1). Alternatively, a thin flat object can be difficult to see when viewed from the side. However, a thin flat disc of sufficient radiopacity to have this appearance on the AP view would appear as a very radiopaque line when viewed from the side on a lateral view.

One characteristic of the object's appearance on the AP view indicates that it is not a radiopaque object contained within the abdomen. The object has very well-defined inferior and lateral margins, but its superior border is indistinct, gradually blending with the soft tissues of the abdomen. This implies that the object is a broad-based soft tissue mass protruding downwards from the anterior abdominal wall. (Alternatively, it could be a soft tissue mass extending from the back of the patient, such as an extremely large lipoma.) If the lateral radiograph is viewed with a very bright light, the soft tissue mass is faintly visible extending from the anterior abdominal wall (Figure 3).

Patient Outcome

This patient had end-stage renal disease that was being managed with peritoneal dialysis. He had developed a large **umbilical hernia** that was mildly tender and nonreducible (Figure 3). There were no clinical or radiographic signs of bowel obstruction. At surgery, the hernia sac was found to contain loculated peritoneal fluid, but no bowel. The fluid collection was drained and the defect in the abdominal wall was repaired.

The abdominal radiograph had been ordered at the request of a surgical consultant to look for evidence of bowel obstruction due to the umbilical hernia. The hernia itself was, of course, obvious on physical examination.

These radiographic principles can have the opposite effect–making a relatively radiopaque region disappear when it does not have a sharp interface with its surroundings (See Chest Radiology, Patient 14B on page 131).

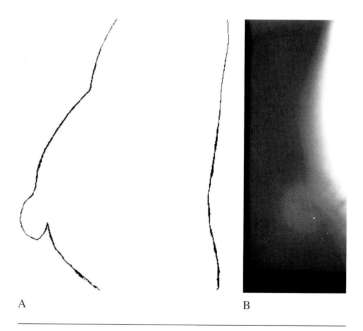

A   B

FIGURE 3

(*A*) The patient's torso in profile.

(*B*) "Bright-light" view of the lateral radiograph.

PRINCIPLES OF SKELETAL RADIOLOGY

CLINICAL DIAGNOSIS OF A FRACTURE

Although radiography is often considered the mainstay of fracture diagnosis, two orthopedic principles must be kept in mind when evaluating patients with extremity trauma:

A fracture is a clinical, not a radiographic, diagnosis
A fracture is a soft tissue injury with skeletal involvement

Radiographic studies serve to confirm the clinical diagnosis of a fracture and define its anatomy. Over-reliance on radiography is a potential pitfall in patient care. In some cases, a fracture may be present without apparent radiographic abnormality, i.e., an occult fracture. Second, soft tissue injuries (neurovascular and ligamentous) can be of greater consequence than the fracture itself and are in general not visible on the radiographs.

The clinical diagnosis of a fracture is based on:

(1) the mechanism of injury,
(2) the findings on physical examination, and
(3) the age of the patient.

Some physical examination findings are highly predictive of a fracture. Definite signs of a fracture include gross deformity, abnormal mobility at the injury site, and crepitus on palpation of the injured part. In the pre-radiographic era, these findings served as diagnostic criteria for a fracture. Bone tenderness is also characteristic of a fracture, although soft tissue tenderness is usually difficult to distinguish from bone tenderness. Other physical examination findings are less specific for a fracture because they are also seen with soft tissue injuries such as sprains, strains, and contusions. These include soft tissue swelling, ecchymosis, pain on motion of the involved joint, limitation of range of motion, and pain on weight bearing.

There are a number of important instances in which a fractures may be difficult or impossible to detect radiographically (see Table 4 on p.232). When such an injury is suspected based on clinical examination, but is not seen radiographically, a fracture should presumed to be present and the patient managed with adequate immobilization and follow-up care. Examples of fractures that have serious consequences if missed include scaphoid fractures and femoral neck fractures. Such fractures

may have normal radiographs ("occult fractures") or have subtle radiographic findings that must be sought when examining the radiographs.

RADIOGRAPHIC DIAGNOSIS OF A FRACTURE

There are **three radiographic signs** that are useful in the diagnosis of a fracture:

(1) identification of the fracture line,
(2) alterations in skeletal contour or alignment, and
(3) changes in adjacent soft tissues.

Visualization of the fracture line is the most obvious sign of a fracture. Usually, a fracture appears as a radiolucent break in the cortex or trabeculae. If a fracture is impacted or the fracture fragments are overlapping, the fracture may appear radiopaque (white).

A minimum of *two views* perpendicular to each other are required to detect and characterize a fracture. Additional radiographs such as oblique views are occasionally needed to demonstrate the fracture, especially if the fracture is nondisplaced and not in a plane parallel to the x-ray beam.

On the other hand, not all lucent breaks in a bone are fractures. Unfused secondary ossification centers (accessory ossicles), growth plates in children, and nutrient artery foramina should not be mistaken for fractures. They usually have smooth, well-corticated margins, lack cortical defects on the adjacent donor site, and are not tender on clinical examination.

Alteration in skeletal contour and alignment is a second radiographic sign of a fracture. Accurate identification depends on knowledge of normal and pathological anatomy. Measurements of radiographic landmarks can serve as a guide to distinguishing normal from abnormal anatomy, but assessment based on recognition of normal and pathological patterns can be more dependable than discrete measurements.

Soft tissue changes are sometimes easier to see than the fracture itself. These include soft tissue swelling or a joint effusion. An abnormal position or obliteration of fat planes between muscle layers by edema or hemorrhage can also be a clue to a nearby fracture. Examples of helpful soft tissue signs include the elbow fat pad sign, cervical spine prevertebral soft tissue swelling, and maxillary sinus air/fluid levels.

RADIOGRAPHIC VIEWS

Knowledge of the standard and supplementary radiographic views is essential for accurate radiograph interpretation (Table 1). A minimum of two views in perpendicular planes are necessary to define an injury. In regions of complex anatomy such as the wrist, hand, ankle and foot, a third view (often an oblique view) is often standard. The views that are included in a standard radiographic series may vary from institution to institution. Clinicians should be familiar with their institutional protocol.

Supplementary views are helpful when there are questionable findings on the standard views or when a particular fracture is suspected based on clinical examination but not seen on the standard views. Supplementary views may include oblique views, views in a third perpendicular plane (such as an axial view), or views with special positioning (such as the scaphoid view of the wrist).

SKELETAL RADIOGRAPH INTERPRETATION

Two complementary approaches are used in the interpretation of skeletal radiographs. A **systematic approach** looks for each of the radiographic signs of a fracture mentioned above: a fracture line, changes in bone contour or alignment, and soft tissue changes. In a **targeted approach,** specific injury patterns are sought (Table 2).

The first step is to assess whether the radiographic series includes all of the standard views and whether the views have been properly performed.

Systematic Approach

The radiographic signs of a fracture can be summarized by the mnemonic device **ABCS** in which **A** stands for **alignment** (and technical adequacy of the radiograph), **B** stands for the *bones* that are examined for fracture lines and deformities, **C** stands for **cartilage** representing the joint spaces between the bones, and **S** stands for **soft tissue changes** that may be associated with a fracture (Table 3).

Targeted Approach

In a targeted approach, the radiographs are first examined for **common sites of injury.** Then, the radiographs are scrutinized for signs of **easily missed fractures** that can have subtle radiographic manifestations. Recognition of subtle radiographic findings is especially important for injuries that can cause significant disability when missed (Table 4).

TABLE 1

Standard and Supplementary Views of the Extremities

	STANDARD VIEWS	SUPPLEMENTARY VIEWS

Shoulder	AP views:
	   External rotation
	   Internal rotation
		Y view (standard for trauma)
		Axillary view

Clavicle	AP Angled AP (15°)	
Elbow	AP Lateral	Oblique views, Capitellum view Olecranon view (axial)
Wrist	PA Lateral Pronation oblique	Scaphoid view (ulnar deviation PA) Supination oblique Carpal tunnel view (axial)
Hand	PA Lateral Pronation oblique	Supination oblique (ball-catcher view)
Finger	PA Lateral Pronation oblique	
Pelvis	AP	CT Judet views (oblique of acetabulum) Inlet and outlet views
Hip	AP (pelvis) "Frog-leg" or external oblique	Cross-table (groin) lateral
Knee	AP Lateral	Oblique views (2) Axial "sunrise" patellar view Intercondylar notch view
Ankle	AP Lateral Mortise (15° internal oblique)	Oblique views (2)
Foot	AP Lateral Internal oblique	Calcaneus axial view External oblique

TABLE 2

An Approach to Interpreting Skeletal Radiographs

SYSTEMATIC INTERPRETATION—ABCS

Adequacy	All views are included Correct positioning and penetration (exposure)
Alignment	Anatomical relationships between all bones are normal
Bones	Look for fracture lines, disruption of cortex or trabeculae Supplementary views may be needed to detect nondisplaced fractures Pseudofractures can mimic a fracture
Cartilage	Joints should be of normal width and have uniform spacing Fracture fragments may be seen within joint space
Soft tissues	Soft tissue swelling, joint effusions and distortion of fat planes can be easier to see than the fracture itself

TARGETED INTERPRETATION

- Common sites of injury
- Easily missed injuries

TABLE 3

Soft Tissue Signs of a Fracture

RADIOGRAPHIC VIEW	SOFT TISSUE SIGN	COMMON FRACTURES

Elbow lateral	Elbow fat pads:
	    Posterior fat pad
	    Anterior "sail" sign
		Radial head (adult)
		Supracondylar humerus, lateral
		    condyle (child)

Wrist lateral	Pronator quadratus fat stripe	Distal radius
Knee cross-table lateral	Knee lipohemarthrosis	Tibial plateau, intercondylar eminence, osteochondral fractures
Ankle lateral	Ankle effusion	Distal tibia or fibula articular surface, talar dome fracture
Cervical spine lateral	Cervicocranial prevertebral soft tissue swelling	Cervicocranial injuries

Face: Waters view (upright)
    (occipitomental view)
	Maxillary sinus air/fluid level	Blow-out fracture (orbital floor or
		    medial orbital wall), tripod fracture,
		    LeFort fractures

Waters view	Orbital emphysema	Fracture into maxillary sinus or ethmoid sinus
Head CT	Scalp swelling	Skull fracture. Also subdural, epidural, or intracerebral hematoma
Head CT (bone windows)	Pneumocephalus Sphenoid sinus air/fluid level	Open skull fracture (basilar, linear, or depressed fracture)

TABLE 4

Easily Missed Fractures and Dislocations

Common injuries that present with subtle clinical and radiographic findings.
Fractures are usually nondisplaced or minimally displaced. Additional radiographic views
    are sometimes needed to visualize these injuries.
Some of these fractures can have particularly serious consequences if missed (*).

Shoulder	Posterior dislocation* Concomitant proximal humeral fracture and posterior dislocation* Distal clavicle fracture or A-C separation
Elbow	Adult—Radial head fracture Child—Supracondylar, lateral condylar, and medial epicondylar fractures*
Forearm	Monteggia and Galeazzi fracture-dislocations*
Wrist	Distal radius fracture Carpal fractures: scaphoid (*), triquetrum, etc. Dislocations/instability: perilunate, lunate, scapholunate dissociation* Metacarpal base fractures
Hand	Tendon and ligament injuries*; phalangeal avulsion fractures
Pelvis	Isolated pubic ramus fracture, iliac wing fracture, avulsions (ischial tuberosity, iliac spine) Acetabular fractures* Posterior pelvic ring fractures (sacral wing fractures)
Hip	Femoral neck fracture (elderly, osteoporosis)* Intertrochanteric fracture* Pubic ramus fracture or other pelvic fracture
Knee	Tibial plateau fracture (lateral plateau)* Patella fractures (vertical or oblique) Osteochondral fractures and ligament or meniscal injuries*
Ankle	Lateral malleolus fracture Ligament tears and instability, tibio-fibular syndesmosis tear* Fifth metatarsal base, navicular and other midfoot fractures
Foot	Calcaneus and talus (hindfoot) fractures* Tarso-metatarsal fracture-dislocation (Lisfranc)*

Fractures in children
    Growth plate fractures (Salter-Harris)*
    Torus (buckle) fractures and acute plastic bowing

Missed fractures in the multiple trauma victim (requires complete secondary survey)*

PSEUDOFRACTURES

A variety of findings can mimic fractures by causing lucent lines across bones and altering skeletal contour. Examples include: growth plates in children, anatomical variants and overlapping shadows (Table 5). Many such anomalies are easily identified. Correlation between an area of questionable radiographic abnormality and findings on clinical examination will usually resolve any uncertainty. When questions remain, reference can be made to an atlas of radiographic variants that can mimic fractures (Keats and Anderson 2001).

TABLE 5

Pseudofractures

Anatomical variants (congenital anomalies)

Developmental findings in children (growth plates, ossification centers)—need comparison views

Degenerative changes (elderly patients), old trauma

Nutrient artery foramina

Imaging artifacts (e.g., Mach band adjacent to overlapping bones)

Suboptimal or incorrect positioning

NONTRAUMATIC EXTREMITY PAIN

Radiography can be helpful in the diagnosis of certain disorders that cause nontraumatic extremity pain. The pain may be acute, subacute and chronic. Skeletal lesions such as tumors osteomyelitis and arthropathies can be detected.

Most nontraumatic skeletal lesions develop gradually and do not cause acute pain. Therefore, a patient's visit to the ED should not be attributed to a skeletal lesion that has been present for a long time. Focal or diffuse bone disease (e.g., osteoporosis) *can*, however, cause acute extremity pain when there is a pathological fracture.

In addition, extremity pain may be referred from a visceral site (intra-abdominal or intrathoracic). Correct diagnosis rests on a careful clinical examination, not radiographic studies of the involved extremity. Extremity pain may also be a manifestation of nerve root compression, even in the absence of back or neck pain. Imaging studies of the spine may help confirm the diagnosis.

Nontraumatic extremity pain is often due to soft tissue disorders such as tendonitis, vascular insufficiency, infection, or cancer. Some soft tissue disorders causing extremity pain have characteristic radiographic findings, for example, calcific tendinitis of the shoulder. Radiographic studies can occasionally be helpful in patients with soft tissue infections of the extremities. Radiopaque (metallic) foreign bodies in soft tissues may be present in patients who inject drugs or have stepped on a foreign body. Gas may be present in patients with severe soft tissue infections, even in the absence of palpable crepitus. Such gas-forming soft tissue infections have a grave prognosis.

WHEN TO ORDER RADIOGRAPHS IN PATIENTS WITH EXTREMITY TRAUMA

Differentiation between isolated soft tissue injuries (sprains, strains, or contusions) and fractures on purely clinical grounds can be difficult. This is especially true for injuries in the regions around the joints. Therefore, to avoid missing skeletal injuries, a large number of radiographs are ordered, most of which will be negative for a fracture. For example, only 15% of ankle and knee radiographs show fractures, and only 3% of cervical spine radiographs show injuries.

In an attempt to reduce the number of negative radiographs, as well as to make the decision to order radiographs more consistent, several **clinical decision rules** have been developed. These are also called "clinical prediction rules" because their goal is to help predict which patients have isolated soft tissue injuries instead of fractures. Rules developed by Stiell et al, in Ottawa for the ankle and midfoot are widely known and have been extensively studied. Similar rules have been developed for the knee (three different sets of rules by three groups of investigators) and the cervical spine (two sets of rules).

The Ottawa Ankle Rules

The Ottawa ankle rules are relatively simple to remember and apply. There are *two sequential questions* (Figure 1). **First,** is there **tenderness** over the posterior margin or tip of the lateral or medial malleolus, or over the navicular or base of the fifth metatarsal? If tenderness is present, radiographs should be ordered (of the ankle or foot, respectively). Tenderness along the anterior margin of the malleoli, in particular the lateral malleolus, is discounted because this is the most common site for ankle sprains (the anterior talofibular ligament); and bone tenderness in this area is impossible to reliably distinguish from soft tissue tenderness.

Second, when there is no bone tenderness in these regions, is the patient was **able to walk** four steps (two steps on the injured ankle) both at the time of injury and in the ED (regardless of the degree of limping)? If the patient has no bone tenderness and is able to walk, radiographs can be omitted. Other factors are not necessary to consider, such as the degree of soft tissue swelling, ecchymosis, or age of the patient. Patients who do not undergo radiography should be managed symptomatically (limited or no weight bearing and adequate immobilization) and be instructed to seek follow-up care should pain persist.

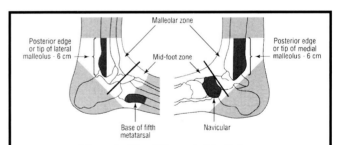

Figure 1. **The Ottawa Ankle Rules**

1. Bone tenderness: ankle — posterior edge (distal 6 cm) or tip of lateral or medial malleolus, or midfoot — navicular or base of the fifth metatarsal
2. Unable to bear weight (four steps) both immediately at the time of injury and in the ED

Malleolar tip avulsion fractures less than 3 mm in breadth are excluded because they are not considered clinically significant. These rules remain secondary to the clinical judgment and common sense of the physician. Altered sensorium, other distracting injuries and underlying bone disorders must be taken into account. Patients under the age of 18 were not studied.
[From: Stiell IG, et al: The "Real" Ottawa ankle rules. Ann Emerg Med 1996; 27:103, with permission.]

Development of Clinical Decision Rule

To be successful, a rule must be relatively easy to apply and have nearly 100% sensitivity (no missed fractures). A rule is often **derived** in one set of patients. However, before being used in clinical practice, the rule must be **validated** in a prospective study using a different group of patients. The validation study should confirm the rule's sensitivity and demonstrate that it can be applied consistently by various practitioners.

Finally, a rule is only worthwhile if it has a beneficial **impact** on clinical practice in comparison to standard clinical practice. Specifically, the rule must effectively reduce the number of radiographic studies ordered without increasing the number of missed fractures. A decision rule could also potentially reduce the number of missed diagnoses in comparison to usual clinical practice, although this is not the usual rationale for developing such rules.

Such **impact studies** (implementation studies) are laborious to conduct. Optimally, they should be conducted in multiple clinical sites, including sites different from the one in which the decision rule was developed and validated. Implementation studies have therefore not been conducted for most clinical decision rules. The Ottawa ankle/midfoot rule is one rule that has been fully studied. The rule has been prospectively validated and its impact on clinical practice has been studied in both a single center and a multicenter trial that included 12,000 patients (Stiell 1995). The rules were found to be nearly 100% sensitive (99.5%). However when compared to standard clinical practice, the reduction in radiograph ordering was less than in the derivation and validation studies. When initially studied, the rules led to a reduction in radiograph ordering of 34%. However, this was in comparison to an artificial setting in which nearly all patients with ankle injuries had radiography. In the multicenter implementation (impact) trial, the reduction in radiography was only 13% (from 91.6% to 78.3%). However, there was a greater reduction in the number of patients who had both ankle and foot radiographs. Nonetheless, for radiographic studies that are ordered frequently, this reduction can amount to substantial cost savings (Stiell et al.: BMJ 1995).

One additional observation can be made from these studies. Despite the use of this decision rule, most radiographs will still be negative. For example, in the control group, 20% of patients with ankle injuries had fractures, whereas in the group using the decision rule, only 27% had fractures. Therefore, even when using a decision rule, most radiographic studies will be negative (nearly three-quarters). In the NEXUS cervical spine study, there was a 12% reduction in radiograph ordering but the number of positive cervical spine radiographs increased only from 2.7% to 3.4%. This observation confirms that a large number of negative radiographs will still need to be obtained to avoid missing significant injuries, and the clinician should not be overly selective in ordering radiographs.

Investigations to develop and test clinical decision rules are also useful by providing prospective information about a large number of patients with a particular clinical problem. These studies reveal the types and frequencies of injuries, as well as range of clinical presentations. These insights can also have a beneficial impact on clinical practice.

SUGGESTED READING

Daffner RH: Skeletal pseudofractures. *Emerg Radiol* 1995;2:96–104.

Field HA, Shields NN: Most frequently overlooked radiographically apparent fractures in a teaching hospital emergency department. *Ann Emerg Med* 1984;13:900–904.

Harris JH, Harris WH: *The Radiology of Emergency Medicine*, 4th ed. Williams & Wilkins, 2000.

Keats TE, Anderson MW: *Atlas of Normal Roentgen Variants that May Simulate Disease*, 7th ed. Mosby, 2001.

Riddervold HO: *Easily Missed Fractures and Corner Signs in Radiology*. Mt. Kisco, NY: Futura, 1991.

Rogers LF: *Radiology of Skeletal Trauma*, 3rd ed. London: Churchill Livingstone, 2002.

Schwartz DT, Reisdorff EJ: Fundamentals of skeletal radiology, in Schwartz DT, Reisdorff EJ, ed. *Emergency Radiology*. New York: McGraw–Hill, 2000.

Clinical Decision Rules

Bachmann LM, Kolb E, Koller MT, Steurer J, ter Riet G: Accuracy of Ottawa ankle rules to exclude fractures of the ankle and mid–foot: Systematic review. *BMJ* 2003;326:417.

Heyworth J: Ottawa ankle rules for the injured ankle. *BMJ* 2003;326:405–406.

McGinn TG, Guyatt GH, Wyer PC, Naylor CD, Stiell IG, Richardson WS: Users' guides to the medical literature: How to use articles about clinical decision rules. *JAMA* 2000;284:79–84.

Stiell IG: Emergency decision making. *Acad Emerg Med* 1994;1: 146–149.

Stiell IG, Greenberg GH, McKnight RD, et al: A study to develop clinical decision rules for the use of radiography in acute ankle injuries. *Ann Emerg Med* 1992;21:384–390.

Stiell IG, Greenberg GH, McKnight RD, et al: Decision rules for the use of radiography in acute ankle injuries: Refinement and prospective validation. *JAMA* 1993;269:1127–1132.

Stiell IG, Greenberg GH, Wells GA, et al: Derivation of a decision rule for the use of radiographs in acute knee injuries. *Ann Emerg Med* 1995;26:405–412.

Stiell IG, McKnight RD, Greenberg GH, et al: Implementation of the Ottawa ankle rules. *JAMA* 1994;271:827–832. McDonald CJ (editorial) 872–873.

Stiell IG, Wells GA. Methodologic standards for the development of clinical decision rules in emergency medicine. *Ann Emerg Med* 1999;33:437–447.

Stiell IG, Wells G, Laupacis A, et al: A multicenter trial to introduce clinical decision rules for the use of radiography in acute ankle injuries. *BMJ* 1995;311:594–597.

Upper Extremity: Patient 1

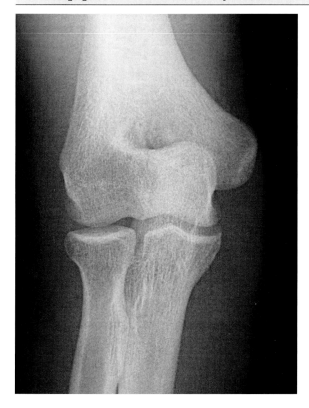

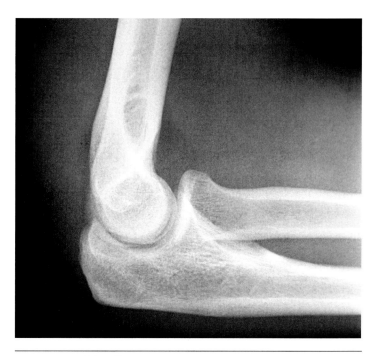

FIGURE 1   Right elbow.

Elbow and forearm injures in a young man hit with a nightstick

A 24-year-old man was hit with a nightstick during an altercation. He held up both his arms to protect himself and received blows to the forearms. He had pain on the ulnar aspect of his left forearm and the extensor surface of his right elbow.

- Are any fractures seen on these radiographs (Figures 1 and 2)?

- What are the radiographic signs of a fracture?

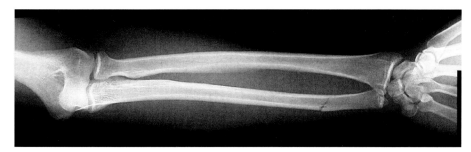

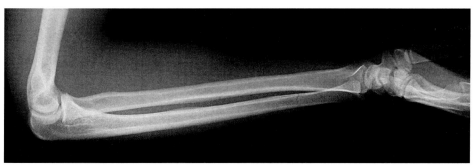

FIGURE 2   Left forearm

235

HOW TO DIAGNOSE A FRACTURE

Fracture diagnosis is based on both clinical and radiographic findings. Three clinical predictors of a fracture are: 1) the mechanism of injury, 2) the findings on physical examination, and 3) age-related common injuries (Table 1). Likewise, there are three radiographic findings of a fracture: 1) visualization of the fracture line; 2) alterations in skeletal contour or alignment (most useful in children); and 3) soft tissue changes. Supplementary views are occasionally needed to visualize the fracture. These principles are illustrated for the elbow in this and the following chapter.

The elbow is a prime example of the usefulness of soft tissue signs in fracture diagnosis. Soft tissue changes can sometimes be easier to see than the fracture itself (see Principles of Skeletal Radiology, Table 3, page 231). Soft tissue changes include swelling, joint effusions, and distortion or obliteration of the fats planes between muscle layers.

Post-traumatic joint effusions can serve as a clue to an intra-articular fracture. An effusion usually appears as an area of fluid density adjacent to the joint. Examples include ankle and knee effusions (although knee effusions are more reliably detected by physical examination).

The elbow anatomy is unusual because there are two collections of fatty tissue contained within the joint capsule (anterior and posterior **fat pads**) (Figure 3A). When the elbow is flexed to 90°, these *fat pads* lie nearly entirely within the coronoid and olecranon fossae of the distal humerus. On a properly performed lateral radiograph, the anterior fat pad may appear as a small lucent area just anterior to the distal humerus. The posterior fat pad is not normally visible (Figure 4A).

If the joint space is filled by blood (due to a fracture) the fat pads are displaced outwards (Figure 3B). The posterior fat pad becomes visible posterior to the olecranon fossa, and the anterior fat pad is displaced anteriorly, forming a radiolucent triangle, the "**sail sign**" (Figure 4B). The elbow fat pad signs are not do to fat entering the joint from bone marrow through an intra-articular fracture, as is the case with a *lipohemarthrosis* of the knee (see Lower Extremity Patient 3, figure 16 on p. 315).

Radiographic technique can obscure or mimic the fat pad signs. If the radiograph is overpenetrated (too dark) with respect to soft tissues, a bright light (or a lightened digital image) may be needed to detect the fat pads (Figure 5). This is often the case because extremity radiographs are generally exposed to show bone detail.

If the lateral view is incorrectly positioned with an oblique orientation, the fat pad signs can be obscured. If the elbow is extended rather than flexed, the posterior fat pad may be visible because it is displaced from the olecranon fossa by the olecranon. Finally, fat pad signs can also caused by nontraumatic elbow effusions such as infectious and inflammatory arthritides.

The Fat Pad Sign in Adults

In adults, the fat pad sign is most frequently associated with a **radial head fracture**. Radial head fractures are by far the most common fracture in adults, accounting for 50% of cases. This fracture can be difficult to see if it is nondisplaced. An oblique view or radiocapitellar view (lateral view taken with an angled x-ray beam) can sometimes reveal the fracture (Figure 6). However, there is little need to obtain this additional view because management is not altered. An adult patient with a fat pad sign and no visible fracture is treated as though a non-displaced radial head fracture were present, i.e., simply using a forearm sling with early mobilization exercises.

A radial head fracture is usually caused by a fall onto an outstretched hand causing the radial head to impact against the capitellum. Tenderness over the radial head can be difficult to elicit because of the thickness of the surrounding muscles. Pain and limited range of motion (flexion–extension and supination–pronation) are reliable clinical signs of a radial head fracture. In fact, these signs are useful criteria in deciding to order elbow radiographs, although this has not been studied in a large clinical trial (Hawksworth and Freeland 1991, Brasher and Macias 2001).

TABLE 1

Common Elbow Injuries

ADULT		CHILD	
Radial head or neck fracture	50%	Supracondylar fracture	60%
Olecranon fracture	20%	Lateral condyle fracture	15%
Elbow dislocation	15%	Medial epicondyle fracture	10%
		Radial neck or head fracture	6-12%
Others		Others	
Distal humerus fracture		Elbow dislocation	
Capitellum fracture		Olecranon fracture	
Coronoid fracture		Monteggia injury	
Monteggia injury		Complete epiphyseal separation (rare)	

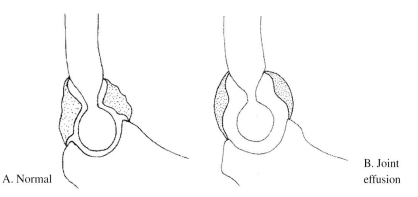

A. Normal

B. Joint
effusion

FIGURE 3 Normally, the anterior and posterior fat pads are within the coronoid and olecranon fossae (*A*). A traumatic hemarthrosis displaces the fat pads outward (*B*).

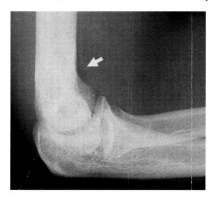
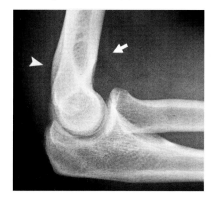

FIGURE 4 (*A*) A normal anterior fat pad is sometimes visible on the lateral radiograph (*arrow*). (*B*) In Patient 1, both the anterior pad sail sign (*arrow*) and posterior fat pad (*arrowhead*) are seen on the lateral radiograph. A fracture is not visible on this view.

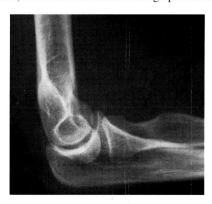
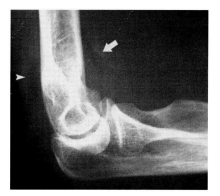

FIGURE 5 A bright light (lighter window level for digital radiographs) may be needed to see the fat pad sign. Skeletal radiographs are usually exposed for bone detail; soft tissues are often overpenetrated (too dark).

(*A*) With standard viewing, the fat pad signs are not well seen

(*B*) With a bright-light, the anterior and posterior fat pad signs are visible; no fracture is seen

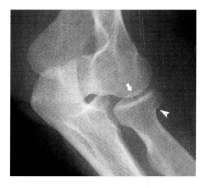

FIGURE 6 In another patient, a radial head fracture is only seen on an **oblique view.**

Patient Outcome

This patient's **lateral elbow radiograph** show both an anterior fat pad sail sign and a small posterior fat pad, meaning that an intra-articular fracture is likely present (Figure 1B and 4B). A radial head fracture is the most common, associated fracture.

However, given this patient's mechanism of injury—a direct blow to the extensor surface of his elbow by a nightstick—and the findings on physical examination (tenderness over the olecranon), a radial head fracture is unlikely. This patient's direct blow mechanism of injury is reflected by the "nightstick" fracture (ulnar shaft fracture) of his left forearm (Figure 2).

Olecranon fractures are the second most common about the elbow in adults (20%). Olecranon fractures are usually transverse or avulsion fractures and are easily seen on the lateral view (Figure 7).

An intra-articular elbow fracture that can be caused by a direct blow to the elbow and which may be difficult to detect radiographically is a longitudinally-oriented olecranon fracture.

In this patient, a supplementary **olecranon view** was necessary to demonstrate the fracture (Figure 8). In retrospect, close examination of the AP view reveals a very faint longitudinal fracture line through the olecranon (Figure 9).

This patient was treated with a padded posterior splint and sling for the olecranon fracture of his right elbow and a long arm cast for the "nightstick fracture" of his left forearm.

Supplementary radiographic views are indicated when a fracture is suspected based on physical examination findings, but is not clearly seen on the standard radiographic views.

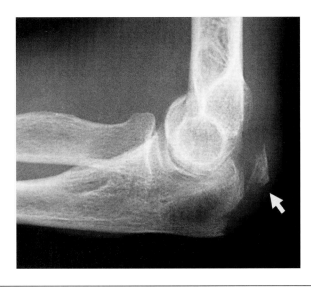

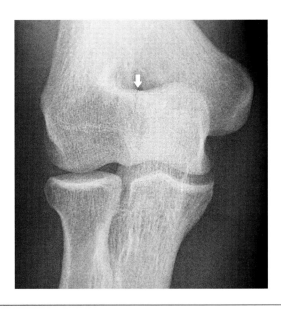

FIGURE 7 Another patient with a more common type of olecranon fracture —an avulsion fracture. Olecranon fractures are usually readily detected on the lateral elbow view (*arrow*).

FIGURE 9 A subtle longitudinal fracture of the olecranon is visible on the patient's AP radiograph (*arrow*).

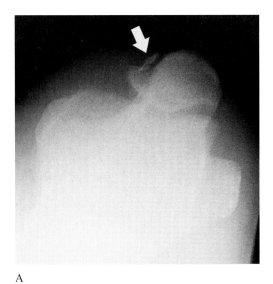

A

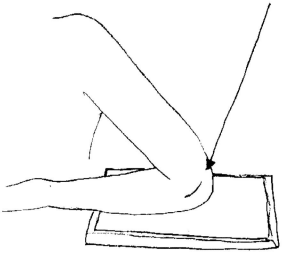

B

FIGURE 8 (*A*) Olecranon view reveals the longitudinal fracture through the olecranon (*arrow*). (*B*) Positioning of the axial olecranon view.

The Fat Pad Sign in Children

In children, the fat pad sign is especially important because it serves as a clue to potentially serious fractures—most commonly a **supracondylar fracture** or a **lateral condylar fracture** (Table 1). When a pad sign is seen in a child, a search should be made for subtle signs of these fractures (Figure 10). If a fracture cannot be found, an occult supracondylar fracture is presumed to be present and the child should be immobilized in a splint or cast.

Supracondylar condylar fractures can cause neurovascular injuries (most commonly median nerve and brachial artery) and growth deformities. Although these complications are usually associated with displaced fractures that are readily apparent on radiography, all supracondylar fractures require specific orthopedic treatment—a posterior splint or cast if nondisplaced, and reduction and pin fixation if displaced—and all patients need close clinical follow-up.

Sensitivity and Specificity of the Fat Pad Sign

Because treatment of children having an elbow fat pad sign requires more prolonged immobilization than in adults, the specificity (positive predictive value) of the fat pad sign for an occult fracture is important to consider in children. In early reports, only a minority of patients with fat pad signs and no demonstrable fracture actually had fractures (6–29%). This calls into question the need to immobilize all children with isolated fat pad signs. However, a larger prospective study (Skaggs 1999) found that 76% of 45 children ultimately had fractures (53% supracondylar, 26% proximal ulnar, 12% lateral condylar, and 9% radial neck). Two studies using MRI in elbow trauma also revealed a high incidence of occult fractures, although treatment was not altered on the basis of the MRI findings (Griffith 2001, Major 2002).

The sensitivity of the fat pad sign (i.e., does the absence of a fat pad sign exclude a fracture) has not been studied in a systematic fashion. However, it is reasonable to assume that when no fracture is visible, the absence of a fat pad sign makes a significant fracture unlikely. Nonetheless, fractures can be present without a visible fat pad sign. In two large series, fat pad signs were seen on only 41-66% of patients with radiographically visible fractures (Kohn 1959, Corbett 1978). A fat pad sign

does not occur if the joint capsule is disrupted or if correct radiographic positioning cannot be attained because of the injury (elbow flexed to 90° on the lateral view).

Ulnar Shaft Fractures

Patient 1 also has a left ulnar shaft fracture (Figure 11). Because the ulna and radius are rigidly bound to each other by the interosseus ligament, a fracture of one of these bones may be accompanied by a fracture or dislocation of the other. With a displaced ulnar shaft fracture, there may be dislocation of the radial head at the elbow. This is called a ***Monteggia lesion*** (Figure 12). Patients with forearm fractures must be carefully examined at the elbow and wrist, and radiographs should be obtained when there is pain or tenderness of either joint.

In this patient, the ulnar shaft fracture is not displaced and the elbow and wrist are normal. This is termed a ***nightstick fracture*** owing to the usual mechanism of injury—a direct blow to the forearm as the patient holds up his forearm to protect himself from an assault. A night-stick fracture is usually managed with cast immobilization, although if the fracture is displaced, reduction can be difficult to maintain and internal fixation may be necessary. A Monteggia fracture is unstable and always needs internal fixation. The mechanism of injury of a Monteggia fracture is either a direct blow to the ulnar aspect of the forearm or a fall on an outstretched arm.

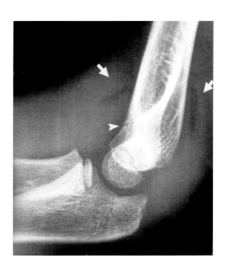

FIGURE 10 Supra-condylar fracture in a 5-year-old child. Anterior and posterior fat pad signs are present (*arrows*). However, the fracture itself is subtle. There is a slight interruption of the anterior cortex of the distal humerus in the supracondylar region (*arrowhead*).

SUGGESTED READING

Chuirazzi DM, Riviello RJ: The elbow and distal humerus. In Schwartz DT, Reisdorff EJ, eds. *Emergency Radiology.* New York: McGraw-Hill, 2000.

Greenspan A, Norman A: Radial head-capitellum view: An expanded imaging approach to elbow injury. *Radiology* 1987;164:272–274.

Hall-Craggs MA, Shorvon PJ, Chapman M: Assessment of the radial head–capitellum view and the dorsal fat-pad sign in acute elbow trauma. *AJR* 1985;145:607–609.

Hawksworth CR, Freeland P: Inability to fully extend the injured elbow: an indicator of significant injury. *Arch Emerg Med* 1991; 8:253.

Fat Pad Signs

Corbett RH: Displaced fat pads in trauma to the elbow. *Injury* 1978;9:297–298.

Goswami GK: The fat pad sign. *Radiology* 2002;222:419–420.

Kohn AM: Soft tissue alterations in elbow trauma. *AJR* 1959;82:867–874.

Major NM, Crawford ST: Elbow effusions in trauma in adults and children: Is there an occult fracture? *AJR* 2002;178:413–418.

Zimmers TE: Fat plane radiological signs in wrist and elbow trauma. *Am J Emerg Med* 1984;2:526–532.

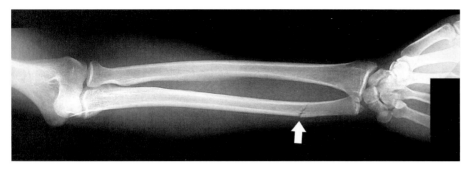

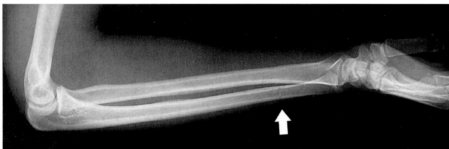

FIGURE 11   Nightstick fracture.

Patient 1 had an isolated nondisplaced fracture of the left ulnar shaft that was caused by a direct blow to the ulnar aspect of the forearm by a nightstick. The elbow and wrist are normal.

This is known as a *nightstick fracture*. The fracture is managed by immobilization in a cylindrical cast.

If the force of impact had been greater and the ulnar fracture was displaced, a concomitant dislocation of the radial head could be present–a Monteggia lesion.

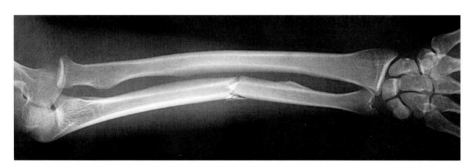

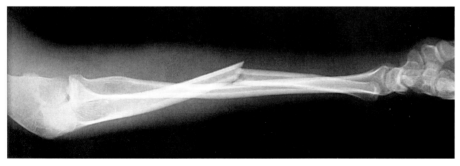

FIGURE 12   When is a nightstick injury not a nightstick fracture?

(*A* and *B*) In another patient who was hit by a nightstick on the ulnar aspect of his forearm, there is a moderately displaced fracture of the ulnar shaft.

A radial head dislocation should be suspected in such cases and the patient should be examined for elbow pain and limited range of motion.

On first glance, the radial head appears to articulate with the distal humeral articular surface. There is, however, significant malalignment. The radial head is actually near the trochlea, not to the capitellum.

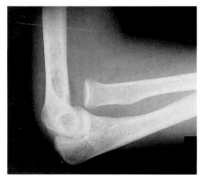

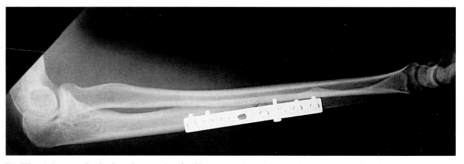

D. The Monteggia lesion is mechanically unstable and requires open reduction and internal fixation

C. The elbow radiograph reveals dislocation of the radial head-a *Monteggia lesion*

Upper Extremity: Patient 2

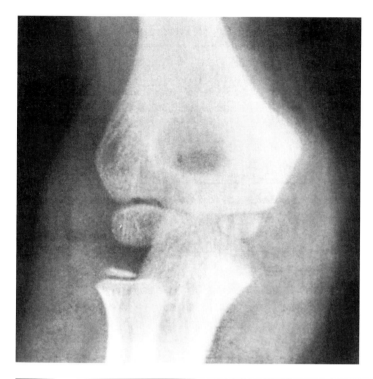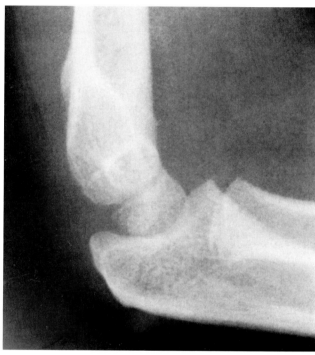

FIGURE 1

An elbow injury in a 7-year-old girl who fell on to her outstretched right hand

A 7-year-old girl fell off "monkey bars" on to her outstretched right hand. She complained of pain localized to the right elbow.

On examination, there was diffuse swelling and tenderness about the elbow. She was unable to flex the elbow more than 30°. The remainder of the right upper extremity was normal.

The elbow radiographs are shown in Figure 1.

- Are any abnormalities present?

- What is the third most common fracture about the elbow in children?

Without a clear understanding of the radiographic landmarks and injury patterns in children, the findings in this patient are difficult to appreciate, even though this child has a major injury that will require surgical treatment.

Although comparison views are often obtained in children, the correct diagnosis can be made in this patient using the radiographs of the injured side alone.

[From: Rogers LF: *The Radiology of Skeletal Trauma*, 3rd ed. Churchill-Livingstone, 2002, with permission.]

CRITOE

Fractures of the elbow are among the most common extremity injuries in children. However, they can be difficult to diagnose due to the complex developmental anatomy of the elbow and the subtle radiographic manifestations of some injuries. Comparison views are often obtained to aid radiograph interpretation, although by knowing the principal anatomical landmarks and injury patterns, the diagnosis can be made in many cases using radiographs of the injured side alone (Table 1).

Fractures are often difficult to detect in young children because much of the elbow is not ossified. In addition, the pliable cortical bone in children may be deformed without a discrete fracture line (acute plastic bowing) or have a fracture on only one side of the cortex (a greenstick fracture). Such fractures can often only be detected by noting malalignment of the bones of the elbow.

There are two key landmarks of alignment that are useful in detecting elbow injuries in children—the **anterior humeral line** and the **radiocapitellar line.** In addition, the location and the sequence of appearance of the six **ossification centers** of the elbow must also be understood because they are often involved in elbow injuries. The growth plates do not fuse until late adolescence and these can be difficult to distinguish from fractures.

There are **three distinctive elbow injuries** in children: *supracondylar fractures, lateral condylar fractures* and *medial epicondylar avulsion fractures* (Table 1). Each of the above mentioned radiographic landmarks has a role in detecting these injures: the anterior humeral line for supracondylar fractures, the radiocapitellar line for lateral condylar fractures, and the sequence of appearance of the elbow ossification centers for medial epicondylar features.

Finally, the **fat pad signs** (posterior fat pad sign and anterior fat pad sail sign) are useful in detecting injuries in children. The fat pad signs are seen in supracondylar and lateral condylar fractures (Figure 2-4). The presence of a fat pad sign should prompt a search for these factures. If a fracture is not seen, the child should be immobilized in a splint for a possible occult fracture and referred for follow-up.

Supracondylar Fractures and the Anterior Humeral Line

The **anterior humeral line** is a feature of alignment seen on the lateral view. A line drawn along the anterior cortex of the humeral shaft should intersect the middle third of the capitellum (Figure 2). The *capitellum* is the rounded ossification center of the distal humerus that articulates with the radial head.

The anterior humeral line is useful in the diagnosis of **supracondylar fractures,** the most common fracture about the elbow in children. In most cases, the fracture is posteriorly displaced and the capitellum is posterior to the anterior humeral line (Figure 3). When a fracture is not visible, this can be an important clue to its presence (Figure 4).

Another radiographic landmark that is helpful in the diagnosis of a supracondylar fractures is the *radiographic teardrop.* It is formed by the cortices of the distal humerus at the olecranon and coronoid fossae (Figure 2). A supracondylar fracture will often deform the radiographic teardrop (Figure 3).

Although called "supracondylar," the fracture actually traverses through the humeral condyles, not above them. For this reason, it is more properly termed a "transcondylar" fracture, i.e., an intra-articular rather than extra-articular fracture (Figure 3B).

Treatment of supracondylar fracture if displaced generally entails closed reduction and then fixation with percutaneous pins (Figure 3C). Percutaneous pin fixation permits early mobilization and avoids complications such as Volkmann's ischemic contracture of the forearm. In the past, forearm ischemia occurred due to compression of the brachial artery caused by swelling in the antecubital fossa while the elbow was immobilized in a flexed position using a cast or splint.

TABLE 1

Common Elbow Injuries in Children

Supracondylar fracture	60%
Lateral condyle fracture	15%
Medial epicondyle fracture	10%
Radial neck or head fracture	8%
Others	
Elbow dislocation	
Olecranon fracture	
Monteggia injury	
Complete epiphyseal separation (rare)	

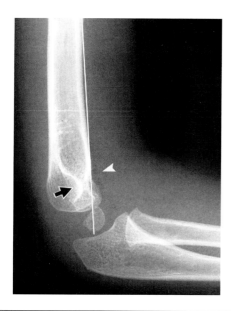

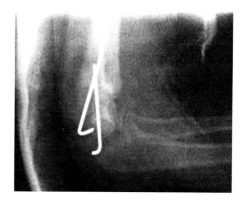

FIGURE 2 Anterior humeral line.

A line drawn along the anterior cortex of the humeral shaft normally intersects the middle third of the capitellum.

A **normal radiographic teardrop** is seen where the cortices of the olecranon and coronoid fossae come together (*black arrow*).

A small **normal anterior fat pad** is visible (*arrowhead*).

FIGURE 3 Supracondylar fracture in a 3-year-old child.

(*A*) On the **lateral view,** there is a fracture through the anterior cortex of the distal humeral metaphysis (*arrowhead*). This disrupts the radiographic teardrop of the distal humerus (see Figure 2). The capitellum is displaced posterior to the anterior humeral line. A posterior fat pad is visible (*arrow*).

(Figure 2 is the comparison view of the opposite normal elbow in this patient.)

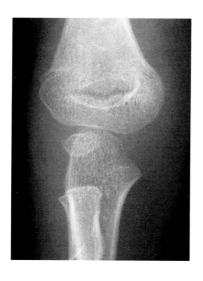

(3B) On the **AP view,** the fracture is seen traversing the humeral condyles.

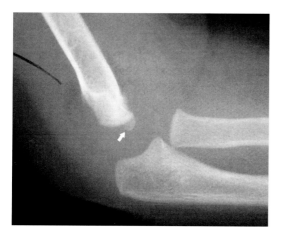

(3C) **Postoperative radiograph** showing fixation with percutaneous pins.

FIGURE 4 Subtle supracondylar fracture in an 18-month-old child.

The capitellum ossification center (*arrow*) is displaced posteriorly in relation to the **anterior humeral line.** The fracture itself is not visible because it involves only noncalcified growth plate.

A **posterior fat pad sign** (*black line*) and faint anterior fat pad sail sign are visible.

Lateral Condylar Fractures and the Radiocapitellar Line

The second elbow alignment feature is the **radiocapitellar line.** A line drawn along the shaft of the radius should intersect the middle of the capitellum. This alignment should be present in both the AP and lateral views (Figure 5).

The radiocapitellar line can be useful in detecting the second most common fracture about the elbow in children—a **lateral condylar fracture.**

In most cases, the fracture is clearly seen (Figure 6). Occasionally, only a thin sliver of the distal humerus is displaced with the fracture (Figure 7). When the fracture is entirely through the growth plate, the only finding is malalignment of the capitellum in relation to the radiocapitellar line (Figure 8). When the fracture is not displaced, the radiocapitellar line is normal and the only radiographic clue to a fracture may be the fat pad sign.

Although most useful in detecting lateral condylar fractures, the radiocapitellar line is also disrupted in elbow dislocations, but is intact with supracondylar fractures (Figure 9).

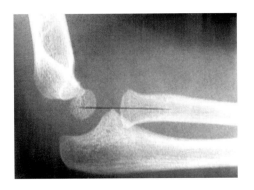
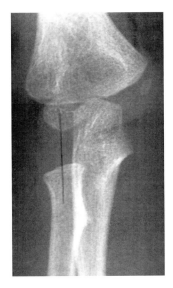

FIGURE 5   Radiocapitellar line.
A line drawn along the long axis of the radial shaft should intersect the middle of the capitellum on each view.

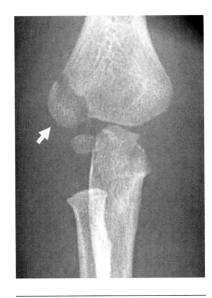

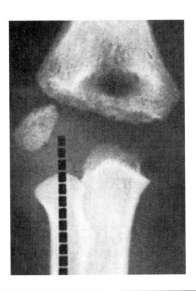

FIGURE 8   Lateral condylar fracture involving only the growth plate of the capitellum. The only indication of the fracture is malalignment of the capitellum with the radiocapitellar line.

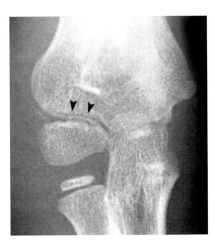

FIGURE 6   Lateral condylar fracture.
A markedly displaced fracture involves a large portion of the distal humeral metaphysis (*arrow*).

FIGURE 7   Lateral condylar fracture.
A subtle fracture in which only a thin portion of the distal numeral metaphysis is involved (*arrows*).

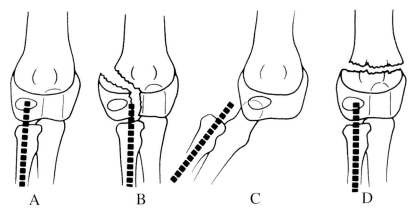

A   B   C   D

FIGURE 9   The radiocapitellar line is disrupted with a lateral condylar fracture (*B*) and elbow dislocation (*C*), but is intact with a supracondylar fracture (*D*).

[From: DeLee JC, et al: Fracture-separation of the distal humeral epiphysis. *J Bone Joint Surg (Am)* 62-A:46 1980, with permission.]

Ossification Centers of the Elbow

The third anatomical feature that should be evaluated on the elbow radiographs is the six **ossification centers** of the distal humerus and proximal ulna and radius (Figure 10). Although the age of appearance of the ossification centers is variable, the sequence of their appearance is constant. The sequence of appearance of the ossification centers can be remembered by using the mnemonic device: **CRITOE,** in which C stands for **capitellum,** R is the **radial head,** I is the **internal (medial) epicondyle,** T is the **trochlea,** O for the **olecranon,** and E is the **external (lateral) epicondyle.** The ossification centers appear roughly at each odd-numbered year of age – 1, 3, 5, 7, 9, and 11 years (Table 2).

Using this mnemonic device, one can estimate the age of a child based on the appearance of the elbow radiograph. For example, in a 6-year-old child, the capitellum, radial head and medial epicondyle are visible (Figure 10). In a 10-year-old, the trochlear and olecranon ossification centers are also present.

Medial Epicondylar Fractures

Of greater clinical significance, the CRITOE mnemonic plays a role in the diagnosis of the third most common fracture of the elbow in children—**medial epicondylar avulsion fracture**—particularly when the avulsed medial epicondyle becomes entrapped within the elbow joint.

With a medial epicondylar fracture, the ossification center is displaced from its normal position adjacent to the distal humerus. Avulsions can range from minimally to markedly displaced fractures (Figures 11 and 12). Comparison views of the opposite uninjured elbow can help assess displacement. The fat pad sign is not present in most cases because the injury is extra-articular.

In some cases, the elbow joint capsule is torn and the medial epicondyle may migrate into and become **entrapped** within the elbow joint (Figure 13). This requires surgical treatment. The entrapped medial epicondyle is usually readily apparent as an abnormal intra-articular fragment of bone (Figure 14).

The appearance of an entrapped medial epicondyle depends on the **age of the patient** (Figure 15). After the age of 7 years, the trochlea is ossified and with an entrapped medial epicondyle, there are two intra-articular bone fragments (Figure 16).

In a child of **age 6–7 years,** such as **Patient 2,** the entrapped medial epicondyle appears as a single intra-articular bone fragment, which could be misinterpreted as the trochlear ossification center. This error can be avoided by considering the sequence of appearance of the ossification centers. In accordance with the CRITOE mnemonic, the medial epicondyle must appear before the trochlear ossification center. If there is no ossification center in the region of the medial epicondyle, the intra-articular bone fragment is an entrapped medial epicondyle (Figure 17A). A comparison view of the opposite elbow, although not necessary to diagnose this injury, demonstrates that the medial epicondyle is not in its correct position (Figure 17B).

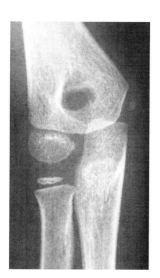

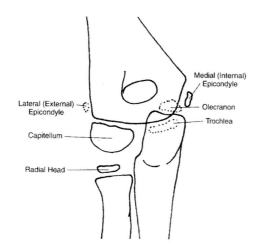

FIGURE 10   Ossification centers of the elbow.
In a 6-year-old child, the capitellum, radial head, and medial epicondyle are ossified.

TABLE 2

CRITOE
Sequence of Appearance of Elbow Ossification Centers and Range of Age of Appearance

Capitellum	1 year	1–8 months
Radial head	3 years	3–6 years
Internal (medial) epicondyle	5 years	3–7 years
Trochlea	7 years	7–10 years
Olecranon	9 years	8–10 years
External (lateral) epicondyle	11 years	11–12 years

Growth plates close at age 14–17 years. Medial epicondyle fuses at age 15–18 years.

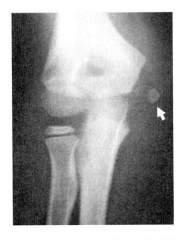 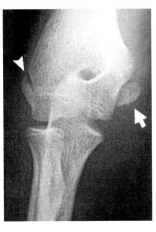 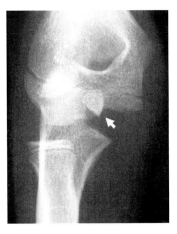 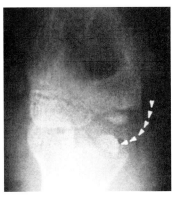

FIGURE 11 Medial epicondylar avulsion.

Marked displacement in a 6-year-old child (*arrow*).

[From: Pizzutillo PD: *Pediatric Orthopaedics in Primary Practice.* McGraw-Hill, 1997.]

FIGURE 12 Medial epicondylar avulsion.

Minimal displacement (*arrow*). Comparison views may be needed to assess the presence of displacement. A partially fused growth plate (*arrowhead*) should not be misinterpreted as a fracture.

FIGURE 14 Entrapped medial epicondyle.

In a 15-year-old child, the intra-articular entrapped medial epicondyle is clearly abnormal (*arrow*).

[From: *Emergency Radiology.* Schwartz DT, Reisdorff EJ: McGraw-Hill 2000.]

FIGURE 16 Entrapped medial epicondyle.

In an 11-year-old child, two intra-articular ossifications are seen, the trochlea and entrapped medial epicondyle (*arrowheads*).

[From: Swichuk LE: *Emergency Imaging of the Acutely Ill or Injured Child,* 3rd ed. Lippincott Williams and Wilkins, with permission.]

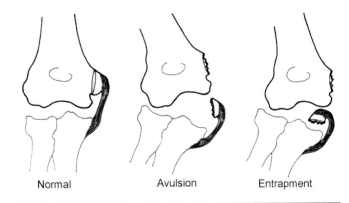

FIGURE 13 Medial epicondylar injuries.

Traction by the flexor-pronator tendon causes an avulsion fracture of the medial epicondyle. When the joint capsule is torn, the medical epicondyle can become entrapped.

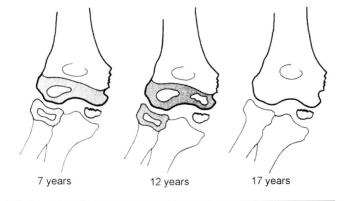

FIGURE 15 Entrapped medial epicondyle.

The appearance depends on the age of the patient and the expected ossification of the growth centers.

[From: Chessare JW, et al: Injuries of the medial epicondylar ossification center of the humerus. *AJR* 1977; 129:49–55, with permission.]

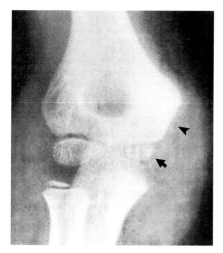 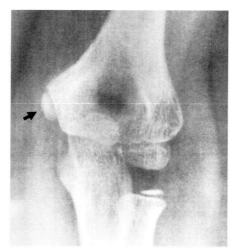 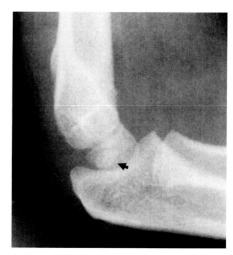

A. AP view   B. Compresion AP view   C. Lateral view

FIGURE 17   Patient 2—Entrapped medial epicondyle.

(*A*) The intra-articular ossification center (*arrow*) is not the trochlea because the medial epicondyle is not present in its usual location (*arrowhead*), i.e., the medial epicondyle normally ossifies before the trochlea. The intra-articular ossification center must therefore be an entrapped medial epicondyle.

(*B*) The comparison view of the opposite uninjured elbow confirms the normal location of the medial epicondyle (*arrow*).

(*C*) Close inspection of the lateral view discloses the entrapped medial epicondyle (*arrow*).

[From Rogers LF: *Radiology of Skeletal Trauma*, 3rd ed. Churchill Livingstone, 2002, with permission.]

In **Patient 2,** close inspection of the **lateral view** reveals the entrapped medial epicondyle (Figure 17C). A fat pad sign was not present in this case even though there was an intra-articular injury because the joint capsule was torn at the time of injury and the intra-articular blood (hemarthrosis) drained into the surrounding soft tissues.

Although the radiograph superficially appears benign, this patient had a major injury that requires open exploration of the elbow joint to retrieve the intra-articular bone fragment and reattach the avulsed medial epicondyle.

Interpretation of radiographs in children with elbow injuries requires a clear understanding of normal anatomical landmarks as well as the changes that occur with common injuries (Table 3).

TABLE 3

How to Interpret Elbow Radiographs in Children

1. Two views properly performed
   Lateral view—elbow flexed to 90° and not rotated

2. Fat pad signs—may need to lighten image to see

3. Three features
   A. Anterior humeral line
   B. Radiocapitellar line
   C. Ossification centers—correct location and sequence of appearance based on child's age

4. Three injuries
   A. Supracondylar fracture
   B. Lateral condylar fracture
   C. Medial epicondylar avulsion fracture
   (also, radial head fracture in older children)

SUGGESTED READING

Chessare JW, Rogers LF White H, Tachdjian MO: Injuries of the medial epicondylar ossification center of the humerus. *AJR* 1977; 129:49–55.

Chuirazzi DM, Riviello RJ: The elbow and distal humerus. In: Schwartz DT, Reisdorff EJ, eds. *Emergency Radiology.* New York: McGraw-Hill, 2000.

DeLee JC, Wilkins KE, Rogers LF, Rockwood CA: Fracture-separation of the distal humeral epiphysis. *J Bone Joint Surg (Am)* 1980; 62-A:46.

Griffith JF, Roebuck DJ, Cheng JCY, et al: Acute elbow trauma in children: Spectrum of injury revealed by MR imaging not apparent on radiographs. *AJR* 2001;176:53–50.

Rogers LF: *Radiology of Skeletal Trauma*, 3rd ed. New York: Churchill Livingstone, 2002.

Skaggs DL, Mirzayan R. The posterior fat pat sign in association with occult fracture of the elbow in children. *J Bone Joint Surg (Am)* 1999;81-A:1429–1433.

Swischuk LE: *Emergency Imaging of the Acutely Ill or Injured Child*, 4th ed. Philadelphia: Lippincott Williams and Williams, 2000.

Wu J, Perron AD, Miller MD, Powell SM, Brady WJ: Pediatric supracondylar humerus fractures. *Am J Emerg Med* 2002;20:544–550.

Upper Extremity: Patient 3

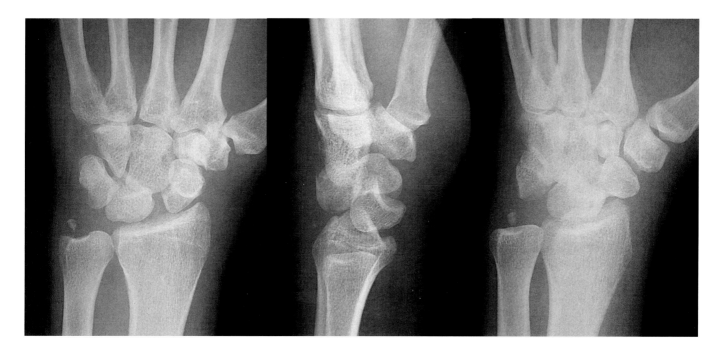

FIGURE 1

Wrist pain after minor trauma in a young man

A 24-year-old man presented to the ED with pain after hitting his wrist on a table.

Five weeks earlier, he had fallen from his bicycle onto his outstretched hand injuring his wrist. He was examined at another hospital where radiographs were obtained and a wrist injury was diagnosed. He was immobilized in a splint and was told to follow-up with a hand surgeon, but he did not do so. The patient continued to have pain and limited mobility of his wrist and so following this minor injury, he decided to have it evaluated again.

On examination, there was tenderness of the volar surface of the wrist. Flexion of the wrist was limited to 10°. He also had limitation of flexion of his middle and ring fingers. Sensation of the hand was intact. Abduction and adduction of the fingers were normal.

- There are four injuries in this patient.

- How are wrist radiographs systematically interpreted?

HOW TO INTERPRET WRIST RADIOGRAPHS

Wrist injuries can be difficult to diagnose because of their complex anatomy and frequently subtle radiographic manifestations. This case illustrates the importance of a **systematic approach** to radiograph interpretation in which each of the radiographic signs of a fracture are sought: cortical interruption or deformity due to a fracture, alterations in skeletal alignment, and changes in adjacent soft tissues. The ***ABCS*** mnemonic works well for wrist radiographs—*A* is for ***adequacy*** and ***alignment,*** *B* is for ***bones*** (fracture lines), *C* is for ***cartilage*** (joint spaces), and *S* is for ***soft tissue changes*** (Table 1).

Efficient and accurate radiograph interpretation also entails a **targeted approach,** looking for *common injury patterns* and *injuries that can easily be missed.* One of the common wrist injury patterns is illustrated in this case.

The **three standard radiographs** of the wrist are the PA, lateral, and pronation oblique views (Figures 2 to 4). On the PA view, the bones of the radial aspect of the wrist are not well seen; the pronation oblique view shows this area to better advantage, particularly the distal pole of the scaphoid.

On the **PA view,** each carpal bone should be examined for evidence of a fracture, paying particular attention to the scaphoid, the most frequently fractured carpal (Figure 2). The distal radius and ulna and metacarpal bases are also examined. Next the **alignment** of the carpal bones is checked. Normally, the articular surfaces of the proximal and distal carpal rows are aligned in three smooth arcs: (1) the proximal articular surfaces of the scaphoid, lunate, and triquetrum; (2) the distal surfaces of these carpals at the midcarpal articulation; and (3) the proximal articular surfaces of the capitate and hamate. Finally, the spaces between the carpal bones are examined, especially the scapholunate joint space. The intercarpal joint spaces should be of uniform width, approximately 1–2 mm.

Next, examine the **lateral view** (Figure 3). Distal radius fractures are common and usually easy to see. The carpal bones overlap on the lateral view and, aside from the dorsal surface of the triquetrum and distal pole of the scaphoid, fracture detection is difficult. There are two landmarks of **alignment.** First, the C-shaped articular surface of the distal radius should articulate with the lunate, and the distal surface of the lunate with the capitate. Second, the axis of the scaphoid makes an angle of 30°–60° with the long axis of the wrist—the *scapholunate angle.* The *pronator quadratus fat stripe* is a thin radiolucent layer of fat tissue overlying the pronator quadratus muscle that normally parallels the volar cortex of the distal radius. If there is a wrist injury, particularly a distal radius fracture, the fat stripe is bowed outward or obliterated.

Finally, examine the **pronation oblique view** (Figure 4). The radial aspect of the wrist is seen without overlap—the distal pole (tuberosity) of the scaphoid, the trapezium, and the bases of the first and second metacarpals.

TABLE 1

Systematic Analysis of Wrist Radiographs—The ABCS

There are two regions of injury: the carpals and the distal radius

	PA	**LATERAL**	**PRONATION OBLIQUE**
Adequacy	No radial deviation	No rotation No flexion or extension	Trapezium seen without overlap
Alignment	3 carpal arches	4 C's (lunate articulations) Scapholunate angle	
Bones	Carpals (scaphoid) Distal radius and ulna Metacarpals (proximal)	Distal radius Triquetrum (dorsal surface)	Scaphoid (distal pole) Distal radius
Cartilage	Intercarpal joint spaces		
Soft tissues		Pronator fat stripe	

[From Schwartz DT, Reisdorff EJ, *Emergency Radiology*. McGraw-Hill, 2000.]

Normal Radiographic Anatomy of the Wrist

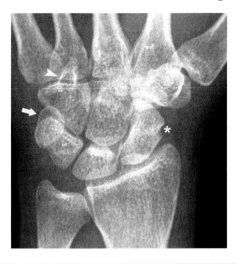 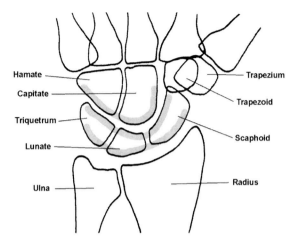

FIGURE 2   PA view showing normal alignment of the proximal and distal carpal rows. The articular surfaces of the carpals form **three smooth arcs** (*curved gray lines*). The intercarpal spaces should be equal in width, approximately 1 mm to 2 mm.
Asterisk—indentation of the radial margin of the scaphoid is a normal variant. A*rrow*—pisiform. *Arrowhead*—hook of hamate.

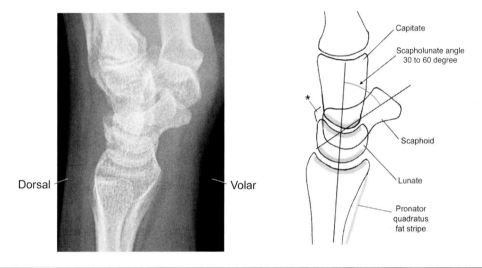

FIGURE 3   Lateral view showing normal carpal articulations. The four C-shaped articular surfaces are in contact, and the axes of the distal radius, lunate and capitate are aligned. The entire capitate is difficult to see because of its overlap with the other carpals. The *scapholunate angle* between the scaphoid and the long axis of the lunate is 30° to 60°. The *pronator quadratus fat stripe* parallels the volar cortex of the distal radius.
Asterisk—triquetrum.

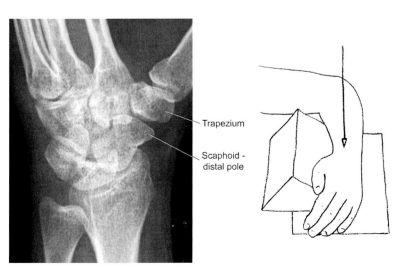

FIGURE 4   Pronation oblique view shows the distal pole of the scaphoid and the trapezium. Positioning is 45° semipronation.

Radiographic Findings—Patient 3—PA View

There are three significant findings (Figure 5).

1. **Ulnar styloid fracture:** This is the most obvious injury (*arrowhead*). An ulnar styloid fracture does not usually occur as an isolated injury. It is most often associated with a distal radius fracture, although not in this patient.
2. **Scapholunate dissociation:** The space between the lunate and the scaphoid is widened due to disruption of the scapholunate ligament (*). This is called the *Terry-Thomas sign,* named for the distinctive grimace of the British comedian who had a gap between his two front incisor teeth; David Letterman has similar dentition (Figure 6).

    When there is a complete tear of the scapholunate ligament, the scaphoid rotates volarly and appears foreshortened on the PA view. Its distal portion is seen end-on—the "*ring sign*" (Figure 5, *arrow*).
3. **Carpal malalignment:** The carpal articular surfaces are not aligned in smooth arcs. Instead, the proximal and distal carpal rows are overlapping. The lunate has a triangular shape like a "*piece of pie*" (L, Figure 5). The cause of these findings is evident on the lateral view.

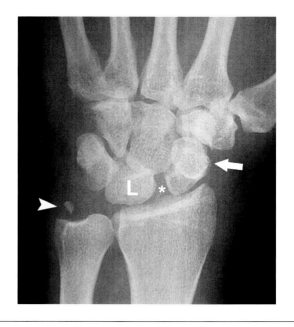

FIGURE 5   PA view—Patient 3 (see text for explanation).

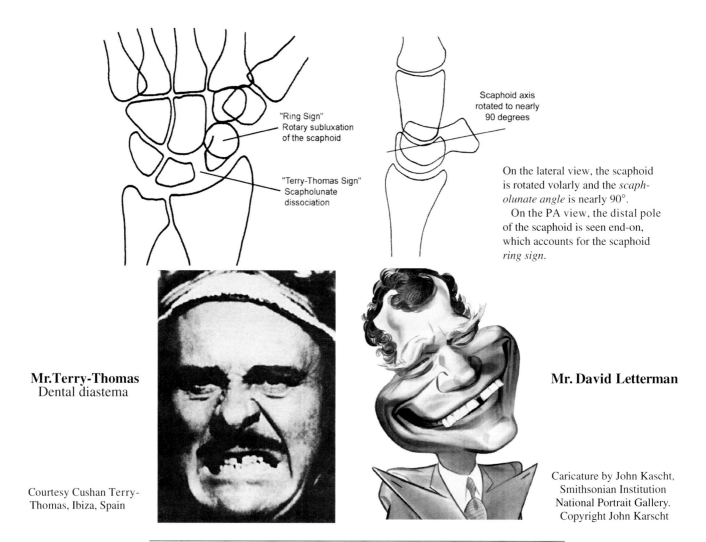

"Ring Sign" Rotary subluxation of the scaphoid

"Terry-Thomas Sign" Scapholunate dissociation

Scaphoid axis rotated to nearly 90 degrees

On the lateral view, the scaphoid is rotated volarly and the *scapholunate angle* is nearly 90°.

On the PA view, the distal pole of the scaphoid is seen end-on, which accounts for the scaphoid *ring sign*.

Mr. Terry-Thomas
Dental diastema

Courtesy Cushan Terry-Thomas, Ibiza, Spain

Mr. David Letterman

Caricature by John Kascht, Smithsonian Institution National Portrait Gallery. Copyright John Karscht

FIGURE 6   Scapholunate dissociation and rotary subluxation of the scaphoid.

Lateral View

The lateral view (Figure 7) clarifies the reason for the carpal malalignment seen on the PA view.

1. In a **dorsal perilunate dislocation,** the capitate is dislocated dorsal to the lunate (Figure 8A). In a **volar lunate dislocation,** the lunate is displaced from the distal radius, rotated volarly, and looks like a "spilled teacup" (Figure 8B). The capitate is re-aligned with axis of the distal radius. Perilunate and lunate dislocations form a spectrum of injury; with lunate dislocation there is greater ligamentous disruption.

   In this patient, the lunate is slightly rotated volarly, which accounts for its triangular shape on the PA view (looks like a "piece of pie"), although it maintains its articulation with the distal radius a perilunate dislocation (Figure 7).

2. **Rotary subluxation of the scaphoid:** The scaphoid is rotated volarly such that the angle between the scaphoid and lunate is nearly 90° (Figure 7, *white lines*). Rotary subluxation of the scaphoid occurs when there is complete disruption of the scapholunate articulation. It is responsible for the scaphoid "ring sign" seen on the PA view (Figure 6).

Pronation Oblique View

The pronation oblique view (Figure 9) reveals a transverse fracture across the body of the triquetrum—the most ulnar carpal of the proximal carpal row.

In summary, this patient has **four injuries**—an ulnar styloid fracture, scapholunate dissociation, perilunate dislocation, and triquetrum fracture.

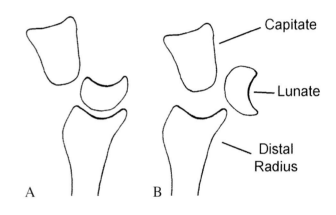

FIGURE 8 (*A*) Dorsal perilunate dislocation (dislocated capitate). (*B*) Volar lunate dislocation—"spilled teacup."

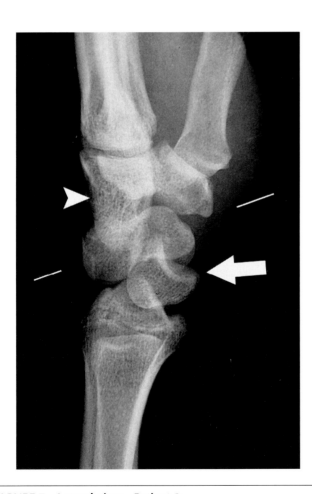

FIGURE 7   Lateral view—Patient 3.
There is a **dorsal perilunate dislocation** with the capitate (*arrowhead*) dislocated dorsal to the lunate. There is slight volar tilt of the lunate (*arrow*).

The scaphoid is rotated volarly such that the scapholunate angle is greater than 60° (*white lines*). This accounts for the "ring sign" seen on the patient's PA radiograph in which the distal pole of the scaphoid is seen end-on.

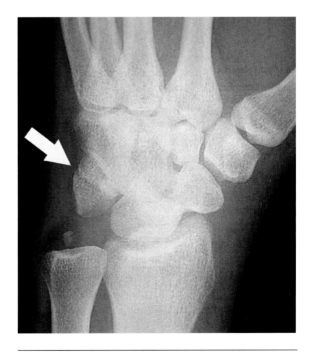

FIGURE 9   Pronation oblique view—Patient 3
There is a transverse fracture through the triquetrum (*arrow*).

Why Does This Patient Have Four Injuries to His Wrist?

1) Ulnar styloid fracture, 2) scapholunate dislocation,
3) perilunate dislocation, and 4) triquetrum fracture.

These four injuries are, in fact, all part of a single injury pattern termed **perilunate injury.** A perilunate injury occurs in an arc surrounding the lunate (Figure 10). The injuries may be in the ligaments attached to the lunate or through the adjacent bones—the scaphoid, capitate or triquetrum. The injury can extend to the radial styloid or ulnar styloid. This patient's injury is termed a **transtriquetral perilunate fracture-dislocation** (Figure 11).

The severity of a perilunate injury can also be classified in four successive stages that extend around the four sides of the lunate (Figure 12). The mechanism of injury is a fall on an outstretched hand. Treatment of perilunate injuries consists of urgent reduction of the dislocation. Kirschner wire fixation is usually needed to stabilize ligament tears and screw fixation for displaced fractures, particularly of the scaphoid.

Patient Outcome

This patient had been inadequately managed during his initial emergency department visit. The dislocation should have been reduced at that time, or if not possible, an appointment to a hand surgeon for the next day should have been made. Delay in treatment lead to formation of extensive scar tissue that prevented reduction, even open reduction during surgery. The patient required complete excision of the proximal carpal row—**proximal row carpectomy**—to restore at least partial function to his wrist (Figure 13).

Perilunate Injury

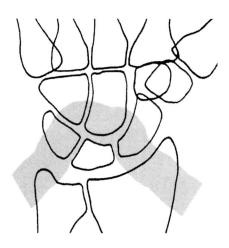

FIGURE 10   Arc of perilunate injury.
Forceful impact on the volar surface of the hyperextended wrist causes injuries in a vulnerable zone surrounding the lunate (shaded area). The injuries may be ligamentous or involve the bones adjacent to the lunate.

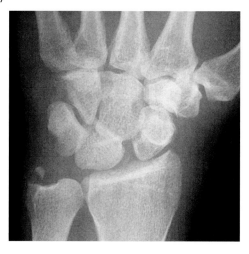

FIGURE 11   Transtriquetral perilunate fracture-dislocation.
There is also scapholunate dissocation and an ulnar styloid fracture.

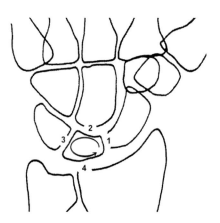

FIGURE 12   Four stages of perilunate injury.

(1) Scapholunate dissociation or scaphoid fracture.
(2) Perilunate dislocation.
(3) Perilunate dislocation with lunate-triquetrum dissociation or triquetrum fracture (this patient).
(4) Lunate dislocation.

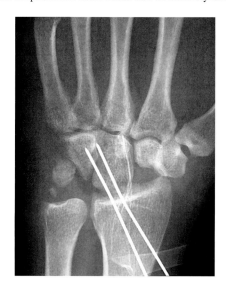

FIGURE 13   Proximal row carpectomy.
Postoperative radiograph showing excision of the proximal carpal row and temporary pin fixation with Kirschner wires. This was necessary because the perilunate dislocation could not be reduced due to extensive scar tissue.

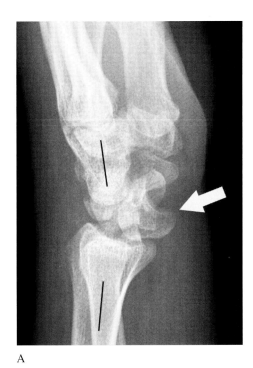

A

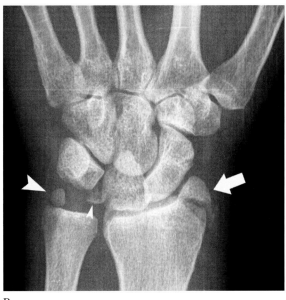

B

FIGURE 14   Another patient with a complex perilunate injury.

(A) The lateral radiograph shows a **volar lunate dislocation.** The lunate is rotated volarly and appears like a **spilled teacup** (*arrow*). The capitate is in alignment with the long axis of the radius (*black lines*).

(B) On the PA view, the proximal carpal row alignment is disrupted and the lunate has a triangular appearance. The lunate-triquetrum articulation is widened and there is a small avulsion fragment within the intercarpal joint space (*small arrowhead*). There are fractures of the radial styloid (*arrow*) and ulnar styloid (*large arrowhead*).

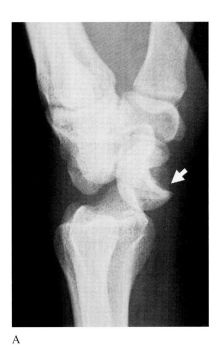

A

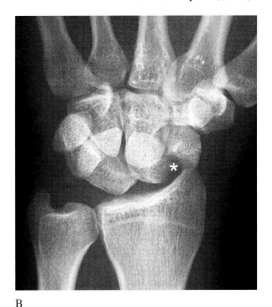

B

FIGURE 15   Combined lunate dislocation and scaphoid fracture.

(A) The lateral view shows a volar lunate dislocation (*arrow*).

(B) On the PA view, there is a markedly displaced scaphoid fracture (*asterisk*).

SUGGESTED READING

Chawla-Mital R, Beeson M: The wrist. In Schwartz DT, Reisdorff EJ, eds. *Emergency Radiology.* New York: McGraw-Hill, 2000.

Chin HW, Visotsky J: Ligamentous wrist injuries. *Emerg Med Clin North Am* 1993;11:717–737.

Frankel VH: The Terry-Thomas sign. *Clin Orthop* 1977;129:321–322.

Meldon SW, Hargarten SW: Ligamentous injuries of the wrist. *J Emerg Med* 1995;13:217–225.

Perron AD, Brady WJ, Keats TE, Hersh RE: Lunate and perilunate injuries. *Am J Emerg Med* 2001;19:157–162.

Rettig ME, Raskin KB: Long-term assessment of proximal row carpectomy for chronic perilunate dislocation. J Hand Surg (Am) 1999:24:1231–1236.

Upper Extremity: Patient 4

Six patients with "negative" wrist radiographs after spraining their wrists.
They had all fallen on their outstretched hands.
PA *(A)*, lateral *(B)* and pronation oblique views *(C)* are shown for each patient (except where noted).

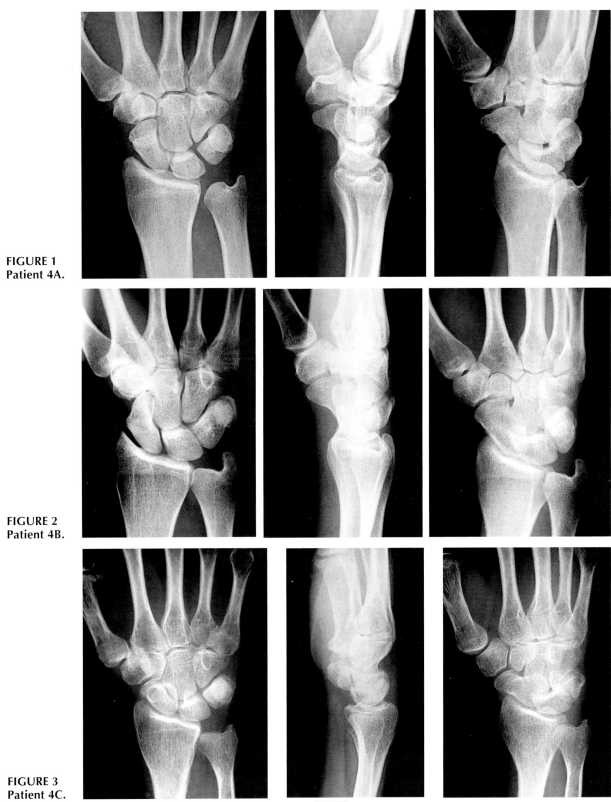

FIGURE 1
Patient 4A.

FIGURE 2
Patient 4B.

FIGURE 3
Patient 4C.

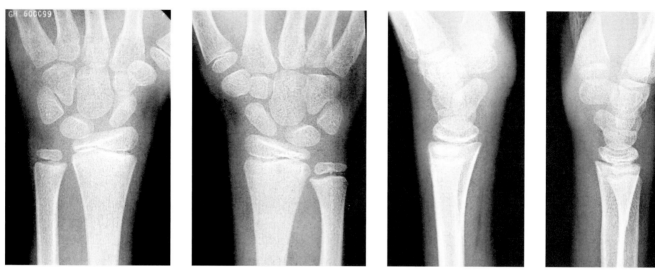

FIGURE 4   **Patient 4D:** *(A)* Left wrist PA. *(B)* Right wrist PA. *(C)* Left wrist lateral. *(D)* Right wrist lateral.

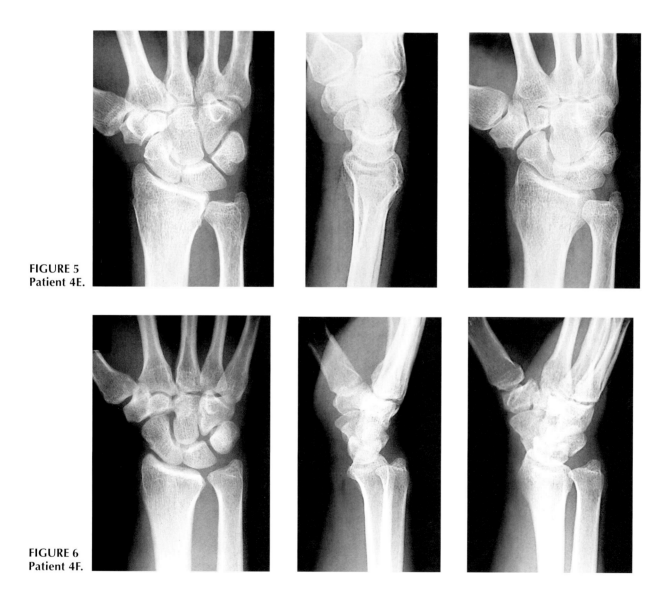

FIGURE 5
Patient 4E.

FIGURE 6
Patient 4F.

A SPRAINED WRIST

Effective interpretation of wrist radiographs is based on the knowledge of typical injury patterns. Simply looking for cortical breaks or irregularities makes the search for injuries laborious and potentially misleading. This **targeted approach** to radiograph interpretation focuses on *common sites of injury* as well as *easily missed injuries* that can have subtle radiographic findings.

There are **two distinct regions** of the wrist: the distal radius and the carpals. **Distal radius fractures** are 10 times more common than carpal fractures. Distal radius fractures are usually obvious on the lateral view. On the PA and pronation oblique views, a distal radius fracture appears as an area of trabecular disruption or impaction. If a fracture is not clearly seen, obliteration or outward bowing of the *pronator quadratus fat stripe* on the lateral view can be a clue to the presence of a fracture (see Figure 16 on p.262).

Among **carpal injuries**, scaphoid fractures are by far the most common, accounting for 60% of radiographically apparent carpal injuries (Table 1). **Scaphoid fractures** are usually seen on the PA view, but may only be visible on the pronation oblique view. In some cases, a "scaphoid view" (PA view with the wrist in ulnar deviation) is needed to visualize the fracture.

The **triquetrum** is the second most commonly fractured carpal, particularly a dorsal chip fracture. **Perilunate injuries** (dislocations, ligament disruptions, and fractures) account for 20% of carpal injures. Other carpal fractures are much less common, accounting for fewer than 1% of carpal injuries. Finally, the metacarpals may be involved in wrist injuries.

Supplementary radiographic views are sometimes needed to visualize a fracture. These views should be obtained when a particular fracture is suspected based on the clinical examination but is not seen on the standard views. The choice of supplementary view depends on the injury suspected (Table 2).

Radiographically occult wrist injuries are common and patients with significant pain and negative radiographs should be splinted and referred to an orthopedist. Later MRI may reveal ligamentous or osseous injuries.

TABLE 1
Frequency of Carpal Injuries

Scaphoid	~60%
Triquetrum	~20%
Perilunate injuries	~20%
Other	~1%

Distal radius fractures are 10 times more common than carpal injuries.

TABLE 2
Supplementary Radiographic Views of the Wrist

RADIOGRAPH	AREA OF TENDERNESS	SUSPECTED FRACTURE
Scaphoid view (PA ulnar deviation)	Anatomical "snuff box"	Scaphoid fracture
Supination oblique view	Ulnar aspect of wrist	Fifth metacarpal base, pisiform, hook of hamate
Carpal tunnel view (axial)	Volar surface of wrist	Hook of hamate, volar tubercle of trapezium

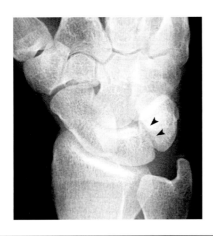

FIGURE 7   Mach band pseudofracture of the triquetrum due to overlap by the lunate (*arrowheads*) (Patient 4B, oblique view).

Pseudofractures   A variety of radiographic findings can mimic fractures. Several of these findings are seen in the radiographs of these patients. Scaphoid irregularities are common and can mimic a fracture. Overlapping bones or soft tissues create radiolucent *Mach bands*—an optical illusion that can appear like the cortical interruption of a fracture (Figure 7). A Mach band can usually be distinguished from a fracture because it extends beyond the margin of the overlapped bone.

Unfused secondary ossification centers and old fractures form accessory ossicles. These small bone fragments have rounded well-corticated margins that distinguish them from fractures. There is no associated defect in adjacent bone. Finally, a thin osseous band extending across the distal radius is a remnant of the growth plate and should not be misinterpreted as an impacted distal radius fracture (see Figure 17 on p.262).

PATIENT 4A   The **scaphoid** is the most commonly fractured carpal and should be examined carefully when reviewing wrist radiographs. In Patient 4A, a small nondisplaced fracture of the distal pole of the scaphoid is seen on the oblique view (Figure 8). Detection of such fractures is the major role of the pronation oblique view. (A slight cortical irregularity is also visible on the lateral view, Figure 1B.)

Scaphoid fractures are clinically significant because they can cause chronic disabling wrist pain. Fractures through the midportion (the "waist") of the scaphoid are most common. The scaphoid arterial supply enters the distal portion of the scaphoid. A scaphoid waist fracture can interrupt the blood supply to the proximal fragment, resulting in *avascular necrosis* (AVN) (Figure 9). Distal scaphoid fractures, as seen in this patient, are at lower risk of AVN. Nonunion is another common complication of scaphoid fractures.

Up to 20% of patients with scaphoid fractures have negative radiographs (occult fractures), although in many cases subtle radiographic signs may have been overlooked (Figures 8 and 13).

A supplementary **scaphoid view** should be obtained in patients with negative radiographs and tenderness in the "anatomical snuff-box" over the scaphoid. On a standard PA view, the distal pole of the scaphoid overlaps the midportion of the scaphoid, whereas on the scaphoid view, the scaphoid is elongated. This aligns the fracture parallel to the x-ray beam and may also slightly distract the fracture making it easier to see (Figure 10). Scaphoid fractures are sometimes missed on the standard PA view because positioning is suboptimal, i.e., the wrist is held in radial deviation due to pain. This further foreshortens the scaphoid and obscures the fracture.

Even when properly performed radiographs are normal, including a scaphoid view, patients with "snuff-box" tenderness may still have an occult fracture and should be immobilized in a splint with thumb spica and warned of the possibility of an occult scaphoid fracture. Immobilization reduces the risk of nonunion and avascular necrosis. Radiographs should be repeated in 10–14 days, at which time osseous resorption adjacent to the fracture makes the fracture more conspicuous. However, only 8–20% of patients immobilized actually have a fracture. Alternative management strategies are to obtain a bone scan after 4 days of immobilization, or MRI or possibly CT at the time of initial presentation (Murphy et al. 1995, Memarsadeghi et al. 2006, Dorsay et al. 2001).

It could be argued that it is unnecessary to obtain a scaphoid view because a patient with "snuff-box" tenderness should be immobilized regardless of the radiographic findings. However, a scaphoid view is beneficial because when a scaphoid fracture is definitely identified, immobilization is different. Most authors recommend a *splint* with thumb spica for a suspected occult scaphoid fracture, whereas a *cast* with thumb spica is used for a definite fracture. If a splint is applied to a scaphoid fracture in the ED, the patient should return in 2 or 3 days for casting, rather than 10–14 days as is the case for a suspected occult fracture. Displaced fractures usually require operative screw fixation.

Pseudofractures of the Scaphoid.   There are two common radiographic findings that should not be misinterpreted as fractures. First, the cortex of the radial side of the scaphoid often has a small irregularity or indentation at the edge of the radioscaphoid articular cartilage (Figures 11–13). Second, the distal pole of the scaphoid overlaps the body of the scaphoid on the PA view. This should not be misinterpreted as an impacted fracture (Figure 14).

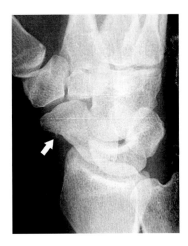

FIGURE 8   Patient 4A—Fracture of the distal pole of the scaphoid seen on the pronation oblique view (*arrow*).

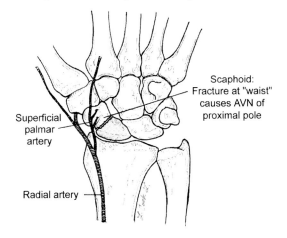

FIGURE 9   The blood supply enters the distal portion of the scaphoid. A fracture through the midportion of the scaphoid interrupts perfusion to the proximal pole causing AVN.

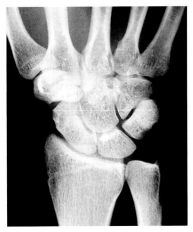

A. PA view

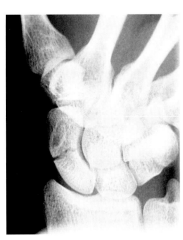

B. Scaphoid view

FIGURE 10   Another patient with a scaphoid fracture that was only visible on the **scaphoid view**— a PA view with the wrist in ulnar deviation (*B*).

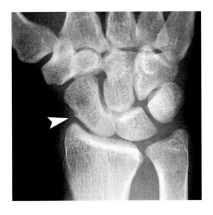

FIGURE 11   Pseudofracture   An indentation of the radial cortex of the scaphoid on the PA and oblique views of Patient 4F is not a fracture but is a common cortical irregularity at the margin of the radioscaphoid articular cartilage (*arrowheads*).

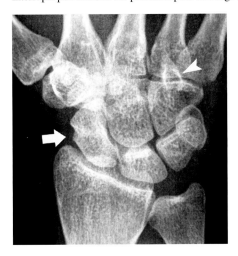

FIGURE 12   Pseudofracture

Indentation of scaphoid is a normal finding, not a fracture (*arrow*).

The hook of the hamate (*arrowhead*) overlies the hamate and the base of fourth metacarpal.

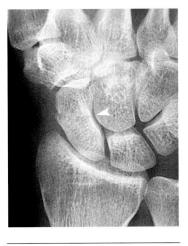

FIGURE 13   A subtle scaphoid fracture.

The fracture can be differentiated from the normal cortical indentation at the radial surface of the scaphoid because the trabecular irregularity extends across the scaphoid and there is a break in the medial cortex (*arrowhead*).

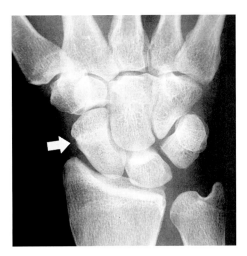

FIGURE 14   Pseudofracture

Overlap of the distal pole of the scaphoid (*arrow*) should not be misinterpreted as an impacted fracture (Patient 4A, PA view). A scaphoid view can be useful in such cases.

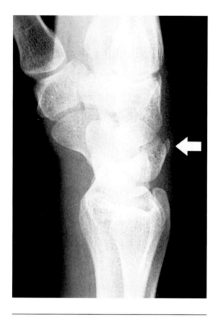

FIGURE 15   Patient 4B—Dorsal avulsion fracture of the triquetrum (*arrow*) is only visible on the lateral view.

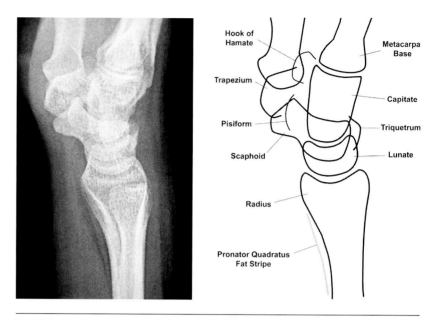

FIGURE 16   Normal lateral view of the wrist.
The *triquetrum* is the most dorsally projecting proximal carpal bone.
The *pronator quadratus fat stripe* is normal (see also Figures 1B and 3B).

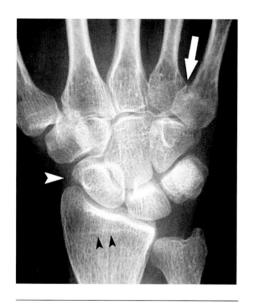

FIGURE 17   Patient 4C—Fracture of the base of the fifth metacarpal (*arrow*).

Two pseudofractures are seen: overlap of the distal pole of the scaphoid (*white arrowhead*) and a fine white line that is a remnant of the distal radius growth plate (*black arrowheads*).

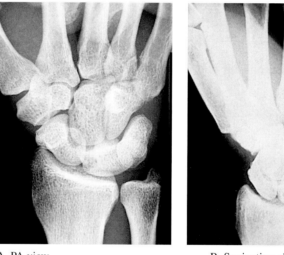
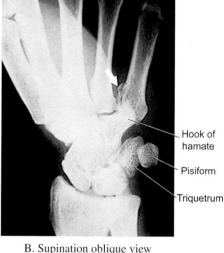

A. PA view   B. Supination oblique view

**FIGURE 18   In another patient, a fracture of the base of the fifth metacarpal is not clearly seen on the PA view (*A*).
The supination oblique view (*B*) shows the fracture (*arrow*).

PATIENT 4B   The **triquetrum** is the second most frequently fractured carpal (20% of carpal fractures). A dorsal avulsion fracture is most common and is visible only on the lateral view (Figure 15). On the lateral view, the triquetrum is the most dorsally projecting proximal carpal bone (Figure 16).

The usual mechanism of injury is a fall on an outstretched hand. The patient presents with tenderness and swelling over the dorsum of the wrist.

PATIENT 4C   Some wrist injuries do not involve the distal radius or carpals. In Patient 4C, there is a minimally displaced fracture at the **base of the fifth metacarpal** (Figure 17).

The fourth and fifth metacarpal bases are sometimes not well seen on the standard PA view. A **supination oblique view** is useful when there is tenderness of the ulnar aspect of the wrist and a fracture is not seen on the standard views (Figure 18). The supination oblique view can also detect fractures of the pisiform and hook of the hamate.

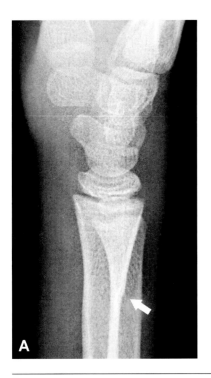
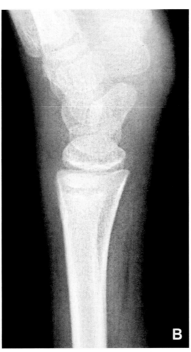

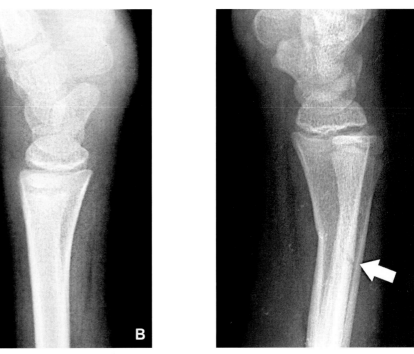

FIGURE 19   **Patient 4D**—A subtle torus (buckle) fracture of the dorsal cortex of the distal radius (*arrow*). The comparison view of the right wrist (*B*) shows a normal distal radial cortex.

FIGURE 21   A "greenstick" fracture of the dorsal cortex of the distal radius (*arrow*) and buckling of the volar cortex.

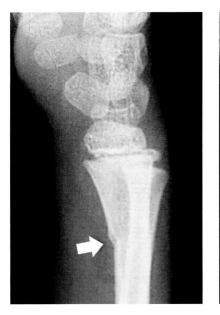
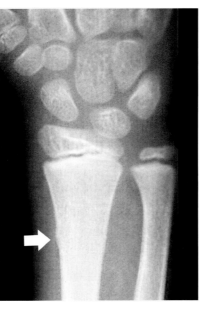

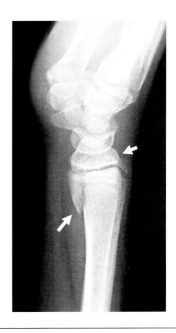

FIGURE 20   A more pronounced torus fracture causes buckling of the volar cortex of the distal radius. It is visible on both the lateral and PA views (*arrows*).

FIGURE 22   A Salter-Harris II fracture involving the growth plate and the adjacent metaphysis (*arrows*).

PATIENT 4D   In children, the distal radius is most vulnerable to injury. There are two types of fractures: one involves the growth plate and the other involves the metaphysis.

Patient 4D is a 9-year-old child with a **torus (buckle) fracture** of the left distal radius. Slight buckling of the dorsal cortex of the distal radius is seen on the lateral view (Figure 19).

A buckle fracture may involve the volar cortex, and, when severe, is also visible on the PA view (Figure 20). When the compressed buckled cortex is broken, the injury is referred to as a *lead pipe fracture*.

Other common distal radius fractures include a distracted fracture of one side of the cortex, called a *greenstick fracture* (Figure 21) and growth plate fractures (*Salter-Harris fractures*) (Figure 22). Carpal fractures are uncommon in young children.

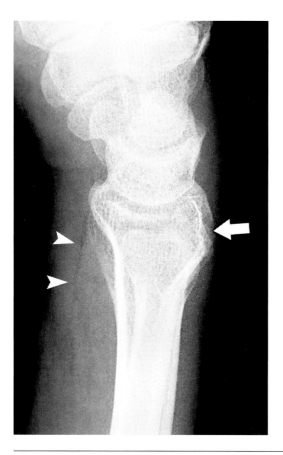 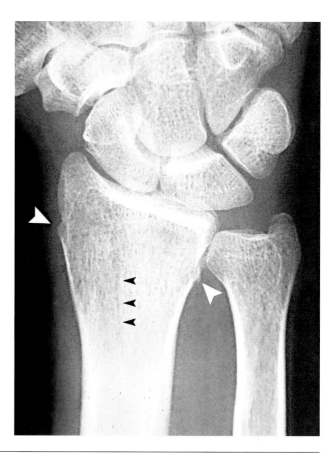

FIGURE 23   Patient 4E—A subtle nondisplaced distal radius fracture (*arrow*).
The pronator quadratus fat stripe is bowed outward and partially obliterated (*white arrowheads*).
On the PA view, there is slight trabecular disruption (*black arrowheads*) and buckling of the cortical
margins (*white arrowheads*).

PATIENT 4E   Distal radius fractures are the most common fractures of the wrist. When nondisplaced, the radiographic findings can be subtle.

In this patient, careful inspection of the lateral view reveals slight disruption and deformity of the dorsal cortex of the distal radius (Figure 23). The pronator quadratus fat stripe is abnormal—volarly displaced and partially obliterated. On the PA view, there is slight trabecular and cortical disruption.

One common radiographic finding that should not be misinterpreted as a distal radius fracture is a thin transverse band extending across the distal radius. It is a remnant of the growth plate (Figure 17).

PATIENT 4F   The ulnar shaft is displaced dorsally relative to the radius (Figure 24). This is due to a **distal radioulnar joint dislocation**. The dislocation is "posterior" (named for displacement of the ulna relative to the radius). When treated soon after the injury, closed reduction is usually successful, and the wrist should be immobilized in supination. When treatment is delayed, open reduction and pinning may be necessary.

Poor radiographic positioning, i.e., a rotated (oblique) rather than a true lateral view, can cause similar malalignment (Figure 25). There are two ways to determine whether apparent malalignment of the distal radius and ulna is due to incorrect (rotated) positioning. First, the ulnar styloid normally "points" to the dorsal surface of the triquetrum, even when the lateral view is rotated. In Patient 4F, the ulnar styloid is directed dorsal to the triquetrum (Figure 24).

Second, on a correctly positioned lateral view, the apex of the radial styloid should be aligned with the long axis of the radius and located midway between the volar and dorsal surfaces of the radial shaft (Figure 24). If the lateral view positioning is rotated, the apex of the radial styloid will be either too volar or too dorsal with respect to the radial shaft (Figure 25). (A correctly positioned lateral view is shown in Figure 1B.) In some cases, CT may be needed to confirm the diagnosis.

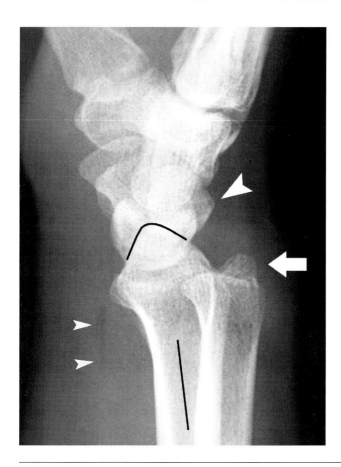

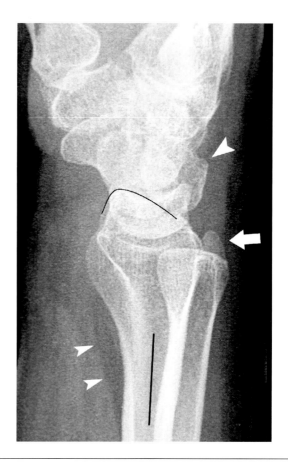

FIGURE 24   Patient 4F—Distal radioulnar joint (DRUJ) dislocation.

The ulna is dorsally displaced relative to the distal radius.

This is not due to poor (rotated) positioning given that (1) the tip of the ulnar styloid (*arrow*) points posterior to the triquetrum (*large arrowhead*), which is abnormal and (2) the tip of the radial styloid is in line with the long axis of the distal radius (*black lines*), i.e., the view is correctly positioned.

The pronator quadratus fat stripe is bowed forward and partly obliterated (*small arrowheads*).

FIGURE 25   A normal but incorrectly positioned (rotated) lateral view.

The ulna appears dorsally displaced relative to the radius mimicking a DRUJ dislocation. Signs that this is due to rotated positioning and not a DRUJ dislocation are (1) the tip of the ulnar styloid (*arrow*) "points" to the triquetrum (*large arrowhead*), as is normal and (2) the tip of the radial styloid is volar relative to the axis of the radius (*black lines*), i.e., the positioning is rotated.

The pronator quadratus fat stripe is normal (*small arrowheads*).

SUGGESTED READING

Chawla-Mital R, Beeson M: The wrist. In Schwartz DT, Reisdorff EJ eds., *Emergency Radiology*. New York: McGraw-Hill, 2000.

Keats TE, Anderson MW: *Atlas of Normal Roentgen Variants that May Simulate Disease*, 8th ed. Mosby, 2006.

Kumar A, Iqbal MJ: Missed isolated volar dislocation of distal radioulnar joint: A case report. *J Emerg Med* 2001;17:873–875.

Murphy DG, Eisenhauer MA, Powe J, Pavlofsky W: Can a day 4 bone scan accurately determine the presence or absence of scaphoid fracture? *Ann Emerg Med* 1995;26:434–438.

Perron AD, Brady WJ, Keats TE, Hersh RE: Scaphoid fractures. *Am J Emerg Med* 2001;19:310–316.

Staniforth P: Scaphoid fractures and wrist pain: Time for new thinking. *Injury* 1991;22:435–436.

Stapczynski JJ: Fracture of the base of the little finger metacarpal: importance of the "ball-catcher" radiographic view. *J Emerg Med* 1991;9:145–149.

Stenstrom RJ: Clinical scaphoid fracture—Overtreatment of a common injury? (abstract) *Acad Emerg Med* 2003;10:498.

Waeckerle JF: A prospective study identifying the sensitivity of radiographic findings and the efficiency of clinical findings in carpal navicular fracture. *Ann Emerg Med* 1987;16:733–737.

MRI and CT for Occult Scaphoid Fractures

Breederveld RS; Tuinebreijer WE: Investigation of computed tomographic scan concurrent criterion validity in doubtful scaphoid fracture of the wrist. *J Trauma* 2004; 57:851–854.

Dorsay TA, Major NM, Helms CA: Cost-effectiveness of immediate MR imaging versus traditional follow-up for revealing radiographically occult scaphoid fractures. *AJR* 2001;177:1257–1263.

Eustace S: Emergency MR imaging of orthopedic trauma. Current and future directions. *Radiol Clin North Am* 1999;37:975–994.

Hobby JL, Dixon AK, Bearcroft PWP, et al. MR imaging of the wrist: Effect on clinical diagnosis and patient care. *Radiology* 2001;220:589–593.

Memarsadeghi M, Breitenseher MJ, Schaefer-Prokop C, et al: Occult scaphoid fractures: Comparison of multidetector CT and MR imaging—Initial experience. *Radiology* 2006;240:169–170.

Upper Extremity: Patient 5

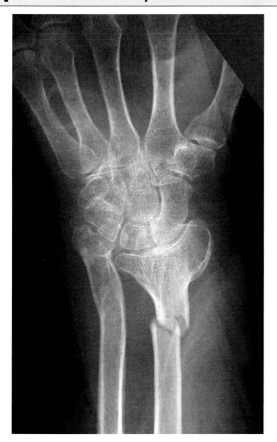

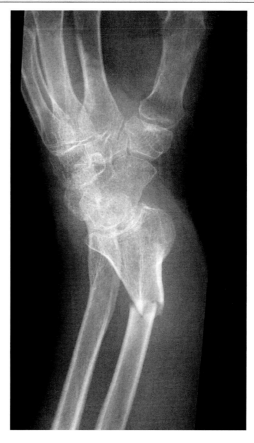

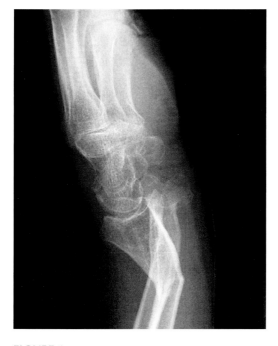

FIGURE 1

A wrist injury in an elderly woman who fell on her outstretched arm

A 78-year-old woman presents with wrist pain after falling on her outstretched arm. There is a dorsally displaced deformity at the area of tenderness (Figure 1). Distal neurovascular function is intact.

- What is this fracture called?
- How is it managed?

Hint: There is an *eponym* associated with this fracture (name of the person credited with the initial description of the injury).

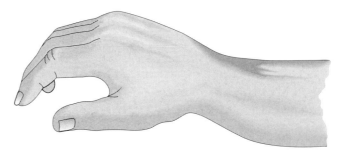

THE FRACTURE OF NECESSITY

The nature of an extremity injury can often be predicted from the mechanism of injury, the age of the patient, and the findings on physical examination. A fall on an outstretched hand is a common mechanism causing wrist injury.

The patient's age determines the weakest part of the extremity, i.e., the part most susceptible to fracture. In children, the growth plate and distal radial metaphysis are the weakest elements and so growth plate (Salter-Harris) fractures and metaphyseal torus (buckle) fractures are most common. In young adults, the distal radius is relatively strong, and so scaphoid fractures and other carpal injuries are more likely. In the elderly with osteoporosis, the distal radius is again the most vulnerable part.

Distal Radius Fractures

A number of eponyms are associated with common fractures of the distal radius: Colles, Smith, Barton, and Hutchinson ("chauffeur's" or "back-fire" fracture) (Figures 3–6).

The **Colles fracture** is the most frequent. This fracture occurs within one and a half inches of the distal end of the radius (according to the original description) and is characterized by dorsal displacement of the distal fragment. On physical examination, there is a characteristic "dinner fork" deformity of the wrist.

Abraham Colles described this fracture in 1814. In the pre-radiographic era, fracture diagnosis depended on physical examination and the principal signs of a fracture were crepitus and abnormal movement during manipulation (very painful). If there was deformity but not crepitus or abnormal mobility, then a dislocation was diagnosed. Colles' great contribution was in noting that an impacted fracture might not show crepitus or abnormal mobility even though the injury was a fracture and not a dislocation (Figure 3). Colles found that by applying traction to the injury, mobility and crepitus could be demonstrated, confirming that this was, in fact, a fracture. Colles also noted that by applying traction, the fracture could be effectively reduced and splinted to allow for proper healing.

Treatment and prognosis of Colles fractures depend on the degree of fragmentation of the fracture (comminution), the presence and extent of articular surface involvement, and the age and level of functioning of the patient. Simple fractures are treated with closed reduction and casting, whereas comminuted intra-articular fractures need stabilization with an external fixation device.

Patient Outcome

In Patient 5, the fracture was through the shaft (diaphysis) of the distal radius. This should not be mistaken for a Colles fracture, which occurs through the metaphysis. (The metaphysis is the portion of a long bone that flares out towards the articular surface.) Management differs significantly.

The radius and ulna are closely bound together by the interosseus ligament. A displaced fracture of one of the forearm bones is almost invariably accompanied by a fracture or dislocation of the other.

In this patient, the displaced fracture of the distal radial shaft is associated with a dislocation of the distal ulna at the distal radio-ulnar and ulnar-carpal joints. This dislocation is evident on all three views (Figures 7 and 8). (The patient also has osteoporosis and chronic deformity of the distal radius and ulna.)

This fracture-dislocation was described by **Riccardo Galeazzi** in 1934. The fracture is usually at the junction of the middle and distal thirds of the radial shaft. It has also been called a "reverse Monteggia" fracture. The Monteggia fracture, described in 1814, is a proximal or mid-ulnar shaft fracture with dislocation of the radial head at the elbow (see Upper Extremity Patient 1, Figure 12, page 240).

The Galeazzi fracture has also been termed the "**fracture of necessity**"—even though closed reduction can usually be accomplished, the reduction is unstable due to the extent of skeletal and ligamentous disruption. Internal fixation using a compression plate and screws is *necessary* for a good result (Figure 9).

Eponyms

Although eponyms are widely used for various orthopedic injuries and are convenient and colorful, they can be a source of confusion and misdiagnosis. It is preferable to accurately describe the anatomy of the injury rather than resort to potentially misleading terminology.

SUGGESTED READING

Colles A: On the fracture of the carpal extremity of the radius. *Edinburgh Med Surg J* 1814;10;182–186

Hunter TB, Peltier Lf, Lund PJ: Radiologic history exhibit. Musculoskeletal eponyms: Who are those guys? Radiographics 2000;20: 819–836.

Lee P, Hunter TB, Taljanovic M: Musculoskeletal colloquialisms: How did we come up with these names? Radiographics 2004;24: 1009–1027.

Pelitier LF: Fractures of the distal radius: An historical account. *Clin Orthop* 1984;187:18–22.

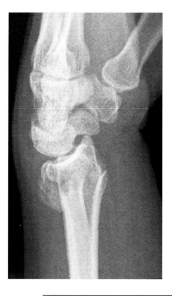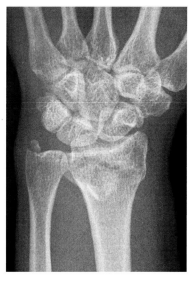

FIGURE 2 Colles fracture.

A fracture through the distal radial metaphysis with dorsal displacement. There is extension of the fracture into the radiocarpal joint as well as a fracture of the ulnar styloid.

On the Fracture of the Carpal extremity of the Radius. By A. Colles, M. D. one of the Professors of Anatomy and Surgery in the Royal College of Surgeons in Ireland.

THE injury to which I wish to direct the attention of surgeons, has not, as far as I know, been described by any author; indeed the form of the carpal extremity of the radius would rather incline us to question its being liable to fracture. The absence of crepitus, and of the other common symptoms of fracture, together with the swelling which instantly arises in this, as in other injuries of the wrist, render the difficulty of ascertaining the real nature of the case very considerable.

This fracture takes place at about an inch and a half above the carpal extremity of the radius, and exhibits the following appearances.

The posterior surface of the limb presents a considerable deformity; for a depression is seen in the fore-arm, about an inch and a half above the end of this bone, while a considerable swelling occupies the wrist and metacarpus. Indeed, the carpus and base of metacarpus appear to be thrown backward so much, as on first view to excite a suspicion that the carpus has been dislocated.

FIGURE 3 Excerpt from Colles' 1814 paper describing the difficulty in determining whether the injury is a fracture or dislocation. Earlier authors had believed it was a dislocation.

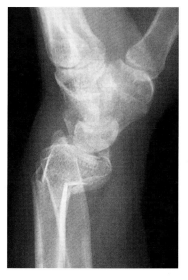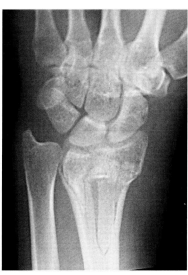

FIGURE 4 Smith fracture.

A distal radius fracture with volar displacement. The mechanism of injury is either a blow to the dorsum of the wrist or a fall onto an outstretched supinated hand.

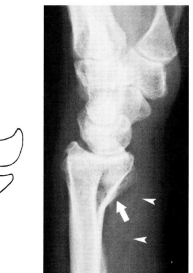

FIGURE 5 Volar Barton fracture.

A fracture of the volar rim of the distal radius with subluxation of the radiocarpal joint (arrow). The dorsal cortex of the distal radius is intact. The pronator quadratus fat stripe is bowed forward (arrowheads). Internal fixation is usually needed. A dorsal Barton fracture is less common. (figure to left)

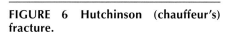

FIGURE 6 Hutchinson (chauffeur's) fracture.

A fracture of the radial styloid (arrow) is due to an impact on the radial aspect of the wrist. This fracture was described in the early days of automobiles when the starter crank could forcefully backfire injuring the chauffeur's wrist. There is also an ulnar styloid fracture (arrowhead). (figure to right)

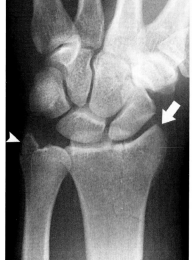

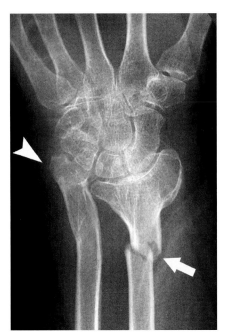 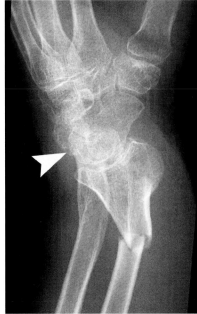 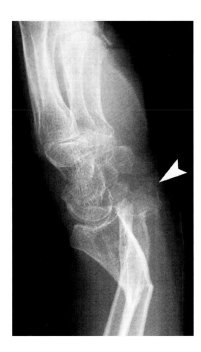

FIGURE 7   Galeazzi fracture–Patient 5.

A fracture of the distal radial shaft (*arrow*) with dislocation of the ulnar-carpal articulation (*arrowhead*). *Not* a Colles fracture!

The injury is unstable so closed reduction alone is insufficient to maintain the reduction.

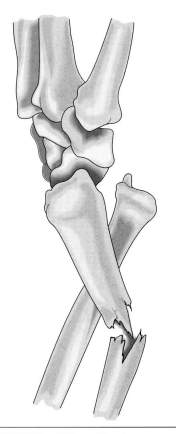 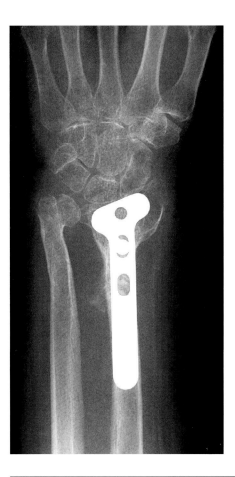 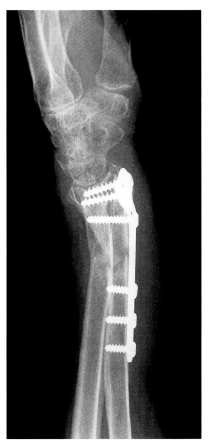

FIGURE 8   Galeazzi fracture.

Fracture of the distal radial shaft and dislocation of the distal ulna.

FIGURE 9   Postoperative radiographs showing reduction and internal fixation with compression plate and screws.

Upper Extremity: Patient 6

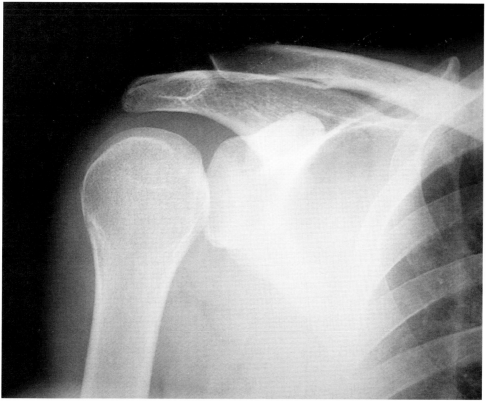

A

A shoulder injury in a young man who fell onto an outstretched arm

A 25-year-old man lost his balance while getting onto his bicycle and fell forward, landing on his outstretched right arm. He complained of pain in his right shoulder. There is no other injury. He presents holding his arm as shown in the photograph. He found it painful to move his shoulder from this position. There was no shoulder deformity or localized tenderness.

- What, if any, abnormalities are present on the shoulder radiograph (Figure 1)?

- How would you manage this patient's shoulder injury ?

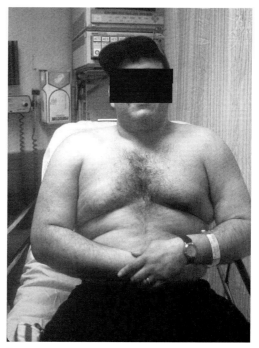

B

FIGURE 1

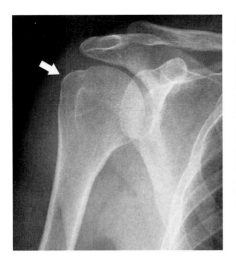 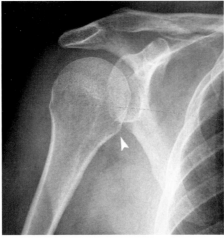 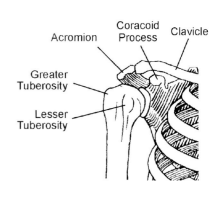

FIGURE 2   Normal AP views of the shoulder.
(A) AP view in external rotation. The greater tuberosity projects laterally (*arrow*).
(B) AP view in internal rotation. The greater tuberosity has rotated anteriorly and is seen en-face. The humeral head has a rounded appearance. The lesser tuberosity projects medially (*arrowhead*).

FIGURE 3   Shoulder anatomy.
[From Pansky B: *Review of Gross Anatomy*, 6th ed. McGraw-Hill, 1996.]

Shoulder Radiographs

When ordering a radiographic study, it is important to know which views are included and whether they have been properly performed. The standard views included in a radiographic study often vary from hospital to hospital. This is especially true of the shoulder. In many hospitals, the standard radiographs of the shoulder are **AP views** of the patient with the arm (humerus) in **external** and **internal rotation** (Figures 2 and 3).

In Patient 6, because of his limited range of motion, only one view was obtained.

• **Which view was this?** (Figure 1A)

The standard AP views of the shoulder may not be sufficient to establish a diagnosis in certain situations.

An additional view was obtained in this patient (Figure 4).

• Which view is this?

• Are any abnormalities present?

• When should you order this additional view?

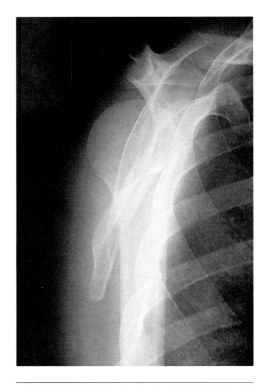

FIGURE 4 Patient 6.

LIGHT BULB ON A STICK

The shoulder is the most frequently dislocated joint owing to the shallowness of the glenoid fossa and the shoulder's great mobility. The vast majority of shoulder dislocations are anterior (>95%). Posterior dislocations are uncommon because the strong muscular and skeletal support prevents posterior displacement of the humeral head.

Posterior shoulder dislocations are frequently misdiagnosed; up to 50% are missed on initial presentation. They are missed because of a lack of familiarity with this uncommon injury, and a failure to appreciate the findings on the standard AP views of the shoulder. The findings on physical examination are, however, quite characteristic and over-reliance on radiography contributes to the high rate of misdiagnosis. Posterior dislocations are also easily missed when there is a concomitant proximal humerus fracture; the fracture is obvious and the dislocation is overlooked. When a posterior dislocation is suspected, additional radiographic views should be obtained to confirm the clinical diagnosis.

There is significant morbidity associated with delayed diagnosis of a dislocation. Reduction of the dislocation becomes increasingly difficult and contractures eventually develop necessitating open reduction and surgical reconstruction of the shoulder.

Radiographic Diagnosis

The standard AP shoulder views are actually oblique views of the glenohumeral joint (Figure 5). This makes a posterior dislocation difficult to visualize because it is impossible to determine on the radiograph whether the humeral head is anterior to (normal) or behind the glenoid fossa (Figure 6).

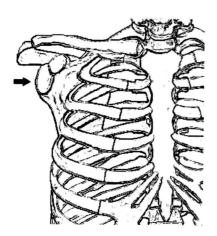

FIGURE 5   The AP shoulder view is an *oblique* view of the glenoid fossa (*arrow*) and glenohumeral joint.

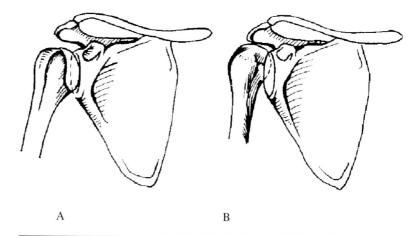

A   B

FIGURE 6   The humeral head is normally anterior to the glenoid fossa (*A*). With a posterior dislocation, the humeral head is posterior to the glenoid fossa (*B*). However, unlike these line drawings, it is impossible to visualize on an AP radiograph whether the humeral head is in front of or behind the glenoid fossa.

[From Simon RR, Sherman SC, Koenigsknecht JJ: *Emergency Orthopedics: The Extremities*, 5th ed. McGraw-Hill, 2006, with permission.]

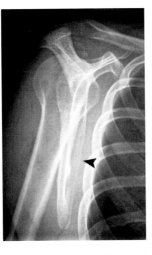

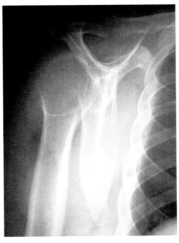

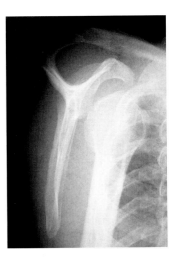

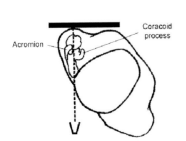

FIGURE 7   Positioning of the scapular Y view.

FIGURE 8A   Normal Y view. (see text for explanation)

FIGURE 8B   Posterior dislocation

FIGURE 8C   Anterior dislocation

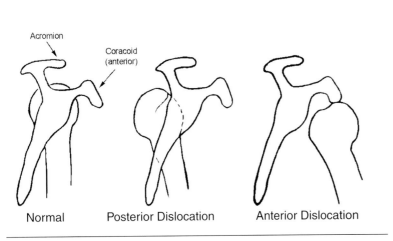

FIGURE 8D   Y view in shoulder dislocations.

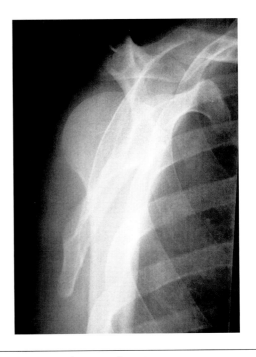

FIGURE 9   Y view—Patient 6.

Posterior displacement of the humeral head is only slight

Scapular Y view

Additional views assist in the diagnosis of a posterior dislocation, namely the scapular Y view and the axillary view.

The **scapular Y view** is a frontal view of the glenohumeral joint (Figure 7). The Y view is standard in many hospitals, especially in patients with shoulder trauma. It is used to better visualize glenohumeral dislocations. Positioning does not require movement of the injured shoulder. Normally, the humeral head is centered in the crux of the Y where the acromion, coracoid process and body of the scapula meet. With a posterior dislocation, the humeral head is displaced posteriorly (Figure 8).

In some instances, the Y view is difficult to interpret either because it is not properly positioned (oblique), or because the amount of displacement is slight, as in Patient 6 (Figure 9). In these cases, the **axillary view** can more clearly show the dislocation.

For example, in the normal Y view shown in Figure 8A, the humeral head is not centered exactly over the glenoid fossa. This is because the positioning of the patient was slightly oblique and the scapular body is not perfectly aligned with the x-ray beam (*black arrowhead*).

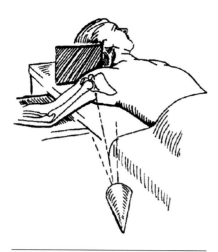

FIGURE 10   Axillary view positioning

[From: Simon RR, et al: *Emergency Orthopedics: The Extremities*, 5th ed. McGraw-Hill, 2006, with permission.]

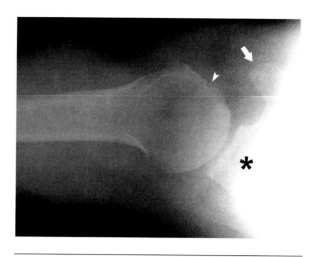

FIGURE 11A   Normal axillary view.

The humeral head articulates with the glenoid fossa (*asterisk*). The coracoid process (*arrow*) is anterior—a feature useful in orienting the radiograph.

This is Patient 6's post-reduction radiograph. A slight indentation of the humeral head (*arrowhead*) is an impacted fracture from the posterior dislocation (see Figure 11B).

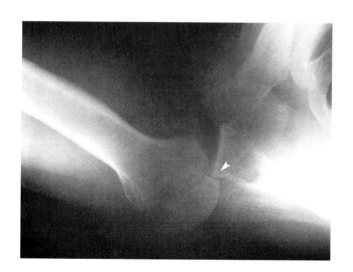

FIGURE 11B   Posterior dislocation—Patient 6.

The humeral head is dislocated posterior to the glenoid fossa. There is a small impacted fracture of the anterior surface of the humeral head by the glenoid rim (*arrowhead*).

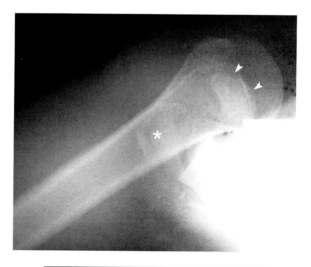

FIGURE 11C   Anterior dislocation

The humeral head is anterior to the glenoid and overlies the coracoid process (*arrowheads*). A bone fragment overlying the proximal humeral shaft is an avulsion fracture of the greater tuberosity (*asterisk*).

Axillary view

The axillary view clearly shows a posterior glenohumeral dislocation (Figures 10 and 11). In fact, the principal role of the axillary view in ED patients with shoulder trauma is to detect a posterior dislocation .

This view must be obtained with caution because it can be painful to abduct the patient's arm and, if the patient has a humeral neck fracture, the fracture can become displaced, which increases the risk of avascular necrosis. Only 15° of abduction is needed to obtain this view.

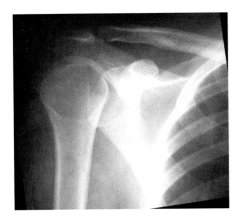

FIGURE 12A   Normal AP view in internal rotation.

The humeral head appears spherical but there is a normal amount of overlap of the humeral head on the glenoid fossa.

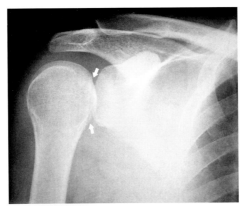

FIGURE   12B   Posterior   dislocation—Patient 6

Light bulb on a stick—the humeral head is internally rotated and has diminished overlap with the glenoid fossa (*arrows*).

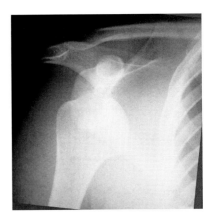

FIGURE 12C   Anterior dislocation.

The humeral head is externally rotated and widely separated from the glenoid fossa. The humeral head is in a *subcoracoid* position, the most common location for an anterior dislocation.

The AP view in posterior dislocation

The AP view is often diagnostic of a posterior dislocation, although the radiographic signs are subtle, as in this patient. There are three characteristic findings (Figure 12, Table 1).

First, there is **diminished overlap** of the humeral head and glenoid fossa. With normal glenohumeral overlap, the distance between the edge of the humeral head and the anterior rim of the glenoid is 6 mm or less, although the anterior glenoid margin is usually not well-defined. The reason for this diminished overlap is that the glenohumeral joint is oblique to the AP view when the humeral head is dislocated posteriorly, it is also displaced laterally (Figures 6 and 13).

Second, the humeral head is **fixed in internal rotation** and an external rotation view cannot be obtained. The humeral head is impacted against the posterior rim of the glenoid fossa, and this prohibits external rotation of the shoulder. The humeral head in internal rotation has a spherical appearance because the greater tuberosity is seen "en-face (Figure 2)."

These two findings, internal rotation of the proximal humerus plus diminished overlap with the glenoid fossa, give the proximal humerus in a posterior dislocation its characteristic appearance—a "**light bulb on a stick.**" (Others see an ice cream cone with a scoop of ice cream.) This *visual analogy* is a more reliable indicator of posterior dislocation than are measurements of the amount of overlap between the humeral head and glenoid fossa.

The **third** finding on an AP view is an impacted fracture of the anterior surface of the humeral head that occurs when it impacts upon the posterior rim of the glenoid fossa. This is seen as a vertical line parallel to the glenoid rim, the **trough line.** The axillary view shows this impacted fracture clearly (Figure 11B). The trough line sometimes called a "*reverse Hill-Sachs deformity*" because it is analogous to the Hill-Sachs deformity (an impacted fracture of the posterior aspect of the

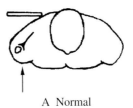
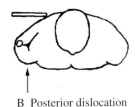

A Normal   B Posterior dislocation

FIGURE 13 Diminished glenohumeral overlap with posterior dislocation.

(*A*) Positioning of the AP shoulder view showing the humeral head in the glenoid fossa (*arrow*). (*B*) With a posterior dislocation, the humeral head is displaced laterally relative to the glenoid fossa resulting in diminished overlap on the AP view (*arrow*).

TABLE 1

Signs of Shoulder Dislocation on an AP Radiograph

Posterior dislocation *Light bulb on a stick*	Anterior dislocation
Diminished glenohumeral overlap	Marked separation of glenohumeral joint
Fixed in internal rotation (proximal humerus appears spherical). No external rotation view.	Fixed in external rotation (greater tuberosity is lateral). No internal rotation view.
Trough line (reverse Hill-Sachs deformity)	Hill-Sachs deformity

humeral head seen with an anterior shoulder dislocation). Larger fractures usually occur in patients with repeated dislocations (Figure 14).

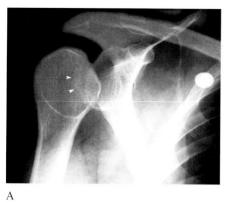 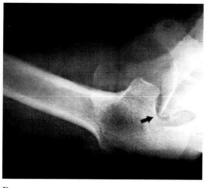 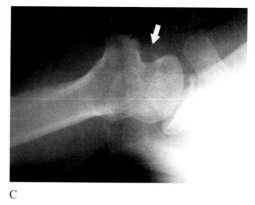

A   B   C

FIGURE 14 **Posterior shoulder dislocation with a large impacted humeral head fracture** ("reverse Hill-Sachs deformity").

The "light bulb on a stick" sign is not evident in this patient.

(A) On the AP view, there is nearly normal glenohumeral overlap because of the large impacted fracture of the humeral head. This patient had a prior posterior shoulder dislocation. In this instance, a posterior dislocation is difficult to detect on the AP view. The fracture is visible as a linear region of increased density of the humeral head and is known as the *trough line* (*arrowheads*). This is a radiographic clue to a posterior shoulder dislocation.

(B) The axillary view shows the posterior dislocation and the large impacted fracture of the anterior aspect of the humeral head at the point of contact with the glenoid rim, a "reverse Hill-Sachs deformity" (*arrow*). This is responsible for the "trough line" seen on the AP view.

(C) Post-reduction axillary view showing the large impacted fracture of the humeral head (*arrow*).

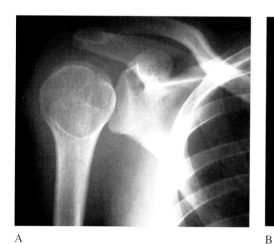 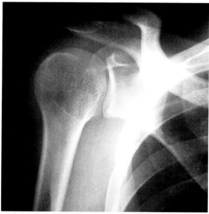 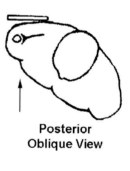

Posterior Oblique View

A   B   C

FIGURE 15 **Attempted external rotation AP view** in a patient with a posterior shoulder dislocation.

(A) The initial AP view shows a typical "light bulb on a stick."

(B) When the patient was instructed to externally rotate his arm, he instead externally rotated his torso because his shoulder was fixed in internal rotation by the posterior dislocation. This resulted in a "posterior oblique view" of the shoulder. The humeral head and glenoid fossa are slightly overlapping because of the posterior dislocation.

(C) Positioning of the posterior oblique view.

There are two instances in which posterior dislocations are more difficult to detect on an AP view.

In one, a deep humeral head impaction fracture ("reverse Hill-Sachs deformity") can cause the glenohumeral overlap to appear normal on the AP view (no "light bulb on a stick" sign) (Figure 14). Detection of posterior dislocation is dependent on

identification of the **trough line.**

Second, a patient who attempts to externally rotate the shoulder as instructed by the radiology technician, may instead rotate the entire torso, which produces an oblique view of the shoulder (Figures 15 and 16).

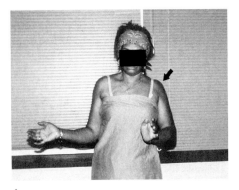
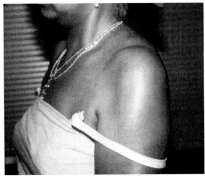
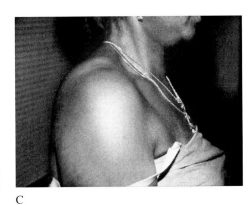

A   B   C

FIGURE 16   Clinical diagnosis of a posterior shoulder dislocation.

(*A*) When asked to externally rotate both arms, the patient was unable to externally rotate her left shoulder because it was fixed in internal rotation (*arrow*). She was able to externally rotate her right arm.

(*B*) There was an anterior concavity of her left shoulder due to the posterior dislocation.

(*C*) The normal right shoulder for comparison.

This patient's posterior shoulder dislocation was misdiagnosed as a "frozen shoulder" (adhesive capsulitis) for six months. She eventually was diagnosed using CT and required extensive shoulder reconstruction surgery. (Courtesy Evan G. Schwartz, MD)

Clinical Diagnosis of a Posterior Shoulder Dislocation

With a posterior dislocation, the shoulder is adducted and internally rotated and the patient is unable to externally rotate the arm (Figure 16). In addition, there may be a visible or palpable concavity of the anterior surface of the shoulder. In Patient 6 (Figure 1B), the shoulder deformity was not evident because of his body habitus. The patient was unable to externally rotate his arm.

The usual **mechanism of injury** responsible for a posterior shoulder dislocation is a forceful impact applied to the anterior aspect of the shoulder either by a direct blow or a fall on an outstretched arm (Figure 17). Forceful contraction of the shoulder muscles during an electrical shock or a seizure can also cause a posterior dislocation. This is because the strongest muscles that act on the shoulder cause internal rotation and posterior displacement—latissimus dorsi, pectoralis major, and subscapularis overpower the infraspinatus and teres minor (Figure 18). Nonetheless, anterior dislocation is the most common dislocation following a seizure or electrical shock because of the associated fall.

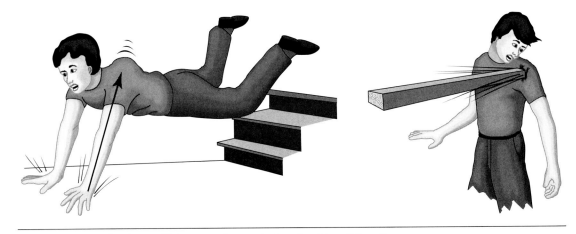

FIGURE 17   Mechanisms of injury causing posterior shoulder dislocation.
A fall on an outstretched hand or direct blow to the shoulder with the arm adducted and internally rotated.

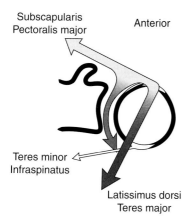

Subscapularis
Pectoralis major

Anterior

Teres minor
Infraspinatus

Latissimus dorsi
Teres major

FIGURE 18 Mechanism of posterior shoulder dislocation due to seizure or electrical shock.

Forceful contraction of the muscles acting on the proximal humerus causes internal rotation and posterior displacement.

Muscles causing internal rotation (subscapularis and pectoralis major) are stronger than the muscles causing external rotation (teres minor and infraspinatus). The latissimus dorsi and teres major cause posterior displacement as well as internal rotation.

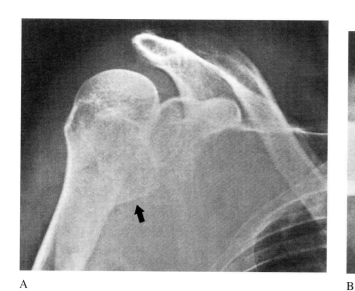

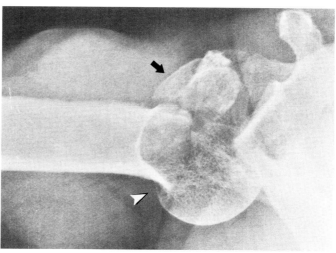

A   B

FIGURE 19 Concomitant proximal humeral fracture and posterior dislocation.

(*A*) The AP view shows only a proximal humerus fracture involving the lesser tuberosity (*arrow*).

(*B*) The dislocation is revealed by the axillary view. A humeral neck fracture (*arrowhead*), as well as the lesser tuberosity fracture (*arrow*), is seen.

[From: Riddervold HO: *Easily Missed Fractures and Corner Signs in Radiology.* Futura, 1991, with permission.]

Posterior Fracture/Dislocation

A posterior dislocation can occur in association with a fracture of the proximal humerus. A posterior dislocation must be excluded in all patients with proximal humeral fractures because it significantly alters management. A proximal humeral fracture without dislocation is treated with simple immobilization (unless it is highly fragmented or displaced), whereas a proximal humeral fracture with posterior dislocation requires reduction (usually in the operating room). Additional radiographic views (in particular, an axillary view) are often needed in patients with proximal humeral fractures to detect a concomitant posterior dislocation (Figure 19). In addition, a lesser tuberosity fracture is associated with posterior dislocation, whereas a greater tuberosity fracture is associated with anterior dislocation.

SUGGESTED READING

Gor DM: The trough line sign. *Radiology* 2002;224:485–486.
Maguire W, Schwartz DT: The shoulder. In: Schwartz DT, Reisdorff EJ eds., *Emergency Radiology.* New York: McGraw-Hill, 2000.
Perron AD, Jones RL: Posterior shoulder dislocation: Avoiding a missed diagnosis. *Am J Emerg Med* 2000;18:189–191.

Sanders TG, Jersey SL: Conventional radiography of the shoulder. *Semin Roentgen* 2005; 40:207–222.
Wadlington VR, Hendrix RW, Rogers LF: Computed tomography of posterior fracture-dislocations of the shoulder. *J Trauma* 1992; 32:113–115.

Upper Extremity: Patient 7

A shoulder injury in an elderly woman

A 65-year-old woman presented to the ED with shoulder pain after falling down. She was pushed and fell onto her outstretched right arm and shoulder. There were no other injuries.

On examination, her vital signs were normal. She was in moderate distress and resisted any attempt to move her shoulder, which had been immobilized in a sling by the ambulance crew in the field. There was loss of the normal shoulder contour with a prominent step-off deformity at the acromion and a palpable concavity of the deltoid region. Neurovascular function was intact.

Parenteral analgesia was administered and radiographs were obtained (Figure 1). (A metal clip from the shoulder sling is seen on the AP view.)

- Why obtain x-rays on a patient with a shoulder dislocation that can be diagnosed by clinical examination?

- How would you reduce this shoulder dislocation?

- What are the significant findings on these radiographs?

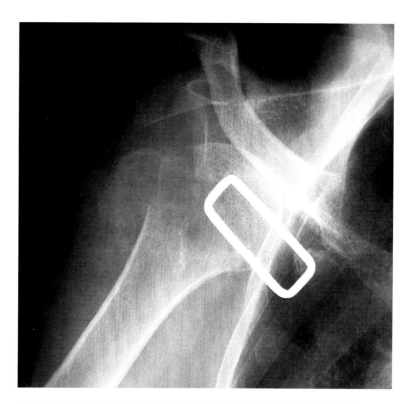

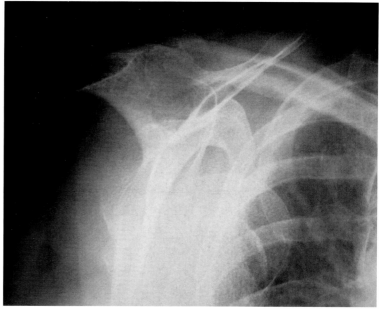

FIGURE 1

WHY OBTAIN RADIOGRAPHS IN PATIENTS WITH SHOULDER DISLOCATIONS?

The standard AP view of the shoulder, in conjunction with the findings on physical examination, is usually sufficient to diagnose an anterior dislocation (Figure 2A).

Although an AP radiograph does not allow direct determination of whether the dislocated humeral head is anterior or posterior to the glenoid fossa, anterior dislocation can be surmised by making two observations. First, with an anterior dislocation, displacement of the humeral head is much greater than is possible with a posterior dislocation. The humeral head is usually in a subcoracoid position, although subglenoid and subclavicular dislocations occasionally occur. With a posterior dislocation, displacement is limited by the muscles of the rotator cuff. Second,

with an anterior dislocation the humerus is fixed in external rotation (greater tuberosity is lateral) and an internal rotation view cannot be obtained. Internal rotation of the shoulder is prevented by impaction of the humeral head on the anterior rim of the glenoid fossa.

To directly demonstrate the proximal humerus dislocation, an additional view such as a *scapular Y view* or a *axillary view* can be obtained (Figure 2B and Patient 6, Figures 8 and 11, pages 274–275). Although these views are frequently obtained in patients with anterior dislocations, they are generally not essential to make that diagnosis. Occasionally, these views will reveal a scapular fracture that was not evident on the AP view.

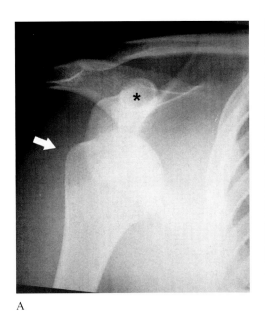

A

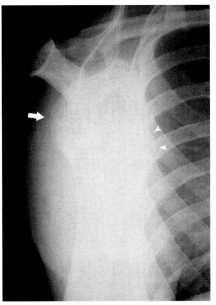

B

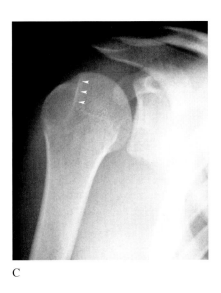

C

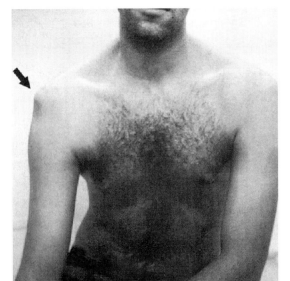

D

FIGURE 2   Anterior shoulder dislocation.

(*A*) **AP view:** The humeral head is in external rotation (greater tuberosity is lateral, *arrow*) and in a subcoracoid location. *Asterisk* = coracoid process.

(*B*) **Scapular Y view:** Interpretation of this view can be difficult when it is slightly oblique and overlying soft tissues obscure the image, as in this patient. The humeral head overlies the ribs (*arrowheads*). *Arrow* = glenoid fossa.

(*C*) **Post-reduction view:** There is a large linear deformity (*arrowheads*) representing an impacted fracture of the humeral head (*Hill-Sachs deformity*). This was not evident on the initial radiographs. This common fracture does not alter emergency management. If large, it predisposes to recurrent dislocation and may need surgical repair.

(*D*) **Clinical findings** include an abrupt step-off deformity due to a prominent acromion (*arrow*), palpably empty glenoid fossa, and the arm held in external rotation and abduction.

[D from: Knoop KJ, Stack LB, Storrow AB: *Atlas of Emergency Medicine*, 2nd ed., McGraw-Hill, 2002, with permission.]

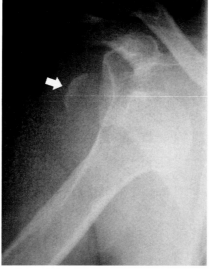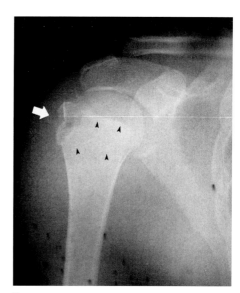

FIGURE 3 Anterior dislocation and avulsion fracture of the greater tuberosity (*arrow*) in an 18-year-old boy who fell off his bicycle.

(*B*) After reduction of the glenohumeral joint in the standard fashion, the greater tuberosity is realigned with the proximal humerus (*arrow*).

(*Arrowheads* = nearly fused growth plate in an 18-year-old is normal)

A   B

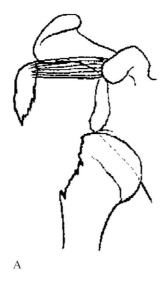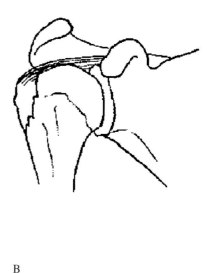

FIGURE 4 Greater tuberosity avulsion is the most common fracture associated with an anterior shoulder dislocation. It does not alter the technique of reduction.

(*A*) The supraspinatus tendon is attached to the greater tuberosity causing avulsion at the time of dislocation.

(*B*) Successful reduction of both the dislocation and the avulsion fracture.

A   B

Because anterior shoulder dislocations are usually obvious on physical examination, radiographs are generally not necessary to make the diagnosis. Instead, the principal role of radiography is to detect associated fractures, which occur in 8–25% of shoulder dislocations (Perron et al. 2003, Emond et al. 2004). (This does not include Hill-Sachs deformities, which occur in up to 25% of dislocations.) However, in most cases, the fracture does not alter emergency management.

The most common fracture associated with an anterior shoulder dislocation is an **avulsion of the greater tuberosity** of the humerus, occurring in 5–19% of cases (Figure 3). Avulsion

occurs because the *supraspinatus tendon* is attached to the greater tuberosity (Figure 4). This fracture does not alter the technique of reduction because when the shoulder is reduced, the avulsed fragment usually returns to its proper position (Figure 3B). If the fracture remains displaced by 1 cm or more, surgical screw fixation is indicated, particularly in younger patients.

Proximal humerus fractures associated with shoulder dislocations occur more commonly in older individuals. Fractures are seen in as many as 40% of shoulder dislocations in patients over age 50 years. The radiographs therefore must be carefully inspected for evidence of a fracture.

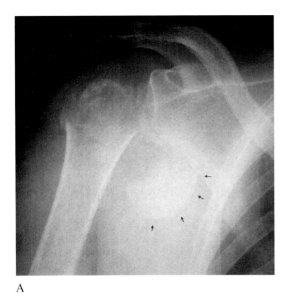

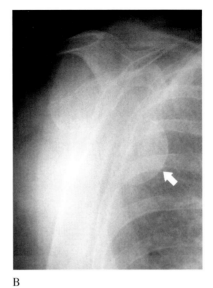

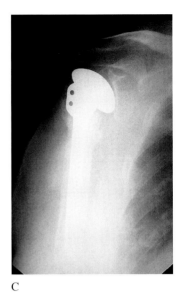

A   B   C

FIGURE 5   Patient 7—Post-reduction radiographs

The AP view (*A*) and Y view (*B*) revealed complete displacement of the humeral head (*arrows*) due to an unsuspected humeral neck fracture. The humeral shaft was "reduced," but the humeral head remained dislocated.

(*C*) Postoperative view showing hemi-arthroplasty of the proximal humerus.

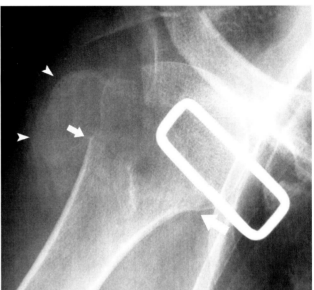

FIGURE 6   Patient 7—Initial AP view

Initial AP view showing an anterior dislocation, avulsion fracture of the greater tuberosity (*arrowheads*) and a subtle fracture through the humeral neck (*arrows*).

(The metallic rectangle is a clip for the shoulder sling.)

Patient Outcome

In Patient 7, a greater tuberosity fracture was recognized, in addition to the anterior dislocation. However, a non-displaced fracture of the humeral neck was not appreciated. Standard closed reduction using traction/counter-traction was performed. Post-reduction radiographs revealed that the attempted reduction caused complete displacement of the humeral head from the humeral shaft (Figure 5).

Because of the risk of avascular necrosis as well as the potential difficulty attaining internal fixation using plates and screws in this elderly woman, the patient was treated with a hemi-arthroplasty (Figure 5C).

Review of the initial AP radiograph reveals a subtle fracture of the humeral neck. It appears as trabecular impaction and cortical disruption at the humeral neck (Figure 6). Had this been recognized, closed reduction should not have been attempted.

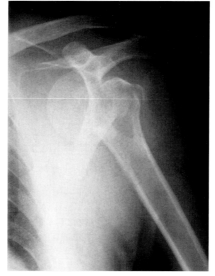
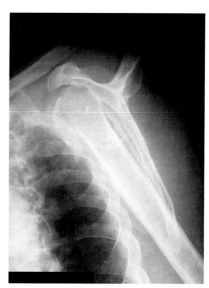

FIGURE 7 A 40-year-old man with an anterior dislocation and displaced humeral neck fracture (*A* and *B*).

(*C* and *D*) During attempted closed reduction, the humeral shaft was re-aligned with the glenoid fossa, but the humeral head remained dislocated. Closed reduction should not have been attempted because it was ineffective and further displaced the fracture.

(*E*) Open reduction was necessary. The humeral neck fracture was treated with plate and screws fixation.

A   B

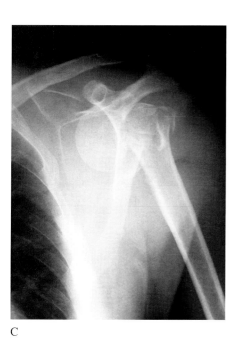
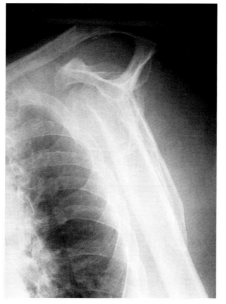
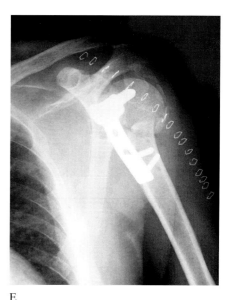

C   D

E

Humeral neck fracture/dislocations

Humeral neck fracture/dislocations are less common than greater tuberosity avulsion fractures, occurring in 2.6–4% of cases (Perron et al. 2003, Emond et al. 2004). However, they are the second most common fracture associated with anterior shoulder dislocations and are the most important reason to obtain radiographs in patients with clinically evident anterior shoulder dislocations because management is substantially altered.

The humeral head cannot be reduced by applying traction on the humeral shaft. Attempted closed reduction can cause further separation of the fracture fragments, increasing the risk of avascular necrosis of the humeral head (Figure 7).

A nondisplaced humeral neck fracture can be difficult to visualize but should be specifically sought, particularly in older individuals with shoulder dislocations.

When a humeral neck fracture is found or suspected, closed reduction can still be attempted, although this should be done either in the operating room under general anesthesia with fluoroscopic guidance (Hersche and Gerber 1994), or possibly in the ED, after consultation with an orthopedic surgeon, using adequate sedation, analgesia and gentle traction while manipulating the displaced humeral head. If unsuccessful, open reduction should be performed. If an inapparent humeral neck fracture is displaced during attempted reduction, immediate open reduction and internal fixation has been suggested, particularly for younger patients, in the hope of decreasing the incidence of later avascular necrosis of the humeral head (Ferkel et al. 1984).

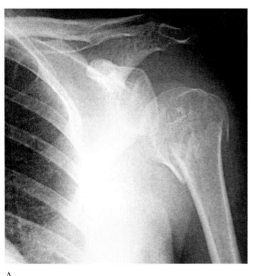

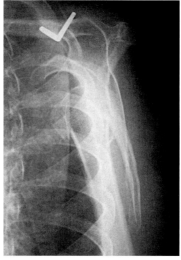

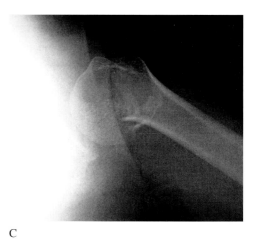

A   B

FIGURE 8   Pseudo-dislocation of the shoulder.

(*A*) The AP view shows a minimally displaced humeral neck fracture with inferior displacement of the humeral head that mimics a dislocation. This is due to a hemarthrosis distending the joint capsule and is known as a pseudo-dislocation.

(*B*) On the Y-view, the humeral head is inferiorly and anteriorly displaced. Although the Y-view can usually distinguish a dislocation,

in this patient, glenohumeral subluxation mimics an anterior shoulder dislocation. This illustrates the limitations of the Y view in this situation.

(*C*) An axillary view confirms that there is no dislocation.

Pseudo-dislocation

An injury that should not be mistakenly interpreted as a fracture-dislocation is a *pseudo-dislocation* (Figure 8). In a patient with a proximal humerus fracture, a hemarthrosis can distend the joint capsule and displace the humeral head from the glenoid fossa. On the AP radiograph, this displacement can mimic dislocation of the glenohumeral joint. A Y-view or axillary view may be needed to show that the humeral head is still in alignment within the glenoid fossa. Traction on the arm in an attempt to reduce this injury should not be attempted because it will further displace the fracture increasing the risk of avascular necrosis of the humeral head.

Indications for radiography in patients with anterior shoulder dislocation

Standard management of a patient with suspected anterior shoulder dislocation is to obtain both pre- and postreduction radiographs. However, because both an anterior dislocation and its successful reduction are usually obvious on clinical examination, the role of radiography is controversial. The two principal roles of radiography are (1) to establish the diagnosis of dislocation when it is uncertain and (2) to detect fractures that have occurred in association with the dislocation.

Pre-reduction radiographs could theoretically be omitted if the diagnosis was certain based on clinical examination. However, when the traumatic force causing the dislocation could also cause a fracture, prereduction radiographs should be obtained whenever possible. In settings where radiography is not

available, such as when the injury occurs on an athletic field, reduction could be attempted without radiography to avoid a prolonged delay in treatment (Shuster 1999). One instance when radiography may not be necessary is in a patient with recurrent shoulder dislocations in whom the dislocation occurred with minimal force such as by simply abducting the arm. In this case, there is clearly insufficient force to cause a fracture.

Emond et al. (2004) identified three factors predictive of a fracture in association with a shoulder dislocation: age 40 years or older, first episode of dislocation, and dangerous mechanism of injury (fall greater than one flight of stairs, fight/assault or motor vehicle crash). Absence of all three features was 98% sensitive at excluding an associated fracture and could potentially be used to omit pre-reduction radiographs, although this has not yet been prospectively validated.

The necessity of **post-reduction radiographs** has been questioned because reduction is usually clinically evident by noting the change in shoulder contour and increased range of motion. Based on a prospective series of 104 patients, Hendey (2000) suggested that in patients without a fracture, when clinicians were confident of the success of reduction (93% of 85 cases), post-reduction radiographs could be omitted because the clinicians were correct in all cases. When the clinicians were not confident of the reduction (6 cases) or there was a concomitant fracture (10 cases), post-reduction radiographs were necessary.

Concern that post-reduction radiographs should be obtained because a fracture could be caused by the force of manipulation is implausible given current nontraumatic techniques of reduction.

Hendey (2000) proposed an **algorithm** defining two circumstances in which radiography could potentially be omitted. First, *pre-reduction* radiographs could be omitted in patients with recurrent dislocation when mechanism of injury was atraumatic (28% of patients). Second, *post-reduction* radiographs could be omitted when there were no associated fractures seen on the prereduction radiographs and the clinicians were confident of the reduction. In his series, this would reduce the use of radiography by 51%. A small prospective series found that the algorithm reduced radiograph utilization by 47%, without missing any clinically significant fractures or persistent dislocations (Hendey et al. 2004).

Post-reduction radiographs may show fractures that were not seen on the prereduction radiographs, although these fractures generally do not alter acute management, such as Hill-Sachs deformities (Figure 2) (Hendey and Kinlaw 1996, Harvey et al. 1992). Nonetheless, the fractures may have long term implications and radiographs would likely be desired by the orthopedist during follow-up of the patient. In addition, if a subtle humeral neck fracture was unrecognized prior to reduction, as in this patient, failure to obtain post-reduction radiographs could result in significant morbidity.

SUGGESTED READING

Beeson MS: Complications of shoulder dislocation. *Am J Emerg Med* 1999;17:288–295.

Emond M, Le Sage N, Lavoie A, Rochette L: Clinical factors predicting fractures associated with an anterior shoulder dislocation. *Acad Emerg Med* 2004;11:853–858.

Ferkel RD, Hedley AK, Eckardt JJ: Anterior fracture-dislocations of the shoulder: Pitfalls in treatment. *J Trauma* 1984;24:363–367.

Harvey RA, Trabulsy ME, Roe L: Are postreduction anteroposterior and scapular Y views useful in anterior shoulder dislocations? *Am J Emerg Med* 1992;10:149–151.

Hendey GW, Chally MK, Stewart VB: Selective radiography in anterior shoulder dislocation: Prospective validation of a clinical decision rule (abstract). *Acad Emerg Med* 2004;11:575.

Hendey GW, Kinlaw K: Clinically significant abnormalities in postreduction radiographs after anterior shoulder dislocation. *Ann Emerg Med* 1996;28:399–402.

Hendey GW: Necessity of radiographs in the emergency department management of shoulder dislocations. *Ann Emerg Med* 2000; 36:108–113.

Hersche O, Gerber C: Iatrogenic displacement of fracture-dislocations of the shoulder. *J Bone Joint Surg (Br)* 1994;76:30–33.

Kahn J: The role of post-reduction x-rays after shoulder dislocation (abstract). *Acad Emerg Med* 2001;8:521.

Ogawa K, Yoshida A, Ikegami H: Isolated fractures of the greater tuberosity of the humerus: Solutions to recognizing a frequently overlooked fracture. *J Trauma* 2003;54:713–717.

Perron AD, Ingerski MS, Brady WJ, Erling BF, Ullman EA: Acute complications associated with shoulder dislocation at an academic Emergency Department. *J Emerg Med* 2003;24:141–145.

Shuster M, Abu-Laban R, Boyd J, et al: Prospective evaluation of a guideline for the selective elimination of pre-reduction radiographs in clinically obvious anterior shoulder dislocation. *Can J Emerg Med* 2002;4:257–262.

Shuster M: Pre-reduction radiographs in clinically evident anterior shoulder dislocation. *Am J Emerg Med* 1999;17:653–658.

Upper Extremity: Patient 8

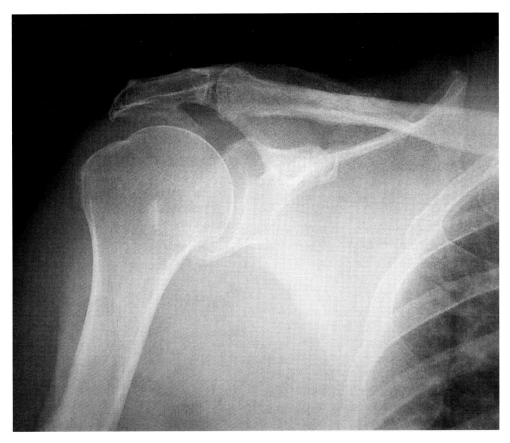

FIGURE 1

Shoulder pain in an elderly woman that radiated down her arm

A 71-year-old woman complained of right shoulder pain that radiated down her arm. The pain began three days earlier. It was persistent, but had gradually improved. Her daughter was finally able to convince her to come to the doctor.

She had had shoulder pain for the past year, which had begun after a motor vehicle collision. The patient had been to several orthopedists, rehabilitation physicians, and physical therapists. Litigation was pending with regard to her injury. Her home health aide was with her when the current episode of shoulder pain began and noted that the patient's arm appeared pale at that time.

The patient denied any recent trauma. Her past medical history included diabetes and hypertension.

On examination, she was elderly and overweight. She ap-

peared fatigued but was in no acute distress. Her vital signs were normal aside from a blood pressure of 180/100 mm Hg in both arms.

The right shoulder had mild diffuse tenderness but no swelling. There was pain on range of motion, which became severe during passive abduction to 70°. Sensation and strength were normal except as limited by pain. Pulses were normal and equal in both arms. A few small ecchymoses were present on the medial aspect of her right upper arm.

A radiograph of the right shoulder was obtained (Figure 1).

- What are the diagnostic possibilities?

- How would you manage this patient?

WHEN NOT TO GET AN X-RAY

The radiograph was interpreted as showing a large **osteophyte** extending from the acromion. Osteophytes are outgrowths of new bone that forms at the margins of a joint injured by degenerative osteoarthritis. Osteophyte formation is an attempted reparative process at the edge of remaining articular cartilage.

The correct interpretation is that the coracoacromial ligament is calcified (Figure 2). This is also a response to wear-and-tear stresses but is a "traction spur" or "bone spur" similar to calcification of the plantar ligament in the foot. The proper name for a bone spur is **enthesophyte.**

Calcification of the coracoacromial ligament may be associated with shoulder *impingement syndrome*. There is painful compression of the supraspinatus tendon between the greater tuberosity of the humeral head and the coracoacromial ligament when the patient abducts the shoulder. This could be the cause of the patient's chronic pain and limited range of motion.

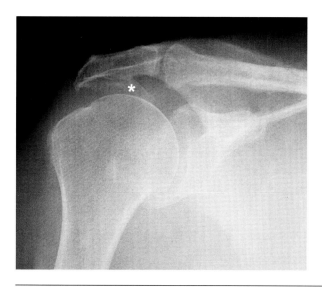
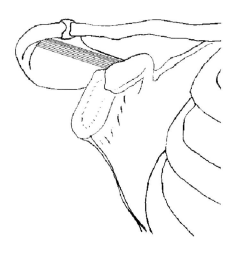

FIGURE 2   The coracoacromial ligament is partially calcified in this patient (*asterisk*).

Differential Diagnosis of Shoulder Pain That Radiates Down the Arm

In a patient with **shoulder pain that radiates down the arm,** there are a large number of diagnostic possibilities (Table 1).

Localized musculoskeletal disorders of the shoulder can cause pain with distal radiation. These include tendonitis, bursitis, and skeletal lesions (neoplasm or osteonecrosis). Disorders of the elbow and wrist (e.g., carpal tunnel syndrome) can cause pain radiating proximally up the arm.

Reflex sympathetic dystrophy, also known as *causalgia* or *shoulder–hand syndrome,* is a chronic disabling condition due to vasomotor instability in the arm. It may occur following a traumatic injury to the shoulder, especially if there has been a period of immobility. There are recurrent episodes of pain, paresthesia, swelling, and hyperemia of the arm. Over 6–12 months cutaneous atrophy, contractures and osteoporosis may develop (*Sudek's atrophy*). Reflex sympathetic dystrophy can also complicate stroke and myocardial infarction. This occurred more frequently in the past when long periods of bedrest were prescribed following a "heart attack."

TABLE 1

Differential Diagnosis of Shoulder Pain That Radiates Down the Arm

1. Musculoskeletal disorders of the shoulder or arm

2. Reflex sympathetic dystrophy

3. Neurological disorders:
   - Spinal root
   - Brachial plexus
   - Spinal cord

4. Thoracic outlet syndrome

5. Vascular occlusion

6. Visceral disorders (referred pain): cardiac, diaphragmatic, abdominal

Various **neurological disorders** can cause pain radiating down the arm. Impingement on a cervical nerve root by a herniated disk or osteophyte is common (*cervical radiculopathy*). This may not be accompanied by neck pain. Disorders affecting the *spinal cord* include intrinsic spinal cord tumors and extrinsic compression of the cord from a herniated cervical disc, vertebral tumor or epidural abscess. Cord compression causes a different neurological picture than nerve root compression, e.g., increased rather than decreased reflexes, and lower extremity involvement with spastic gait and a Babinski sign. Finally, there could be *brachial plexus* involvement by, for example, a tumor at the lung apex. Hence, it is important to carefully examine the patient for signs of neurological dysfunction, such as weakness, muscular atrophy, sensory deficits, and abnormal reflexes.

Impingement of the neurovascular supply to the arm can occur at the thoracic outlet (between the first rib and clavicle). **Thoracic outlet syndrome** occurs in persons with anomalies such as a cervical rib, and in overweight women with poor posture and large, pendulous breasts. The *Adson maneuver* is useful to diagnose this disorder. The examiner raises the patient's arm in abduction and extension, and the neck is rotated to the opposite direction. This will reproduce the patient's pain and paresthesia and can also cause a diminished radial pulse.

The disorders mentioned above generally cause chronic symptoms. The clinician must therefore first search for acute disorders to account for the patient's emergency department visit before attributing it to any of the above mentioned disorders. For example, **visceral disorders** can cause referred pain to the shoulder and arm, particularly cardiac ischemia and diseases causing diaphragmatic irritation such as a subphrenic abscess, hepatic or splenic disorders, or cholecystitis. Usually, there is pain at the primary site (chest or abdomen) in addition to the referred shoulder pain.

Patient Outcome

In this patient, the relatively rapid onset of pain and the initial pallor of the extremity suggest an acute vascular event. After this history was elicited, the patient was re-examined for signs of arterial insufficiency. These were not evident: color, warmth, pulse, and blood pressure of both arms were equal. However, the event had occurred 3 days earlier and so objective signs of diminished perfusion could have resolved. The only diagnostic clues that remained were the history of initial pallor of the arm and the small ecchymoses on the medial aspect of the upper arm, possibly embolic. To add to the uncertainty, an *impingement sign* was positive—abduction of the shoulder caused pain when the greater tuberosity moved under the acromion.

The patient was referred for *Doppler studies* of the arm, which revealed a diminished pulse waveform on the right, suggesting arterial insufficiency. A thoracic *aortogram* revealed an aneurysm at the origin of the inominate artery with a large intraluminal filling defect, the probable source of the embolism (Figure 3). (Auscultation of this region for a bruit might have been revealing.) Possible etiologies of the aneurysm include atherosclerosis or a post-traumatic pseudoaneurysm that developed following the motor vehicle collision one year earlier.

Prior to the planned thoracotomy and aortic reconstruction surgery, the patient suffered another embolic event — emboliztion to the right carotid artery caused left arm paralysis. (Paradoxically, the patient presented with right arm symptoms and then developed left arm weakness.) The patient's neurological deficit eventually improved, but she then refused surgery.

Summary

Without a clear idea of the information desired from a diagnostic test, its result could confuse rather than clarify the diagnosis. "Geographic" test ordering—obtaining radiographs of the region that is symptomatic without regard to the potential diagnoses—should be avoided. Positive findings could be irrelevant and negative results falsely reassuring. The patient's degenerative changes could account for shoulder pain and an impingement syndrome. However, these r adiographic abnormalities were long-standing and, totally *unrelated* to the patient's emergency department visit. The clinicians were almost mislead by the radiographic findings into thinking that they had found a benign cause for this patient's shoulder pain. One must always be hesitant to ascribe an emergency department visit to a chronic disorder such as degenerative arthritis.

SUGGESTED READING

Resnick D, Niwayama G: Degenerative disease of extraspinal locations. In: Resnick D, ed. *Diagnosis of Bone and Joint Disorders*, 4th ed. Philadelphia, WB Saunders, 2000.

Fisher RG, Chasen MH, Lamki N: Diagnosis of injuries of the aorta and brachiocephalic arteries caused by blunt chest trauma: CT vs. aortography. *AJR* 1994;162:1047–1052.

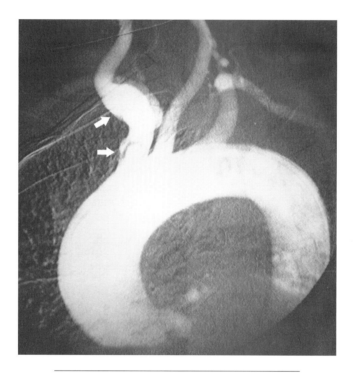

FIGURE 3   Aortogram—Patient 8.
Innominate artery aneurysm with an intimal flap *(arrows)*, the source of the patient's embolism.

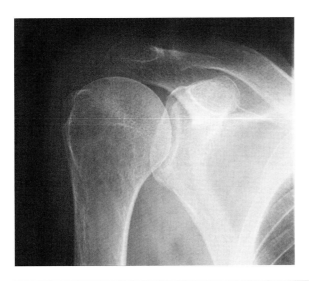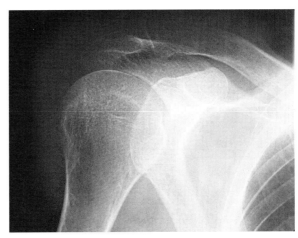

FIGURE 4

PATIENT 7B

A 65-year-old man presented with shoulder pain of six week's duration. He had visited several other doctors on three occasions and had had two sets of radiographs which, he was told, were normal. Ibuprofen was prescribed, but the pain persisted. He now presented for a "fourth opinion."

- Should you repeat the radiographs of the shoulder, accept that they were negative, or attempt to retrieve the images or reports from the other hospitals?

(Shoulder radiographs were obtained and are shown above)

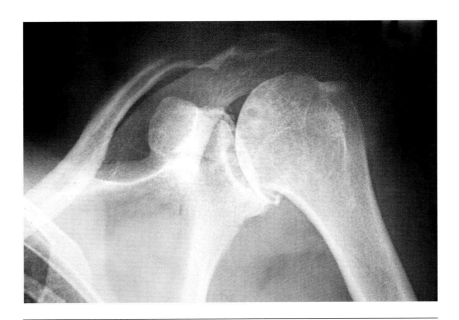

FIGURE 5

PATIENT 7C

A 62-year-old man presented to the urgent care clinic with bilateral shoulder pain, greater on the left than the right. He had pain when moving his shoulders but no limited range of motion. The patient did not speak English and the family member with him spoke only limited English so details of his history were not obtained.

Radiographs of the shoulder (Figure 5) showed typical findings of **degenerative osteoarthritis:** joint space narrowing, osteophyte formation, subchondral sclerosis (eburnation), and subchondral cyst formation.

Ibuprofen was prescribed and the patient was discharged from the ED.

Patient 7B Outcome

A careful history and physical examination should first be performed. On examination, the patient was able to move his right shoulder with only minimal pain. The area of pain was actually localized to the supraclavicular region. On neurological examination, there was weakness of the forearm and hand, and wasting of the thenar muscles. Cranial nerve function was normal and, specifically, there was no Horner's syndrome.

Shoulder radiographs were negative (Figure 4), but the radiograph of the chest (Figure 6) revealed a tumor of the lung apex with erosion of the adjacent ribs (*arrow*)—a Pancoast tumor.

Despite our trepidation about informing the patient of these findings, he was, in fact, thankful that the cause of his pain had finally been determined after having been told on several occasions that "nothing was wrong."

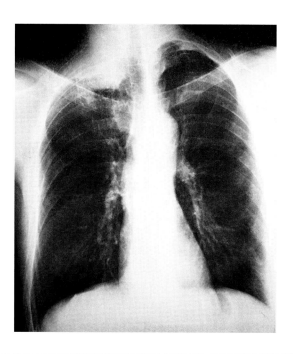

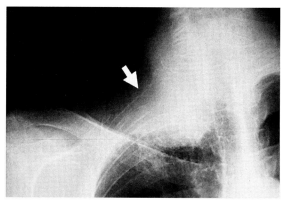

FIGURE 6

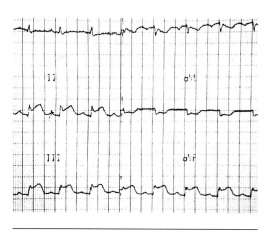

FIGURE 7

Patient 7C Outcome

The following day, the patient returned to the ED complaining of increased chest and shoulder pain. An EKG showed an acute inferior wall myocardial infarction (Figure 7).

As in Patient 7, an acute ED visit should not be attributed to a chronic medical condition without a cogent explanation. An inadequate history, coupled with "geographic" ordering of radiographs, is a recipe for disaster.

Lower Extremity: Patient 1

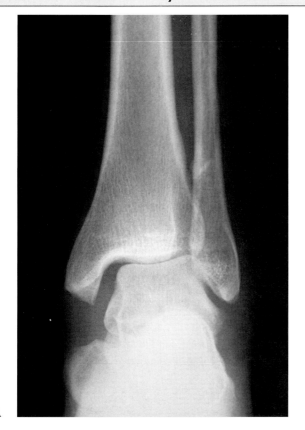

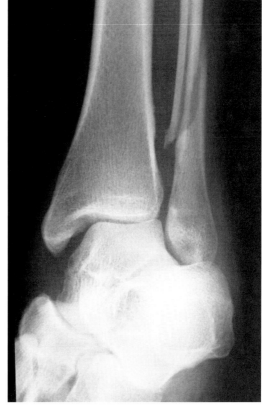

A

B

FIGURE 1

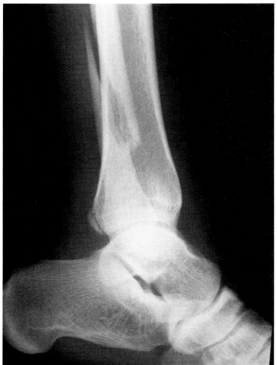

C

An ankle injury in a middle-aged woman

A 44-year-old woman who worked as an emergency medical technician (EMT) presented to the ED with ankle pain after she twisted her ankle stepping out of the back of an ambulance. Her ankle radiographs are shown in Figure 1.

- Is this a single malleolar fracture, a bimalleolar fracture, or a trimalleolar fracture?

- In which way did the patient twist her ankle to cause this injury?

HOW FRACTURES ARE CLASSIFIED

There are many types of fracture classification systems. The simplest schemes describe the injury anatomically. Other classification systems elucidate the mechanism of injury or are based on treatment and prognosis.

Even though the ankle is a relatively simple hinge joint, there are a number of different classification systems for ankle injuries. The most basic classification scheme simply describes the number of fractures about the ankle—either one, two, or three malleoli. (The third malleolus is the posterior margin of the distal tibia.) Although this classification system is straightforward, it oversimplifies ankle injuries and has little relevance to mechanism of injury or treatment. In addition, the term "bimalleolar fracture" is ambiguous because it can be used for fractures of any two of the three malleoli.

By contrast, the **Lauge-Hansen classification** system includes 13 separate injuries divided into four groups (Table 1).

This classification system is based on the mechanical forces responsible for various ankle injuries. Each injury is classified by two terms: the *position of the foot* at the time of injury (either supinated or pronated), and the *direction of the force* applied to the ankle (Figure 2).

The force applied is either **adduction** (commonly called "inversion"), **external rotation,** or rarely abduction (commonly called "eversion"). External rotation, by convention describes the motion of the foot relative to the leg, although clinically, the patient's foot is stationary on the ground and the patient's body rotates internally with respect to the foot.

This classification system does not include fractures of the tibial plafond, known as *pylon fractures*, which are due to axial compression.

TABLE 1

Lauge-Hansen Classification—Based on mechanism of injury

Injuries occur in sucessive stages as listed

Supination–external rotation, 60%	SER 1	Tear of the anterior–inferior tibiofibular ligament (AITFL)
	SER 2	Spiral fracture of the lateral malleolus at or above the mortise
	SER 3	Tear of the posterior–inferior tibiofibular ligament (PITFL) or fracture of the posterior malleolus
	SER 4	Fracture of the medial malleolus or deltoid ligament tear
Pronation–external rotation, 20%	PER 1	Tear of the AITFL
	PER 2	Fracture of the medial malleolus or deltoid ligament tear
	PER 3	Tear of the PITFL or fracture of the posterior malleolus
	PER 4	High fracture of the lateral malleolus above mortise
Supination–adduction (inversion), 20%	SAD 1	Low fracture of the lateral malleolus or lateral ligament tear.
	SAD 2	Oblique fracture of the medial malleolus
Pronation–abduction (eversion), <0.5%	PAB 1	Fracture of the medial malleolus or deltoid ligament tear
	PAB 2	Tear of the inferior tibiofibular ligaments (syndesmosis)
	PAB 3	Oblique fracture of the lateral malleolus at mortise

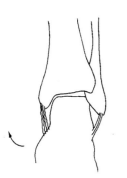
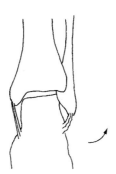
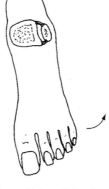
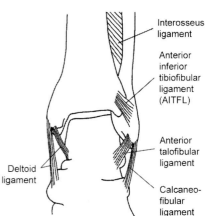

Position: Supination
Force: Adduction
Alternate term: Inversion

Position: Pronation
Force: Abduction
Alternate term: Eversion

Force: External Rotation

Interosseus ligament

Anterior inferior tibiofibular ligament (AITFL)

Anterior talofibular ligament

Deltoid ligament

Calcaneo-fibular ligament

FIGURE 2   Terminology of positions, injury forces and ligaments of the ankle.
Injury forces are indicated by the curved arrows.

The Lauge-Hansen classification system was derived from cadaver experiments. The foot was held in either the supination or pronation position and then a force (adduction or external rotation) was applied to produce various injuries. Although clinically the patient cannot usually recall their foot position and the direction of the force of injury, this classification scheme provides a clear explanation of the mechanisms responsible for injuries to the ankle.

Adduction is the most frequent mechanism of ankle injury. However, in most cases, adduction causes a *sprain* to the anterior talofibular ligament rather than a fracture. Adduction is responsible for 20% of fractures. First, there is an avulsion-type horizontal fracture cf the lateral malleolus below the level of the mortise (stage 1) followed by an oblique fracture of the medial malleolus (stage 2) (Figure 3).

External rotation is responsible for 80% of malleolar fractures, as in this patient. External rotation causes a sequence of fractures and ligament disruptions about the ankle mortise. The specific sequence of injuries depends on the position of the foot at the time of injury, whether it is supinated or pronated (Figure 2).

In 60% of fractures; the foot is supinated at the time of external rotation (**supination-external rotation**), the lateral ligaments are under tension, and lateral injuries occur before medial injuries (Figure 4).

First, there is a tear of the anterior–inferior tibiofibular ligament or, less commonly, a fracture of the anterior margin of the distal tibia, known as a *Tillaux fracture*. Second, torsional forces cause a spiral fracture of the lateral malleolus at and above the level of the mortise (Figure 5). Third, there is tearing of the posterior inferior tibiofibular ligament or a avulsion fracture of the posterior margin of the distal tibia ("posterior malleolus"). In some cases, there is a large intra-articular posterior malleolar fracture, which is caused by axial compression with the foot in plantar flexion and may require operative fixation. Fourth, there is a medial malleolar fracture or deltoid ligament tear.

This fourth stage, in which all three malleoli are fractured, is common and is referred to as a **"trimalleolar fracture"** (Figure 6).

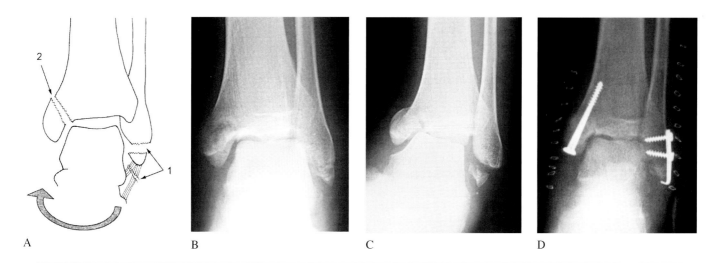

A   B   C   D

FIGURE 3   Supination–Adduction injury (inversion).

(A) Stage 1. Transverse fracture of the lateral malleolus below the level of the mortise *or* lateral ligament tear (the common ankle sprain).
       Stage 2. Oblique fracture of the medial malleolus.

Supination–Adduction stage 2 injury (SAD-2)—AP (*B*) and stress views (*C*).
Because both malleoli are fractured, it is mechanically unstable and requires surgical fixation (*D*).

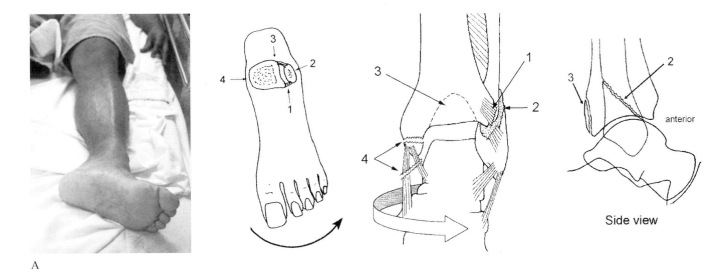

A

FIGURE 4   Injuries produced by external rotation of the ankle.

Supination–External rotation—The foot is supinated at the time of injury and the lateral side is injured first

On physical examination (*A*), the foot is externally rotated reflecting the mechanism of injury.

Stage 1:   Tear of the anterior-inferior tibiofibular ligament (AITFL) or avulsion of anterior tibia.

Stage 2:   Spiral fracture of the lateral malleolus at and above the level of the mortise.

Stage 3:   Tear of the posterior-inferior tibiofibular ligament (PITFL) or avulsion of the posterior malleolus.

Stage 4:   Transverse fracture of the medial malleolus or tear of the deltoid ligament (trimalleolar fracture).

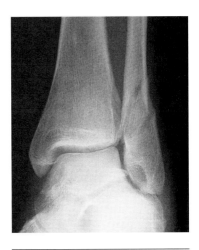

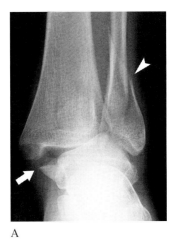

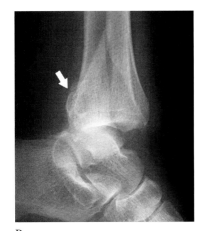

A   B

FIGURE 5   Supination–External rotation, stage 2—SER 2.

Isolated spiral fracture of the lateral malleolus originating at the level of the mortise.

This single malleolar fracture is stable and does not require surgical fixation.

FIGURE 6   Supination–External rotation, stage 4—SER 4 (Trimalleolar fracture).

AP view (*A*) shows a spiral fracture of the lateral malleolus at the level of the mortise (*arrow*) and a transverse fracture of the medial malleolus (*arrowhead*).

The lateral view (*B*) and post-reduction lateral view (*C*) show a posterior malleolar fracture (*arrow*).

These radiographs are of the patient shown in Figure 4A. If there had been a diminished pulse or excessive tenting of the skin, reduction of the injury and splinting would have been performed prior to radiography.

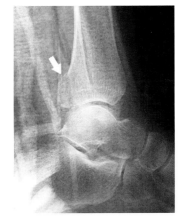

C

In 20% of fractures, the foot is pronated at the time of external rotation (**pronation-external rotation**), the medial ligaments are under tension and the sequence of injuries is reversed—first anterior, then medial, then posterior, and finally lateral (Figure 7). The fracture of the lateral malleolus occurs above the level of the mortise because the distal tibiofibular joint is disrupted before the fibular fracture occurs.

Danis-Weber Classification

A second classification scheme, **Danis-Weber,** is based on the level of the lateral malleolar fracture and correlates with the need for surgical treatment (Figure 8).

Type A is below the level of the mortise and usually does not need surgical treatment, unless the medial malleolus is fractured (Figure 3). **Type B** is at the level of the mortise and requires surgery in about half the cases (Figures 4–6). **Type C** is above the mortise and nearly always requires surgery because the distal tibiofibular joint is disrupted (Figure 8C).

The correlation between the Danis-Weber and Lauge-Hansen systems is that: Danis-Weber type A injuries are due to supination–adduction, Danis-Weber B injuries are due to supination-external rotation, and Danis-Weber C injuries are due to pronation–external rotation.

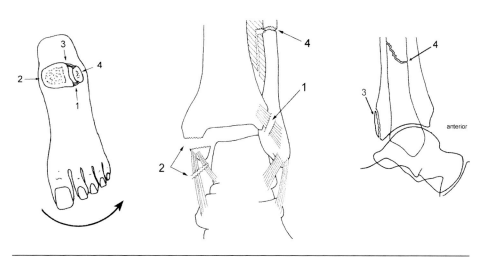

FIGURE 7   Pronation–External rotation.

When the ankle is pronated, the medial ligaments are taught and therefore injured first.

Stage 1: Tear of the anterior–inferior tibiofibular ligament (AITFL).

Stage 2: Transverse fracture of the medial malleolus or tear of the deltoid ligament.

Stage 3: Tear of the posterior–inferior tibiofibular ligament (PITFL) or avulsion of the posterior malleolus.

Stage 4: Fracture of the distal fibular shaft above the level of the mortise (also a "trimalleolar fracture").

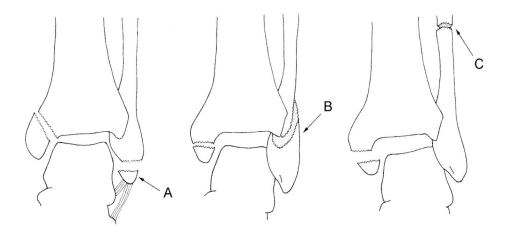

FIGURE 8   Danis-Weber classification.

(*A*) Lateral malleolar fracture below the level of the mortise = Supination–Adduction, SAD.

(*B*) Lateral malleolar fracture at and above the level of the mortise = Supination–External rotation, SER.

(*C*) Lateral malleolar fracture entirely above the level of the mortise = Pronation–External rotation, PER.

Patient Outcome

This patient's most obvious injury was a **spiral fracture of the fibula** (lateral malleolus) above the level of the mortise (Figure 9). Whenever one malleolar fracture is found, the radiographs should be carefully examined for other injuries. By understanding the mechanisms underlying various ankle injuries, specific fractures or ligament tears can be predicted (Table 1).

A lateral malleolar fracture above the level of the mortise is the hallmark of a **pronation–external rotation injury**, in particular a stage 4 injury (PER 4). With this fracture, there must be anterior, medial, and posterior injuries (Table 1).

In this patient, there is no medial malleolar fracture. The medial injury is instead a **deltoid ligament tear.** This causes widening of the medial side of the mortise and is seen on both the AP and mortise views (Figures 9A and B).

Third, there is a small **posterior malleolar fracture** (Figure 9C, *arrow*). This represents an avulsion fracture associated with disruption of the PITFL.

In accordance with the external rotation mechanism of injury, there must also be a tear of the AITFL (stage 1 injury) and concomitant **disruption of the distal tibiofibular joint** (DTFJ), the ankle *syndesmosis*. This is evident radiographically by widening of the DTFJ on the mortise view, i.e., no overlap of the distal tibia and fibula (Figure 9B, *arrowhead*). Disruption of the distal tibiofibular joint causes mechanical instability and necessitates surgical treatment.

Using the **Danis-Weber** classification scheme, this patient has a **type C** injury—a lateral malleolar fracture above the level of the mortise. This is mechanically unstable due to the associated injuries and requires surgical treatment.

This analysis demonstrates the limitations of the terminology: "single malleolar," "bimalleolar," and "trimalleolar" fracture. It is uncertain which term best describes this patient's injury. Only one malleolus, the lateral malleolus, is clearly fractured. Usually, single malleolar fractures are mechanically stable, although this is not the case in this patient. There is a second small posterior malleolar fracture. However, the term "bimalleolar fracture" is imprecise since this would encompass medial and lateral fractures, lateral and posterior fractures, and medial and posterior fractures, which are all very different injuries. A "trimalleolar fracture" is perhaps the most suitable description, even though this patient has only two fractures among her four injuries. Thus, better descriptors for this patient's injury are **pronation–external rotation injury, stage 4** (PER 4) and "Danis-Weber type C injury."

The patient's ankle was immobilized in a splint and she was admitted to the hospital. Operative repair consisted of plate and screw fixation of the distal fibular fracture and a long screw across the syndesmosis to stabilize the mortise (Figure 9D).

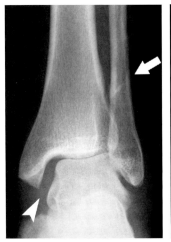 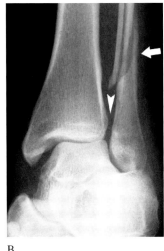 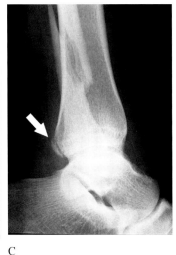 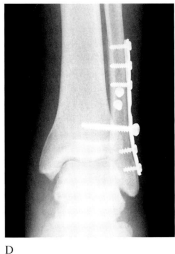

A   B   C   D

FIGURE 9   Pronation–External rotation, stage 4—Danis-Weber C—Patient 1.

(*A*)   AP view shows widening of the medial joint space due to medial (deltoid) ligament tear (*arrowhead*). The fibular fracture is barely visible (*arrow*).

(*B*)   Mortise view shows a fibular fracture above the mortise (*arrow*). There is separation of the tibiofibular syndesmosis due to disruption of the anterior and posterior tibiofibular ligaments (*arrowhead*).

(*C*)   Lateral view shows the posterior malleolus fracture (*arrow*) and the fibular fracture.

(*D*)   Postoperative view. The fibular fracture is fixed with a compression plate and screws. A longer syndesmosis screw is used to stabilize the distal tibiofibular joint.

SUGGESTED READING

Williamson B, Schwartz DT: The ankle. In Schwartz DT, Reisdorff EJ, eds. *Emergency Radiology*. McGraw-Hill, 2000.

Lower Extremity: Patient 2

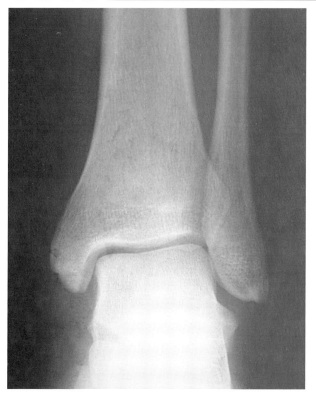

A

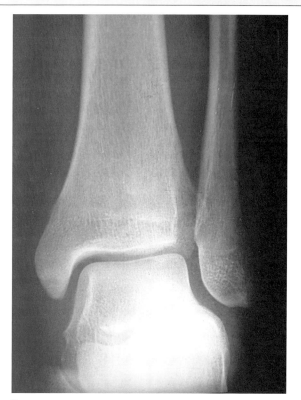

B

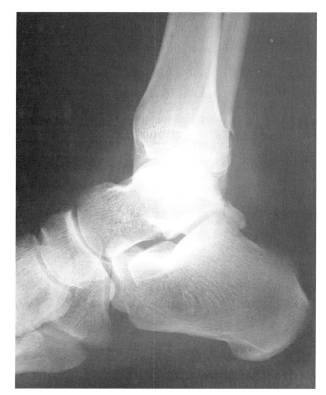

C

FIGURE 1

301

An ankle sprain in a young man

A 26-year-old man twisted his left ankle while sliding into home plate during a baseball game.

The ankle swelled immediately. He was able to bear weight, but could walk only two steps without assistance.

On **examination**, the ankle was moderately swollen and tender. The swelling and tenderness were greater on the medial than the lateral side of the ankle. There was ecchymosis over the medial malleolar area, but no deformity. Plantar and dorsiflexion were limited due to pain. There was no tenderness over the mid-foot (navicular or base of the fifth metatarsal).

Ankle radiographs were obtained (Figure 1).

• How would you manage this patient's ankle sprain?

THE FRENCHMAN'S FIBULAR FRACTURE

Three radiographic views are included in a standard ankle series: AP and lateral views and a mortise view (AP view with 15° internal rotation).

The mortise view shows the entire mortise joint space between the talar dome and the medial malleolus, tibial plafond and lateral malleolus (Figures 1B and 2). On the AP view, the lateral malleolus overlaps and obscures the lateral joint space (Figure 1A).

The **mortise view** is key to assessing the structural integrity of the ankle. The entire **mortise joint space** adjacent to the talar dome should be of uniform width. The **distal tibiofibular joint space** should be only slightly wider than the mortise joint space. Tibiofibular overlap should be at least 1 mm on the mortise view (Figure 2). Lack of overlap implies disruption of the distal tibiofibular joint. The distal tibiofibular joint is also referred to as the ankle **syndesmosis.**

The tibia and fibula are held rigidly together by the distal and proximal tibiofibular joints and the *interosseus ligament.* Separation of the distal tibiofibular joint, even if slight, must therefore be accompanied by a second injury, usually a fibular fracture. If a fibular fracture is not seen on the ankle radiographs, radiographs of the entire fibula should be obtained because a proximal fibular fracture is likely to be present.

Clinically, all patients with ankle injuries should be examined for tenderness along the length of the fibula, up to the knee. The "squeeze test" (mediolateral compression of the tibia and fibula at the mid-calf level) may reveal tenderness due to an interosseous ligament sprain.

In Patient 2's mortise view, the space between the distal tibia and fibula is slightly widened implying that there is separation of the ankle syndesmosis—a "syndesmosis sprain" (Figure 3A). Widening of the distal tibiofibular joint is also responsible for the slight widening of the space between the lateral malleolus and talar dome (the lateral clear space), i.e., the width of the mortise joint space is not entirely uniform. These changes are evident in comparison to the opposite normal ankle (Figure 3B).

On the **lateral view,** there are several small bone fragments at the posterior cortex of the distal tibia. These are small avulsion fragments at the insertion of the posterior–inferior tibiofibular ligament (PITFL), another sign of distal tibiofibular joint disruption (Figure 4).

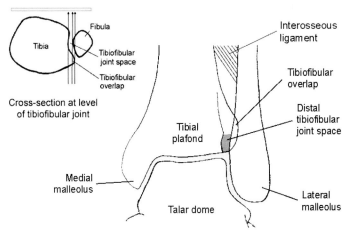

FIGURE 2   Normal mortise view.

The entire **mortise joint space** should be of uniform width, ≤4 mm (*light gray*).

The **distal tibiofibular joint** (*dark gray*) should be only slightly wider than the mortise joint space, ≤5.5 mm.

The **tibiofibular overlap** should be > 1 mm on the mortise view.

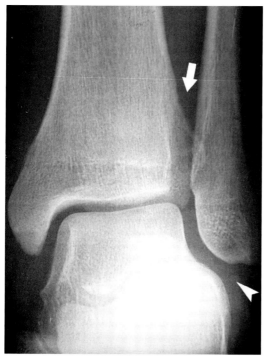
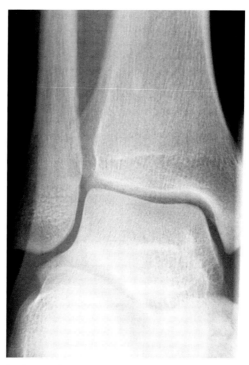

A. Left ankle

B. Comparison view of uninjured right ankle

FIGURE 3   Mortise view—Patient 2.

(A) There is slight widening of the distal tibiofibular joint (arrow) indicative of disruption of the tibiofibular syndesmosis. In addition, the lateral joint space is slightly widened (arrowhead) relative to the medial joint space. This is due to the separation of the distal tibiofibular joint, and not an injury to the lateral ankle ligaments.

(B) Mortise view of the opposite uninjured ankle shows a uniform mortise joint space and normal distal tibiofibular joint space.

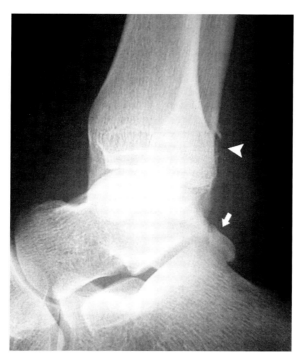

FIGURE 4   Lateral View—Patient 2.

There are several small bone fragments along the posterior surface of the distal tibia (arrowheads) that are caused by an injury to the posterior–inferior tibiofibular ligament (PITFL).

A common accessory ossicle, the os trigonum (arrow), is an unfused secondary ossification center of the posterior tuberosity of the talus. It should not be misinterpreted as a fracture. The margins of the ossicle are smooth and well corticated.

Patient Outcome

After the initial radiographs were reviewed, the patient was re-examined and tenderness was noted over the proximal fibula.

Radiographs of the tibia and fibula were then obtained revealing a spiral fracture of the proximal fibular shaft (Figure 5). This is known as a **Maisonneuve fracture.**

Stress views of the ankle under anesthesia demonstrated further widening of the distal tibiofibular joint confirming disruption of the ankle syndesmosis. There was no abnormal talar tilt, i.e., deltoid and lateral ligaments were intact. A **syndesmosis screw** was inserted to stabilize the ankle joint (Figure 6).

Maisonneuve Fractures

Occasionally misdiagnosed as a "sprained ankle," the **Maisonneuve fracture** can present with subtle clinical and radiographic findings even though the ankle joint is significantly disrupted. The Maisonneuve fracture is a fracture of the proximal third of the fibula that occurs in association with ankle injuries. If unrecognized or inadequately treated, there may be progressive instability of the ankle. Detection of a Maisonneuve fracture is the reason that all patients with ankle injuries should be examined for tenderness over the proximal fibula.

The Maisonneuve fracture is, in fact, not uncommon. It occurs in approximately 5% of all ankle fractures. In most instances, the Maisonneuve fracture is associated with displaced fractures of the ankle and the severity of injury is obvious. When there are no fractures and minimal joint space widening, the severity of injury can be underestimated.

The **mechanism of injury** was deduced by Maisonneuve from cadaver experiments in the preradiographic era (1840). Forceful **external rotation of the foot** causes the talus to wedge apart the distal tibiofibular joint and fracturing the proximal fibula (Figure 7). Maisonneuve likened this injury to the rotation of a ruler (measuring stick) placed between two books. As the ruler rotates, it separates the two books. This is analogous to the splitting apart of the mortise as the talus rotates within the ankle joint.

External rotation is the most common mechanism causing ankle fractures (see Patient 1, Table 1, page 296). As the talus rotates and splits apart the mortise, a sequence of injuries occurs involving the lateral and medial malleoli and the distal tibiofibular joint.

In some cases, the lateral fracture occurs at the proximal fibula (a Maisonneuve fracture). The factors that cause the fibular fracture to occur proximally rather than at the ankle are unclear, but probably relate to the forces of weight bearing and position of the foot at the time of injury. Patients with a Maisonneuve fracture may not complain of knee or calf pain because of the greater pain caused by the ankle injury.

Clinically, Patient 2's presentation differed from that of a typical ankle sprain. The most common mechanism causing ankle sprain is **adduction (inversion),** which tears the lateral collateral ligaments. This patient had tenderness and swelling over the *medial,* rather than lateral, aspect of the ankle. The mechanism of injury was **external rotation** that caused stretching of the medial (deltoid) ligaments rather than the lateral ligaments. Of greater significance, was the tear of the distal tibiofibular joint ligaments. This injury is sometimes referred to as a *syndesmosis sprain.*

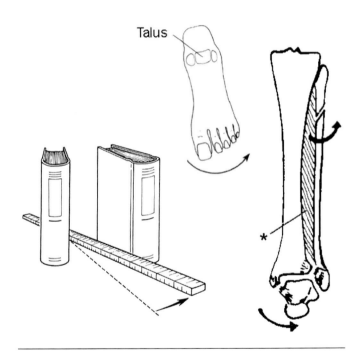

FIGURE 7 Maisonneuve's analogy of external rotation injury. Rotation of the talus within the ankle mortise wedges apart the medial and lateral malleoli like the rotation of a measuring stick separating two books. This can cause a fracture of the proximal fibula. *Asterisk* = interosseus ligament.

[From Rogers LF: *Radiology of Skeletal Trauma*, 3rd ed. Churchill–Livingstone, 2002, with permission.]

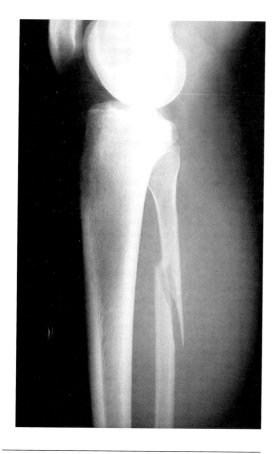

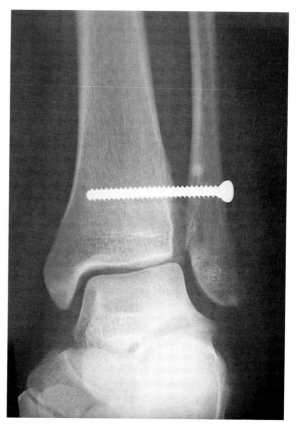

FIGURE 5 Patient 2.
Maisonneuve fracture of the proximal fibula.

FIGURE 6   Postoperative radiograph—Patient 2.
A syndesmosis screw stabilizes the ankle mortise.

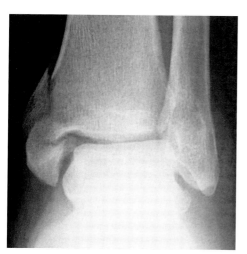

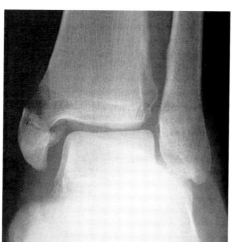

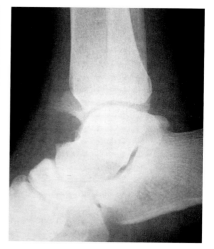

FIGURE 8

Patient 2B.   Another patient who twisted his ankle and complained of severe ankle pain.
His ankle radiographs are shown in Figure 8.

- How should this injury be described and classified?
  (see Patient 1, Table 1, *Lauge-Hansen classification of ankle injuries,* on page 296)

- What is the mechanism of injury?

Patient 2B Outcome

There is an obvious comminuted fracture of the medial malleolus and widening of the distal tibiofibular joint (Figure 9).

According to the **Lauge-Hansen classification,** this injury is due to external rotation while the foot is pronated, which tears the anterior and posterior tibiofibular ligaments and fractures the medial malleolus—a **pronation–external rotation, stage 3 injury** (PER 3) (see Patient 1, Table 1 page 296). However, despite the inclusion of the PER 3 injury in the classification, it does not occur clinically. Widening of the distal tibiofibular joint cannot occur without a fibular fracture due to the rigid nature of the tibiofibular articulation.

This patient's ankle injury has features suggestive of a **Maisonneuve fracture**—a medial malleolar fracture and widening of the distal tibiofibular joint without a lateral malleolar fracture. When the patient was re-examined, he had tenderness over the proximal fibula. Tibia/fibula radiographs were obtained which revealed the expected proximal fibular fracture (Figure 10). (A Maisonneuve fracture could be considered a variant of the PER 4 injury.)

A Maisonneuve fracture should be suspected whenever there is a fracture or ligamentous injury to the medial aspect of the ankle or widening of the distal tibiofibular joint without a fracture of the lateral malleolus (Table 1). Some authors recommend radiography of the entire tibia and fibula in all patients with displaced fractures about the ankle because a proximal fibular fracture can occur even when there is a distal fibular fracture (Pankovich 1976). Finally, all patients with ankle sprains should be examined for tenderness over the entire length of the fibula to look for clinical evidence of a Maisonneuve fracture, even when the ankle radiographs are normal.

TABLE 1

When to Suspect a Maisonneuve Fracture

1. Medial malleolar fracture or deltoid ligament tear (wide medial joint space) without a distal fibular fracture.

2. Widening of the distal tibio-fibular joint without a distal fibular facture.

3. Tenderness over the proximal fibula in a patient who has sprained their ankle—radiographs may be normal.

4. Displaced fractures about the ankle, including distal fibular fractures, when there is tenderness over the proximal fibula.

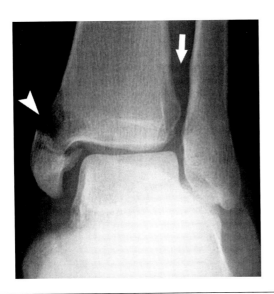

FIGURE 9   Mortise view—Patient 2B.
There is a comminuted medial malleolar fracture (*arrowhead*) and widening to the distal tibiofibular joint (*arrow*).

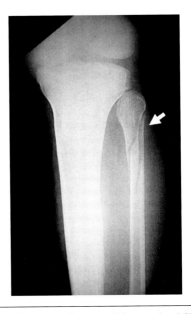

FIGURE 10   Maisonneuve fracture of the proximal fibula (*arrow*).

SUGGESTED READING

Babis GC, Papagelopoulos PJ, Tsarouchas J, et al.: Operative treatment for Maisonneuve fracture of the proximal fibula. *Orthopedics* 2000;23:687–690.

Del Castillo J, Geiderman JM: The Frenchman's fibular fracture (Maisonneuve fracture). *JACEP* 1979;8:404–406.

Duchesneau S, Fallat LM: The Maisonneuve fracture. *J Foot Ankle Surg* 1995;34:422–428.

Hensel KS, Harpstrite JK: Maisonneuve fracture associated with a bimalleolar ankle fracture-dislocation. *J Orthop Trauma* 2002; 16:525–528.

Lock TR, et al.: Maisonneuve fracture: Case report of a missed diagnosis. *Ann Emerg Med* 1987;16:805–807.

Pankovich AM: Maisonneuve fracture of the fibula. *J Bone Joint Surg* 1976;58A:337–342.

Lower Extremity: Patient 3

Knee pain in two patients following minor trauma

PATIENT 3A A 62-year-old woman twisted her knee two days earlier while moving a sofa at her home. Her pain persisted and she needed a cane to walk.

On examination, the lateral aspect of her knee was tender and there was a small effusion. Flexion was limited to 60°. There was no tenderness over the patella. Her quadriceps strength was good and there was no ligamentous instability.

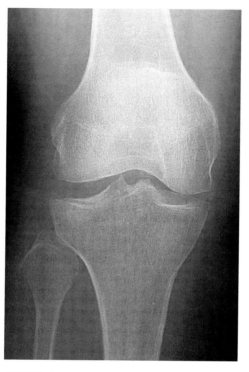 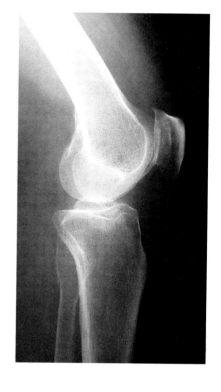

FIGURE 1

PATIENT 3B A 24-year-old woman was struck on the lateral aspect of her right knee by the fender of a slow moving car and fell to the ground. Swelling of the knee occurred immediately. The patient had no other injuries aside from several minor bruises.

Examination revealed tenderness of the anterior and lateral aspects of her knee. There was a moderate joint effusion and flexion was limited to 45°. There was no ligamentous instability to valgus and varus stress, and the anterior drawer and Lachman tests were normal.

- Are there any abnormalities on these patients' knee radiographs (Figures 1 and 2)?

- What is the most frequently missed radiographically apparent fracture in the ED?

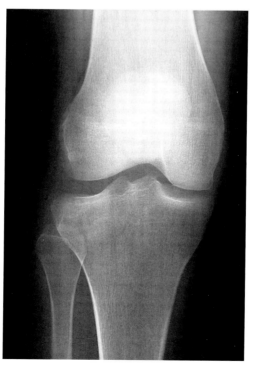 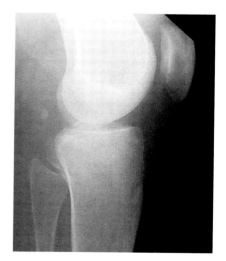

FIGURE 2

FENDER FRACTURE

Compared to the wrist and ankle, the radiographic anatomy of the knee is relatively simple and the range of potential fractures is small (Table 1). However, some fractures can have subtle radiographic findings and substantial morbidity if missed.

A **targeted approach to radiograph interpretation** looking for common and easily missed injuries works well for knee injuries. It is more effective and efficient than a systematic approach in which all of the bone contours are traced looking for cortical breaks or deformities.

Most fractures are apparent on the standard AP and lateral radiographs. In some cases, supplementary views are needed to detect an injury. These include: oblique views, an axial patellar ("sunrise") view, or intercondylar notch ("tunnel") view (AP view with knee flexed).

Tibial plateau fractures are common, second in frequency only to patellar fractures (Table 1). Markedly displaced fractures can be identified without difficulty. However, minimally displaced fractures often have subtle radiographic findings and can easily be missed. In one series, tibial plateau fractures were the most frequently missed radiographically apparent fracture in the ED, missed in 16% of 19 cases (Table 2) (Freed and Shields 1984). Another investigator also found tibial plateau fractures to be among the most frequently missed radiographic findings in the ED. Distal radius fractures, radial head fractures, and chest findings were also frequently missed (Sprivulis et al. 2001).

TABLE 1

Relative Frequencies of Various Fractures About the Knee in Adult ED Patients

Patella	40%
Tibial plateau	32%
Fibular head	9%
Distal femur	8%
Tibial spine	7%
Tibial tuberosity	2%
Osteochondral junction (articular cartilage) fracture	1%

Data from 192 patients
(Stiell 1996, Weber 1995, Bauer 1995)

TABLE 2

The Most Frequently Overlooked Radiographically Apparent Fractures in an ED

	PERCENT MISSED	NUMBER MISSED/TOTAL
Tibial plateau	16%	3/19
Radial head	14%	12/84
Elbow—child	14%	5/35
Scaphoid	13%	7/53
Calcaneus	10%	5/50
Patella	6%	3/53
Ribs	4%	23/548

3%, ankle, metacarpals, metatarsals, phalanges.
(Data from Freed and Shields 1984.)

Tibial plateau fractures are classified as vertically oriented, locally compressed, or combined split-compression (Figure 3).

The **lateral tibial plateau** is involved in 85–90% of cases. This is because trauma to the lateral aspect of the knee is common, and because the lateral tibial plateau is weaker than the medial plateau. A valgus (medially-directed) force to the lateral side of the knee drives the lateral femoral condyle into the lateral tibial plateau.

Tibial plateau fractures have a wide range of severity. Markedly displaced comminuted fractures destroy the articular surface of the knee and can injure the popliteal artery and the tibialis and peroneal nerves.

Minimally displaced fractures are difficult to detect radiographically. Delayed diagnosis of these milder injuries can cause significant morbidity if the fracture becomes displaced, disrupting knee's articular surface and requiring operative repair.

There are two reasons why minimally displaced tibial plateau fractures can be difficult to detect radiographically. First, the fracture often lies in an oblique plane and is therefore not parallel to the x-ray beam in either the AP or lateral view. Second, the tibial plateau surface slopes inferiorly, going from anterior to posterior (Figure 4). This makes localized compression fractures difficult to see because the cortical surface is not parallel to the x-ray beam. In addition, accurate assessment of the depth of depression of a tibial plateau fracture is not possible on an AP radiograph.

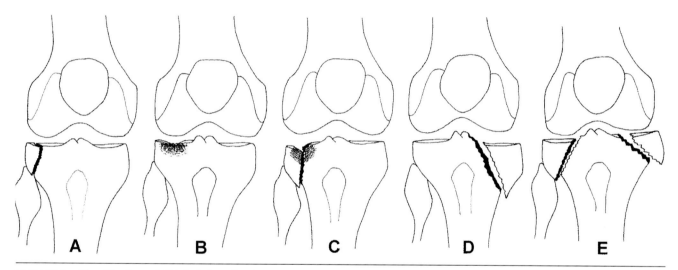

FIGURE 3   Classification of tibial plateau fractures.
(*A*) Split. (*B*) Local compression. (*C*). Split-compression. (*D*) Medial condyle (10–15%). (*E*) Bicondylar.

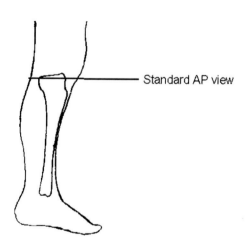

Standard AP view

FIGURE 4 The standard AP view is slightly oblique (15°) to the surface of the tibial plateau.
[From Simon et al: *Emergency Orthopedics,* 3rd ed. McGraw-Hill, 1995, with permission.]

AP View

Knowledge of the **normal radiographic anatomy of the knee** is important in detecting subtle tibial plateau fractures. Because most of the body's weight is borne on the medial side of the knee, the trabecular density of the medial tibial plateau is greater than that of the lateral plateau (Figure 5). (In Figure 5, osteoporosis accentuates the primary trabeculae due to loss of secondary bridging trabeculae.)

Increased trabecular density of the lateral tibial plateau relative to the medial plateau is a sign of a compression fracture of the lateral tibial plateau (Figures 6 and 7). This increased trabec-

ular density is termed "sclerosis," although it actually represents trabecular compaction due to the fracture rather than increased bone production, as the term "sclerosis" implies.

The tibial plateau surface may appear interrupted or deformed. In addition, the fracture can cause lateral displacement of the tibial plateau relative to the femoral condyle (Figure 7B), although that can also be seen in norml knees (Figure 5).

Widening of the joint space on the injured side would seem to be a sign of injury. However, because the joint space of the knee can only be reliably assessed when the patient is standing, a standard (non-weight-bearing) AP view cannot be used to assess the knee joint space.

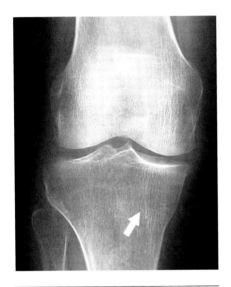

FIGURE 5   AP view—Osteoporosis.
The trabeculae are normally more dense on the medial side (*arrow*) than the lateral side.

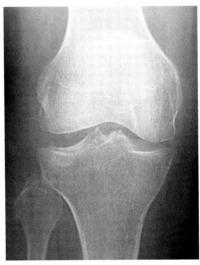

FIGURE 6A   AP view—Patient 3A.

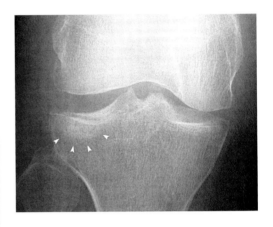

FIGURE 6B   AP view—Patient 3A (detail).
A compression fracture of the lateral tibial plateau causes increased trabecular density (sclerosis) (*arrowheads*).

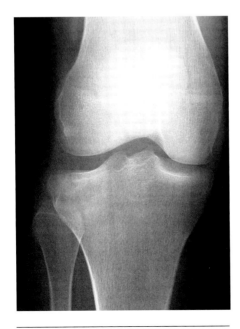

FIGURE 7A   AP view—Patient 3B.

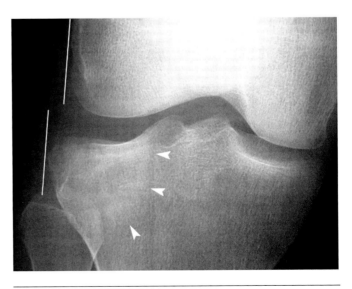

FIGURE 7B   AP view—Patient 3B (detail).
A compression fracture causes irregularity of the cortical surface and increased trabecular density (*arrowheads*). The tibial plateau is laterally displaced relative to the femoral condyle (*lines*).

Lateral View

On a lateral radiograph, the lateral and medial tibial plateau surfaces should be smooth and continuous. When the view is perfectly aligned, the two cortical surfaces are superimposed (Figure 8A). When not superimposed, each tibial plateau surface should be equidistant from the respective femoral condyle articular surface (Figure 8B).

Interruption, deformity, or displacement of a portion of the tibial plateau surface is indicative of a fracture (Figure 9).

Knee effusions can be detected on the lateral radiograph. Normally, the quadriceps tendon has a slender appearance and is out-lined by fat tissue. An effusion appears as fluid in the suprapatellar bursa located just posterior to the quadriceps tendon (Figure 9). Knee effusions are a nonspecific indicator of a knee injury.

However, when there is an intra-articular fracture such as a tibial plateau fracture, the effusion will contain fat from bone marrow, as well as blood—a **lipohemarthrosis.** A fat fluid level, can be seen on a **cross-table lateral** radiograph (see Figure 16 on p. 315). A cross-table lateral view is performed with the patient supine and using a horizontally directed x-ray beam. The standard lateral view is obtained with the patient lying on the injured side, extending the knee, and using a vertically oriented x-ray beam. It cannot detect a lipohemarthrosis.

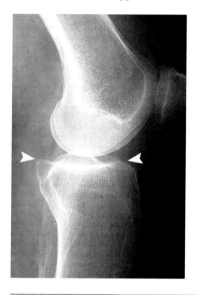

FIGURE 8A   Normal lateral view.
The medial and lateral tibial plateaus are superimposed (*arrowheads*). The femoral condyles are also superimposed.

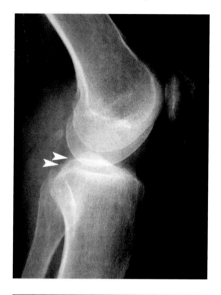

FIGURE 8B   Normal lateral view.
The view is slightly tilted and the tibial plateaus and femoral condyles are not superimposed (*arrowheads*).

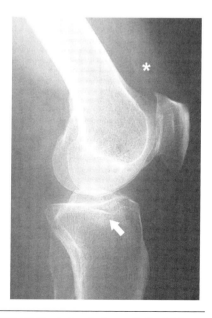

FIGURE 9   Lateral view—Patient 3A.
A fracture causes depression of the cortical surface and trabecular compression (*arrow*).
Asterisk = suprapatellar knee effusion.

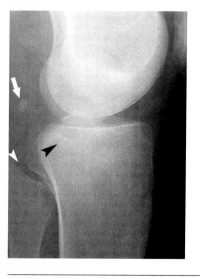

FIGURE 10   Lateral view—Patient 3B.
The fracture is not visible, aside from a questionable cortical interruption (*black arrowhead*).
Arrow = fabella or "little bean," an accessory ossicle (sesamoid) within the semimembranosus tendon.
White arrowhead = proximal tibiofibular joint.

Oblique Views

Oblique views are useful in demonstrating tibial plateau fractures. In an oblique view, the fracture line is often aligned with the x-ray beam (Figure 11). Oblique views should be ordered when there is clinical suspicion of a tibial plateau fracture and the standard AP and lateral views are negative or have questionable findings. Oblique views also show the margins of the patella and can detect a fracture in that area (Daffner 1987).

Computed Tomography

When CT, particularly MDCT with coronal and sagittal reformatted images, is readily available, it can be used instead of oblique views to confirm that a fracture is present when the radiographs are equivocal. CT is mainly used in patients with tibial plateau fractures to define the extent of injury and degree of displacement, factors that are important in planning orthopedic treatment.

Clinical Features and Treatment

The **mechanism of injury** most commonly associated with a tibial plateau fracture is a **"bumper"** or **"fender" injury.** The anterolateral aspect of the knee suffers a direct impact from an automobile bumper, and the impact on the lateral femoral condyle drives it into the lateral tibial plateau. This mechanism is responsible for 25–50% of these fractures. **Axial compression** such as occurs during a fall from height are responsible for most of the others.

Osteoporosis is a major risk factor for tibial plateau fractures. Elderly patients, especially women, can have tibial plateau fractures following minor trauma such as stepping off a sidewalk curb, as in Patient 3A. Long-term functional outcome is often suboptimal in these patients (Schwartsman et al. 1998, Keating 1999).

Two factors are important for the treatment of tibial plateau fractures: (1) the degree of displacement and (2) associated ligamentous or meniscal injuries. The **depth of depression** of a tibial plateau fracture must be accurately assessed. Depression greater than 8 mm is usually treated with surgical elevation and restoration of the articular surface.

Because of the downward slope of the tibial plateau surface, the depth of depression cannot be accurately assessed on an AP radiograph (Figure 4). CT with coronal and sagittal reformatted images is the test of choice to assess depth of depression (Martin 2000, Wicky et al. 2000, Liow et al. 1999, Rafii et al. 1987).

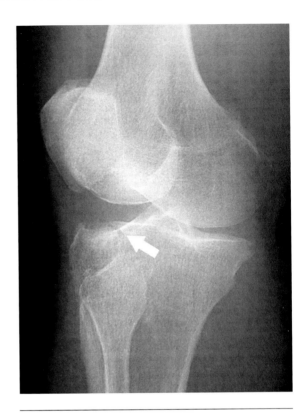

FIGURE 11   Oblique view—Patient 3A.
The fracture is visible (*arrow*).

Formerly, a 15° inferiorly directed view (tibial plateau view) or conventional tomography was used. CT need not be performed in the ED so long as the patient does not bear weight on the injured knee and has ready access to outpatient care.

Ligamentous and meniscus injuries occur in many patients with tibial plateau fractures. Assessment depends on a complete physical examination, although this can be difficult to perform in an acutely injured patient. MRI is the preferred imaging test to diagnose soft tissue injuries of the knee (not in the ED) (Oei 2003, Eustace 1999). Both MRI and arthroscopy demonstrate a high rate (up to 90%) of meniscus and ligamentous injuries even when the fracture is minimally displaced (Shepard et al. 2002, Yocoubian et al. 2002, Bennett and Browner 1994).

Markedly displaced proximal tibial fractures can injure the **popliteal artery,** in a fashion similar to knee dislocations. Emergency angiography should be considered when an arterial injury is suspected.

Patient Outcome

PATIENT 3A: The AP view shows slight "sclerosis" (an impacted fracture) of the lateral tibial plateau (Figure 6). On the lateral view, there is depression of the tibial plateau surface with trabecular impaction (Figure 9). An oblique view readily demonstrates the fracture (Figure 11).

The depression was less than 8 mm and ligamentous function was intact. The patient was treated with a compressive dressing and kept non-weight-bearing with crutches. Active non-weight-bearing exercises were prescribed to maintain quadriceps strength. Light weight-bearing began after 6 weeks, when fracture healing started to become evident.

PATIENT 3B: This patient had a classic "fender fracture," although the car must have been going slowly because this mechanism of injury usually results in more severe injuries. On the AP view, the lateral tibial plateau surface is poorly defined and the adjacent trabeculae are compacted (Figure 7). The lateral view is essentially normal (Figure 10). An intercondylar notch view demonstrated a break in the cortex near the lateral tibial spine (Figure 12).

Joint aspiration yielded 100 mL of blood with fat globules. Range of motion improved and ligamentous function could then be better evaluated. This patient was managed with a bulky dressing and non-weight-bearing and referred for orthopedic follow-up and CT.

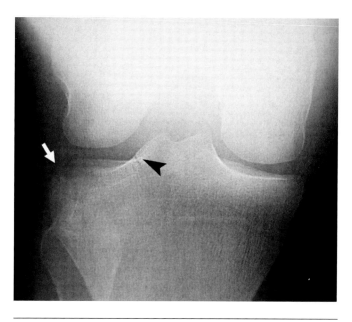

FIGURE 12. Intercondylar notch view—Patient 3B.
Arrowhead = fracture near the lateral tibial spine.
Arrow = depressed fragment of lateral aspect of tibial plateau.

PATIENT 3C

A 35-year-old man was knocked down by a slow moving automobile as he was crossing the street. He presented to the ED with right-sided chest pain and right knee pain. Chest radiography revealed a right fifth rib fracture. The knee radiographs were initially interpreted as normal (Figure 13). The patient was discharged with analgesic medications, a knee immobilizer, and crutches.

The following day, the radiographs were reread as showing a tibial plateau fracture and the patient was recalled. Repeat radiographs revealed greater displacement of the fracture (Figure 14). The patient was advised that he would need operative repair of his knee (Figure 15). Although the initial depth of depression of the tibial plateau may have necessitated surgery, the patient was upset that he had been misdiagnosed

and had been in so much pain while trying to use the knee immobilizer.

Patients with knee injuries that are associated with pain on weight bearing should be managed with crutches so that there is no additional damage to the knee. Such injuries include an occult tibial plateau fracture, a loose intra-articular fragment of articular cartilage, or a meniscal tear. Any of these could result in additional damage to the knee if the patient were to bear weight. In these circumstances, a simple compressive dressing may be preferable to a knee immobilizer because it permits the patient to bend the knee slightly, facilitating the use of crutches. The patient should be referred for follow-up within the next several days and, if pain persists, have additional imaging studies to determine the extent of the injury.

Patient 3C

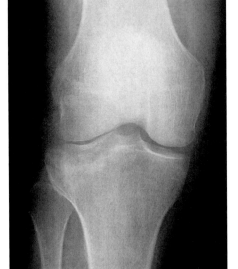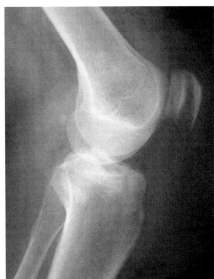

FIGURE 13 Radiographs obtained during the first ED visit were initially interpreted as normal, although there is a moderately displaced fracture of the lateral tibial plateau.

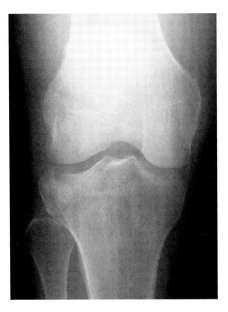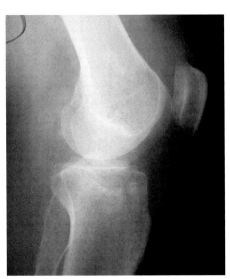

FIGURE 14 Repeat radiographs after the patient was recalled showing a markedly displaced fracture. Surgical repair was necessary to restore the articular surface.

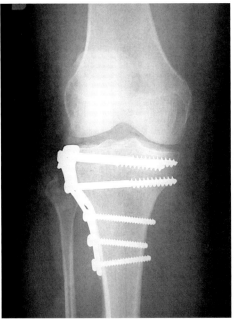

FIGURE 15 Postoperative radiograph showing fracture repair and fixation with buttress plate and screws.

[Courtesy Evan G. Schwartz, MD.]

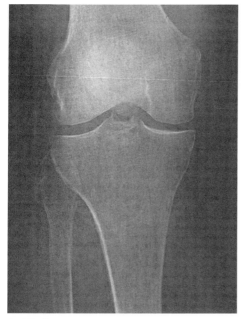

A. AP view

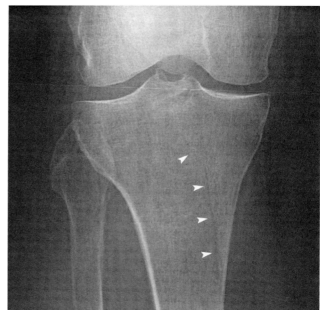

B. AP view (detail)

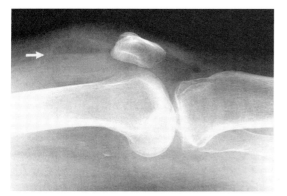

C. Cross-table lateral view

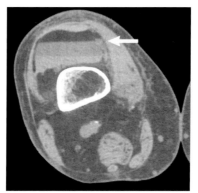

E. CT suprapatellar region

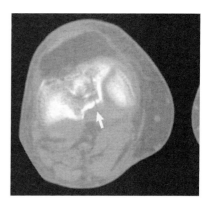

F. CT tibial plateau surface

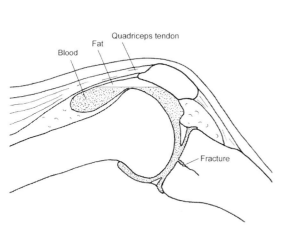

D. A knee effusion with a fat-fluid level in the suprapatellar bursa

FIGURE 16   A subtle tibial plateau fracture disclosed by a lipohemarthrosis.

A 60-year-old woman tripped and fell on the sidewalk landing on her knee. On examination, there was a large effusion. She had limited range of motion and was unable to bear weight.

The AP view initially was interpreted as normal (*A*), although close inspection revealed a subtle nondisplaced medial tibial plateau fracture (*B*).

A large **lipohemarthrosis** in the suprapatellar bursa was visible on the cross-table lateral view (*C*). This is indicative of an intra-articular fracture with blood and fat entering the joint from the bone marrow (*D*).

A standard lateral view (knee positioned on its side and x-ray beam directed vertically) would not show a fat/fluid level. A cross-table lateral view is therefore preferred in patients with knee trauma.

CT showed the fat/blood level in the suprapatellar bursa (*E, arrow*) and a subtle nondisplaced tibial plateau fracture (*F, arrow*).

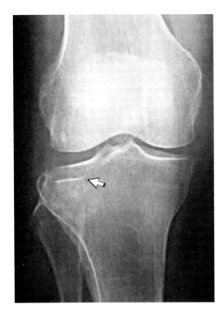

FIGURE 17 Missed tibial plateau fracture.

An 80-year-old woman injured her knee while stepping off a bus on to the curb.

The radiographs were initially read as normal, aside from osteoporosis. However, a fragment of the tibial plateau is depressed below the plateau surface (*arrow*) and there is increased trabecular density of the lateral plateau.

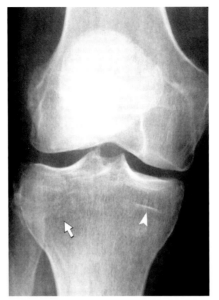

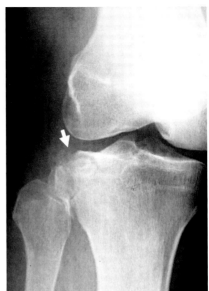

A. AP view   B. Oblique view

FIGURE 18 Tibial plateau fracture seen only on an oblique view.

A 43-year-old man fell on to his right knee.

A fracture was not evident on the AP (*A*) and lateral views, although the lateral tibial plateau trabeculae are irregular (*arrow*). A fine line below the medial tibial plateau surface is a remnant of the growth plate and not a fracture (*arrowhead*).

(*B*) Oblique views were obtained, which showed a mildly displaced split fracture of the lateral tibial plateau (*arrow*).

SUGGESTED READING

Bennett WF, Browner B: Tibial plateau fractures: A study of associated soft tissue injuries. *J Orthop Trauma* 1994;8:183–188.

Capps GW, Hayes CW: Easily missed injuries around the knee. *Radiographics* 1994;14:1191–1210.

Daffner RH, Tabas JH: Trauma oblique radiographs of the knee. *J Bone Joint Surg Am* 1987;69:568–572.

Dennan S: Difficulties in the radiological diagnosis and evaluation of tibial plateau fractures. *Radiography* 2004;10:151–158.

Freed HA, Shields NN: Most frequently overlooked radiographically apparent fractures in a teaching hospital emergency department. *Ann Emerg Med* 1984;13:900–904.

Keating JF: Tibial plateau fractures in the older patient. *Bull Hosp Jt Dis* 1999;58:19–23.

Kowalenko T, Schwartz DT: The knee. In Schwartz DT, Reisdorff EJ: *Emergency Radiology*. New York: McGraw-Hill, 2000.

Schwartsman R, Brinker MR, Beaver R, Cox DD: Patient self-assessment of tibial plateau fractures in 40 older adults. *Am J Orthop* 1998;27:512–519.

Shepherd L, Abdollahi K, Lee J, Vangsness CT: The prevalence of soft tissue injuries in nonoperative tibial plateau fractures as determined by magnetic resonance imaging. *J Orthop Trauma* 2002;16:628–631.

Sprivulis P, Frazer A, Waring A: Same-day X-ray reporting is not needed in well-supervised emergency departments. *Emerg Med (Fremantle)* 2001;13:194–197.

CT and MRI for Tibial Plateau Fractures

Chan PS, Klimkiewicz JJ, Luchetti WT, et al.: Impact of CT scan on treatment plan and fracture classification of tibial plateau fractures. *J Orthop Trauma* 1997;11:484–489.

Kode L, Lieberman JM, Motta AO, et al.: Evaluation of tibial plateau fractures: efficacy of MR imaging compared with CT. *AJR* 1994;163:141–147.

Liow RY, Birdsall PD, Mucci B, Greiss ME: Spiral computed tomography with two- and three-dimensional reconstruction in the management of tibial plateau fractures. *Orthopedics* 1999;22:929–932.

Rafii M, Lamont JG, Firooznia H: Tibial plateau fractures: CT evaluation and classification. *Crit Rev Diagn Imaging* 1987;27:91–112

Wicky S, Blaser PF, Blanc CH, et al.: Comparison between standard radiography and spiral CT with 3D reconstruction in the evaluation, classification and management of tibial plateau fractures. *Eur Radiol* 2000;10:1227–1232

Yacoubian SV, Nevins RT, Sallis JG, et al.: Impact of MRI on treatment plan and fracture classification of tibial plateau fractures. *J Orthop Trauma* 2002;16:632–637.

Lower Extremity: Patient 4

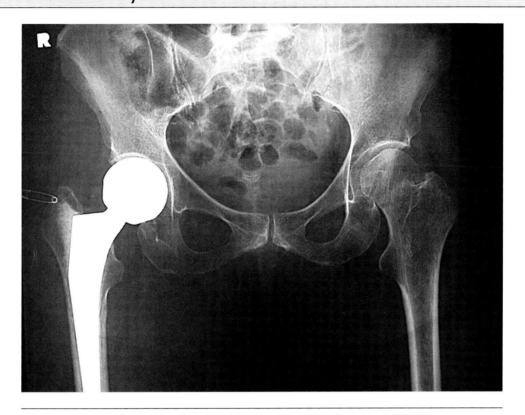

FIGURE 1A   AP pelvis view—Patient 4A.

Hip injuries in elderly women who fell from standing

PATIENT 4A   A 77-year-old woman standing at a bus stop was accidentally pushed and fell, landing on her left side.

She was able to get up, but noted pain in the left groin when standing. The pain persisted over several hours and therefore she came to the ED. She was able to ambulate with a cane, but noted pain in the left hip on weight bearing.

On examination, there was no foreshortening or external rotation of the left hip. Range of motion was full with pain on internal rotation. There was slight tenderness over the greater trochanter but no ecchymosis.

Radiographs of the left hip and pelvis were obtained and interpreted as showing degenerative changes (Figure 1). She had previously had a fracture and hemiarthroplasty of her right hip.

The patient was discharged on ibuprofen, with instructions to rest, and referred to an orthopedist if her pain persisted.

• What would you have done?

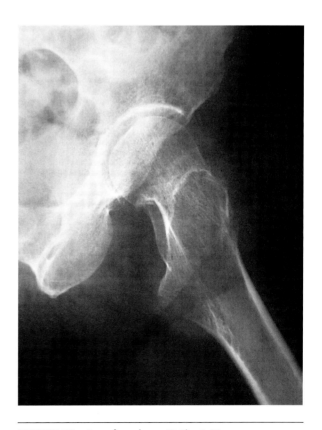

FIGURE 1B   Frog-leg view—Patient 4A.

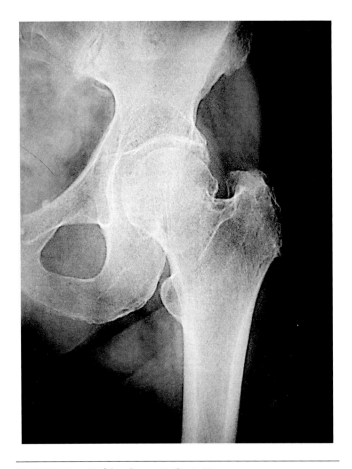

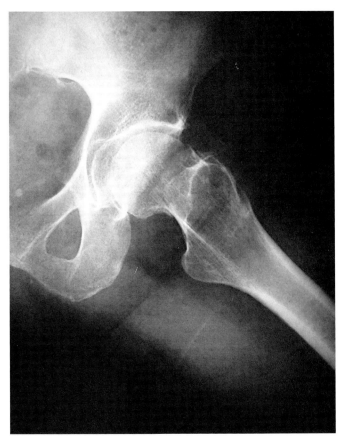

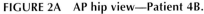

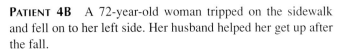

FIGURE 2A   AP hip view—Patient 4B.

FIGURE 2B   Frog-leg view—Patient 4B.

PATIENT 4B   A 72-year-old woman tripped on the sidewalk and fell on to her left side. Her husband helped her get up after the fall.

She was able to walk, but had a limp due to left hip pain. The pain persisted and therefore, on the following day, she decided to come to the ED. On examination, there was localized tenderness over the hip and pain on internal and external rotation. She was able to fully flex and extend the hip without pain.

Radiographs of the hip were reported as negative for a fracture (Figure 2) and the patient was discharged with the diagnosis of hip contusion. She was instructed to limit weight bearing, take a mild pain reliever, and contact her doctor if pain persisted.

• Do you agree with this management?

HIP FRACTURE OR CONTUSION—NOT CONFUSION

The typical patient with a fractured hip (proximal femoral fracture) is an elderly individual who has fallen from a standing position. The patient presents lying on the stretcher with the involved leg externally rotated and foreshortened. However, a patient with a **nondisplaced fracture** can present with subtle clinical and radiographic findings (2–9% of cases), and the diagnosis can be missed on initial evaluation (Perron et al. 2002, Dominguez et al. 2005). In some instances, the radiographs are entirely negative for a fracture (an "occult fracture") and other imaging modalities such as bone scan, MRI, or CT are needed.

The consequences of delayed diagnosis of a hip fracture are substantial, particularly when a nondisplaced femoral neck fracture becomes displaced necessitating a more extensive surgical procedure. Caution should therefore be exercised before diagnosing a "hip contusion" as opposed to a fracture in an elderly patient. Even with timely diagnosis and prompt surgical treatment, mortality within one year of the fracture ranges from 14% to 36% (Zuckerman 1996).

The **diagnosis** of a fracture is based on (1) clinical findings, (2) patient risk factors, (3) results of the radiographs, and (4) other imaging studies. **Patients at risk** for this injury are elderly persons, usually women, with **osteoporosis.** The injury commonly follows minor trauma such as a fall from standing.

Clinical signs of a nondisplaced proximal femoral fracture can be difficult to distinguish from a muscle strain, sprain, or contusion. The patient may complain only of mild pain about the hip or inguinal region, or have pain referred to the knee. Inability to bear weight is suggestive of a fracture. However, some patients may be able to walk, although most will have an antalgic gait (avoiding full weight bearing on the injured leg). Range of motion of the hip may be only slightly limited or painful. Internal and external rotation should be specifically tested, although such manipulation should not be attempted if there is excessive pain, because it may displace a fracture.

Because the clinical findings of a nondisplaced hip fracture can be equivocal, it is important to carefully scrutinize the radiographs for signs of a fracture.

Fracture Classification

There are two main types of proximal femoral fractures: **femoral neck** and **intertrochanteric fractures** (Figure 3). These are similar in frequency and clinical presentation. Surgical fixation is used for both types of fractures because it permits early mobilization of the patient and avoids the complications of prolonged bed rest. However, surgical treatment differs significantly for these two types of fractures largely because of the anatomy of the blood supply to the femoral head.

Most of the **blood supply** of the femoral head originates from the circumflex artery which encircles the base of the femoral neck just outside the insertion of the joint capsule. The ascending cervical and epiphyseal arteries branch from the circumflex artery and course along the femoral neck to the femoral head (Figure 4).

Femoral neck fractures occur within the joint capsule and are termed "*intracapsular.*" When displaced, they interrupt the blood supply to the femoral head, leading to avascular necrosis (AVN). Displaced fractures therefore usually require replacement of the proximal femur with a prosthesis. Nondisplaced femoral neck fractures can be treated by simple screw fixation. Delay in diagnosis of a nondisplaced fracture substantially increases morbidity because the fracture often becomes displaced, which necessitates a more extensive surgical procedure.

Intertrochanteric fractures are *extracapsular* and do not interrupt the blood supply to the femoral head. Therefore, even when displaced, intertrochanteric fractures can be treated with surgical fixation using a plate and screws.

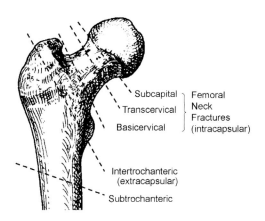

FIGURE 3 Proximal femoral fractures.
Femoral neck and intertrochanteric fractures have equal frequencies (45–50% each). Most femoral neck fractures are subcapital. Subtrochanteric fractures are 5–10% of proximal femoral fractures.

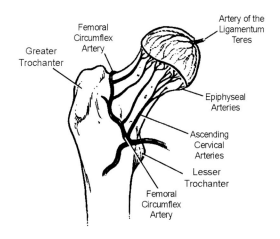

FIGURE 4 Blood supply of the proximal femur.
The circumflex arterial ring encircles the base of the femoral neck distal to the insertion of the hip joint capsule and supplies most of the blood to the femoral head. The artery of the ligamentum teres supplies a small amount of blood to the femoral head.
[From: Dee R, et al. *Principles of Orthopedic Practice,* 2nd ed. McGraw-Hill, 1997, with permission.]

Radiographic Diagnosis of a Nondisplaced Femoral Neck Fracture

Radiographic signs of a nondisplaced (or slightly impacted) femoral neck fracture include: disruption of the cortex or trabeculae; impaction or separation of bone along the fracture line; and foreshortening or malalignment between the femoral neck and head (Table 1). Accurate radiograph interpretation is essential to avoid misdiagnosis and to reduce the reliance on advanced imaging studies such as bone scan, MRI, or CT.

Interruption of the trabecula of the proximal femur is a key finding of a femoral neck fracture. In patients with **osteoporosis,** the interconnecting secondary trabeculae are resorbed and so the primary trabeculae are, paradoxically, accentuated on the radiographs. The *primary compressive trabeculae* extend vertically from the medial cortex of the femoral shaft. The *primary tensile trabeculae* arch across the superior aspect of the femoral neck (Figure 5). (Cortical thinning is also present in patients with osteoporosis, although there are no definite measurements to discriminate normal from abnormal cortical bone.)

Detection of a nondisplaced femoral neck fracture depends on using correct radiographic technique. In a **properly positioned AP view** of the hip, the patient's leg is rotated 15° internally such that the great toes are touching. This elongates the femoral neck and may reveal a fracture that was not visible on an improperly positioned view (Figure 6).

Normally, when lying supine, the hips tend to rotate externally, which makes the femoral neck appear *foreshortened.* Such foreshortening makes visualization of a femoral neck fracture difficult. When positioning is suboptimal, the radiograph should be repeated with 15° internal rotation of the hip.

TABLE 1

Radiographic Signs of a Nondisplaced Femoral Neck Fracture

1. Discontinuity or abrupt angulation of the normally smooth contour of cortical bone

2. Disruption of the normal trabecular architecture of the femoral neck (see Figure 5)

3. Altered bone density along the fracture line.
   A transverse band of increased bone density ("sclerosis") where the fracture fragments are impacted together, and/or diminished bone density ("rarefaction") where the bone fragments are separated

4. Foreshortening of the femoral neck due to impaction of the fracture—the AP view must be properly performed (see Figure 6)

5. Abnormal angle between the femoral neck and femoral head

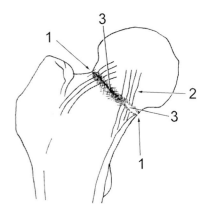

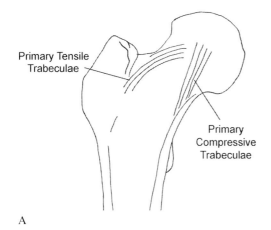

A

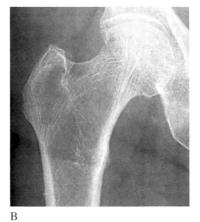

B

FIGURE 5 Normal trabecular architecture of the proximal femur.
(*A*) The primary compressive and tensile trabeculae.
(*B*) Radiograph of a patient with osteoporosis showing the normal trabecular pattern.

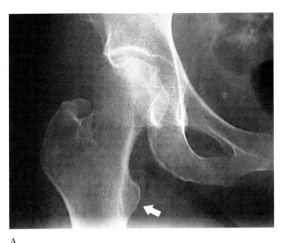 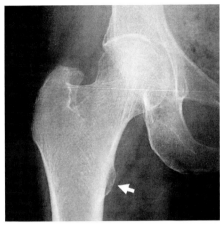 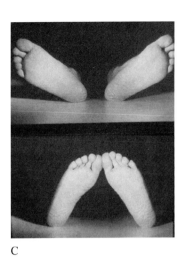

A   B   C

FIGURE 6   Positioning of the AP hip radiograph.

(*A*) Improper positioning with the hip in a neutral position (slight external rotation). The femoral neck appears foreshortened and the lesser tuberosity is prominent (*arrow*).

(*B*) Correctly positioned AP view with the hip rotated 15° internally (great toes touching). This elongates the femoral neck and improves fracture detection. The lesser tuberosity appears smaller (*arrow*).

(*C*) At rest, the legs tend to rotate externally. For correct positioning, the great toes should be touching (internal rotation of the legs).

[C from Ballinger PW, Frank ED: *Merrill's Atlas of Radiographic Positions and Radiologic Procedures,* 10th ed. Mosby, 2003, with permission.]

Radiographic Views of the Hip

Standard views include an AP view and a second view of the femoral neck at an angle perpendicular to the AP view. Due to overlap by the opposite hip, a true lateral view is not useful.

An **AP view of the pelvis** is preferred to a hip view because fractures of the adjacent portions of the pelvis are common and may not be visible on an AP hip view. In addition, the pelvis view shows the opposite uninjured hip, which can be compared to the injured side. An **AP view of the hip** is centered on the involved hip and therefore provides slightly better radiographic detail of the hip. However, if only one AP view is obtained, the AP pelvis is preferred. The patient should be positioned with 15° internal rotation of the legs, as mentioned above.

The **"frog-leg" view** is the second view that is most easily obtained and interpreted. This is an AP or oblique view with the hip abducted and externally rotated (Figure 7). This should not be used in patients with significant hip pain because the movement needed to position the patient could displace a fracture.

If the patient cannot assume the frog-leg position, a **cross-table lateral view** or "groin lateral view" should be obtained. The opposite (uninjured) leg is raised and the x-ray beam directed toward the groin (Figure 8). The injured hip does not need to be moved. However, interpretation of this view is difficult because overlapping structures can obscure anatomical landmarks and make it difficult to orient the image.

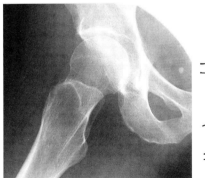 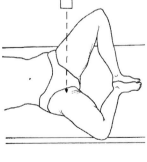 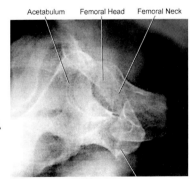

FIGURE 7   Frog-leg view of the hip.
The hip is abducted and externally rotated. The radiograph shows an AP view with patient supine, whereas the line drawing shows oblique positioning of the patient's pelvis; both are acceptable.

FIGURE 8   Cross-table lateral (groin lateral) view of the hip.
The uninjured leg is raised and the x-ray beam is directed as shown.

Patient 4A Outcome

The radiographs show typical signs of a nondisplaced (slightly impacted) femoral neck fracture (Figure 9). When the radiographs were re-read the following morning, the fracture was identified and the patient was recalled to the ED. Repeat radiographs revealed that the fracture was now displaced. The patient was treated with a prosthetic hip replacement. Her recovery was uneventful.

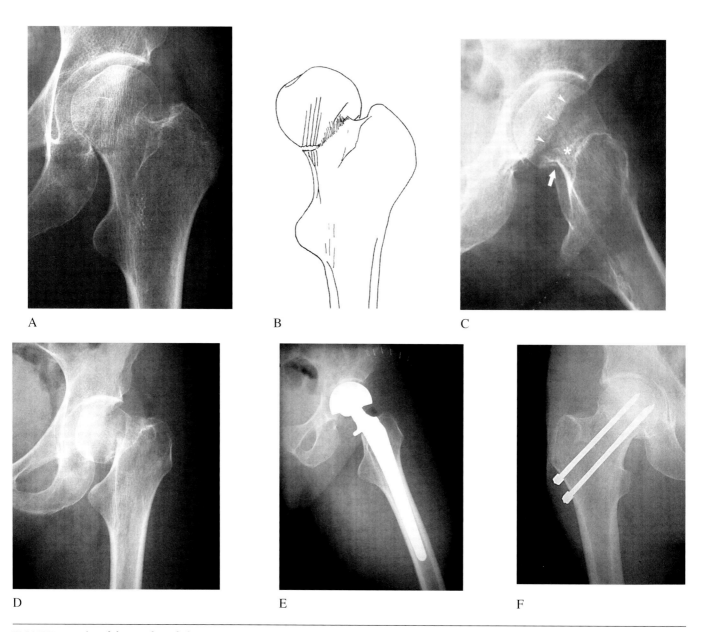

A   B   C

D   E   F

FIGURE 9   Missed femoral neck fracture—Patient 4A.

(*A* and *B*) Initial AP view shows typical signs of a femoral neck fracture. The normal trabecular pattern is interrupted. Along the fracture line, there is distraction (rarefaction) of trabeculae, medially, and impaction (sclerosis) laterally. The angle between the femoral neck and head is abnormal—a *valgus* deformity (i.e., the distal part, femoral shaft, is displaced laterally).

(*C*) On the frog-leg view, there is an abrupt angulation of the medial cortex (*arrow*) and impaction of the fracture (*asterisk*). The acetabular rim overlies the femoral head, which is normal (*arrowheads*).

(*D*) Repeat radiograph when the patient was recalled to the ED shows that the fracture became displaced.

(*E*) Replacement of the proximal femur was now necessary due to the risk of avascular necrosis of the femoral head as a consequence of fracture displacement. A "bipolar" prosthesis, which replaces the acetabulum as well as the proximal femur, was used. It reduces wear on the acetabulum that occurs with a hemiarthroplasty (proximal femoral prosthesis alone), although long-term studies have not shown a definite advantage.

(*F*) In another patient, screw fixation of a nondisplaced femoral neck fracture shows the likely treatment of Patient 4A if the nondisplaced fracture had been diagnosed during her initial ED visit.

Patient 4B Outcome

The findings on the initial radiographs in this patient are more subtle than in the preceding case (Figure 10). A fracture cannot be identified on the AP view. On the frog leg view, there is interruption of the cortex and slight impaction of the femoral neck. The fracture had become displaced when the patient was recalled to the ED. This patient was treated with a hemiarthroplasty.

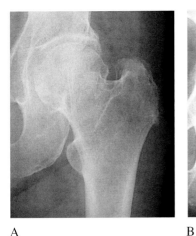 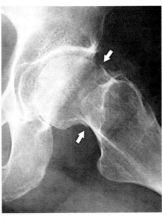 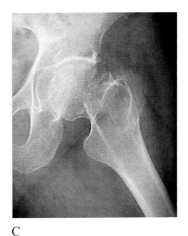 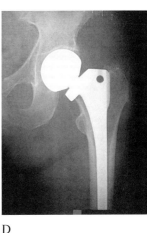

A   B   C   D

FIGURE 10   Missed femoral neck fracture—Patient 4B.

(*A*) The initial AP view was negative for signs of a femoral neck fracture. However, positioning of the view was suboptimal (the hip is not internally rotated) and the foreshortening obscured any signs of the fracture. Degenerative changes cause irregularity of the margin of the femoral head articular surface.

(*B*) On the frog-leg view, there was interruption of the medial and lateral cortices (*arrows*).

(*C*) Repeat radiograph when the patient was recalled to the ED showed that the fracture was now displaced.

(*D*) The patient was treated with a hemiarthroplasty (replacement of the proximal femur with a prosthesis).

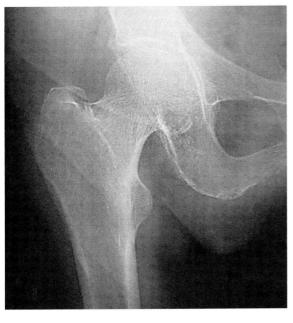 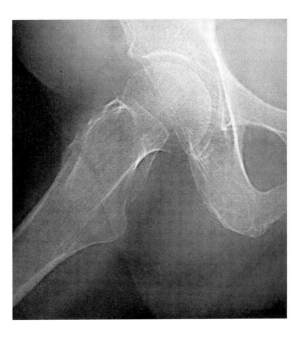

FIGURE 11

PATIENT 4C   An 85-year-old woman fell while getting out of bed. She had extreme pain of her right hip while walking. On examination, there was pain with flexion and internal rotation of the right hip, but no deformity.

The radiographs were initially interpreted as negative for a fracture (Figure 11) and the patient was discharged home.

• Can you find the fracture?

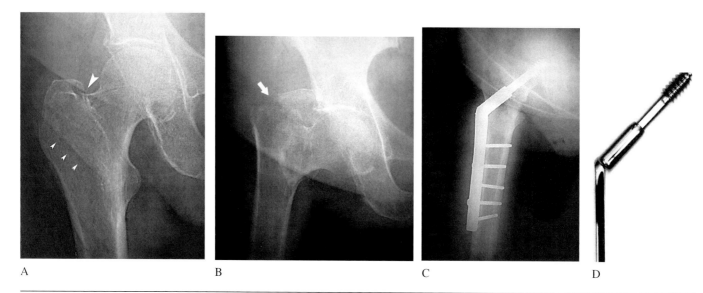

A   B   C   D

FIGURE 12   Missed intertrochanteric fracture—Patient 4C.

(A) Minimal cortical interruption and abrupt angulation is seen where the greater trochanter intersects the superior cortex of the femoral neck (*arrowhead*). This is obscured by an overlapping skin fold. The femoral neck is normal. Another soft tissue skin fold overlies the trochanters (*small arrowheads*). This should not be misinterpreted as a fracture.

(B) When recalled to the ED, the patient had a markedly displaced intertrochanteric fracture (*arrow*).

(C) Despite this displacement, treatment differs little for a displaced versus nondisplaced intertrochanteric fracture. In both cases, the patient is treated with fixation using a plate and sliding screw device. Unlike femoral neck fractures, intertrochanteric fractures are *extracapsular* meaning that the blood supply to the femoral head is not disrupted by the fracture. There is little risk of avascular necrosis of the femoral head and hemiarthroplasty is not needed.

(D) **Sliding screw device.** The femoral neck screw is mounted in a cylindrical collar through which it can slide. The sliding screw allows the fracture fragments to collapse together in a controlled fashion strengthening the repair. With a fixed screw, there is risk of screw breakage or of the screw tip protruding through the femoral head as the fracture becomes compressed.

[From Dee R, et al.: *Principles of Orthopedic Practice*, 2nd ed. McGraw-Hill, 1997, with permission.]

This fracture is very subtle and could easily be missed. However, the presence of severe hip pain suggests that a fracture might be present and that, if a radiographic abnormality is not identified, additional imaging, either MRI or CT, is needed (see below).

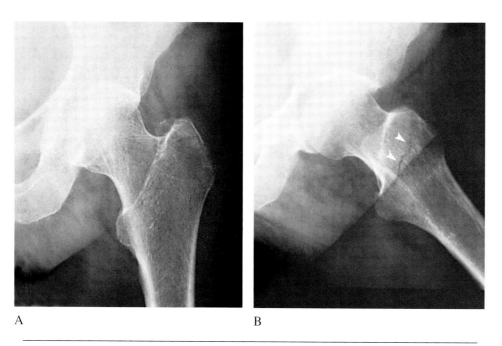

A   B

FIGURE 13   Another patient with a nondisplaced intertrochanteric fracture that was visible only on the frog-leg view (*arrowheads*).

[Courtesy Mahvash Rafii, MD, Department of Radiology, New York University Medical Center.]

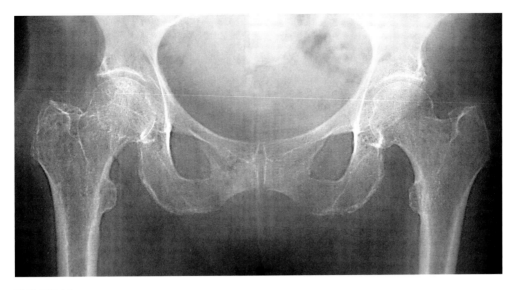

FIGURE 14

PATIENT 4D   An elderly woman who had fallen down. No fracture was identified on the initial radiograph interpretation. She was later recalled to the ED because of an abnormality suspicious for a fracture (Figure 14).

• Is there a fracture?

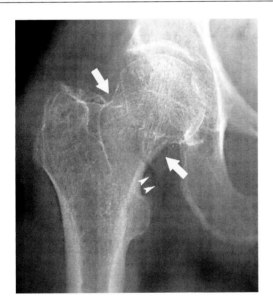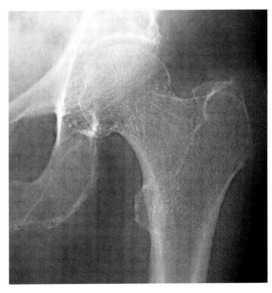

FIGURE 15   Degenerative changes mimic a femoral neck fracture—Patient 4D.

PATIENT 4D   Degenerative changes of the hip can mimic an impacted fracture (Figure 15). This contributes to the difficulty in radiograph interpretation.

In this patient, there is a sclerotic band across the femoral neck that has an appearance similar to an impacted fracture (*arrows*). In addition, a skin fold overlies the medial cortex of the femoral neck, which can simulate a fracture (*arrowheads*). A skin fold is distinguished from a fracture by noting that it has smooth margins and extends beyond the cortex of the bone.

This patient had had a pelvis radiograph because of pain at the left iliac crest and lower back after falling down. There was no pain in the right hip and the patient was able to walk without difficulty. When recalled to the ED, the physical examination and repeat radiographs were unchanged.

Radiographic findings that can be mistaken for a fracture include degenerative changes of the hip, osteophytes extending from the margin of the acetabulum or femoral head, or a skin fold overlying the femoral neck. Ultimately, the clinical findings should determine patient care.

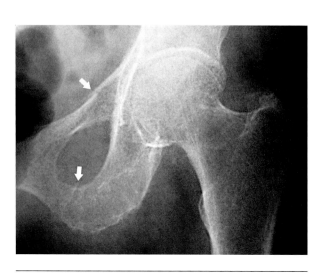

FIGURE 16   Pubic rami fractures.

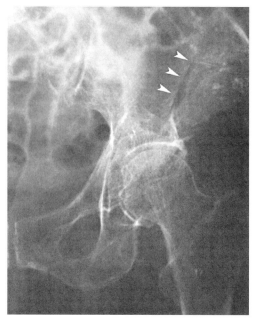

FIGURE 17   Iliac wing fracture.

Pelvic Fractures in Patients with Trauma to the Hip

Fractures of the pelvis are common in elderly patients following falls injuring the region of the hip. These include pubic rami fractures (Figure 16), acetabular fractures, and iliac wing fractures (Figure 17). Iliac wing fractures can be difficult to detect because this region of the radiograph is often overpenetrated (dark).

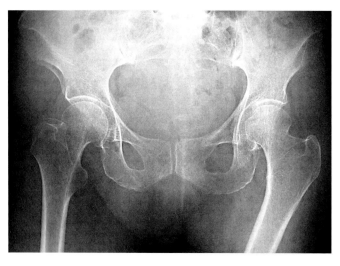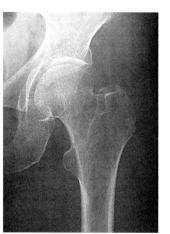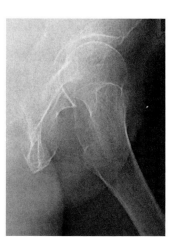

FIGURE 18

PATIENT 4E

A 77-year-old woman slipped and fell in her kitchen and was unable to get up. Her nephew helped her into her bed. She was unable to bear weight due to left hip pain.

She remained in bed for 5 days and finally came to the hospital because of persistent hip pain and inability to walk.

Her examination was notable for extreme pain on internal rotation of her hip.

The radiographs were interpreted as negative for a fracture (Figure 18).

• How would you manage this patient?

OCCULT FRACTURES

Occasionally, a patient will have a fracture of the proximal femur in which the radiographs are truly negative. These *occult fractures* have a similar risk of complications as radiographically visible fractures if not diagnosed and treated appropriately. Such complications include fracture displacement and avascular necrosis of the femoral head.

Diagnostic Strategy

Various diagnostic strategies have been proposed for managing patients suspected of having an occult hip fracture.

In the **traditional approach,** the patient is kept at bed rest and non-weight-bearing for 3–5 days, and then, if still symptomatic, has repeat radiography. If the radiographs are again negative, a **bone scan** is performed. Many authors recommend hospitalization to minimize movement of the hip, although others suggest sending the patient home so long as strict bed rest can be maintained.

Radionuclide **bone scan** had been used in the past to detect occult fractures (Figure 19). It has high sensitivity for fracture detection (90–95%). The major limitation is that the scan does not become positive until three to five days following the injury. This is because the radionuclide-labeled tracer is only taken up as new bone is formed during fracture healing. In older patients with osteoporosis, bone deposition may take even longer. In addition, a bone scan has limited specificity—abnormal uptake can occur with arthritis, tumors, and infections. CT or MRI is sometimes needed after the bone scan to distinguish these disorders.

MRI is currently used in the diagnosis of radiographically occult fractures and has several advantages over other imaging modalities (Figure 20). MRI does not, however, directly visualize bone. Instead, it detects edema and hemorrhage within the marrow that is associated with a fracture. MRI accurately defines the location and extent of the injury, and can detect adjacent soft tissue abnormalities. In addition, MRI can be performed on the day of injury, unlike bone scan. Although MRI is more expensive and often not readily available on an emergency basis, its expense is offset by the reduced length of hospital stay. Use of an abbreviated scan protocol (coronal T1-weighted images only) can reduce the cost of MRI, although T2-weighed images can help identify other injuries (see below).

CT is more sensitive than conventional radiography, although *less sensitive* than MRI and missed cases have been reported (Lang et al. 1992, Conway et al. 1996, Hayes and Balkisson 1997). On CT, the fracture may be visible on only one or two slices (Figure 19).

Multidetector CT (MDCT) with coronal and sagittal reformatted images has not been extensively studied for this use. In one small series of six patients with occult fractures, CT was able to detect fractures in all six cases (Lubovsky 2005). However, MRI was more accurate in depicting the anatomy of the fracture. In two cases, CT showed only greater rochanteric fractures when intertrochanteric fractures were present on MRI. The treatment of these two injuries differs substantially. In general, CT may miss subtle fractures involving predominantly the trabeculae with only minor cortical deformity, whereas MRI is able to detect these injuries.

CT is perhaps most useful when the radiographs are equivocal (i.e., have questionable signs of a fracture). However, if CT does not reveal a fracture, MRI may still be needed.

Although MRI, bone scan, and CT are more sensitive at detecting hip fractures than conventional radiography, such advanced imaging modalities should not be used as a substitute for accurate radiograph interpretation. It is more efficient to correctly interpret the radiographs and identify subtle signs of a fracture than to obtain an MRI or CT in the ED when a fracture is, in fact, visible on the radiographs (Figures 22 and 23).

Patient 4E Outcome

This patient was admitted to the hospital and had a bone scan the next day (several days had elapsed since her injury). It showed increased uptake in the region of the femoral neck. A CT scan showed only a small cortical interruption on one slice, representing an incomplete femoral neck fracture. The patient was treated with screw fixation of the femoral neck (Figure 19).

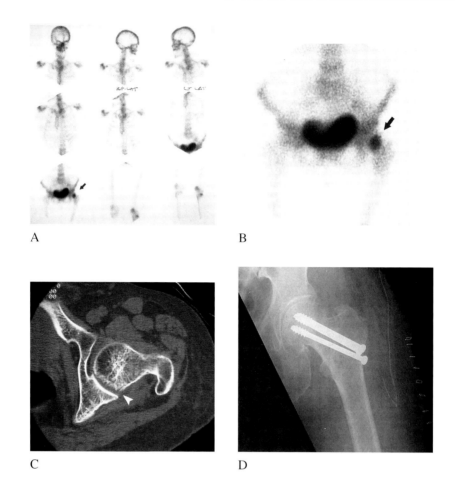

FIGURE 19 Occult femoral neck fracture revealed by bone scan—Patient 4E.

(*A* and *B*) Bone scan reveals abnormal uptake at the left femoral neck (*arrow*). The radioactive tracer also collects in the urinary bladder.

(*C*) CT shows questionable signs of a fracture. On one slice, there is a small cortical interruption representing an incomplete subcapital femoral neck fracture. In addition, there is slight cortical impaction of the femoral head articular surface (*arrowhead*). The diagnosis of an occult fracture was based on the bone scan, not CT findings.

(*D*) Stabilization of the femoral neck fracture with screw fixation.

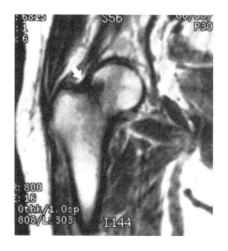
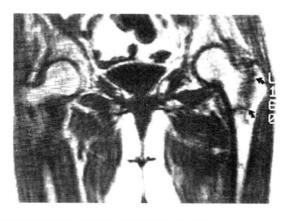

FIGURE 20 MRI of radiographically occult proximal femoral fractures.

In these T1-weighted images, normal bone marrow produces high signal intensity and appears white. Edema and hemorrhage within the marrow along the fracture causes low signal intensity and appears dark. Cortical bone produces little MR signal and appears black; the cortical fracture is not directly visualized by MRI.

(*A*) Femoral neck fracture (*arrow*). (*B*) Intertrochanteric fracture (*arrows*).

[From Dee R, et al: *Principles of Orthopedic Practice*, 2nd ed. McGraw-Hill, 1997, with permission.]

Frequency of Occult Hip Fractures

Occult factures about the hip are not rare. In one series of 764 ED patients with hip trauma, 219 (29%) had fractures on radiography, 65% of which were proximal femoral fractures (Dominguez et al. 2005). Among 545 patients with negative radiographs, 62 (11%) had MRI for a suspected occult fracture.

Twenty-four of the patients that underwent MRI had fractures (38%). (Ten percent of fractures were radiographically occult.) Seven of the occult fractures (24%) were proximal femoral fractures; the others were pubic ramus, acetabular or sacral fractures (see Figure 23).

There were no missed fractures among the 483 patients with negative radiographs who did not have MRI.

Conclusion

Never diagnose a "hip contusion" in an elderly patient unless a fracture has been definitively excluded. The diagnosis of a fracture is based on the clinical examination (pain on weight bearing and range of motion of the hip), risk factors (chiefly osteoporosis), and radiographic findings (Figure 21).

A nondisplaced fracture can have subtle radiographic findings that should be specifically sought. However, negative radiographs do not entirely exclude a fracture, particularly in patients at high risk due to osteoporosis. Therefore, when the clinical findings are suggestive of a fracture, and the radiographs are negative or equivocal, further investigation with MRI, bone scan or possibly CT should be under taken.

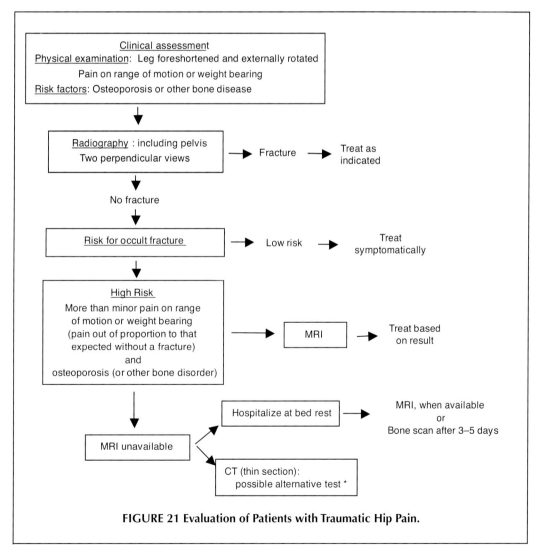

FIGURE 21 Evaluation of Patients with Traumatic Hip Pain.

*CT is most useful when the radiographs are equivocal (show questionable signs of a fracture)

[Adapted from Perron AD, Miller MD, Brady WJ: Orthopedic pitfalls in the ED: Radiographically occult hip fracture. Am J Emer Med 2002:20:234–237, with permission.]

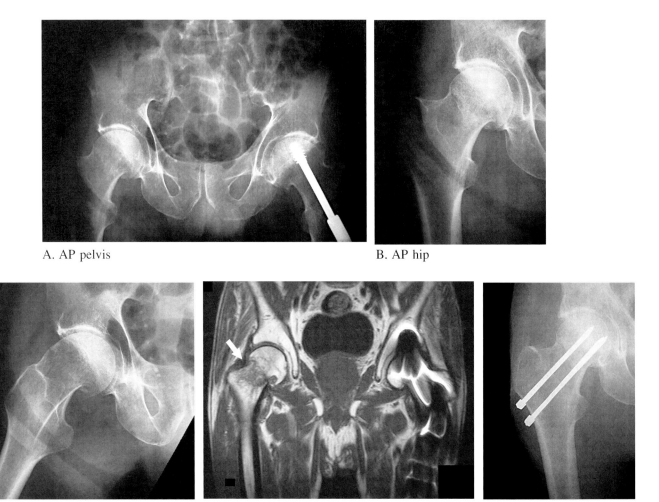

A. AP pelvis   B. AP hip

C. "Frog-leg" view   D. MRI   E. Postop view

FIGURE 22   A "non-occult" hip fracture diagnosed using MRI.

A 78-year-old man tripped and fell fracturing the humeral shaft of his right arm. He could not walk due to hip pain and was admitted to the hospital. The hip and pelvis **radiographs** were initially interpreted as negative for a fracture (A–C). He previously had an intertrochanteric fracture of his left hip that was treated with a plate and sliding screw device (A).

MRI the next day revealed a right subcapital femoral neck fracture (D) (arrow). Metallic orthopedic hardware causes MRI artifacts of the left hip. The fracture was stabilized using screw fixation (E).

Close inspection of the **initial radiographs** reveals that the fracture was, in fact, visible. On the AP pelvis and hip radiographs (A, B, and F), there is impaction (asterisk) and cortical interruption (arrowhead) of the femoral neck. On the frog-leg view (C and G), there is an abnormal angle between the femoral head and neck, as well as cortical interruption on both the lateral and medial sides of the femoral neck (arrowheads).

Accurate radiograph interpretation is important to reduce the need for advanced imaging studies such as MRI, which is

costly and often difficult to obtain in the emergency department, as well as to reduce the chances of misdiagnosis. CT would have demonstrated the fracture, although CT was unnecessary because the fracture was visible on the radiographs.

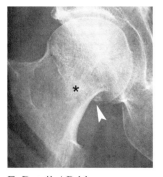

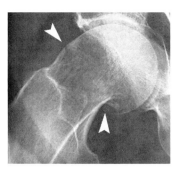

F. Detail AP hip   G. Detail frog view

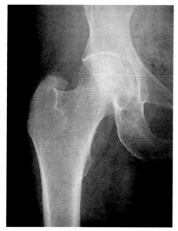

A. AP hip view

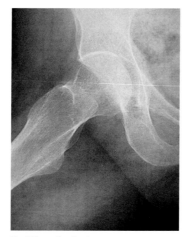

B. "Frog-leg" view

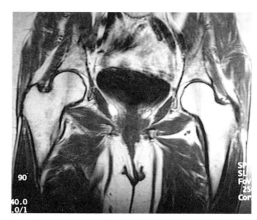

C. T1-weighted MRI is negative for proximal femur fracture

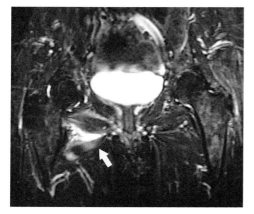

D. T2-weighted MRI shows edema is muscles adjacent to the right public rami (*arrow*). This finding calls attention to an injury in this region and prompts further inspection of the TI-weighted images (E).

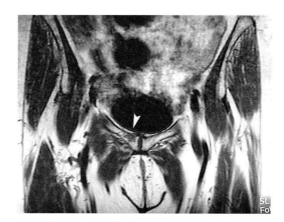

E. T1-Weighted MRI shows a right superior public ramus fracture (*arrowhead*).

FIGURE 23   Injuries other than proximal femoral fractures can be detected by MRI.

An elderly woman could not walk due to hip pain after falling. Her **hip radiographs** were normal (A and B). An **MRI** was obtained which was negative for a proximal femoral fracture (C). However, the MRI did reveal a fracture of the superior pubic ramus (D and E). This region was not included on her initial hip radiographs, and a pelvis radiograph had not been ordered. The pubic rami are common sites of fractures and should always be examined in such patients, i.e., by obtaining an AP pelvis radiograph.

On the other hand, experience with MRI has shown that *occult pubic rami fractures* (negative pelvis radiographs) are sometimes seen in patients suspected of having femoral neck fractures (Table 3).

The high incidence of injuries other than proximal femur fractures argues against the use of limited MRI (coronal T1-weighed images focusing on only the proximal femur). Even though none of the other injuries required surgical intervention, management was modified by the MRI results. For example, a pubic ramus fracture is managed with early mobilization, whereas an acetabular fracture needs more prolonged bed rest (Bogost et al. 1995, Dominguez et al. 2005 Oka and Monu 2004).

MRI scanning protocols. This case illustrates the usefulness of different MR imaging sequences. *T1-weighted* images show fine anatomical detail but do not clearly show edema in soft tissues—a sign of injury (C and E). *T2-weighted* images provide less anatomical detail than T1 images, but fluid collections (e.g., urine in the bladder and CSF) and soft tissue edema have very high signal intensity (appear white), and are therefore more easily seen on T2-weighted images (D).

TABLE 3

Occult Fractures and Soft Tissue Injuries Diagnosed by MRI

70 patients with negative radiographs, 56 (80%) positive MRI

Proximal femoral fracture	26 (37%)
Femoral neck	11 (41%)
Intertrochanteric	14 (52%)
Pelvic fractures alone	11 (16%)
Pubic ramus, acetabulum, sacrum	
Soft tissue injury alone	16 (23%)

(Data from Bogost 1995)

SUGGESTED READING

Alba E, Youngburg R: Occult fractures of the femoral neck. *Am J Emerg Med* 1992;10:64–68.

Bogost GA, Lizerbram EK, Crues JV: MR imaging in evaluation of suspected hip fracture: Frequency of unsuspected bone and soft-tissue injury. *Radiology* 1995;197:263–67.

Campbell SE: Radiography of the hip: Lines, signs, and patterns of disease. *Semin Roentgen* 2005;40:290–319.

Conway WF, Totty WG, McEnery KW: CT and MR imaging of the hip. *Radiology* 1996;198:297–307.

Deutsch AL, Mink JH, et al.: Occult fractures of the proximal femur: MR imaging. *Radiology* 1989;170:113–116.

Dominguez S, Liu P, Roberts C, et al.: Prevalence of traumatic hip and pelvic fractures in patients with suspected hip fracture and negative initial standard radiographs. *Acad Emerg* Med 2005;12:366–370.

Hanlon D, Evans T: The hip and proximal femur. In Schwartz DT, Reisdorff EJ: *Emergency Radiology*. New York: McGraw-Hill, 2000.

Hayes CW, Balkissoon ARA: Current concept in imaging of the pelvis and hip. *Orthop Clin North Am* 1997;28:617–642.

Hofman A, Wyatt R: Missed subcapital fractures. *Ann Emerg Med* 1984;13:951–955.

Lang P, Genant HK, Jergesen HE, Murray WR: Imaging of the hip joint: Computed tomography versus magnetic resonance imaging. *Clin Orthop Related Research* 1992;274:135–153.

Lubovsky O, Liebergall M, Mattan Y, et al.: Early diagnosis of occult hip fractures: MRI versus CT scan. *Injury* 2005;36:788–792.

May DA, Purins JL, Smith DK: MR imaging of occult traumatic fractures and muscular injuries of the hip and pelvis in elderly patients. *AJR* 1996;166:1075–1078.

Mlinek EJ, Clark KC, Walker CW: Limited magnetic resonance imaging in the diagnosis of occult hip fractures. *Am J Emerg Med* 1998;16:390–392.

Oka M, Monu JUV: Prevalence and patterns of occult hip fractures and mimics revealed by MRI. *AJR* 2004;182:283–288.

Pandey R, McNalley E, Ali A, Bulstrode C: The role of MRI in the diagnosis of occult hip fractures. *Injury* 1998;29:61–63.

Perron AD, Miller MD, Brady WJ: Orthopedic pitfalls in the ED: Radiographically occult hip fracture. *Am J Emerg Med* 2002; 20:234–237.

Rizzo PF, Gould ES, Lyden JP, Asnis SE: Diagnosis of occult fractures about the hip: Magnetic resonance imaging compared with bone scanning. *J Bone Joint Surg (Am)* 1993;75:395–401.

Rubin SJ, Marquardt JD, Gottleib RH, et al.: Magnetic resonance imaging: A cost-effective alternative to bone scintigraphy in the evaluation of patients with suspected hip fractures. *Skel Radiol* 1998;27:199–204.

Rudman N, McIlmail D: Emergency department evaluation and treatment of hip and thigh injuries. *Emerg Med Clin North Am* 2000;18:29–66.

Zuckerman JD: Hip fracture. *New Engl J Med* 1996;334:1519–1525.

Lower Extremity: Patient 5

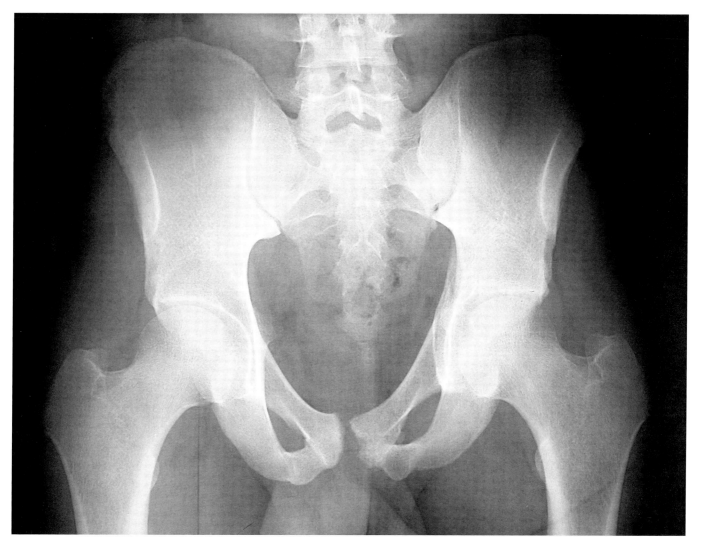

FIGURE 1

Pelvic pain in a young man who fell from a scaffolding

A 27-year-old construction worker fell from a 6-feet high scaffolding. He was hemodynamically stable and had no signs of head, chest, or abdominal trauma. His pelvis was stable but tender to compression. There was an obvious fracture of his wrist.

- Are there any abnormalities on his pelvis radiograph?

TEARDROP

Because the pelvis has a rigid ring-like structure, a single break in the pelvis, especially if displaced, is nearly always associated with a second break elsewhere in the ring. If not immediately obvious, a second fracture must be carefully sought. The same principle holds true for fractures of the **obturator ring** (Figure 2). A single break in the obturator ring must be accompanied by another break elsewhere in the ring. For example, a superior pubic ramus fractures is often associated with an inferior pubic ramus fracture.

In Patient 5, there is deformity of the left side of the **pubic symphysis** (Figure 3A). This is due to a fracture through the body of the left pubic bone. The fracture is better seen on an "outlet" view (Figure 3B). This is an unusual location for a fracture; most obturator ring fractures occur through the superior or inferior pubic rami.

With a pubic bone fracture, a typical site for the second fracture is the **acetabulum.** Detection of fractures in this region requires knowledge of radiographic anatomy of the acetabulum. Interpretation of the radiograph is aided by the symmetry of the pelvis, which provides an opposite side for comparison.

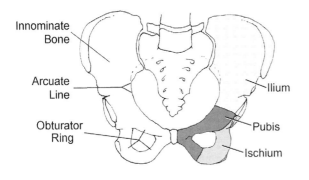

FIGURE 2A   The pelvic ring.

The pelvis is a nearly rigid osseus ring made up by the sacrum and the two innominate bones.

The **innominate bone** is formed from the fused ilium, ischium, and pubic bones.

The **arcuate line** forms the inner circumference of the pelvic ring.

The **obturator ring** is made up by the superior and inferior pubic rami and the ischial ramus.

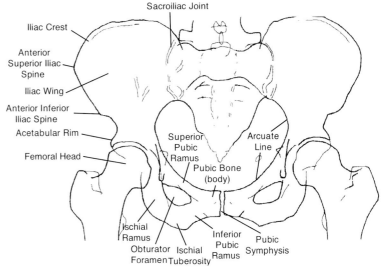

FIGURE 2B   Anatomical landmarks of the pelvis.

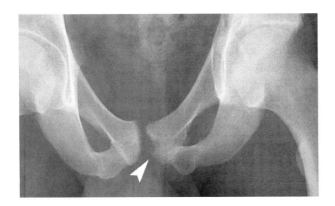

FIGURE 3A   In Patient 5, irregularity of the left pubic bone is due to a fracture (*arrowhead*).

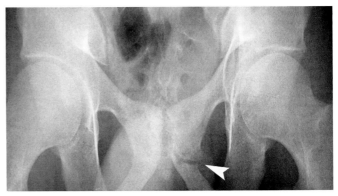

FIGURE 3B   An AP view with cranial angulation of the x-ray beam (an "outlet view," see Figure 15 on p. 340) shows the pubic bone en-face and clearly demonstrates the pubic fracture (*arrowhead*).

The Radiographic Teardrop

There are several radiographic landmarks that are important in identifying acetabular fractures (Figures 4 and 5). The **iliopubic line** extends from the ilium to the pubic bone along the superior pubic ramus. It is the anterior portion of the **arcuate line.** The **ilioischial line** runs vertically from the ilium to the ischial ramus. It lies along the **quadrilateral plate,** which forms the medial wall of the acetabulum.

The curved **articular surface of the acetabulum** parallels the surface of the femoral head. The acetabular articular surface ends inferiorly in a U-shaped curve.

On the AP view, the ilioischial line, the acetabular articular surface, and the radiographic "U" coincide to form an elongated **teardrop** (Figure 4). In some instances, the acetabular contours do not align to form a teardrop (Figure 6).

The left and right sides of the pelvis should be compared to assist in injury detection.

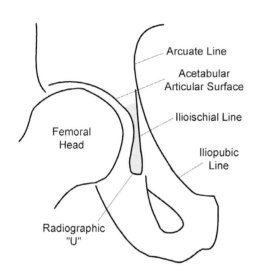

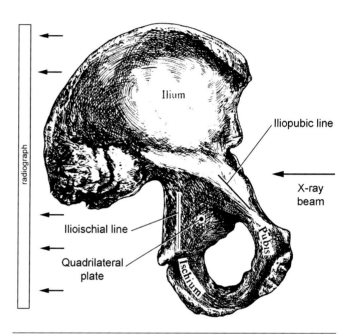

FIGURE 5   Medial view of the left innominate bone.
This shows the correlation between the anatomy of the acetabulum and, the contours seen on an AP pelvis radiograph.

Iliopubic line is continuous with the superior pubic ramus.

Ilioischial line is the vertical portion of the quadrilateral plate and is continuous with the ischial ramus.

Quadrilateral plate is the surface of the innominate bone that forms the medial wall of the acetabulum.

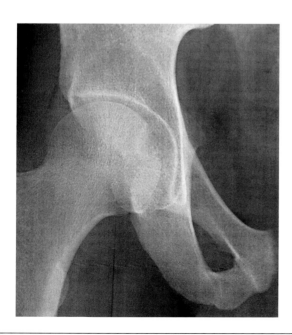

FIGURE 4   The radiographic teardrop.
Radiographic teardrop (*gray*) is composed of the ilioischial line, the acetabular articular surface, and the radiographic "U."
Radiographic "U" is the inferior lip of the anterior articular surface of acetabulum.

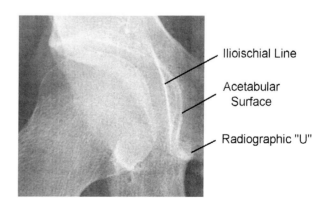

FIGURE 6   When positioning of the patient is slightly rotated, the ilioischial line projects lateral to the acetabular articular surface and a radiographic "teardrop" is not formed.

In Patient 5, a normal teardrop is seen on the right side of the pelvis (Figure 7A). On the left, the radiographic teardrop is disrupted by medial displacement of the iliopubic line (Figure 7B). The fracture itself is not visible because it lies in the coronal plane. (The fracture was visible on an oblique view—see Figure 18 on p. 340.)

CT confirmed that this was a slightly displaced fracture of the anterior acetabular column (Figure 8). It did not involve the weight bearing portion of the acetabulum, the acetabular dome (Figures 7C and 8B). The patient was therefore managed nonoperatively, initially with traction, then partial weight-bearing over the next 4 weeks.

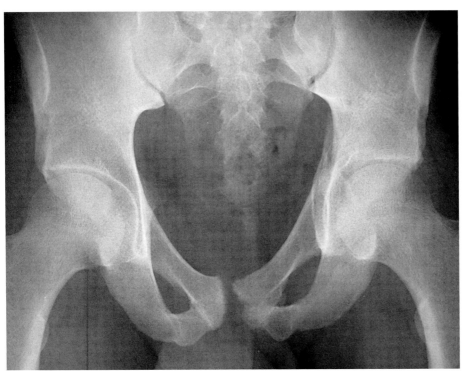

A. AP pelvis view—Patient 5

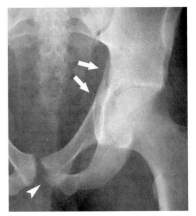

B. Detail of AP pelvis view

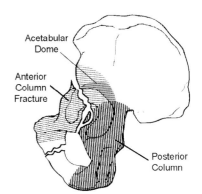

C. Anterior column fracture.

FIGURE 7   The AP radiograph in Patient 5 shows a fracture of the pubic bone (*arrowhead*) and medial displacement of the iliopubic line (*arrows*). These findings indicate a fracture of the anterior column of the acetabulum (*C*).

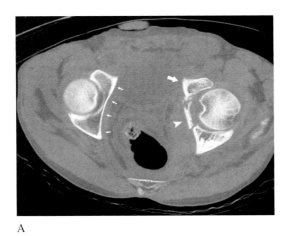

A

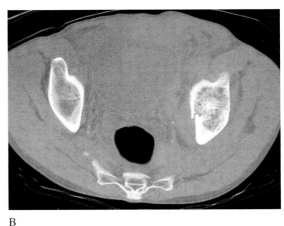

B

FIGURE 8   CT scan—Patient 5.

(*A*) CT slice at the level of the femoral head shows the acetabular fracture (*arrow*). There is a separate small fracture of the medial wall of the acetabulum (*arrowhead*). A normal quadrilateral plate is seen on the right acetabulum (*small arrows*).

(*B*) A CT slice superior to *A* shows that the fracture extends to, but does not disrupt, the acetabular dome. The fracture is not displaced and therefore does not need operative fixation.

Acetabular Fractures

Acetabular fractures are caused by both high-energy and low-energy forces. The usual mechanism of injury is an impact to the lateral aspect of the hip that drives the femoral head into the acetabulum. High-energy injuries occur in motor vehicle collisions, pedestrians struck by motor vehicles, and falls from great heights. "Low-energy" acetabular fractures occur in elderly patients following relatively minor trauma such as a fall from standing. Acetabular fractures are associated with substantial morbidity and mortality, including "low-energy" injuries in the elderly.

When the fracture is markedly **displaced,** it is obvious radiographically. In some cases, the femoral head is medially displaced and the injury is termed a "central dislocation of the hip."

When the fracture is **nondisplaced** or minimally displaced, the radiographic findings are more subtle. Occasionally, the fracture cannot be identified on an AP pelvis radiograph, and additional views (oblique views) or CT is needed.

Acetabular fractures are **classified anatomically** based upon the involvement of the structural elements of the acetabulum. The acetabulum is supported by two osseous columns (Figure 9). The **anterior column** extends from the anterior portion of the acetabulum anteriorly along the superior pubic ramus. Radiographically, it is the *iliopubic line* (Figures 4 and 5). The **posterior column** extends inferiorly from the posterior portion of the acetabulum to the ischial ramus. Radiographically, it is

the *ilioischial line*. The anterior and posterior columns converge superiorly at an angle of approximately 60° and insert on the **acetabular dome**. The acetabular dome is the weight-bearing portion of the acetabulum.

Acetabular fractures can involve the anterior column, the posterior column, both anterior and posterior columns forming a Y-shaped or T-shaped fracture, or bisect the acetabulum (a transverse fracture) (Figure 10). Fractures involving the anterior column disrupt or displace the iliopubic line. Posterior column fractures disrupt the ilioischial line (Figures 7 and 11–13).

Fractures limited to the anterior or posterior acetabular rim are associated with hip dislocations. If the rim fragment is large, hip reduction will be unstable and the fracture requires surgical fixation (Figure 14). Fractures that involve the rim and adjacent portion of the innominate bone are termed acetabular "wall" fractures.

Acetabular fractures that disrupt the **acetabular dome** compromise the structural integrity of the hip and require operative fixation. Fractures that spare the acetabular dome or are displaced less that 2–5 mm (depending on the location of the fracture and patient characteristics) can be treated nonoperatively. An additional indication for surgical treatment is the presence of an intra-articular bone fragment. Such fragments are usually detected only by CT and must be removed to prevent further injury to the acetabular articular surface.

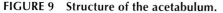

FIGURE 9   Structure of the acetabulum.

The **anterior column** corresponds to the radiographic iliopubic line.

The **posterior column** corresponds to the ilioischial line.

The anterior and posterior columns converge superiorly to the **acetabular dome.**

[From Dee R, et al. *Principles of Orthopedic Practice,* 2ed. McGraw-Hill, 1997, with permission.]

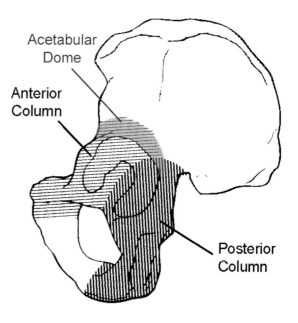

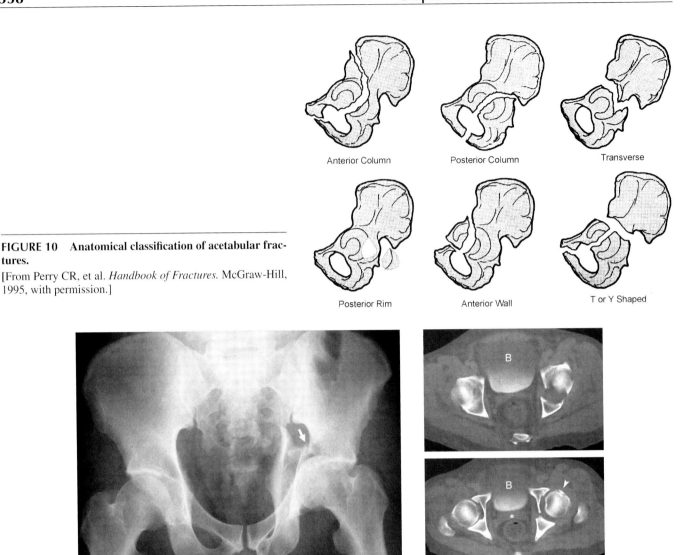

Anterior Column   Posterior Column   Transverse

Posterior Rim   Anterior Wall   T or Y Shaped

FIGURE 10   **Anatomical classification of acetabular fractures.**

[From Perry CR, et al. *Handbook of Fractures.* McGraw-Hill, 1995, with permission.]

FIGURE 11   Y-shaped acetabular fracture.

The posterior column of the acetabulum (ilioischial line) is displaced medially. The femoral head is also displaced medially; this is termed a "central dislocation" of the hip. A mildly displaced anterior column fracture disrupts the iliopubic line (*arrow*). There is a concomitant fracture of the pubic bone (*arrowhead*).

CT confirmed the acetabular fracture with extension into and displacement of the acetabular dome. Surgical fixation with plate and screws was necessary. There is also a small femoral head fracture (*arrowhead*).

A small amount of blood is present between the bladder and rectum (*asterisk*). Intravenous contrast is just beginning to be excreted into the bladder (*B*).

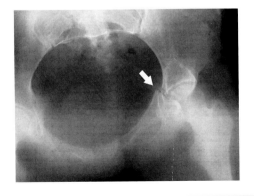

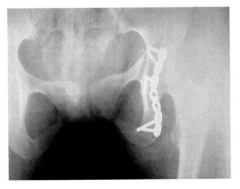

FIGURE 12   Transverse fracture of the acetabulum.

The patient was an automobile driver who was not wearing a seat belt and had a head-on collision. The fracture crosses both the anterior and posterior columns. Surgical fixation of the acetabulum was necessary.

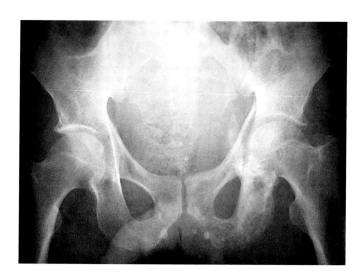
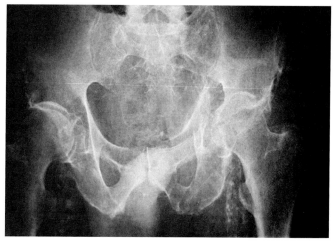

FIGURE 13   Acetabular fractures in elderly patients who fell from standing ("low-energy" injuries).

(A) Anterior column fracture with a second medially displaced fragment of the quadrilateral plate. Paget's disease of the bone causes the irregularly thickened trabecular pattern and was a predisposing factor for this fracture.

(B) An 80-year-old man fell at home causing a displaced acetabular fracture. The patient was taking coumadin for anticoagulation and as a result suffered major pelvic and retroperitoneal hemorrhage. The patient had osteoporosis and extensive vascular calcification.

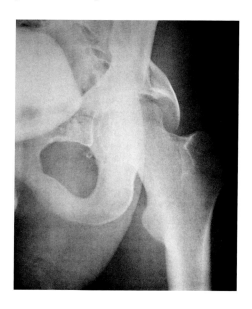

FIGURE 14   Posterior acetabular rim fracture.
This was presumably due to a posterior dislocation that had reduced spontaneously. This large fracture fragment required surgical fixation.

Supplementary Radiographic Views of the Pelvis

Supplementary views are helpful in defining the anatomy of a pelvic fracture, although they have been largely superseded by CT. Supplementary views are now used by orthopedists to clarify the anatomy of an acetabular fracture in concert with CT. Supplementary views are occasionally used in the ED when there are equivocal findings on the AP view. For example, an oblique view may show a nondisplaced acetabular fracture that is not clearly visible on the AP view. However, this use has also been supplanted by CT.

Supplementary views include angled AP views (inlet and outlet views) and oblique views.

An AP view with the x-ray beam directed caudally (**inlet view**) provides a direct view of the circumference of the pelvic ring and is useful in revealing displacement of a fracture. The cranial-angled view (**outlet view**) shows the sacrum

and anterior pelvis en-face and can better reveal fractures in these areas (Figures 15 and 16).

Oblique views of the pelvis are obtained by raising one side of the pelvis to a 45° angle (Figures 17 and 18). Positioning can be painful and potentially injurious if the patient has a significant fracture. The **external oblique view** is also known as the *iliac oblique view* because it shows the iliac wing en face. Its primary role is to detect fractures of the posterior acetabular column. The **internal oblique view,** also called the *obturator oblique view*, shows fractures of the anterior acetabular column and the obturator ring.

Oblique views are also known as **Judet views** in honor of the physician who originally described their usefulness in the diagnosis of acetabular fractures.

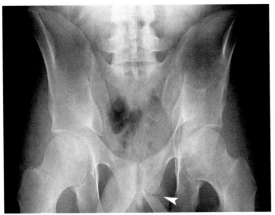

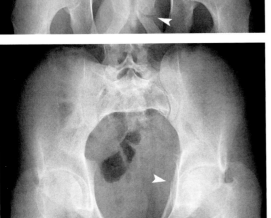

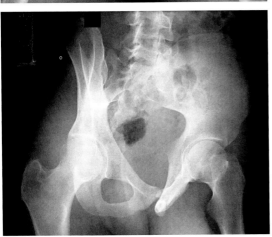

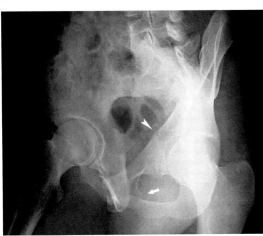

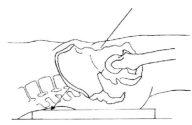

FIGURE 15 Outlet view.

Cranial angulation of the x-ray beam shows the sacrum and pubic bone en face.

In Patient 5, there is a pubic bone fracture (*arrowhead*).

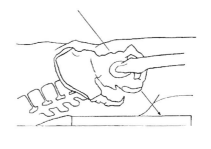

FIGURE 16 Inlet view.

Caudal angulation shows entire circumference of the pelvic ring. Displacement of a pelvic fracture is often better seen on this view.

In Patient 5, there is slight medial displacement of the anterior column fracture (*arrowhead*).

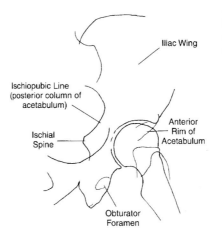

FIGURE 17 Left external (iliac) oblique view shows the posterior column of the acetabulum.

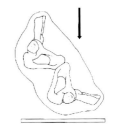

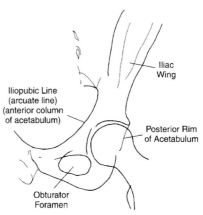

FIGURE 18 Left internal (obturator) oblique view shows the anterior column and obturator ring.

In Patient 5, the anterior column fracture is seen as a break in the iliopubic line (*arrowhead*). The pubic bone fracture is also visible (*arrow*).

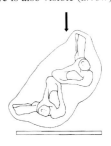

SUGGESTED READING

Brandser EA, El-Khoury GY, Marsh JL: Acetabular fractures: A systematic approach to classification. *Emerg Radiol* 1995;2:18–28.

Durkee NJ, Jacobson J, Jamadar D, et al.: Classification of common acetabular fractures: Radiographic and CT appearances. *AJR* 2006;187:915–925.

Falchi M, Rollandi GA: CT of pelvic fractures. Europ J Radiol 2004; 50: 96–105.

Harris JH, Coupe KJ, Lee JS, Trotscher T: Acetabular fractures revisited: Part 2. A new CT-based classification. *AJR* 2004;182:1367–1375.

Harris JH, Lee JS, Coupe KJ, Trotscher T: Acetabular fractures revisited: Part I. Redefinition of the Letournel anterior column. *AJR* 2004;182:1363–1366.

Hustey F, Moettus Wilber L: The pelvis. In Schwartz DT, Reisdorff EJ: *Emergency Radiology.* New York: McGraw-Hill, 2000.

Judet R, Judet J, Letournel E: Fractures of the acetabulum: Classification and surgical approaches for open reduction. *J Bone Joint Surg (Am)* 1964;46:1612–1646.

Kickuth R, Laufer U, Hartung G, et al.: 3D CT versus axial helical CT versus conventional tomography in the classification of acetabular fractures. *Clinical Radiology* 2002; 7: 140–145.

Ohashi K, El-Khoury GY, Abu-Zahra KW, Berbaum KS: Interobserver agreement for Letournel acetabular fracture classification with multidetector CT: Are standard Judet radiographs necessary? *Radiology* 2006;241:386–391.

Lower Extremity: Patient 6

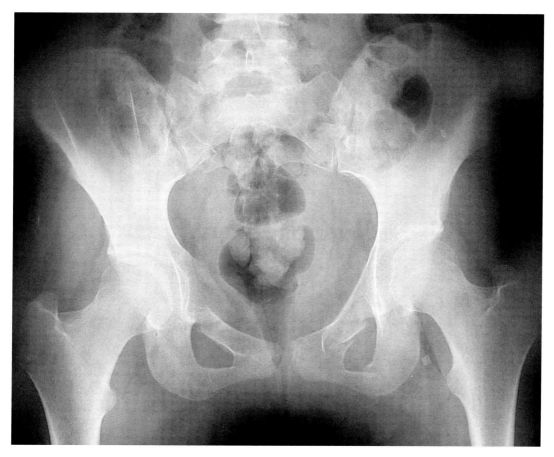

FIGURE 1

Pelvic pain in a young woman following a motor vehicle collision

An 18-year-old woman was an unrestrained back seat passenger of a car that was struck on the passenger side by another vehicle. The automobile was significantly damaged on the side of the impact. None of the other occupants of the car were injured. She was removed from the vehicle and immobilized by the ambulance crew.

In the ED, she was alert and oriented, although anxious and crying. The patient did not think she had lost consciousness, although she could not recall all of the details of the collision. Her only complaint was of lower back pain.

Her blood pressure was 110/70 mm Hg and pulse 100/min. There were several superficial abrasions and glass fragments

on her forehead. Her neck, chest and abdomen were nontender. There was tenderness over the lower lumbar spine. Compression of her pelvis caused pain but there was no abnormal mobility.

- What fractures are seen on her pelvis radiograph (Figure 1)?

- What was the mechanism of injury responsible for these fractures?

- What other injuries would you suspect in this patient?

LIFE SAVER

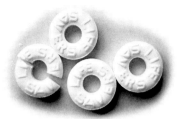

Because the pelvis is a nearly rigid ring-like structure, any single break in the pelvis, especially if displaced, should be accompanied by another break elsewhere in the pelvis. If a second break is not immediately obvious, it must be carefully sought.

In Patient 6, there are **bilateral pubic rami fractures** (Figure 2). This anterior fracture fragment, owing to its characteristic appearance, is sometimes referred to as a **butterfly fracture** (Figure 3). One mechanism that can cause this injury is anterior impact to the perineal area by an object that is straddled by the patient's legs—a **straddle fracture** (Figure 4). These bilateral pubic rami fractures constitute the two breaks in the pelvic ring; an additional fracture need not be present. However, anterior impact is not the mechanism of injury in many butterfly-shaped pelvic fractures and was not the mechanism of injury in this patient.

There is also a fracture through the right **sacral wing** (Figure 5).

- **Why are there three breaks in the pelvic ring?**

  (bilateral pubic rami fractures and sacral wing fracture)

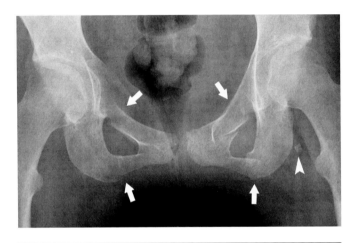

FIGURE 2   Detail of the patient's pelvis radiograph showing bilateral pubic rami fractures (*arrows*). Slight irregularity at the pubic symphysis is normal. *Arrowhead*–fragment of windshield glass lying on the stretcher.

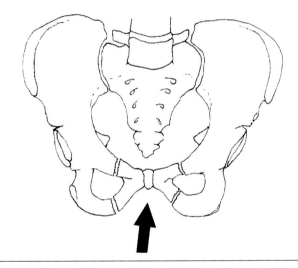

FIGURE 3   A "butterfly" fracture fragment (bilateral pubic rami fractures) produced by an anterior impact on the pubic bone.

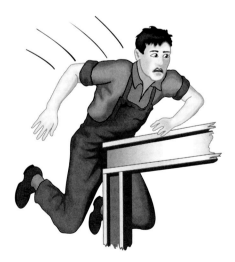

FIGURE 4   Straddle fracture. This mechanism of bilateral pubic rami fractures is actually uncommon.

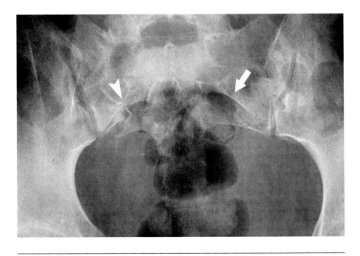

FIGURE 5   Detail of the pelvis radiograph showing disruption of the sacral neuroforaminal lines on the right (*arrowhead*). *Arrow*–normal neuroforaminal lines on the left form smooth arcs.

Why Are There Three Breaks in the Pelvic Ring?

Most pubic rami fractures, including bilateral fractures, are not due to a direct impact on the anterior portion of the pelvis. This patient was seated in a car that was struck on its side by another vehicle. The **laterally directed force** displaced the right side of the pelvis inward. This caused coronally-oriented fractures through the pubic rami due to shearing forces, as well as an impacted fracture of the right sacral wing (Figures 6 and 7). The sacral wing is fractured because it is the weakest part of the sacrum due to perforations by the sacral neuroforamina.

Lateral compression (LC) injuries to the pelvis are usually mechanically stable because the strong *sacrospinous* and *sacrotuberous ligaments* of the pelvic floor remain intact (Figure 8). This injury has been called a **"closed book"** **pelvis** to distinguish it from an "open book" pelvis, which is due to an anteriorly directed force causing pubic symphysis separation (see Figures 11 and 13 on p. 348–349). Because LC forces reduce the pelvic volume, these injuries are not usually associated with severe bleeding, in contrast to injuries that increase pelvic volume, such as open book pelvis and vertical shearing injuries.

Injuries to the anterior pelvis are frequently associated with lower urinary tract injuries. With LC, the sharp ends of the pubic rami fracture fragments can pierce the bladder. This is the usual mechanism of an **extraperitoneal bladder rupture.**

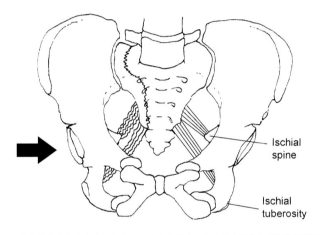

FIGURE 6 **Lateral compression** (*arrow*) causes coronally oriented fractures of the pubic rami and inward buckling of the sacral wing—a "closed book pelvis."

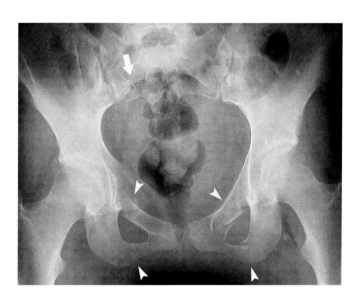

FIGURE 7 Lateral compression injury in this patient causes both anterior and posterior injuries: bilateral pubic rami fractures (*arrowheads*) and a right sacral wing fracture (*arrow*).

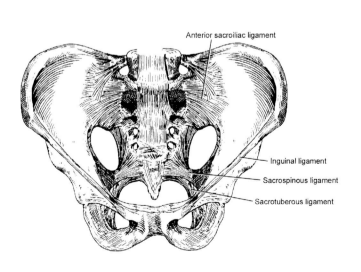

FIGURE 8 The base of the pelvis is supported by two strong ligaments: the sacrospinous (sacrum to ischial spine) and sacrotuberous (sacrum to ischial tuberosity) ligaments.

[From Pansky B: *Review of Gross Anatomy,* 6th ed. McGraw-Hill, 1996]

Patient Outcome

In this patient, the magnitude of her injuries was not fully appreciated until the pelvic fractures were seen on the initial radiograph. Her vital signs remained stable. A Foley catheter was inserted, and the urine obtained was grossly bloody.

A **cystogram** revealed *extraperitoneal bladder rupture* with extravasation of contrast around the bladder neck (Figure 9). An abdominal CT performed after the cystogram did not reveal other injuries (Figure 10).

Her LC injuries were stable and operative fixation was not needed. The patient was allowed out of bed on the fourth hospital day with weight bearing as tolerated on the left and partial weight bearing on the right. The extra-peritoneal bladder laceration was treated with Foley catheter drainage.

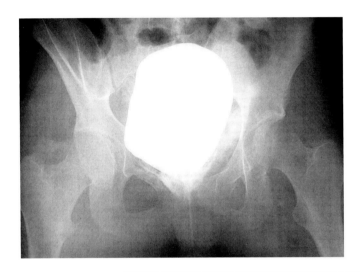
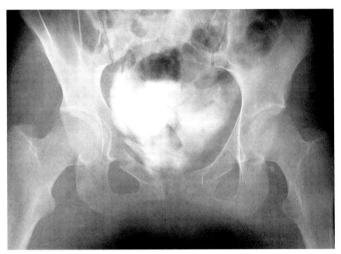

FIGURE 9 Extraperitoneal bladder rupture–Retrograde cystogram.
Retrograde cystogram showing extravasation of contrast into the perivesical tissues. The bladder is otherwise intact. Postvoid radiograph shows contrast in the pelvic soft tissues.

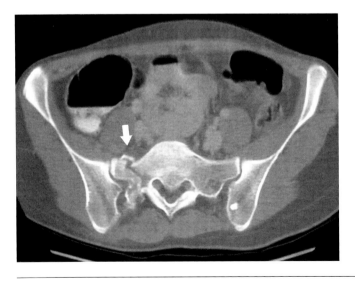
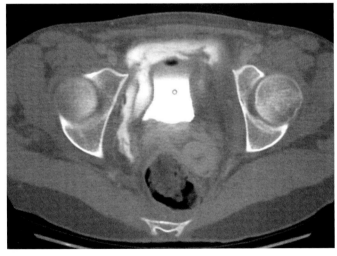

FIGURE 10 Abdominopelvic CT—Patient 6

(*A*) The impacted fracture of the right sacral wing (*arrow*) was confirmed by CT.

(*B*) CT of extraperitoneal bladder rupture.

Extravasated contrast surrounds the bladder. (The tip of the Foley catheter is seen within the bladder.) No contrast was seen within the peritoneal cavity, which excluded an intraperitoneal bladder rupture.

Bladder Injuries Associated With Pelvic Trauma

Urinary bladder injuries associated with blunt trauma include bladder wall contusions, extraperitoneal bladder rupture, and intraperitoneal rupture.

Extraperitoneal rupture is more common (85% of major bladder injuries) and can usually be managed nonoperatively with Foley catheter drainage. **Intraperitoneal bladder ruptures** must be repaired surgically. They occur when the patient's bladder is full at the time of an impact to the lower abdomen. The increased hydraulic pressure ruptures the bladder at its weakest point—the dome. There may only be minor pelvic fractures (Figure 11).

Retrograde cystography was, until recently, the standard diagnostic test. The bladder is filled with 250–300 mL of water-soluble contrast material.

When a urethral injury is suspected, a **retrograde urethrogram** should be performed prior to Foley catheter insertion to avoid converting a partial urethral tear to a complete tear—a particular problem in men. Clinical findings that suggest a urethral injury are blood at urethral meatus, a high-riding prostate, perineal or scrotal hematoma, and a displaced anterior pelvic fracture.

Patients with severe pelvic fractures who may have pelvic arterial bleeding that might require angiography should not undergo cystography prior to angiography because extravasation of bladder contrast into the pelvis will obscure the angiographic images.

With the current widespread use of abdominal CT in the assessment of hemodynamically stable blunt trauma victims, CT protocols have been developed to detect bladder injuries. The bladder must be filled with contrast for CT to be effective. This is not the case with standard abdominal CT. **CT cystography** entails repeating the pelvic CT after a delay of 5–7 minutes to allow filling of the bladder with contrast (the Foley catheter, if present, should be clamped). Alternatively, 250–300 mL of contrast can be instilled into the bladder through the Foley catheter. (Standard abdominal CT is performed 90 seconds after the start of the intravenous contrast bolus and contrast is not present in the urinary tract or bladder.)

The primary indication for cystography (either conventional or CT) is **gross hematuria.** Other criteria for cystography are less well established. These include: displaced anterior pelvic fractures, and intraperitoneal fluid detected on CT that is of water density (possibly urine) rather that blood density.

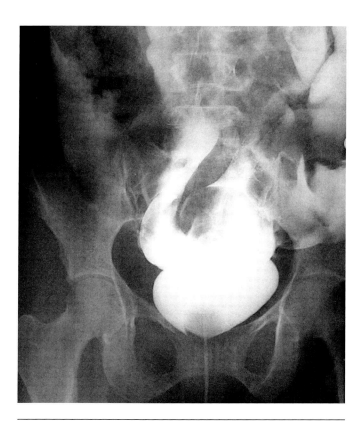

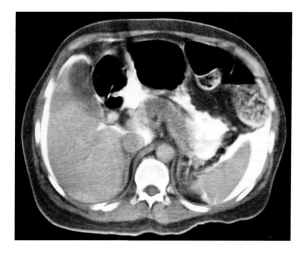

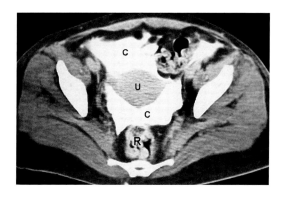

FIGURE 11   Intraperitoneal bladder rupture.

A 36-year-old woman was in a head-on motor vehicle collision. She was hemodynamically stable and had gross hematuria.

Retrograde cystogram and subsequent abdominal CT showed extravasation of contrast throughout the peritoneal cavity.

The patient had only a single nondisplaced pubic ramus fracture, which is typical of intraperitoneal bladder rupture.

C-intraperitoneal contrast in extravasated urine; U-uterus. R-rectum.

Classification of Pelvic Fractures

The spectrum of pelvic injuries ranges widely from minor fractures, which can be treated symptomatically, to severe pelvic disruptions that are associated with life-threatening visceral or vascular injuries. The **Kane classification** system encompasses the entire spectrum of pelvic fractures, which are grouped into four categories (Table 1).

Pelvic ring disruptions (double breaks in the pelvic ring—Kane class 3) have been classified by Young according to the direction of the force of injury (Table 2). LC injuries are the most common. AP compression (APC) and vertical shear (VS) are mechanically unstable because they tear the major pelvic ligaments. They are associated with arterial and other pelvic visceral injuries (Figures 12–14).

TABLE 1

Kane Classification of Pelvic Fractures

1. Fractures of individual bones without disruption of the pelvic ring
    Avulsion fractures (e.g., anterior superior iliac spine); single pubic ramus, iliac wing, transverse sacrum, and coccyx fractures.

2. Single breaks in the pelvic ring
    Ipsilateral pubic rami fractures, symphysis pubis or sacroiliac joint disruption

3. Pelvic ring disruptions–two or more breaks in the pelvic ring

4. Acetabular fractures

TABLE 2

Young Classification of Pelvic Ring Disruptions

Lateral compression (LC)	Pubic rami fractures Compressive posterior injury, e.g., sacral wing fracture
LC-I	Compression of sacroiliac region on the side of impact
LC-II	Compression of sacroiliac region with tear of posterior sacroiliac ligament or iliac wing fracture
LC-III	LC-II on side of impact and external rotation of opposite side ("wind swept pelvis")
AP compression (APC)	Widening of symphysis pubis or pubic rami fractures Widening of posterior elements (unilateral or bilateral)
APC-I	Slight widening of pubic symphysis (0.5–2.5 cm) Posterior elements intact
APC-II	Anterior sacroiliac, sacrotuberous and sacrospinous ligaments disruption. Posterior sacroiliac ligaments intact
APC-III	Posterior sacroiliac ligament disruption plus APC II
Vertical shear (VS)	Vertical displacement at anterior and posterior pelvis
Mixed injury	Combination of above injury patterns

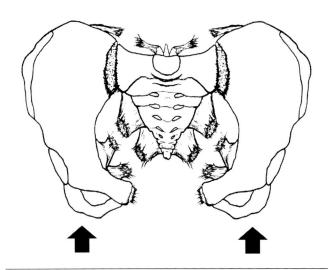

FIGURE 12   APC injury (bilateral). This is called an "open book" pelvis or "sprung" pelvis.
[From Schwartz DT, Reisdorff EJ: *Emergency Radiology.* New York: McGraw-Hill, 2000.]

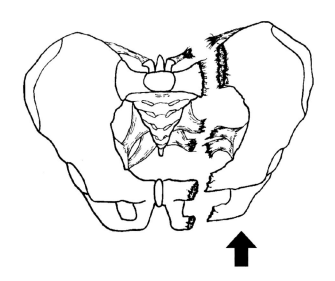

FIGURE 13   Vertical shear injury.

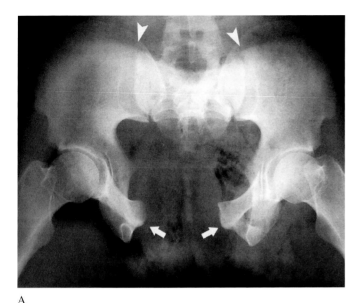

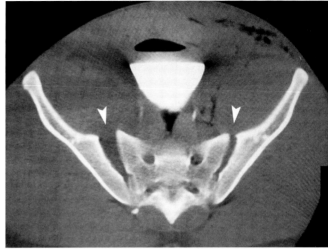

B

A

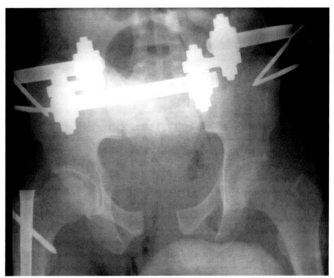

FIGURE 14   APC—Open book pelvis.

A 25-year-old bicyclist was struck by a car. There was marked separation of the pubic symphysis (*arrows*) and both sacroiliac joints (*arrowheads*). The patient was hemodynamically stable.

CT revealed, in addition to the APC pelvic injury, a grade 2 liver laceration, a small hemoperitoneum, and a moderate pelvic hematoma without active arterial extravasation.

The patient has persistent blood loss and required several transfusions over the next 24 hours. He underwent pelvic angiography and embolization of multiple pelvic arterial lacerations. No active bleeding was found in the liver on angiography.

An external fixator was applied to stabilize the pelvis (*C*).

C

Pelvic Fractures in the Hemodynamically Unstable Trauma Victim

In a hemodynamically unstable blunt trauma victim, the immediate objective is to identify and treat major sites of blood loss. In a patient with a markedly displaced pelvic fracture, it must be determined whether hemorrhage is occurring in the pelvis or abdomen. Intra-abdominal exsanguination requires laparotomy to repair the source of bleeding, usually a solid organ or major vascular injury. Exsanguination into the pelvis requires angiography to identify arterial bleeding sites that can be treated with embolization.

First, a **bedside test** (either abdominal sonography or diagnostic peritoneal lavage) is performed to identify intraperitoneal bleeding. If intra-abdominal blood is found, the patient should undergo immediate laparotomy. If intra-abdominal blood is not found, the presumed site of hemorrhage is in the pelvis, and the patient should undergo to pelvic angiography. (A hemodynamically stable patient with a pelvic fracture would undergo CT, which can identify specific organ injuries and sources of bleeding.)

The traditional test to detect intra-abdominal hemorrhage in an unstable patient is **diagnostic peritoneal lavage (DPL)**. A lavage catheter is inserted and then aspirated looking for gross blood. In a patient with a severe pelvic fracture, the catheter should be inserted in a *supraumbilical* location to avoid introducing the catheter into a pelvic hematoma that has extended up the anterior abdominal wall to the umbilicus. DPL using the standard infraumbilical insertion site could introduce the catheter into an abdominal wall hematoma resulting in a false-positive DPL (incorrectly suggesting that blood is present in the abdomen).

DPL is being performed only to look for gross blood and is therefore better termed "diagnostic peritoneal aspiration." The older technique of instilling and then draining one liter of normal saline through the lavage catheter and then performing a cell count looking for greater than 100,000 erythrocytes per mm^3 is outmoded. This dates to the time before CT was routinely used in stable patients with blunt abdominal trauma to decide about performing an exploratory laparotomy.

A newer diagnostic strategy is to perform bedside abdominal sonography looking for intraperitoneal blood–**focused abdominal sonography in trauma (FAST).** Intraperitoneal blood can be detected between the liver and right kidney (Morison pouch), between spleen and left kidney (spleno-renal fossa), or in the pelvis posterior to the bladder (retrovessicle fossa). In addition, a subxyphoid view of the heart is obtained to look for hemopericardium causing tamponade which may be the cause of a patient's hypotension.

One potential shortcoming of FAST is that a pelvic hematoma due to a pelvic fracture can be impossible to distinguish from intraperitoneal blood that has tracked into the pelvis

(retrovessicle fossa). In addition, intraperitoneal urine from a ruptured bladder is indistinguishable from blood on ultrasonography (Jones et al. 2003, Neilsen et al. 2004). Distinguishing between pelvic and intraperitoneal exsanguination in an unstable trauma victim with a displaced pelvic fracture is the most critical role for abdominal sonography in blunt trauma patients. However, pelvic blood due to a pelvic fracture cannot be distinguished from pelvic blood due to an intra-abdominal injury, DPL may therefore still have a role when the FAST shows fluid only in the retrovessicle fossa (Figures 15 and 16) (Tayal et al. 2006, Friese et al. 2007).

During ED management, pelvic fractures should be stabilized to avoid further displacement and reduce the risk of further bleeding. This can be accomplished simply by tying a bed sheet around the patient's pelvis (Simpson et al. 2002). Placement of an external fixator in a widely displaced pelvic fracture can also help reduce pelvic blood loss, although this is time consuming, and should not delay laparotomy or angiography if the patient is hemodynamically unstable.

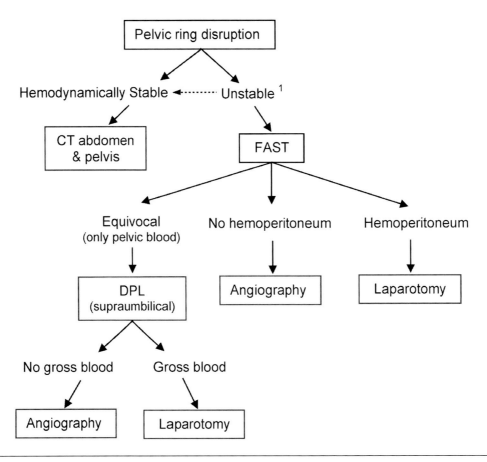

FIGURE 15   Management of a Hemodynamically Unstable Patient with a Pelvic Fracture

The goal is to distinguish intra-abdominal from pelvic exsanguination. Bedside abdominal sonography is performed first. If the results are equivocal, supraumbilical DPL is needed looking for gross intraperitoneal blood. An external fixator can be applied to stablize the pelvis during or after lapartomy, angiography or CT.

1 – Fluid resuscitation, bind pelvis in sheet, and consider thoracic causes of shock (massive hemothorax, tension pneumothorax, cardiac tamponade). If the patient becomes stable, CT can be performed.

FAST – focused abdominal sonography in trauma. DPL - diagnostic peritoneal lavage

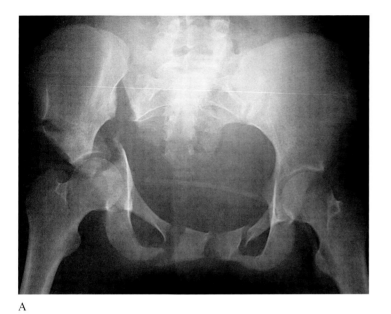

A

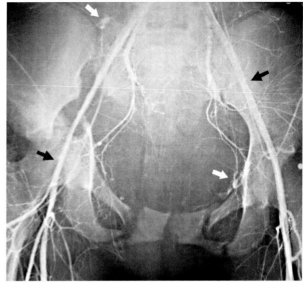

B

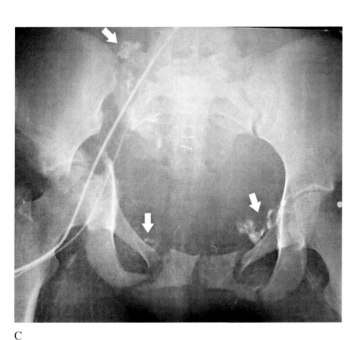

C

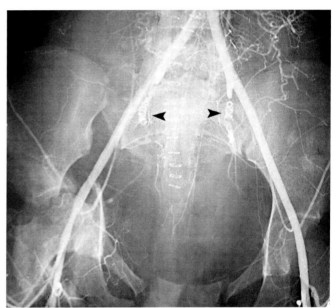

D

FIGURE 16   Mixed pelvic injury—"Pelvic smash."

A complex pelvic fracture occurred in a young woman who fell two stories from a window (*A*). She was hemodynamically unstable on arrival in the ED—blood pressure 80/50 mm Hg and pulse 130 beats/min. Rapid fluid resuscitation was initiated but there was no improvement in her vital signs.

A bedside sonogram found no blood in the hepatorenal fossa (Morison pouch), the splenorenal fossa was poorly visualized, and free-fluid appeared to be present in the pelvis (retrovesicle recess). To confirm the presence or absence of intraperitoneal hemorrhage, a supraumbilical DPL was performed which did not detect gross intraper-itoneal

blood. The pelvis was stabilized by external compression using a bed sheet.

The patient was taken immediately to angiography, which revealed bilateral active arterial extravasation (*white arrows* in *B* and *C*). This was treated with coil embolization of both hypogastric (internal iliac) arteries (*black arrowheads* in *D*). (The external iliac arteries and femoral arteries are indicated by the *black arrows* in *B*).

The patient survived thanks to the timely and accurate diagnosis and treatment of her life-threatening injuries.

SUGGESTED READING

Cisek J, Wilkinson K: Imaging priorities in trauma. In: Schwartz DT, Reisdorff EJ. *Emergency Radiology*. New York McGraw-Hill, 2000.

Demetriades D, Karaiskakis M, Toutouzas K, et al.: Pelvic fractures: Epidemiology and predictors of associated abdominal injuries and outcomes. *J Am Coll Surg* 2002;195:1–10.

Falchi M, Rollandi GA: CT of pelvic fractures. *Europ J Radiol* 2004; 50:96–105.

Guillamondegui OD, Pryor JP, Gracias VH, et al.: Pelvic radiography in blunt trauma resuscitation: A diminishing role. *J Trauma* 2002;53:1043–1047.

Hammel J, Legome E: Pelvic fracture. *J Emerg Med* 2006;30:87–92.

Hustey F, Moettus Wilber L: The pelvis. In: Schwartz DT, Reisdorff EJ. *Emergency. Radiology*. New York McGraw-Hill, 2000.

Niedens BA, Gross EA: Validation of a decision instrument to limit pelvic radiography in blunt trauma. *Acad Emerg Med* 2003;10: 475–476.

Simpson T, Krieg JC, Heuer F; Bottlang M: Stabilization of pelvic ring disruptions with a circumferential sheet. *J Trauma* 2002;52: 158–161.

Stambaugh LE, Blackmore CC: Pelvic ring disruptions in emergency radiology. *Europ J Radiol* 2003;48:71–87.

Theumann NH, Verdon JP, Mouhsine E, et al.: Imaging of pelvic fractures. *Eur Radiol* 2002; 12:1312–1330.

Weishaupt D, Grozaj AM, Willmann JK, et al.: Imaging of abdominal and pelvic injuries. *Eur Radiol* 2002;12:1295–1311.

Cystography and Bladder Injuries

Aihara R, Blansfield JS, Millham FH, et al.: Fracture locations influence the likelihood of rectal and lower urinary tract injuries in patients sustaining pelvic fractures. *J Trauma* 2002;52: 205–209.

Morgan DE, Nallamala LK, Kenney PJ, et al.: CT cystography: radiographic and clinical predictors of bladder rupture. *AJR* 2000; 174:89–95.

Peng MY, Parisky YR, Cornwell EE, et al.: CT cystography versus conventional cystography in evaluation of bladder injury. *AJR* 1999; 173:1269–1272.

Quagliano PV, Delair SM, Malhotra AK: Diagnosis of blunt bladder injury: A prospective comparative study of computed tomography cystography and conventional retrograde cystography. *J Trauma* 2006;61:410–422.

Rehm CG, Mure AJ, O'Malley KF, Ross SE: Blunt traumatic bladder rupture: The role of retrograde cystogram. *Ann Emerg Med* 1991;20:845–847.

Vaccaro JP, Brody JM: CT cystography in the evaluation of major bladder trauma. *RadioGraphics* 2000;20:1373–1381.

Pelvic Hemorrhage

Metz CM, Hak DJ, Goulet JA, Williams D: Pelvic fracture patterns and their corresponding angiographic sources of hemorrhage. *Orthop Clin North Am.* 2004;35:431–437.

Sarin EL, Moore JB, Moore EE, et al.: Pelvic fracture pattern does not always predict the need for urgent embolization. *J Trauma.* 2005;58:973–977.

Yoon W, Kim JK, Jeong YY, et al.: Pelvic arterial hemorrhage in patients with pelvic fractures: Detection with contrast-enhanced CT. *RadioGraphics* 2004;24:1591–1606.

FAST

Blaivas M, DeBehnke D, Phelan MB. Potential errors in the diagnosis of pericardial effusion on trauma ultrasound for penetrating injuries. *Acad Emerg Med* 2000;7:1261–1266.

Bode PJ, Edwards MJ, Kruit MC, van Vugt AB. Sonography in a clinical algorithm for early evaluation of 1671 patients with blunt abdominal trauma. *AJR* 1999; 172:905–911.

Boulanger BR, McLellan BA, Brenneman FD, et al.: Prospective evidence of the superiority of a sonography-based algorithm in the assessment of blunt abdominal injury. *J Trauma* 1999;47:632–637.

Brown MA, Casola G, Sirlin CB, Patel NY, Hoyt DB: Blunt abdominal trauma: Screening US in 2,693 patients. *Radiology* 2001;218: 352–358.

Dolich MO, McKenney MG, Varela JE, et al.: 2576 ultrasounds for blunt abdominal trauma. *J Trauma* 2001;50:108–112.

Farahmand N, Sirlin CB, Brown MA, et al.: Hypotensive patients with blunt abdominal trauma: Performance of screening US. *Radiology* 2005;235:436–443.

Friese, RS, Malekzadeh S, Shafi S, et al: Abdominal ultrasound is an unreliable modality for the detection of hemoperitoneum in patients with pelvic fracture. *J Trauma* 2007;63:97–102.

Jones AE, Mason PE, Tayal VS, Gibbs MA: Sonographic intraperitoneal fluid in patients with pelvic fracture: two cases of traumatic intraperitoneal bladder rupture. *J Emerg Med* 2003;25: 373–377.

Lingawi S, Buckley A: Focused abdominal US in patients with trauma. *Radiology* 2000;217:426–429.

Ma OJ, Mateer JR, Ogata M, et al.: Prospective analysis of a rapid trauma ultrasound examination performed by emergency physicians. *J Trauma* 1995;38:879–858.

Mandavia DP, Joseph A: Bedside echocardiography in chest trauma. *Emerg Med Clin North Am* 2004;22:601–619.

McGahan JP, Richards J, Fogata MLC: Emergency ultrasound in trauma patients. Radiol Clin North Am 2004;42:417–425.

McGahan JP, Richards JR, Gillen M: The focused abdominal sonography for trauma scan: Pearls and pitfalls. *J Ultrasound Med* 2002; 21:789–800.

McKenney M, Lentz K, Nunez D, et al.: Can ultrasound replace diagnostic peritoneal lavage in the assessment of blunt trauma? *J Trauma* 1994;37:439–441.

Miller MT, Pasquale MD, Bromberg WJ, et al.: Not So FAST. *J Trauma* 2003;54:52–60.

Nielsen A, Tayal VS, Jones A, et al.: Accuracy of US in major pelvic injury. *Acad Emerg Med* 2004;11:580.

Plummer D, Brunette D, Asinger R, Ruiz E: Emergency department echocardiography improves outcome in penetrating cardiac injury. *Ann Emerg Med* 1992;21:709–712.

Poletti PA, Kinkel K, Vermeulen B, et al.: Blunt abdominal trauma: Should US be used to detect both free fluid and organ injuries? *Radiology* 2003;227: 95–103.

Rose JS: Ultrasound in abdominal trauma. *Emerg Med Clin North Am* 2004;22:581–599.

Sirlin CB, Brown MA, Andrade-Barreto OA, et al.: Blunt abdominal trauma: Clinical value of negative screening US scans. *Radiology* 2004;230:661–668.

Sirlin CB, Brown MA, Deutsch R, et al.: Screening US for blunt abdominal trauma: Objective predictors of false-negative findings and missed injuries. *Radiology* 2003;229:766–774.

Tayal VS, Nielsen A, Jones AE, et al: Accuracy of trauma ultrasound in major pelvic injury. J Trauma 2006;61:1453–1457.

Lower Extremity: Patient 7

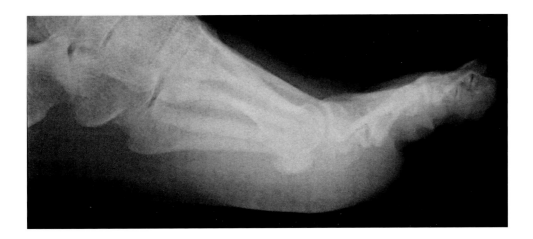

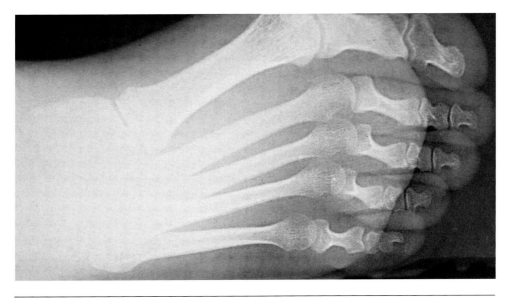

FIGURE 1

A puncture wound to the foot in a young woman

A 20-year-old woman sustained a puncture wound to the sole of her foot from a wooden splinter while walking barefoot on the hardwood floor of her home. She removed the splinter that protruded from her foot. She believed that she had pulled out the entire splinter, but the pain persisted so she came to the ED next morning.

A small puncture wound in the region of the metatarsal heads was cleaned superficially. No foreign body was visible or palpable at the site of the puncture wound. There was tenderness but no swelling, redness, or drainage from the wound. Radiographs were obtained and reported as negative for a foreign body (Figure 1).

The patient was instructed to limit weight bearing, elevate the foot, and to return to the ED if there was persistent or increasing pain, swelling, redness, or fever.

- Do you agree with this management?

THE RADIOLUCENT FOREIGN BODY

Failure to detect retained foreign bodies is a major pitfall in wound management. In one series, 38% of foreign bodies in hand wounds were missed on initial presentation (Anderson et al. 1982). In a large series of ED malpractice litigation claims, wound care cases accounted for 24% of malpractice claims, and failure to detect or treat a foreign body accounted for 44% of wound care litigation cases (Karcz et al. 1990).

Reasons for failure to detect a foreign body include (1) incomplete or inadequate history of the injury; (2) misleading history (e.g., the patient does not recall stepping on a needle); (3) inadequate wound exploration; (4) failure to obtain radiographs; or (5) radiolucency of the foreign body.

The diagnosis of **radiolucent soft tissue foreign bodies** can be a vexing problem. Conventional radiography has a limited ability to distinguish soft tissues and organic wound contaminants such as wood, thorns, soil, and fabrics, which have a high rate of infectious complications. (NB. The terms "radiolucent" and "radiopaque" do not relate to the object itself but are only meaningful when an object's radiographic density is compared to that of its surrounding.)

Imaging Modalities

Conventional radiography will, in a small number of cases, demonstrate a wood foreign body. Therefore, after adequate wound exploration, some authors suggest that radiographs should be obtained when a retained foreign body is suspected. This recommendation is supported by one series of hand wounds in which 15% of wood foreign bodies were visible on the radiographs (Anderson et al. 1982). When the wood is dry, it has the radiographic density of air and might therefore be detectable as a radiolucent foreign body. However, in most studies, wood and other radiolucent foreign bodies were not visible on conventional radiographs (Peterson et al. 2002).

Xerography, mammography, and, more recently, **digital radiography** with image manipulation to enhance edges can potentially make soft tissue foreign bodies appear more conspicuous. However, experimental studies have shown that these techniques do not increase the detection rate of soft tissue foreign bodies over that of conventional radiography. Mammographic equipment provides better soft tissue detail than conventional radiography. Xerography is an antiquated technology that provides edge enhancement but requires an extremely high radiation dose.

Ultrasound imaging depends on differences in acoustic impedance rather than x-ray attenuation and therefore offers distinct advantages in detecting "radiolucent" foreign bodies. Ultrasonography also provides visualization in three dimensions and in real-time—properties that make it useful in localizing foreign bodies and assisting wound exploration. Ultrasonography performs best when the foreign body is located close to the surface and embedded in relatively homogenous tissue (muscle, fat, or inflammatory exudate). In regions of complex anatomy (such as the hand or foot) or where there is overlying or adjacent air, tendon, bone, or fibrotic tissue, sonographic identification of a foreign body can be difficult.

The sensitivity of sonography for soft tissue foreign bodies has a range of 50–95% and specificity of 70–90% depending on the study. Larger quantitative studies have used in vitro models (beef cubes, chicken legs, or cadaver feet or hands) which may not be clinically relevant. Clinical series have included only small numbers of patients that do not allow a precise assessment of sensitivity or specificity.

The sonographic signs of a foreign body are: a bright echogenic focus representing the foreign body itself, an acoustic shadow deep to the foreign body, and a hypoechoic rim surrounding the foreign body due to soft tissue edema and exudate (Figure 2).

A high-frequency ultrasound transducer must be used to provide detailed images of small objects close to the skin surface. In addition, the focal zone of the transducer must be short enough to visualize objects as close as 1–2 cm. A vascular "small objects" transducer is designed for this use. If the transducer has a longer focal zone (e.g., an endovaginal probe), a sonolucent spacer could be placed between the transducer and the skin surface to improve sonographic visualization of the foreign body (Figure 3).

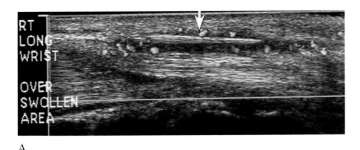

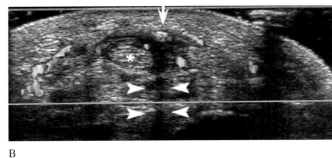

A   B

FIGURE 2   Bamboo splinter detected using a high-resolution, 10-MHz linear array ultrasound transducer.

The patient presented one month after a bamboo splinter pierced the skin of his wrist. He had consulted physicians on two prior occasions.

(A) Longitudinal image of the wrist showing a 2-cm hyperechoic splinter *(arrow)* that is 0.3 cm deep to the skin surface. There is hypoechoic rim surrounding the splinter, which represents edema.

(B) Transverse image showing the splinter with its surrounding hypoechoic rim *(arrow)* and acoustic shadow *(arrowheads)*. The splinter is adjacent to a tendon *(asterisk)*.

[From Lakshmi MV, Gooding GAW: Bamboo splinter: Ultrasound localization. *Emerg Radiol* 2003;10:67–68, with permission.]

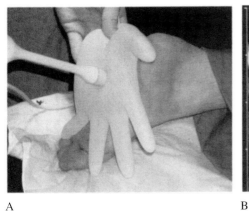

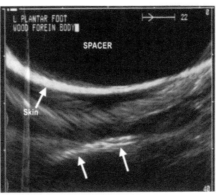

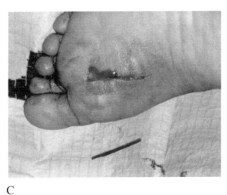

A   B   C

FIGURE 3   Use of an endovaginal ultrasound transducer and an improvised spacer to detect a wood foreign body.

A 13-year-old boy sustained a puncture wound to the sole of his foot while running on a wood floor. A small piece of wood was removed but the patient had a persistent foreign body sensation.

(A) Endovaginal ultrasound transducer and water-filled latex glove spacer.

(B) Ultrasound image of the foreign body *(unlabeled white arrows)*.

(C) Patient's foot after removal of the foreign body, showing the incision and splinter.

[From Dean AJ, Gronczewski CA, Costantino TG: Technique for emergency medicine bedside ultrasound identification of a radiolucent foreign body. *J Emerg Med* 2003;24:303–308, with permission.]

CT is able to distinguish different soft tissue densities with far greater sensitivity than conventional radiography and is therefore useful in detecting "radiolucent" soft tissue foreign bodies. In addition, CT is able to localize objects in three dimensions and can guide surgical removal of an embedded object. CT can also detect more deeply embedded foreign bodies that are beyond the range of ultrasonography. Most reported cases that used CT have been in patients with delayed clinical presentations.

There are several **potential sources of error with CT**. First, the foreign body might be mistaken for an anatomical structure such as a tendon. This can be avoided if both the normal and injured extremity are included in each CT image. Second, if the foreign body has a radiographic density similar to soft tissue, even CT may be unable to distinguish a foreign body from normal structures. Third, if the foreign body is small, such as a piece of rubber from the sole of a tennis shoe or a thread, and has similar radiopacity to the surrounding tissue, CT may fail to detect the foreign material. Detection of very small foreign bodies can be improved using thin CT slices (1.5–3 mm).

MRI has been shown in several case reports to be useful in detecting soft tissue foreign bodies. MRI has generally been used for patients with chronic infection or a soft tissue mass (Peterson et al. 2002).

Patient Outcome

Two days after her initial ED visit, the patient returned with worsening pain and marked swelling of her foot involving both the plantar and dorsal surfaces. A CT was obtained revealing a radiopaque foreign body with surrounding inflammatory reaction that extended along the flexor tendon of the

fourth toe. At the time the CT was performed, a marker was placed on the skin overlying the foreign body. This was used as a guide to locate the foreign body during its surgical removal. A 4.4-cm long wooden splinter was removed and the wound healed uneventfully (Figure 4).

Management of Patients Suspected of Having Soft Tissue Foreign Bodies

In reviewing the **management** of this patient, two issues arise. First, some authors recommend that all plantar puncture wounds be extended, "cored-out," and probed with a blunt metal instrument to determine the depth of penetration, as well as the possible presence of a foreign body. However, this procedure is controversial, as its benefits are unproven, and it is relatively invasive and destructive to normal tissues.

A second issue is whether CT or sonography should have been obtained at the time of the patient's initial ED visit. Either test could have provided an earlier diagnosis and reduced the potential for infection. Because the possibility of a retained foreign body was deemed unlikely on the first presentation, the clinical strategy was to warn the patient about the possibility of a retained foreign body and to stress the importance of returning if signs of infection developed.

Clinical clues to the presence of a retained foreign body are (1) a history suspicious for probable retained material, as in this patient; (2) a high-risk mechanism of injury (stepping on a nail that penetrated to sole of a shoe); (3) pain out of proportion to the apparent size of the wound; (4) pain on the dorsum of the foot or otherwise remote from the wound; and (5) signs of infection. In such cases, imaging evaluation with CT, sonography or MRI, and possibly wound exploration are indicated.

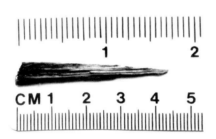

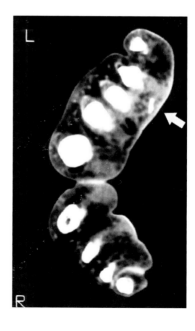

FIGURE 4 Splinter removed from patient's foot.

CT showing the radiopaque splinter in the plantar surface of the left foot (*arrow*). Note the adjacent inflammatory exudate (gray) and diffuse swelling of the left foot in comparison to the right foot.

(Note: the right foot is positioned with the little toe out of this CT slice.)

SUGGESTED READING

Anderson MA, Newmeyer WL, Kilgore ES: Diagnosis and treatment of retained foreign bodies in the hand. *Am J Surg* 1982;144:63–67.

Bodne D, Quinn SF, Cochran CF: Imaging foreign glass and wooden bodies of the extremities with CT and MRI. *J Comput Assist Tomogr* 1988;12:608–611.

Boyse TD, Fessell DP, Jacobson JA, et al.: US of soft-tissue foreign bodies and associated complications with surgical correlation. *RadioGraphics* 2001;21:1251–1256. Clinical cases describing US appearance.

Chisholm CD, Schlesser JF: Plantar puncture wounds: Controversies and treatment recommendations. *Ann Emerg Med* 1989;18: 1352–1357.

Dean AJ, Gronczewski CA, Costantino TG: Technique for emergency medicine bedside ultrasound identification of a radiolucent foreign body. *J Emerg Med* 2003:24:303–308.

DePue S, Bokhari J: A comparison of the accuracy of helical CT, scout CT, digital radiography, plain film radiography, fluorography and film-screen mammography for the diagnosis of radiolucent foreign bodies using a chicken leg model (abstract). *Acad Emerg Med* 2003;10:541–542.

Dewitz A, Frazee BW: Soft tissue applications. In: Ma OJ, Mateer JR: *Emergency Ultrasound.* McGraw-Hill, 2003.

Flom LL, Ellis GL: Radiologic evaluation of foreign bodies. *Emerg Med Clin North Am* 1992;10:163–177.

Graham DD: Ultrasound in the emergency department: Detection of wooden foreign bodies in the soft tissues. *J Emerg Med* 2002;22: 75–79.

Horton KL, Jacobson JA, Powell A, Fessell DP, Hayes CW: Sonography and radiography of soft-tissue foreign bodies. *AJR* 2001; 176:1155–1159. Cadaver heal; glass, wood, metal foreign bodies studied.

Jacobson JA, Powell A, Craig JG, Bouffard JA, van Holsbeck MT: Wooden foreign bodies in soft tissue: Detection at US. *Radiology* 1998;206:45–48. In vitro cadaver feet—sensitivity 90%, specificity 95%.

Karcz A, et al.: Preventability of malpractice claims in emergency medicine: A closed claims study. *Ann Emerg Med* 1990;19: 865–873.

Lakshmi MV, Gooding GAW: Bamboo splinter: Ultrasound localization. *Emerg Radiol* 2003;10:67–68.

Lammers RL, Magill T: Detection and management of foreign bodies in soft tissue. *Emerg Med Clin North Am* 1992;10:767–781.

Lammers RL: Soft tissue foreign bodies. *Ann Emerg Med* 1988;17: 1336–1347.

Mizel MS, Steinmetz ND, Trepman E: Detection of wooden foreign bodies in muscle tissue: experimental comparison of computed tomography, magnetic resonance imaging and ultrasonography. *Foot Ankle Int* 1994;15:437–443.

Peterson JJ, Bancroft LW, Kransdorf MJ: Wooden foreign bodies: Imaging appearance. *AJR* 2002;178:557–562. Twelve cases imaged using radiography, *MRI*: 8, US: 9, CT: 3.

Verdile VP, Freed HA, Gerard J: Puncture wounds to the foot. *J Emerg Med* 1989;7:193–199.

SECTION V

CERVICAL SPINE RADIOLOGY

The diagnosis of cervical spine injuries presents a challenge in emergency practice. The anatomy of the cervical spine is complex, the spectrum of injuries is broad, and the consequences of injury, particularly spinal cord injury, can be devastating. Most serious cervical spine injuries are caused by high-energy forces. However, unstable injuries can occur following relatively minor trauma, such as a fall from a standing position, particularly in the elderly.

Although most cervical spine fractures are radiographically obvious, 10% have subtle radiographic manifestations or even normal radiographs (Mower et al. 2001). Patients at high risk of injury (e.g., severe trauma victims) and those with signs of neurologic injury require imaging with CT and possibly MRI (see Appendix).

WHEN TO ORDER CERVICAL SPINE RADIOGRAPHS

Because of the potentially serious consequences of a missed injury, cervical spine radiographs are ordered whenever there is a chance of an injury, even if the risk is small. In fact, fewer than 3% of cervical spine radiographs will reveal injuries.

Two groups of investigators have developed clinical decision rules with the aim of reducing the number of cervical spine radiographs ordered, as well as to objectively validate clinical criteria useful in the decision to order radiographs.

NEXUS LOW-RISK CRITERIA The National Emergency X-Radiography Utilization Study Group developed the NEXUS Low-Risk Criteria to guide the clinician in "clearing" the cervical spine without radiography (Table 1) (Hoffman et al. 2000). In prior empirically derived clinical practice, the "absence of neck pain" was the major criterion used to clinically clear the cervical spine. With the NEXUS rule, the more selective criterion "no midline cervical tenderness" is employed instead.

The concept of the NEXUS criteria is that in the absence of factors that interfere with pain perception, patients without midline cervical tenderness do not need radiography. This holds true irrespective of the mechanism of injury or the age of the patient.

The NEXUS criteria are not explicitly defined, but instead depend on the judgment of the clinician. Although this creates imprecision, it avoids the complexity of a list of items defining each criterion. Because of the lack of exact definitions, the NEXUS criteria could be applied differently by different clinicians. The reduction in radiography could thereby vary considerably.

The safety of using the NEXUS rule was prospectively validated in a large multicenter trial that included 34,069 patients. A total of 818 patients had injuries (2.4%), of which 578 (71%) were clinically significant. The decision rule identified all but 8 of the 818 injured patients and all but 2 of the clinically significant injuries. The sensitivity of the rule for all injuries was 99.0% (lower 95% confidence interval [CI]: 98.0%). For clinically significant injuries, the sensitivity was 99.6% (lower CI: 98.6%).

Use of the NEXUS criteria would have reduced the number of radiographs by 12.6% (4309 patients out of 34,069). Although this was a more modest reduction than in the pilot study (1992), which showed a 37% reduction in radiography, it still represents significant savings in cost, time, and radiation exposure because of the large number of cervical spine radiographs obtained in emergency practice. Nonetheless, even when using the NEXUS criteria, the proportion of positive radiographs is still very small (2.8% using the NEXUS criteria versus 2.4% without), i.e., over 97% of radiographs will still be negative.

Now that CT is widely used as the initial imaging test in high-risk patients, the frequency that injuries will be found on cervical spine radiography will be even lower (<1%) (Hanson et al. AJR 2000). Selective use of radiography in such patients is warranted.

TABLE 1

NEXUS Low-Risk Criteria

Cervical spine radiography can be omitted when a patient exhibits *all* of the following:

1. No posterior midline cervical tenderness

2. Normal level of alertness

3. No evidence of intoxication

4. No focal neurologic deficit

5. No painful distracting injuries

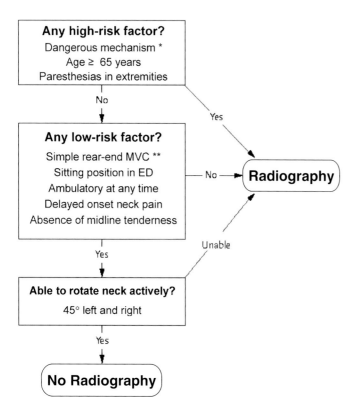

* – Dangerous mechanism of injury:
    Motor vehicle collision (MVC) at high speed (>100 Km/h), rollover, ejection from vehicle
    Fall from > 3 ft or 5 stairs
    Axial load to head (diving)
    Collision involving a motorized recreational vehicle
    Bicycle collision

** – Simple rear–end MVC excludes: being pushed into oncoming traffic, hit by a bus or large truck, rollover, hit by a high speed vehicle.

Inclusion Criteria: Adults with acute trauma to the head or neck who are both alert (Glasgow Coma Scale score of 15) and in stable condition (systolic blood pressure > 90 and respiratory rate 10–24/min) and who either have neck pain or no neck pain but all of the following three features: a visible injury above the clavicles, are nonambulatory, and a dangerous mechanism of injury.

Exclusion criteria: altered mental status (GCS score < 15), unstable vital signs, age < 16 years, acute paralysis, known vertebral disease, previous cervical spine surgery, non-trauma cases.

FIGURE 1   The Canadian Cervical Spine Rule—CCR.

For alert (CGS=15) and stable trauma patients where cervical spine injury is a concern

[From Stiell IG, Grimshaw J, Wells GA, et al.: A matched-pair cluster design study protocol to evaluate implementation of the Canadian C-spine rule in hospital emergency departments: Phase III. Implementation Science 2007, 2:4 doi:10.1186/1748-5908-2-4. © 2007 Stiell et al.]

CANADIAN CERVICAL SPINE RULE   A second group of investigators have developed another clinical decision instrument for cervical spine radiography: the **Canadian Cervical Spine Rule** (CCR) (Stiell et al. 2001 and 2003).

The CCR entails **three steps** (Figure 1): (1) if any one of three **high-risk features** is present (dangerous mechanism of injury, age ≥ 65 years, or paresthesias), cervical spine radiography should be performed; (2) if any one of five **low-risk features** is present, it is safe to check neck rotation; and (3) if the patient is able to actively **rotate his or her neck** 45° to the left and right, cervical spine radiography can be omitted. If no low-risk features are present or if the patient is unable to rotate his or her neck, cervical spine radiography is needed. Neck rotation is therefore always tested before the decision to omit cervical spine radiography is made.

The CCR is relatively complex: three steps including nine individual items. Nine additional features are given which describe mechanisms of injury.

Mechanism of injury is a key criterion in the CCR; both high-risk and low-risk features are specified. **Age ≥ 65 years** is also a high-risk factor for injury. The rationale is that fractures can occur in elderly patients who have sustained less severe mechanisms of injury. Interestingly, the NEXUS criteria were found to be effective in the elderly, despite the frequency of injury being twice as high in the elderly compared to younger patients (Touger et al. 2002).

In the Canadian rule, the presence of midline **neck tenderness** does not mandate radiography, so long as another low-risk factor is present and the patient is able to perform neck rotation. This should reduce the need for cervical spine radiography (make the decision rule more specific) since not all patients with neck tenderness need radiography. In addition, the Canadian rule is potentially more sensitive than the NEXUS criteria because certain injures, e.g., odontoid fractures, may not cause midline neck tenderness, but are likely to limit neck mobility and thereby meet Canadian criteria for radiography. Nonetheless, the NEXUS rule has demonstrated an exceedingly high sensitivity in a large prospective trial.

SUMMARY   Both clinical decision rules have been carefully studied and validated in large numbers of patients and either rule can be used confidently. The NEXUS rule is simpler but the criteria depend more on the subjective assessment of the clinician. Although this does not result in decreased sensitivity, it could have the effect of reducing specificity, i.e., less reduction in radiography. In addition, only one feature is provided to clinically clear the cervical spine, namely, the absence of midline neck tenderness. The Canadian rule is more complex but provides more factors to consider in deciding to obtain or omit radiography, such as the mechanism of injury, various low-risk features, and the testing of neck mobility.

One possible approach would be to use portions of each rule depending on the clinical circumstances. For instance, the Canadian rule does not allow clinical clearance of any patients older than 65 years, whereas the NEXUS rule does and could be applied to older patients, so long as there is an appreciation of the increased incidence of cervical spine fractures in the elderly, particularly persons older than 75 years (Lomoschitz et al. 2002). In patients who seem at low risk of injury, but do have mild midline neck tenderness, the Canadian criteria could be applied, which could allow clinical clearance in some cases.

Finally, testing of neck mobility (both rotation and flexion) would be prudent before a patient is cleared of cervical spine injury both when radiographs are not being obtained and when radiography is obtained and is normal so as not to miss an occult injury that might only be evident when there is excessive pain with motion of the neck (D'Costa 2005).

Computed Tomography

With the advent of rapid helical CT, particularly multidetector CT (MDCT) with sagittal and coronal reformatted images, some trauma centers use CT as the initial test in high-risk major trauma victims (see Appendix) (Hanson et al. 2000, Blackmore 2003). CT has greater sensitivity compared to conventional radiography at detecting injuries and requires little additional time when the patient is also undergoing CT of the head or abdomen.

Formerly, CT was obtained *after* conventional radiography in patients with cervical spine fractures to fully define the anatomy of the injury. CT also had a role when the radiographs are inadequate (usually at the cervicocranium or cervicothoracic junction) or to clarify suspicious but questionable radiographic findings.

Certain injuries can be missed on axial CT images. These include fractures that are in a transverse plane (e.g., fractures through the base of the dens), mild vertebral body wedge compression fractures, and mild vertebral malalignment. These injuries can be detected using sagittal and coronal reformatted images.

Hanson et al. (AJR 2000) studied the use of CT in cervical spine imaging. In a prospective study of 4146 patients, 11% (462) had screening CT. Nine percent of the patients undergoing CT had cervical spine injuries, which is cost-effective. On the other hand, among the 3684 patients judged at low-risk and therefore having initial cervical spine radiography, only 7 (0.2%) had injuries. More selective use of radiography in such patients is warranted.

MRI

MRI is the test of choice for imaging soft tissue injuries of the cervical spine, although it is not generally indicated in the emergency department. MRI can directly visualize: (1) spinal cord injury, (2) ligamentous injury, (3) cervical disk herniation, and (4) vertebral artery injury.

The principal indication for MRI is a neurological deficit referable to the spinal cord. MRI can distinguish spinal cord hemorrhage from edema, of which hemorrhage has a worse prognosis. MRI can also detect intervertebral disk herniation that is causing spinal cord compression which may require surgical intervention. Finally, MRI is useful in obtunded major trauma victims who cannot be clinically evaluated for spinal cord or ligamentous injuries, although the incidence of such injuries is low (Hogan et al. 2005).

CERVICAL SPINE ANATOMY

There are two anatomically distinct regions of the cervical spine: the **cervicocranium** (C1 and C2) and the **lower cervical spine** (C3 to C7).

The *atlas* (C1) is an osseus ring with two lateral masses that articulate superiorly with the occipital condyles and inferiorly with the *axis* (C2) (Figure 2). C1 has no vertebral body. The *odontoid process* (the dens) projects superiorly from the C2 vertebral body and articulates with the anterior portion of C1. This articulation is maintained by the *transverse atlantal ligament*.

Each of the **lower cervical vertebrae** (C3 to C7) consists of a vertebral body, two lateral masses with superior and inferior articular facets, pedicles (connect the lateral masses to the vertebral body), paired laminae, and a spinous process (Figure 3).

The spinal cord is located within the *vertebral canal* that is made up by the posterior aspect of the vertebral body, the pedicles, and the laminae. The *transverse processes* project laterally from the pedicles. The transverse processes form U-shaped channels for the spinal nerve roots and have a perforation for the vertebral artery.

The *vertebral bodies* are joined together by the fibrocartilaginous *intervertebral discs*. The *lateral masses* articulate via the facet joints and form lateral supportive columns of the cervical spine.

Vertebral alignment is maintained by **four strong ligaments**: the anterior longitudinal ligament, the posterior longitudinal ligament, the ligamentum flavum, and the interspinous ligament (Figure 4).

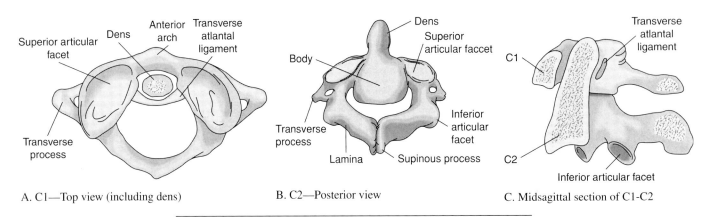

A. C1—Top view (including dens)   B. C2—Posterior view   C. Midsagittal section of C1-C2

FIGURE 2   Anatomy of the cervicocranium.

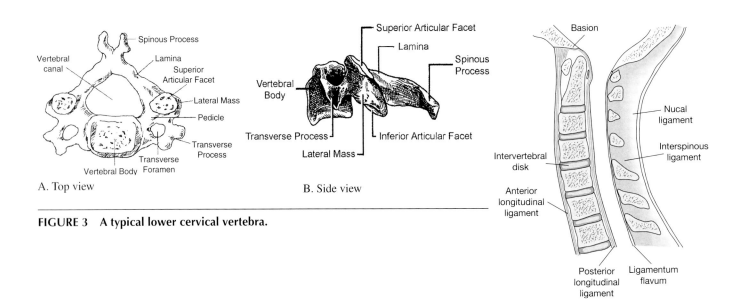

A. Top view   B. Side view

FIGURE 3   A typical lower cervical vertebra.

FIGURE 4   Ligaments of the cervical spine.

[Adapted from Galli et al: *Emergency Orthopedics: The Spine.* McGraw-Hill, 1989, with permission.]

CERVICAL SPINE RADIOGRAPHY

The standard cervical spine radiographic series includes three views: (1) the **lateral view,** (2) the **open mouth view** (an AP view of the cervicocranium), and (3) the **AP view** of the lower cervical spine. In the trauma patient, a **cross-table lateral view** is performed with the patient supine and the neck immobilized.

The **lateral view** must show all seven cervical vertebrae as well as the superior surface of the first thoracic vertebra (cervicothoracic junction). If C7 is not visualized, the lateral view should be repeated with greater traction applied to the patient's arms (pulling inferiorly). If this is not successful, a **swimmer's view** can be obtained in patients at low risk for a spinal injury. For this view, the patient is positioned with one arm fully abducted above the patient's head and the x-ray beam directed toward the axilla and lower cervical spine. The swimmer's view usually shows alignment of the cervicothoracic vertebral bodies, but does not provide complete visualization of the C7 vertebra. CT of the cervicothoracic junction should be performed in patients at high risk for injury.

The lateral view reveals approximately 85% of cervical spine injuries and should therefore never be used alone to "clear" the cervical spine. Most of the remaining 15% of injuries are detected on the open mouth view. A small number of injuries are visible only on the AP view.

In some centers, **oblique views** are included in the cervical spine series. However, the frequency that oblique views detect an injury not seen on the three standard views is very low and, in many institutions, oblique views are no longer obtained routinely in the trauma patient. Oblique views were used in the past to better define certain injuries seen on the three standard views, for example, lateral mass fractures, pedicle or laminar fractures, and unilateral facet dislocations. The use of oblique views in the trauma patient has been largely supplanted by CT.

How Accurate are Cervical Spine Radiographs?

Analysis of the radiographs of the 818 patients with cervical spine injuries in the NEXUS study provides information about the diagnostic sensitivity of cervical spine radiography (Mower et al. 2001). A complete three-view radiographic series was obtained in 570 patients with cervical spine injuries. (The other patients had a lateral view only, followed by CT or MRI.)

Sixty patients (10.5%) had "occult" cervical spine injures. Subtle but suggestive radiographic findings were seen in 37 patients (6.5%) and 23 patients (4.1%) had negative radiographs (three of whom had potentially unstable cervical spine injuries). An additional 24 patients had spinal cord injury without radiographic abnormality (SCIWORA). The overall *sensitivity* of cervical spine radiography (ability to detect at least one lesion in an injured patient) was therefore 89%.

The implications of these observations are: (1) subtle radiographic signs such as prevertebral soft tissue swelling must be recognized in order to avoid missing injuries; and (2) a negative three-view radiographic series does not fully exclude an injury, particularly in patients at high risk due to severe mechanisms of injury. Cervical spine immobilization must therefore be maintained in high-risk patients despite negative initial radiographs until further definitive evaluation (clinical and radiologic) can be accomplished. In current practics, however, such patients would have CT in the ED (when it is readily available), which can detect nearly all injuries.

HOW TO READ CERVICAL SPINE RADIOGRAPHS

Interpretation of cervical spine radiographs entails both systematic and targeted approaches that are based on knowledge of normal radiographic anatomy and common injury patterns. The **systematic approach** provides a stepwise review of important radiographic landmarks. Such a systematic approach is needed because of the anatomical complexity of the cervical spine and relatively low frequency of injuries. A **targeted approach** involves identification of specific injury patterns and enables accurate and efficient radiograph interpretation.

Systematic Approach

This is a *two step process*. First, the overall appearance of the cervical spine is reviewed. Second, each individual vertebra is then examined to avoid missing more subtle injuries (Table 2).

Overall Review   This uses an **ABCS** mnemonic device—assessing the **adequacy** of the radiograph, vertebral **alignment**, the **bones** (for fractures or deformity), **cartilage** (spaces between adjacent vertebral bodies and between the spinous processes), and prevertebral **soft tissues** (especially important for the cervicocranium).

ADEQUACY   A properly performed lateral radiograph demonstrates all seven cervical vertebrae and the C7-T1 interface (see Figure 6 on p. 369). It is preferable to count each of the vertebrae to be certain that all seven are visible, rather than simply on the overall visual appearance. Second, when the patient is in a true lateral position without rotation, the left and right lateral masses of each vertebra are superimposed.

ALIGNMENT   There are **four curves** of alignment: the *anterior vertebral body line* maintained by the anterior longitudinal ligament, the *posterior vertebral body line* maintained by the posterior longitudinal ligament, the *spinolaminar line* maintained by the ligamentum flavum, and the *tips of the spinous processes*. The posterior vertebral body line is the most accurate way to assess alignment. The cervical spine normally has a smooth lordotic curvature. *Straightening* is common in cross-table lateral radiographs because the patient is supine and the neck is immobilized. It is therefore not a useful sign of injury.

PREVERTEBRAL SOFT TISSUES   Swelling of the prevertebral (retropharyngeal) soft tissues is an important clue to cervical injuries, particularly of the cervicocranium. Studies of normal radiographs in uninjured patients have established the upper limits of normal at various levels of the cervical spine (see diagram in Table 2). A recent analysis has shown that the contour of the cervicocranial soft tissues is a more sensitive indicator of injury than are measurements at discrete levels (Harris 2001). Nonetheless, injuries may be present without prevertebral soft tissue swelling, and therefore the absence of swelling does not exclude an injury. In the lower cervical spine, the esophagus is interposed within the prevertebral soft tissues and swelling is rarely seen with spinal injuries.

Detailed Examination   In the second step of the systematic approach, **each individual vertebra** is inspected (see Figure 7 on p. 369). Important radiographic landmarks are identified for the **cervicocranium** (Table 3) and for each of the **lower cervical vertebrae** (Table 4).

Targeted Approach

In the targeted approach, typical injury patterns are identified (see Tables 7 and 8 on p. 367). This is followed by a search for injuries that can easily be missed. Anatomical variants and other radiographic findings that can mimic injuries must also be recognized.

AP and Open Mouth Views

A similar analysis is performed for the **open mouth view** (Table 5) and the **AP view** (Table 6).

TABLE 2

How to Read a Lateral Cervical Spine Radiograph

Systematic approach (two steps): (1) Overall review (ABCS); then (2) examine each individual vertebra.

Targeted approach: Look for specific injury patterns and easily missed injuries (see Tables 7 and 8).

Overall Review—ABCS

    Adequacy
        All 7 vertebrae seen
        No rotation (lateral masses superimposed)

    Alignment
        Four smooth lordotic curves (*drawing*)

    Bones
        Fractures of vertebral bodies, lateral masses,
        laminae, spinous processes

    Cartilage
        Intervertebral disk spaces
        Interspinous process distances

    Soft tissues
        Prevertebral soft tissues (especially C1-C3)
        (upper limits of normal are shown)

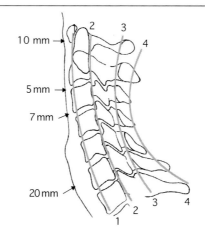

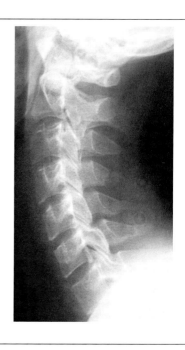

Four Curves of Alignment
1. Anterior vertebral body line
2. Posterior vertebral body line
3. Spinolaminar line
4. Tips of spinous processes

Prevertebral soft tissues (*arrows*)

TABLE 3

Radiographic Landmarks of the Cervicocranium

Basion-dental interval (<12 mm)
Predental space (<3 mm)
C1 posterior arch
Base of dens
"Ring of C2"
C2 vertebral body
C2 posterior arch
Posterior cervical line:
    Spinolaminar junctions of C1-2-3
    align in straight line (within 2 mm)
Prevertebral soft tissues:
    Follow contour of vertebrae

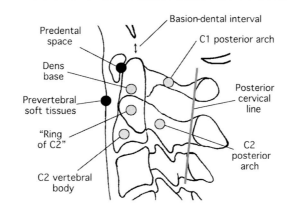

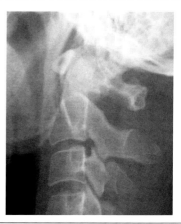

TABLE 4

Radiographic Landmarks of the Lower Cervical Spine

Examine each individual vertebra:
    Vertebral body
    Alignment with adjacent vertebrae
    Intervertebral disk spaces
    Lateral masses and facet joints
    Laminae
    Alignment of spinolaminar junctions
    Spinous process
    Interspinous process spaces

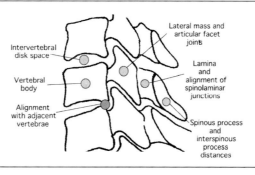

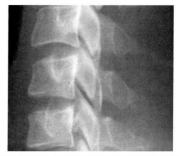

TABLE 5

The Open Mouth View

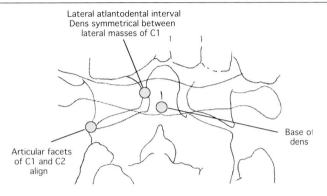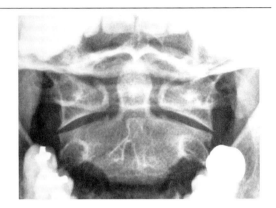

Useful for: fractures of the dens, Jefferson burst fractures of C1, and C1 lateral mass fractures.

Adequacy:

　Lack of head tilt or rotation

　Limited overlap of teeth and base of skull on dens

Radiographic landmarks:

　Base of dens

　Dens symmetrical between lateral masses of C1

　Articular surfaces of C1 and C2 aligned

TABLE 6

The AP View

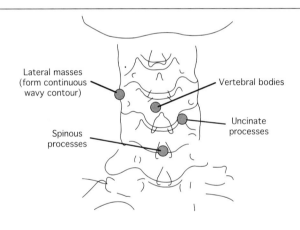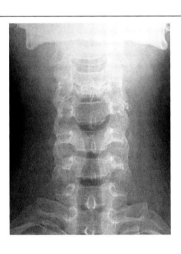

Useful for:

　Vertebral body fractures

　Pedicolaminar and lateral mass (pillar) fractures

　Rotation injuries (unilateral facet dislocation)

　Spinous process fractures (C7)

Radiographic landmarks:

　Lateral masses form continuous wavy line

　Vertebral bodies and uncinate processes intact

　Intervertebral disk spaces uniform

　Spinous processes aligned and evenly spaced

CLASSIFICATION OF CERVICAL SPINE INJURIES

The two regions of the cervical spine—the cervicocranium and the lower cervical spine—sustain different types of injuries and are best described using different injury classification schemes.

　Cervicocranial injuries are classified anatomically based on the particular vertebra involved (Table 7).

　Lower cervical spine injuries are classified by their mechanism of injury (Table 8, Figure 5). Lower cervical spine injuries are divided between those due to flexion and those due to extension. However, a better understanding of these injuries is achieved by considering associated forces of distraction (the head thrown forward or backward) or compression (axial loading). The four main mechanisms of injury are *distractive-flexion*, *compressive-flexion*, *distractive-extension*, and *compressive-extension*. To these four categories are added *isolated axial compression* and *lateral bending*. This mechanistic classification scheme provides an understanding of the forces responsible for a given injury, as well as the associated ligamentous and neurological injuries.

TABLE 7

Cervicocranial Injuries—Anatomical Classification

Occiput	Occipitoatlantal dissociation—wide basion-dental interval. Occipital condyle fracture (CT only)
C1	Jefferson burst fracture—axial compression Isolated posterior arch fracture. Anterior arch avulsion fracture.
Dens	Type II—"high" (through base of dens) (common) Type III—"low" (into C2 vertebral body)
C2	Hangman fracture ("traumatic spondylolisthesis")—bilateral posterior arch fractures C2 vertebral body fractures—compression, hyperextension "teardrop"

TABLE 8

Lower Cervical Spine Injuries—Classified by Mechanism of Injury (Six Types)

Bones fail in compression, ligaments fail in distraction.

Distractive-flexion (35%)—Posterior ligament tear
Hyperflexion sprain ("anterior subluxation"). Bilateral "perched" facets.
Bilateral facet dislocation (causes *complete cord injury*) = bilateral interfacetal dislocation.
Unilateral facet dislocation (with rotational component) (causes *nerve root injury*).

Compressive-flexion (20%)—Anterior fracture (vertebral body)
Wedge compression fracture.
Flexion teardrop (causes *anterior cord syndrome* due to retrolisthesis of the vertebral body into the anterior
portion of the spinal canal).

Axial compression (10%)
Vertebral body burst fracture.

Distractive-extension (6%)—Anterior ligament tear
(Causes *central cord syndrome* due to compression of the spinal cord within the spinal canal).
Hyperextension sprain. Hyperextension teardrop.

Compressive-extension (25%)—Posterior fracture (pedicles, lateral masses, laminae)
Unilateral or bilateral fractures of the lamina, lateral masses (pillar fractures) or spinous process.
Pedicolaminar fractures result in separation of the lateral mass from the vertebra. When bilateral, there may
be anterolisthesis of the vertebral body, called "hyperextension fracture-dislocation."

Lateral bending (3%) usually combined with other injuries
Uncinate process fracture. Unilateral vertebral body or posterior element fracture.

Clay shoveler's fracture—Isolated spinous process fracture of C7 (or C6 or T1)
Pull by shoulder muscles (scapular rhomboid muscle) or direct impact to spinous process

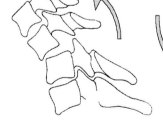

Distractive-Flexion

Flexion sprain
Bilateral "perched" facets
Bilateral facet dislocatior

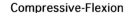

Compressive-Flexion

Wedge compression fracture
Flexion "teardrop"

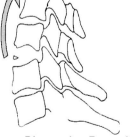

Distractive-Extension

Extension sprain
Extension "teardrop"
Extension dislocation

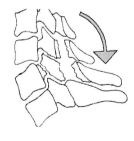

Compressive-Extension

Laminar fracture
Pillar fracture
Pedicolaminar fracture
Hyperextension fx-disloc.

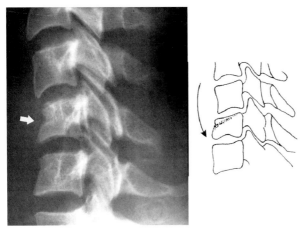

Wedge compression fracture—Mild compressive-flexion

There is buckling of the anterior vertebral body cortex (*arrow*) and loss of anterior vertebral body height

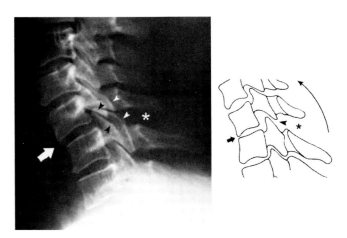

Flexion sprain—Mild distractive-flexion

Posterior ligament tear causes fanning of the spinous processes (*asterisk*), subluxation of the facet joints (*arrowheads*), and anterior slippage and angulation of the vertebral body (*arrow*)

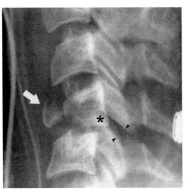
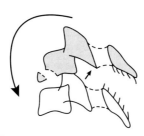

Flexion teardrop—Severe compressive-flexion

Anterior compression on the vertebral body creates a triangular fracture fragment (*arrow*) and retropulsion of the posterior portion of the vertebral body into the spinal canal (*asterisk*), as well as separation of the facet joints (*arrowheads*)

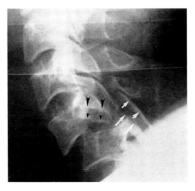
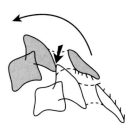

Bilateral facet dislocation—Severe distractive-flexion

The superior vertebral body is displaced anteriorly more than 50% of the vertebral body width, and the facet joints are dislocated (*arrows*)

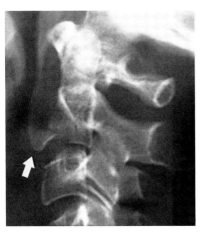
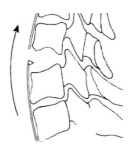

Extension teardrop—Distractive-extension

A triangular fragment has been avulsed from the anterior-inferior corner of the vertebral body (*arrow*) by traction on the anterior longitudinal ligament.

Although both distractive-extension and compressive-flexion create "teardrop" fractures, the causative forces and concomitant injuries are very different

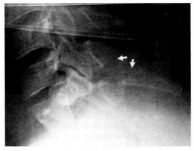
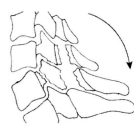

Posterior element fracture—Compressive-extension

Fracture of the C7 spinous process (*arrows*) extends into the laminae. This injury should not be mistaken for the less consequential isolated C7 spinous process fracture, known as a clay shoveler's fracture.

FIGURE 5   Lower cervical spine injuries

Classified by mechanism of injury.

[From Ruoff BE, West OC: The cervical spine, in Schwartz DT. Reisdorff EJ, eds. *Emergency Radiology*, McGraw-Hill, 2000.]

Easily Missed Cervical Spine Fractures

Nondisplaced or minimally displaced fractures can be difficult to detect radiographically because there is no malalignment or deformity of the involved vertebra. The cervicocranium and C7 are the two regions where injuries are most commonly missed. The **cervicocranium** is anatomically complex and is often obscured by overlap of the base of the skull (mastoid region). The C7 **cervicothoracic junction** is often poorly visualized on the lateral radiograph due to overlap by the shoulders and upper thorax (Figures 6 and 7).

The two principal causes of missed cervical spine injuries are failure to recognize subtle signs of cervical spine injury and technically inadequate cervical spine radiographs. (Davis et al. 1993). Inadequate radiographs fail to visulize C7, exhibit poor patient positioning, under- or overpenetration, or are obscured by overlying objects. Concomitant degenerative changes, osteoporosis or congential anomalies can also obscure injuries (Anbari and West 1997).

Radiographic Variants

Radiographic variants that can mimic injuries must be correctly identified to avoid mistaking them as injuries. However, significant injuries can be hidden or obscured by these anomalous radiographic findings.

Radiographic variants include congential anomalies, degenerative changes, old injuries, variations due to suboptimal positioning (rotation or head tilt), and overlapping skeletal or soft tissue shadows. An atlas of radiographic variants that can mimic skeletal injuries is a useful reference to assist in correctly identifying these radiographic findings (Keats and Anderson 2001).

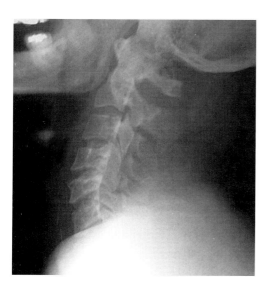
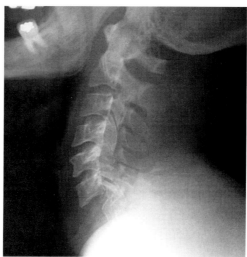

FIGURE 6 All seven cervical vertebrae must be seen in the lateral cervical spine radiograph.

With inadequate visualization, a C6–C7 "hyperextension fracture-dislocation" is missed in a patient who presented with quadriparesis after a fall. In addition to the marked anterior vertebral body displacement, there are multiple posterior element fractures of C5–C7 due to compressive forces.

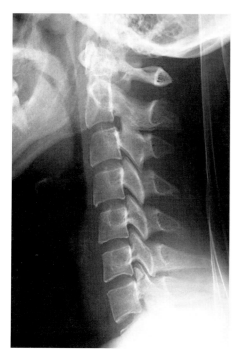
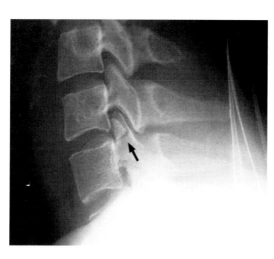

FIGURE 7 After an ABCS review of the entire cervical spine, each vertebra should be examined individually to avoid missing a subtle injury.

Without such a stepwise examination, the facet fracture of C7 could have been missed (*arrow*).

CERVICAL SPINE CT

MDCT allows rapid acquisition of thin axial sections (less than 1 mm) of the entire cervical spine. From these data, high-resolution reformatted images can be generated in sagittal, coronal or curved planar (follow the curvature of the spine) sections (Figure 8).

The sagittal images are analyzed in a fashion similar to the lateral cervical spine view. The midsagittal section shows the vertebral bodies and spinous processes, and the parasagittal sections are used to visualize the lateral masses and facet joints. The coronal sections are analogous to the AP and open mouth views. Finally, the axial images are reviewed from the occipital condyles to C7 and T1. Injuries to the neural arch (pedicles, laminae, and transverse processes) are more easily seen on the axial images.

How Accurate Is Cervical Spine CT?

The sensitivity of helical CT with reformatted images appears to be in the range of 98–99% (cervical spine radiograph sensitivity is 90–95%). Ptak et al. (2001) studied 676 high-risk patients, 60 of which had fractures (9%). One odontoid fracture was missed on CT, yielding a sensitivity of 98% (lower 95% CI: 95%).

Hanson et al. (Emerg Radiol 2000) studied 601 high-risk patients, 81 of which had injuries (13.5%). There were two missed extension-type ligamentous injuries, yielding a sensitivity of 97.5%. Other case series report occasional patients with injuries missed by helical CT, such as a type II dens fracture disclosed by flexion–extension views (Bollinger et al. 2004) and various ligamentous injuries detected by MRI (Benedetti et al. 2000). Among high-risk patients (10% risk of cervical spine injury), the likelihood of an injury after a negative CT is 0.2%.

Hogan et al. (2005) studied 366 obtunded trauma patients with normal MDCT that had MRI. There were no missed osseous or unstable ligamentous injuries. However, seven patients had otherwise unsuspected spinal cord injuries. Therefore, it remains prudent to protect the cervical spine from undue movement until such patients can be clinically evaluated or have MRI.

SUGGESTED READING

Clark CR, Benzel EC, Currier BL, et al.: *The Cervical Spine (The Cervical Spine Research Society Editorial Committee),* 4th ed. Lippincott, 2004.

Errico TJ, Bauer RD, Waugh T: *Spinal Trauma.* Lippincott, 1991.

Galli RL, Spaite DW, Simon RR: *Emergency Orthopedics: The Spine.* McGraw-Hill, 1989.

Harris JH, Mirvis SE: *The Radiology of Acute Cervical Spine Trauma,* 3rd ed. Williams and Wilkins, 1996.

Keats TE, Anderson MW: *Atlas of Normal Roentgen Variants that May Simulate Disease,* 7th ed. Mosby, 2001.

Ruoff BE, West OC: The cervical spine. In Schwartz DT, Reisdorff EJ, ed. *Emergency Radiology.* McGraw-Hill, 2000.

Clinical Features
Davis JW, Phreaner DL, Hoyt DB, et al.: The etiology of missed cervical spine injuries. *J Trauma* 1993;34: 342–346.

D'Costa H, George G, Parry M, et al.: Pitfalls in the clinical diagnosis of vertebral fractures: A case series in which posterior midline tenderness was absent, *Emerg Med J* 2005;22:330–332 (see case 5).

Demetriades D, Charalambides K, Chahwan S, et al.: Nonskeletal cervical spine injuries: Epidemiology and diagnostic pitfalls. *J Trauma* 2000;8:724–727.

Goldberg W, Mueller C, Panacek E, Tigges S, et al.: Distribution and patterns of blunt traumatic cervical spine injury. *Ann Emerg Med* 2001;38:17–21.

Lomoschitz FM, Blackmore CC, Mirza SK, Mann FA: Cervical spine injuries in patients 65 years and older. *AJR* 2002;178:573–577.

Clinical Decision Rules
Hoffman JR, Mower WR, Wolfson AB, et al.: Validity of a set of clinical criteria to rule out injury to the cervical spine in patients with blunt trauma. *New Engl J Med* 2000;343:94–99.

Panacek EA, Mower WR, Holmes JF, Hoffman JR: Test performance of the individual NEXUS low-risk clinical screening criteria for cervical spine injury. *Ann Emerg Med* 2001;38:22–25.

Stiell IG, Clement CM, McKnight RD, et al.: The Canadian C-spine rule versus the NEXUS low-risk criteria in patients with trauma. *N Engl J Med* 2003;349:2510–2518.

Stiell IG, Wells GA, Vandemheen KL, et al.: The Canadian C-Spine rule for radiography in alert and stable trauma patients. *JAMA* 2001;286:1841–1848.

Touger M, Gennis P, Nathanson N, et al.: Validity of a decision rule to reduce cervical spine radiography in elderly patients with blunt trauma. *Ann Emerg Med* 2002;40:287–293.

Clinical Spine Radiography
Anbari MM, West OC: Cervical spine trauma: Sources of false-negative diagnoses. Emerg Radiol 1997;4:218–224.

Harris JH: The cervicocranium: Its radiographic assessment. *Radiology* 2001;218:337–351.

Kim KS, Rogers LF, Regenbogen V: Pitfalls in plain film diagnosis of the cervical spine injury: False-positive interpretation. *Surg Neurol* 1986;25:381.

Lin JT, Lee JL, Lee ST: Evaluation of occult cervical spine fractures on radiographs and CT. *Emerg Radiol* 2003;10:128–134.

Mower WR, Hoffman JR, Pollack CV, et al.: Use of plain radiography to screen for cervical spine injuries. *Ann Emerg Med* 2001;38:1–7.

Mower WR, Oh JY, Zucker MI, Hoffman JR: Occult and secondary injuries missed by plain radiography of the cervical spine in blunt trauma patients. *Emerg Radiol* 2001;8:200–206.

Singh A, O'Connor RE, Mascioli S, Tinkoff GH: The incidence of false negative initial cervical spine radiographs for patients admitted to a level-I trauma center. *Acad Emerg Med* 2003;10:497.

Woodring JH: Limitations of cervical radiography in the evaluation of acute cervical trauma. *J Trauma* 1993;34:32–39.

Flexion-Extension Views
Bolinger B, Shartz M, Marion D: Bedside fluoroscopic flexion and extension cervical spine radiographs for clearance of the cervical spine in comatose trauma patients. *J Trauma* 2004;56:132–136.

Midsagittal section— Analogous to the lateral radiograph. Shows the vertebral bodies, dens, spinous processes and prevertebral soft tissues

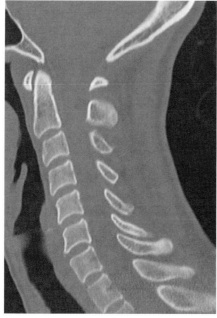

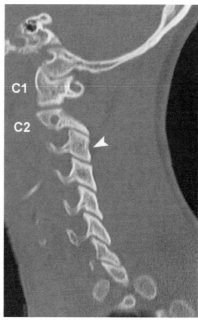

Parasagittal section— shows the lateral masses and facet joints (*arrowhead*)

Coronal section locator— Curved linear sections traced on the midsagittal section

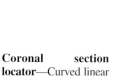

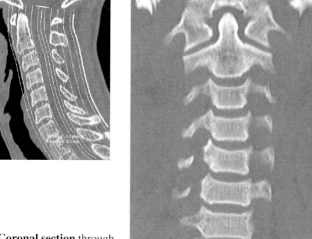

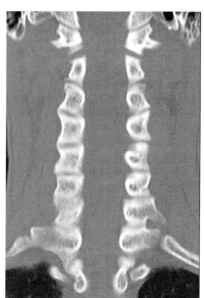

Coronal section throught the lateral masses and facet joints of C1 to C7.

Coronal section through the vertebral bodies, the dens, and the lateral masses of C1.

Axial image of the cervicocranium. (C1 and dens)

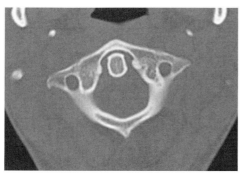

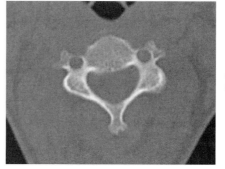

Axial image of a lower cervical vertebra

FIGURE 8 Multidetector helical CT (MDCT) with sagittal and coronal reformatted images.

A normal CT in a 42-year-old woman.

The coronal sections have been curved to follow the contour of the cervical spine. In this way, the same section of each vertebra is seen on each coronal image.

APPENDIX: CERVICAL SPINE IMAGING STRATEGY FOR TRAUMA PATIENTS

Assess risk of cervical spine injury (four categories):

1) **Minimal risk**—Clinically clear without radiography (NEXUS and/or Canadian C-Spine rules)

2) **Low risk**—Three-view cervical spine radiography (CSR).

Very low incidence of injury (0.2%), i.e., 99.8% of radiographs are negative (Hanson 2000). Selective radiography is warranted.

CSR is adequate and normal—Cervical spine is cleared (practically all cases).

CSR is inadequate (C7 not seen)—Swimmer's view or CT should be obtained.

CSR is equivocal (questionable injury)—CT should be obtained through the area in question.
Questionable finding suggestive of **ligamentous injury** (slight malalignment)—**Flexion–extension views,** after CT (patient having significant pain). If neck movement is limited, delayed flexion–extension views after the neck is immobilized in a cervical collar for several days. MRI is an alternative test to detect ligamentous injury.

CSR normal but patient having **excessive pain** (suspect nondisplaced ligamentous injury or occult fracture)—**CT** and possibly **flexion–extension views.** Injuries are rare and this recommendation is controversial. If neck motion is limited by pain, delayed flexion–extension views can be obtained. Alternatively, the patient could be instructed to avoid significant physical activity, to seek immediate medical attention if increased pain or neurological symptoms develop, and return for a follow-up in several days (Mower 2001).

Patients at increased risk for an occult injury are those that are difficult to examine due to a clouded sensorium or have underlying factors that predispose to injury, e.g., elderly patients with degenerative changes or osteoporosis.

3) **High risk**—patients with greater than 5% incidence of injury based on high-energy mechanism of injury or high-risk clinical features (severe head injury, pelvic or multiple extremity fractures).

MDCT of entire cervical spine with sagittal and coronal reformatted images; radiography is omitted.
MDCT also used in less severely injured patients who are undergoing CT of the head, abdomen, or chest.

Hemodynamically unstable patients—Cross-table lateral view of cervical spine obtained to identify markedly displaced injuries that need expeditious reduction and stabilization.

CT is normal—the incidence of injury is very low (CT sensitivity 98–99%). **Cervical immobilization** should be maintained in the ED in major trauma victims.

Alert patients can be clinically cleared (no neck pain or neurological deficits) once they have been stabilized. If neck pain is excessive, further imaging may be needed (MRI or flexion–extension views).

Obtunded patients with normal CT should remain immobilized in a cervical collar. **MRI** can be used to detect occult spinal cord or ligamentous injury and should be performed as soon as feasible. **Flexion–extension views** using fluoroscopic guidance have been advocated to detect isolated occult ligamentous injury, although MRI is a safer.

4) **Neurologic injury** referable to the spinal cord or nerve roots

Helical CT of entire cervical spine—Look for a skeletal lesion impinging on the spinal canal or neuroforamina that needs operative intervention.

MRI, as soon as feasible—Visualizes spinal cord injury directly as well as soft tissue lesions that can injure the spinal cord such a herniated cervical disk or spinal epidural hematoma.

CT and MRI

Bagley LJ: Imaging of spinal trauma. Radiol Clin North Am 2006;44:1–12.

Benedetti PF, Fahr LM, Kuhns LR, Hayman LA: MR imaging findings in spinal ligamentous injury. *AJR* 2000;175:661–665.

Blackmore CC: Evidence-based imaging evaluation of the cervical spine in trauma. *Neuroimaging Clin North Am* 2003;13:283–291.

Hanson JA, Blackmore CC, Mann FA, Wilson AJ: Cervical spine injury: A clinical decision rule to identify high-risk patients for helical CT screening. *AJR* 2000;174:713–717.

Hanson JA, Blackmore CC, Mann FA, Wilson AJ: Cervical spine injury: Accuracy of helical CT used as a screening technique. *Emerg Radiol* 2000;7:31–35.

Hogan GJ, Mirvis SE, Shanmuganathan K, Scalea TM: Exclusion of unstable cervical spine injury in obtunded patients with blunt trauma: Is MR imaging needed when multi-detector row CT findings are normal? *Radiology* 2005;237:106–113.

Ptak T, Kihiczak D, Lawrason JN, et al.: Screening for cervical spine trauma with helical CT: Experience with 676 cases. *Emerg Radiol* 2001;8:315–319.

Rybicki F, Nawfel RD, Judy PF, et al.: Skin and thyroid dosimetry in cervical spine screening: Two methods for evaluation and a comparison between a helical CT and radiographic trauma series. *AJR* 2002;179:933–937.

Cervical Spine: Patient 1

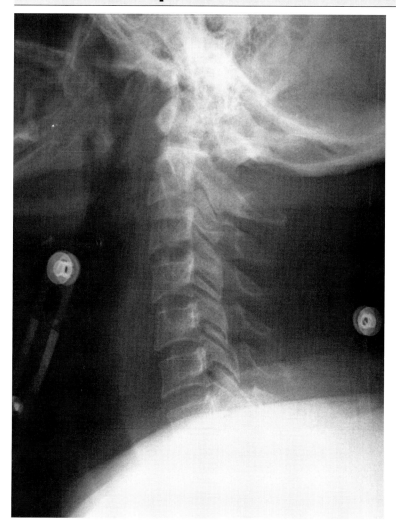

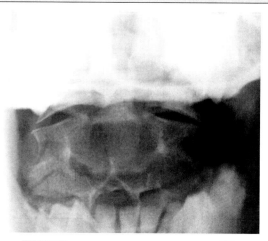

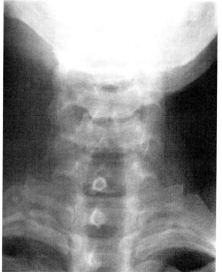

FIGURE 1

Neck pain in a middle-aged man who was struck by a slow-moving motor vehicle

A 43-year-old man was crossing the street when he was struck by a car that, he estimated, was going about 10 miles per hour. He was unsure which part of his body was hit, but he fell to the ground landing on his right shoulder. He hit his head on the pavement and may have had a brief loss of consciousness. He was able to stand up and walk after the injury and came with his family to the hospital. He complained of pain in his neck, back and right shoulder.

In the ED, the patient was placed on a stretcher and immobilized with a hard plastic cervical collar. On examination, he appeared well, fully alert, and in no distress. His vital signs were normal. There was a small abrasion on the right occipital area and mild local tenderness over C7. There was no hemotympanum. The chest, abdomen, and pelvis were nontender. There was tenderness of the right deltoid region, but the shoulder had full range of motion without pain. The neurological examination, including upper and lower extremity strength, sensation, and reflexes, was normal.

- Cervical spine radiographs were obtained and are shown above (Figure 1).

- How would you interpret the radiographs?

- Are there any signs of an injury?

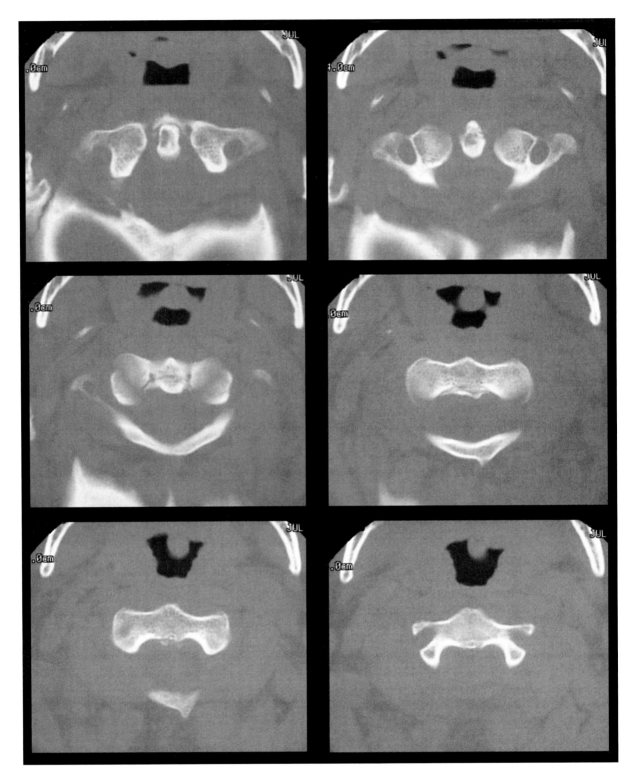

FIGURE 2

Good visualization of C1 and C2 could not be obtained with the open mouth view. This was because the cervical collar was left in place due to concern about moving the patient's neck before all of the radiographs were taken. The open mouth view was repeated, but it was also suboptimal. A CT scan through C1 and C2 was therefore performed.

The CT was read as normal and the patient was discharged home.

Several CT slices are shown in Figure 2.

- Is there a problem with this management?

- Are any additional studies needed?

REMEMBER THE ABCS

The regions of the cervical spine where fractures are most often missed are C7 and the cervicocranium. Injuries to the cervicocranium are problematic due to their complex anatomy, the frequency that radiographs are suboptimal in this region, the difficulty in localizing pain or tenderness to that area, and the frequent lack of neurological deficits—76% of patients with dens fractures have no neurological deficits (Mower et al. 2000). Injuries to C7 are missed because of poor visualization due to overlap by the shoulders.

After noting any obvious injuries, the radiographs must be systematically examined to avoid overlooking subtle abnormalities. The mnemonic device **ABCS** provides an easily remembered scheme: "**A**" stands for adequacy and alignment, "**B**" stands for bones (examined for fractures or deformity), "**C**" stands for cartilage (spaces between the vertebrae), and "**S**" stands for soft tissue changes that can provide clues to injuries that are not otherwise visible (Table 1). The entire spine is assessed first, and then each vertebra is examined individually.

Lateral View—Patient 1

In Patient 1, all seven vertebrae are seen (the C7–T1 junction was faintly visible on the original radiograph) (Figure 3). The patient's neck is slightly tilted such that the left and right lateral masses and facet joints do not overlap exactly (*asterisks*). Because the patient's head is tilted, the base of the skull (S) obscures the posterior portion of C1.

The alignment of the vertebrae is normal: four smooth lordotic curves are formed by the anterior and posterior vertebral body surfaces, the bases of the spinous processes (spinolaminar junctions), and the tips of the spinous processes.

No obvious fractures or skeletal deformities are seen. The spaces between the vertebral bodies, laminae, and spinous processes are all equal.

The critical finding is an abnormal contour of the prevertebral soft tissues of the upper cervical spine (*arrow*). In nondisplaced fractures of the cervicocranium, soft tissues swelling may be the only radiographic sign of a fracture.

TABLE 1

ABCS of the Lateral Cervical Spine Radiograph

A	Adequacy	All seven vertebrae seen Minimal rotation or tilt (facet joints aligned)
	Alignment	Four smooth curves: vertebral bodies (anterior and posterior surfaces), spinolaminar line, and spinous processes
B	Bones	Fractures of vertebral bodies, lateral masses, lamina, and spinous processes
C	Cartilage	Spaces between vertebrae are equal: intervertebral disks, laminae, and spinous processes
		Predental space less than 3 mm (between dens and anterior arch of C1)
S	Soft Tissues	Prevertebral soft tissue swelling

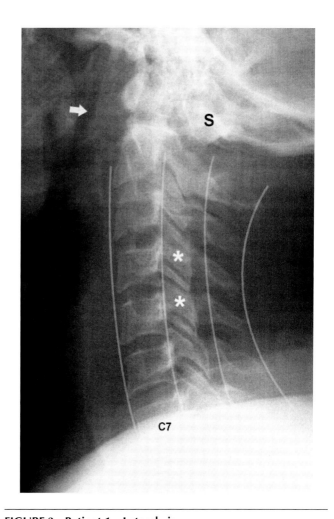

FIGURE 3   Patient 1—Lateral view.
(See text for explanation)

Prevertebral soft tissue swelling

Assessment of prevertebral soft tissues is an important part of cervical spine radiograph interpretation. However, when formally investigated, the presence of soft tissue swelling has been found to have limited sensitivity and specificity for fractures, and its usefulness has therefore been questioned.

The **normal thickness** of the prevertebral soft tissues has been determined by studying large numbers of normal radiographs. Penning found the upper limits of normal to be 10 mm at C1, 5 mm at C2, 7 mm at C3, and 20 mm at C5 to C7 (Figure 4). The greater permissible width at C1 is due to the presence of adenoidal tissue within the retropharyngeal soft tissues, most commonly in younger patients. In the lower cervical spine, interposition of the esophagus within the prevertebral soft tissues makes soft tissue swelling a much less reliable indicator of injury than in the cervicocranium.

In five studies, soft tissue swelling was found in only 50–60% of patients with fractures (Penning, Miles, DeBehnke, Templeton, Herr). Some authors studied upper and lower cervical spine injuries separately. DeBehnke found soft tissue swelling >6 mm at C2 in only 59% of patients with cervicocranial injuries. In the lower cervical spine, soft tissue swelling at C6 was present in only 5% of injuries. Injuries to the lower cervical spine can, however, cause soft tissue swelling that extends up to the cervicocranium. In addition, soft tissue swelling was found to have only moderate specificity (76–84%); i.e., 16–24% of patients with swelling did not have fractures (Miles, DeBehnke).

Templeton et al found considerable overlap in soft tissue measurements between patients with and without fractures. A width of >5mm at C3 or C4 had a sensitivity of 75% and specificity of 44%, whereas a width >8 mm at C3 or C4 had a sensitivity of 33% and specificity of 87%. A width of >7 mm at C2 had a sensitivity of 18% and specificity of 95%. They concluded that prevertebral soft tissue measurements have limited usefulness in detecting injuries. A width >10 mm at C2, C3, or C4, although infrequently seen, should be considered highly suggestive of a fracture, whereas a width of 7–10 mm is "possibly abnormal" (i.e., indeterminate). Approximately 20% of patients with fractures had normal soft tissue thickness (≤5 mm).

To increase the usefulness of prevertebral soft tissue assessment, Harris has suggested that alteration in **cervicocranial soft tissue contour** is a more reliable indicator of injury than are measurements at discrete levels (Harris 1994, 2001, Harris and Mirvis 1996). Normally, the contour of the soft tissues parallels the contour of the anterior surfaces of the bones. There is slight convexity anterior to C1 and anterior to the C2 vertebral body, and slight concavity or straightening above C1 and anterior to dens (Figure 5).

In many children and young adults, enlargement of **retropharyngeal adenoidal tissue** widens the soft tissues between C1 and the skull base (Figure 6). Adenoidal tissue has a lobular contour that ends inferiorly with either an abrupt angular or rounded junction. When there is an abrupt angular transition,

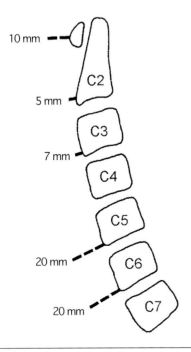

FIGURE 4   Normal width of the prevertebral soft tissues as measured at discrete points.
[From Galli RL, Spaite DW, Simon RR: *Emergency Orthopedics: The Spine.* McGraw-Hill, 1989, with permission.]

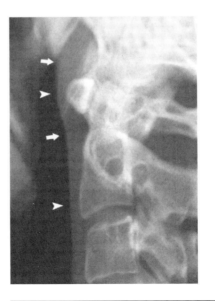
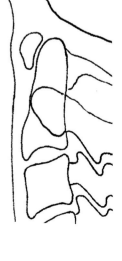

FIGURE 5   Normal cervicocranial soft tissue contour.
There is slight convexity anterior to C1 and the body of C2 *(arrowheads)*, and slight concavity or straightening superior to C1 and anterior to the base of the dens *(arrows)*.

adenopathy is easier to distinguish from traumatic swelling; a smooth rounded transition is more difficult to distinguish from swelling due to trauma.

Certain factors can interfere with the assessment of the prevertebral soft tissue contour. These include: (1) swallowing at the time the radiograph is taken, (2) neck flexion, (3) endotracheal and nasogastric tubes, and (4) blood or secretions pooling in the oropharynx. Accurate soft tissue visualization therefore depends on proper radiographic technique. ED trauma radiographs are often suboptimal with regard to visualization of the soft tissues.

There are **two patterns of traumatic soft tissue swelling** described by Harris: (1) an abnormal convexity (either a focal or diffuse bulge) and (2) a straight anterosuperior upward oblique pattern (see Figure 14 on p. 380).

The **accuracy of cervicocranial soft tissue contour** assessment has not been studied in a well-controlled trial. Harris (1994) found soft tissue contour abnormalities in all 32 patients with subtle fractures of the cervicocranium. In a later report (2001), he found that swelling was present in all but one patient with a fracture, yielding a false-negative rate of <1%. However, in some of the patients illustrated, soft tissue swelling was very subtle, i.e., this high sensitivity was achieved at the expense of a very low specificity (only 16% of patients with swelling had fractures). Nonetheless, this 16% rate of injury is sufficient to justify performing CT scans in patients with isolated soft tissue contour abnormalities.

It should also be noted that Harris used a "**contact lateral view**" (in addition to the standard lateral view) which improves visualization of the cervicocranium. In the contact lateral view,

the x-ray cassette is positioned directly beside the patient's neck rather than next to the shoulder. To assure proper pharyngeal aeration, the patient is instructed to inspire deeply or exhale against pursed lips like a trumpet player at the time the radiograph is exposed.

Summary

Although the usefulness of prevertebral soft tissue abnormalities has been questioned because of their limited sensitivity and specificity, assessment of the cervicocranial prevertebral soft tissues *can* provide important information.

When either the contour or measured thickness is *abnormal*, a cervical spine injury must be definitely excluded by careful examination of the radiographs and additional testing, such as CT. Soft tissues that are *clearly normal* in contour are reassuring, although this alone cannot definitely exclude an injury in a patient at high risk. When the radiographs are suboptimal or the soft tissue findings are equivocal, the radiograph could be repeated or CT obtained depending on the clinical risk of cervical spine injury.

In Patient 1, even though the measured soft tissue width is "normal"—10 mm at C1 and 5 mm at the base of C2—there is a prominent convexity anterior to the base of the dens (Figure 7). This contour abnormality is highly suggestive of an injury in this region. However, no definite fracture can be identified on the lateral view, and so the other views must be carefully inspected for signs of injury.

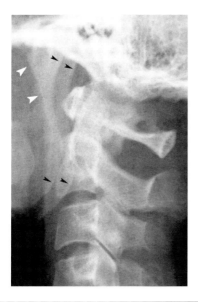

FIGURE 6 Enlarged retropharyngeal adenoidal tissue widens the prevertebral soft tissues at and above C1 *(white arrowheads)*. There is a smooth transition to a normal contour at C2.
The posterior margins of the mandible are indicated by black arrowheads.

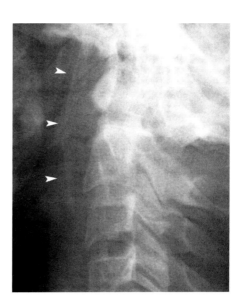

FIGURE 7 Patient 1—Prevertebral soft tissue swelling causes an abnormal convex contour anterior to the base of the dens *(arrowheads)*.

PATIENT 1

AP View

This patient's AP view is normal (Figure 8). The spinous processes (S) lie in the midline and are equally spaced. The lateral masses appear as a continuous undulating contour (*arrowheads*). The vertebral bodies, uncinate processes (*black arrow*), and intervertebral disk spaces do not show fracture, deformity, or disk-space narrowing. The calcified thyroid cartilage overlies the left lateral masses of C5 and C6 (*white arrow*).

Open Mouth View

In this patient, the dens (D) is largely obscured by overlying skeletal structures (Figure 9). Optimal views were not obtained because of concern about opening the cervical collar and repositioning the patient's neck. However, in a cooperative and alert patient without excessive neck pain, slight movement under supervision should be permitted to ensure adequate images.

Despite the suboptimal technique, a fracture through the base of the dens is not seen in this patient. However, even with optimal positioning, a nondisplaced fracture might not be visible if the fracture line is sloping rather than transverse and therefore not parallel with the x-ray beam.

The C1-C2 facet joints are not perfectly aligned (*arrowheads*) and the dens is not located exactly between the lateral masses of C1. These effects are due to slight tilting of the patient's head. If such malalignment was of concern the open mouth view could be repeated with proper positioning of the patient. Notches between the base of the dens and the medial margins of the superior articular facets are normal and should not be mistaken for fractures (*arrows*).

Computed Tomography

CT is highly sensitive at detecting most fractures and is used in patients at high risk of injury and in patients with equivocal or suggestive radiographic findings, e.g., prevertebral soft tissue swelling. Nonetheless, axial CT may fail to detect fractures that lie in the plane of the CT slices such as transverse fractures through the base of the dens (Woodring and Lee 1992). To visualize these fractures, coronal and sagittal reformatted images may be necessary. Nonetheless, cases missed by reformatted images have been reported (Ptak et al. 2001, Bolinger et al. 2004).

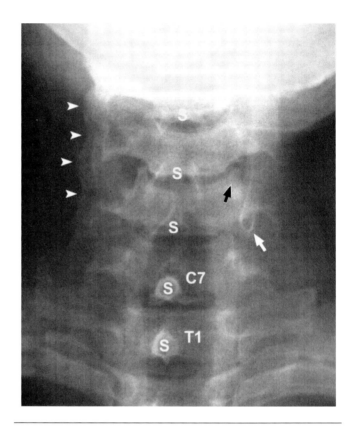

FIGURE 8   Patient 1—AP view.

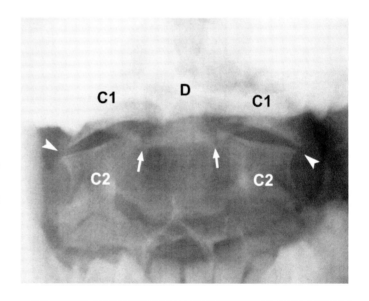

FIGURE 9   Patient 1—Open mouth view.

In Patient 1, the initial CT images were interpreted as normal (Figure 2). In one slice, there is discontinuity of the trabecular pattern at the base of the dens (Figure 10). This was misinterpreted as normal trabecular irregularity.

The next morning, coronal and sagittal reformatted images were generated which revealed a fracture through the base of the dens (Figures 11 and 12). These fractures are mechanically unstable because they can become displaced when the patient moves.

The patient was contacted and an ambulance was dispatched to transport him back to the ED. Fortunately, the patient remained neurologically intact, and he was admitted to the neurosurgery service. The patient was immobilized in a rigid Halo-vest device and was discharged from the hospital two days later.

Dens Fractures

Dens fractures are among the most common cervical spine fractures: 11.5% in the NEXUS series (94 of 818 fractures) (Mower et al. 2000). There are three types (Figure 12). Type II is the most common.

Treatment of nondisplaced type II odontoid fractures usually consists of immobilization in a rigid Halo-vest. Displaced or angulated fractures may be treated with surgical screw fixation because of the high incidence of nonunion.

Dens fractures are also among the most commonly missed fractures and the radiographs must be scrutinized for subtle signs of this injury.

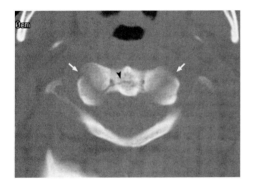

FIGURE 10 Trabecular irregularity *(arrowhead)* was initially misinterpreted as a normal variant, but was actually a sign of fracture at the base of the dens.
The atlantoaxial joint spaces are seen tangentially *(arrows)*.

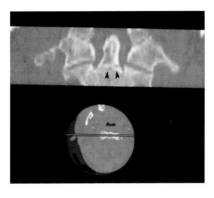 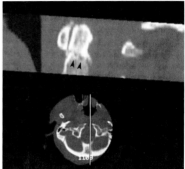

FIGURE 11 Coronal and sagittal CT images reveal a fracture through the base of the dens *(arrowheads)*.
Because a type II dens fracture lies in the transverse plane, axial CT may fail to visualize this fracture.

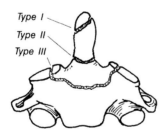

FIGURE 12 **Classification and frequency of odontoid fractures**

Type I—Tip of dens (6%)

Type II—Base of dens, "high" fracture (64%)

Type III—"Low" fracture into body of C2 (29%)

[From Galli RL, Spaite DW, Simon RR: *Emergency Orthopedics: The Spine.* McGraw-Hill, 1989, with permission.]

Summary

1. Cervicocranial prevertebral soft tissue swelling is an important clue to a fracture. If a fracture is not seen on the radiographs, CT is necessary.
2. Changes in the contour of the cervicocranial prevertebral soft tissues are a more accurate indicator of injury than are measurements of soft tissue thickness at discrete points.
3 The absence of soft tissue swelling does not exclude an injury in patients at high risk.
4. The open mouth view can detect cervicocranial fractures not visible on the lateral view. If suboptimal, the patient should be repositioned and the view repeated or obtain a CT.
5. CT can miss fractures in the axial plane. Coronal and sagittal images may be necessary to detect such fractures.
6. Lower cervical spine soft tissue swelling is rarely seen and is not a reliable indicator of injury.

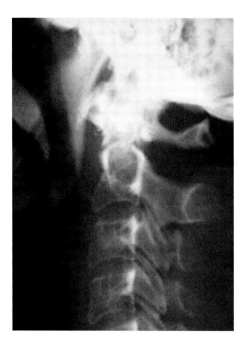
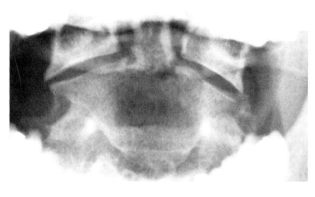

FIGURE 13

PATIENT 1B   A SECOND PATIENT IN WHOM AN ODONTOID FRACTURE WAS MISSED

A 26-year-old woman pedestrian was struck on her leg by a motor vehicle and knocked to the ground. She had a displaced tibial fracture, but denied having neck pain. Her neurological examination was normal.

The radiographs were initially interpreted as normal even though a definite fracture was visible, particularly on the open mouth view (Figure 13). The clinical suspicion for a neck injury seemed low despite the mechanism of injury because her injuries appeared to be limited to the lower extremity and she did not have neck pain. However, the lack of neck pain was a consequence of her tibial fracture, which served as a "distracting injury."

On the initial **lateral view** (Figure 14A), the posterior cortex of the C2 vertebral body (*white arrowheads*) is not continuous with the posterior cortex of the dens (*black arrowheads*). The prevertebral soft tissues are nearly normal. Although there is loss of the normal concavity superior to C1 and anterior to the base of the dens (*arrows*).

The initial **open mouth view** (Figure 14B) clearly shows the fracture through the base of the dens (*arrowheads*).

The fracture was identified the next day on the final radiography report. The radiographs were repeated (Figure 14C) and showed that the fracture was displaced anteriorly and there was definite soft tissue swelling (*arrows*). Fortunately, the patient had no additional injury despite her delayed diagnosis.

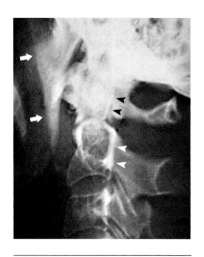

FIGURE 14A   Initial lateral view.

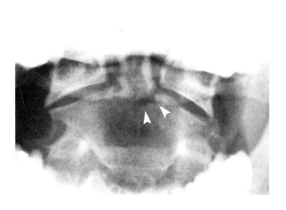

FIGURE 14B   Initial open mouth view.

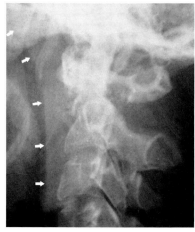

FIGURE 14C   Second lateral view

PATIENT 1C A 90-year-old woman fell backward from standing and injured her neck. She had marked neck pain and stiffness. Her neurological examination was normal.

The initial radiograph interpretation noted degenerative changes and osteoporosis, but no definite fracture (Figure 15).

Degenerative changes cause facet joint narrowing and slight anterior slippage (anterolisthesis) of the C3, C4, and C5 vertebral bodies.

The prevertebral soft tissues are diffusely widened without a focal convexity.

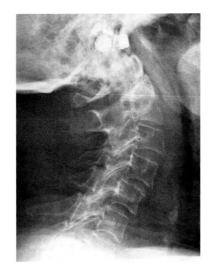
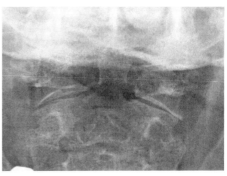

FIGURE 15

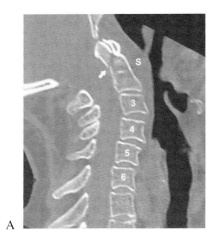
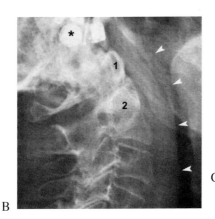
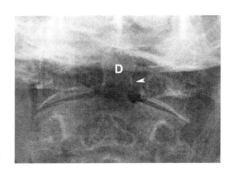

FIGURE 16—Patient 1C

Patient Outcome

Because of the patient's marked neck pain, as well as the suspicious radiographic findings (soft tissue swelling), a CT scan was obtained (Figure 16A). This revealed an oblique fracture through the base of the dens with slight posterior displacement (*arrow*). The prevertebral soft tissues (**S**) have a focal convexity anterior to the dens. Degerative anterolisthesis of C3, C4, and C5 is seen.

The fracture was, in fact, evident on the initial radiographs. On the **lateral view** (Figure 16B), there is posterior displacement of the dens and anterior arch of C1 (**1**) relative to the C2 vertebral body (**2**). The soft tissues are diffusely swollen (*arrowheads*) (*asterisk* = hearing aide). On the **open mouth view** (Figure 16C), there is an indistinct lucency through the base of the dens (**D**) with slight leftwards displacement (*arrowhead*).

The patient was treated with immobilization in a hard plastic cervical collar.

Dens Fractures in the Elderly

The frequency of odontoid fractures increases with age. In patients less than 65 years old, 6% of cervical spine fractures involve the dens (43/683); whereas in those aged 65 and older, 33% involve the dens (44/135) (Mower et al. 2000). The C1–C2 region is especially vulnerable in the elderly because degenerative changes stiffen the lower cervical spine and increase the force of injury on the cervicocranium. Osteoporosis increases the risk of fracture.

Additional fractures were present in almost half the patients with dens fractures, nearly all of which involved C1 or C2. Neurological injuries occurred in 23% of patients.

In a series of 149 patients older than 65 years of age (60% were over 75 years), Lomoschitz found that odontoid fractures were the most common injury (45% of patients) and were especially common in patients older than 75 years. The mechanism of injury was usually a fall from standing or sitting rather than a high-energy impact.

SUGGESTED READING

Odontoid Fractures

Lomoschitz FM, Blackmore CC, Mirza SK, Mann FA: Cervical spine injuries in patients 65 years and older. *AJR* 2002;178:573–577.

Mower WR, Hoffman JR, Zucker MI, for the NEXUS group: Odontoid fractures following blunt trauma. *Emerg Radiol* 2000;7:3–6.

Ngo B, Hoffman JR, Mower WR: Cervical spine injury in the very elderly. *Emerg Radiol* 2000;7:287–291.

Prevertebral Soft Tissue Swelling

Clark WM, Gehweiler JA, Laib R: Twelve significant signs of cervical spine trauma. *Skeletal Radiol* 1979;3:21–205.

DeBehnke DJ, Havel CJ: Utility of prevertebral soft tissue measurements in identifying patients with cervical spine fractures. *Ann Emerg Med* 1994;24:1119–1124.

Gopalakrishnan KC, El Masri W: Prevertebral soft tissue shadow widening—an important sign of cervical spine injury. *Injury* 1986;17:125–128.

Harris JH: Abnormal cervicocranial retropharyngeal soft-tissue contour in the detection of subtle acute cervicocranial injuries. *Emerg Radiol* 1994;1:15–23.

Harris JH: The cervicocranium: Its radiographic assessment. *Radiology* 2001; 218:337–351.

Harris JH, Mirvis SE: *The Radiology of Acute Cervical Spine Trauma*, 3rd ed. Williams and Wilkins, 1996: 475–500.

Herr CH, Ball PA, Sargent SK, Quinton HB: Sensitivity of prevertebral soft tissue measurement of C3 for detection of cervical spine fractures and dislocations. *Am J Emerg Med* 1998;16:346–349.

Matar LD, Doyle AJ: Prevertebral soft-tissue measurements in cervical spine injury. *Australas Radiol* 1997;41:229–237.

Miles KA, Finlay D: Is prevertebral soft tissue swelling a useful sign in injuries of the cervical spine? *Injury* 1988;17:177–179.

Paakkala T: Prevertebral soft tissue changes in cervical spine injury. *Crit Rev Diagn Imaging* 1985;24:201–236.

Penning L: Prevertebral hematoma in cervical spine injury: Incidence and etiologic significance. *AJR* 1981;136:553–561.

Templeton PA, Young JW, Mirvis SE, Buddemeyer EU: The value of retropharyngeal soft tissue measurements in trauma of the adult cervical spine. *Skeletal Radiol* 1987;16:98–104. (Erratum: 435.)

Waeckerle JF: Occult c-spine injuries. *Ann Emerg Med* 1994; 24:1168–1170. Editorial.

Missed Cervical Spine Fractures

Bolinger B, Shartz M, Marion D: Bedside fluoroscopic flexion and extension cervical spine radiographs for clearance of the cervical spine in comatose trauma patients. *J Trauma* 2004; 56:132–136.

Davis JW, Phreaner DL, Hoyt DB, et al.: The etiology of missed cervical spine injuries. *J Trauma* 1993;34: 342–346.

Kirshenbaum KJ, Nadimpalli SR, Fantus R, et al.: Unsuspected upper cervical spine fractures associated with significant head trauma: Role of CT. *J Emerg Med* 1990;8:183–188.

Lin JT, Lee JL, Lee ST: Evaluation of occult cervical spine fractures on radiographs and CT. *Emerg Radiol* 2003;10:128–134.

Ptak T, Kihiczak D, Lawrason JN, et al.: Screening for cervical spine trauma with helical CT: Experience with 676 cases. *Emerg Radiol* 2001;8:315–319.

Woodring JH, Lee C: The role and limitations of computed tomographic scanning in the evaluation of cervical trauma. *J Trauma* 1992;33:698–708.

Mach Bands

Chasen MH: Practical applications of Mach band theory in thoracic analysis. *Radiology* 2001;219:596–610.

Daffner RH: Pseudofractures of the dens: Mach bands. *AJR* 1977;128:176–177.

Friedman AC, Lautin EM, Rothenberg L: Mach bands and pneumomediastinum. *J Can Assoc Radiol* 1981;32:233–235.

Lane EJ, Proto AV, Phillips TW: Mach bands and density perception. *Radiology* 1976;121:9–17.

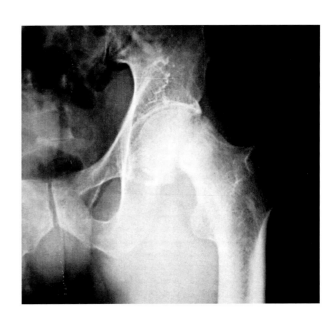

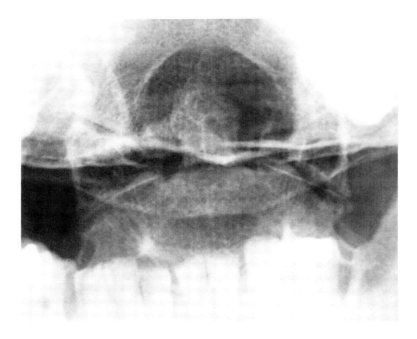

FIGURE 17

PATIENT 1D A 48-year-old man slipped and fell down several steps in the subway. He complained of severe pain in his left hip. There was no other evident trauma.

Hip radiographs revealed a femoral neck fracture (Figure 17).

Because of the mechanism of injury and the fact that the painful hip fracture could mask pain due to a neck injury, a cervical spine series was obtained.

The lateral view was normal. The open mouth view is shown in Figure 17.

• What does it show?

Patient 1D Outcome

On the open mouth view, there is a distinct lucent line across the base of the dens that appears to be a fracture (Figure 18). However, there are several horizontal overlapping shadows in this region caused by the bones of the base of the skull. The apparent fracture line is, in fact, an optical illusion caused by these overlapping shadows. It is due to a visual phenomenon that occurs at the border between two areas of different density.

A dark area adjacent to a light area appears slightly darker than it actually is, increasing the perceived contrast at the border between two areas of *slightly* differing density (Figure 19A). This optical effect results in apparent edge-enhancement and has the benefit of making the edges of objects appear more conspicuous. The effect can also create the illusion of a dark line adjacent to a lighter area (Figure 19B).

This illusory line is termed a **Mach band** in honor of the neurophysiologist who described this phenomenon. In skeletal radiography, this dark line can be misinterpreted as a fracture (Figure 18). On the other hand, when a Mach band is superimposed over a fracture, it can mask or obscure the fracture.

A common site for a Mach band is across the base of the dens on the open mouth view. It is caused by overlying bones such as the base of the skull and posterior arch of C1. When a Mach band is suspected, the open mouth view should be repeated with the head in a slightly different position to move the overlapping shadows away from the base of the dens.

In this patient, when the open mouth view was repeated, the overlapping bones and the Mach band moved up from the base of the dens to the middle of the dens (Figure 20). This proved that the apparent fracture line was actually a Mach band.

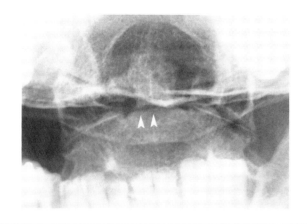

FIGURE 18   Initial open mouth view showing a dark Mach band across the base of the dens that mimics a fracture.

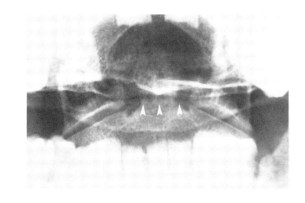

FIGURE 20   Don't get a CT scan, just repeat the open mouth view. A second open mouth view with slightly different positioning shows the dark Mach band in a different position across the dens *(arrowheads)*. In addition, the Mach band extends beyond the margins of the dens.

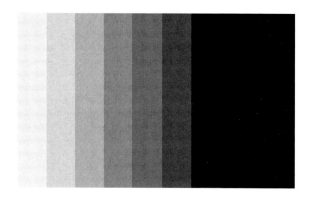

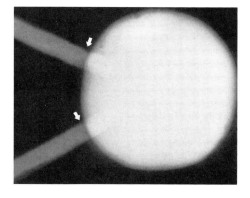

FIGURE 19   Mach bands—An optical effect at the margin between areas of slightly different density.

(*A*) sequence of increasingly dark but uniform gray rectangles. The Mach effect creates the illusion of a "scalloped" appearance—at the border between two gray areas, the left side appears lighter and the right side appears darker creating an edge enhancement effect.

(*B*) Radiograph of a solid sphere into which two sticks have been inserted. The Mach effect causes an apparent darkening of the background adjacent to the edge of the sphere. This dark zone extends across the base of the sticks where they enter the sphere, producing a Mach band *(arrows)*.

[From Felson B: *Chest Roentgenology.* WB Saunders, 1973, with permission.]

Cervical Spine: Patient 2

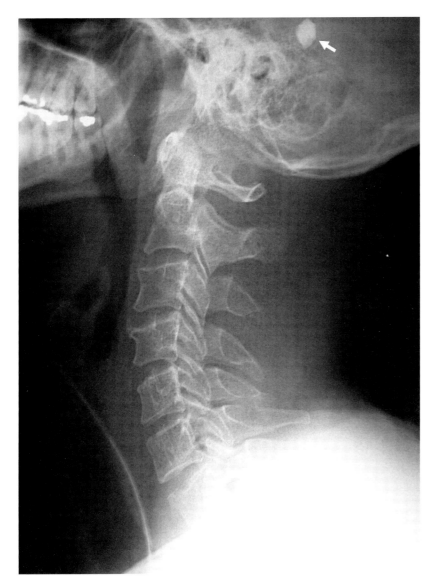
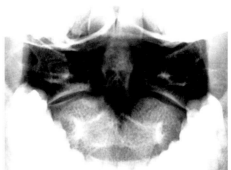
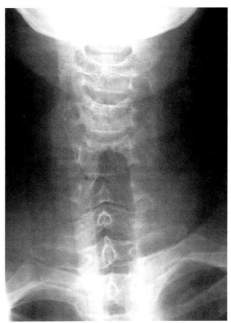

FIGURE 1

A neck injury sustained in a high-speed motor vehicle collision by a middle-aged man

A 41-year-old man was brought to the ED following a motor vehicle collision in which he was an unrestrained driver whose vehicle hit a roadway median divider. The automobile driver's air bag deployed. At the scene, the patient was confused and "oriented times two." Upon his arrival in the ED, his mental status was normal and he admitted to having had "a few beers." He complained of lower back and neck pain.

The patient was hemodynamically stable. The only evident trauma was a left parietal scalp laceration and hematoma. His neurological examination was normal.

The chest and pelvis radiographs were negative for an acute injury. The cervical spine radiographs are shown in Figure 1.

- Are there any abnormalities?

Note: Loss of anterior vertebral body height at C4 is not an acute fracture. However, there is a second finding that represents an unstable cervical spine injury.

(*Arrow* = windshield glass lying next to the patient's scalp.)

THE RING OF C2

Lateral view—ABCS approach

All seven vertebrae are visible (Figure 2). The patient's position is slightly rotated, as evident by the lack of perfect overlap of the left and right articular facets at each vertebra.

The overall **alignment** of the vertebral bodies and spinolaminar line appears normal. The intervertebral *disk spaces* and the spaces between the spinous processes are uniform.

The **prevertebral soft tissues** are less than 5 mm at C1, C2, and C3. However, close examination of the *contour* of the prevertebral soft tissue reveals a slight focal convexity (bulge) anterior to the base of the dens (*white arrowhead*).

Examination of the **bones of the lower cervical spine** reveals narrowing of the anterior aspect of the C4 vertebral body (*arrow,* Figure 2). However, based on the radiographic findings and subsequent evaluation with CT and flexion/extension views, this represents an old injury rather than an acute fracture.

When examining the **bones of the cervicocranium,** several radiographic landmarks should be noted. These include the predental space, the posterior arch of C1, the dens, the C2 vertebral body, and the posterior arch of C2 (Figure 3).

A distinctive radiographic landmark overlies the body of C2—the "**ring of C2**" (Figures 3 and 4). This oblong-shaped ring is formed by cortical bone projecting laterally from the C2 vertebral body (Figures 5 and 6).

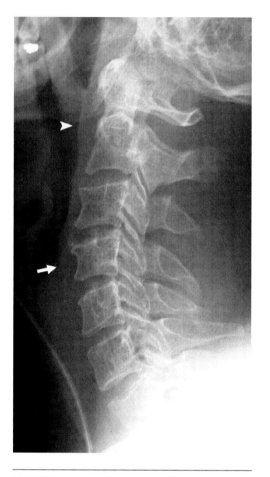

FIGURE 2   Lateral view—Patient 2.

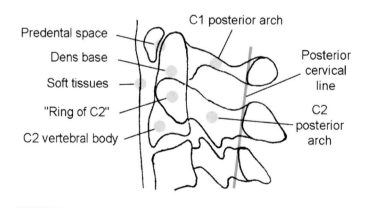

FIGURE 3   Radiographic landmarks of the cervicocranium.

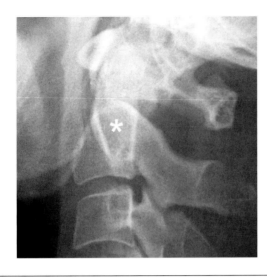

FIGURE 4   Normal Ring of C2.
Both the left and right rings of C2 are exactly superimposed *(asterisk)*. The slight indistinctness of the inferior portion of the ring of C2 is due to the overlying transverse processes.

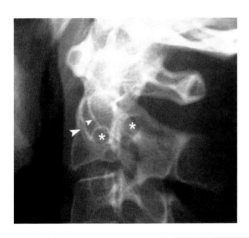

FIGURE 7   Normal Rings of C2—Rotated lateral view.
The left and right sides are not overlapping *(arrowheads)*. The small circles overlying the inferior portions of the rings of C2 are the foramina of the transverse processes *(asterisks)*.

There is a ring of C2 on both sides of the C2 vertebral body. When the positioning of the patient is rotated, the left and right rings of C2 are not superimposed (Figure 7).

A small circle representing the foramen of the transverse process is often superimposed on the inferior aspect of the ring of C2 (Figure 7).

Disruption of the ring of C2 occurs with a fracture known as a **type III** or **"low" odontoid fracture** (Figure 8). Despite this name, it is actually a fracture through the superior portion of the C2 vertebral body. The fracture line usually slopes anteriorly and inferiorly, which is indicative of a flexion mechanism of injury.

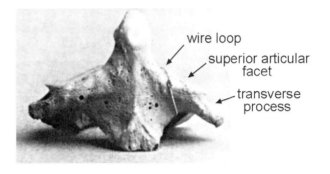

FIGURE 5   Wire loop around the ring of C2.
[From Van Hare: *Ann Emerg Med* 1992, with permission.]

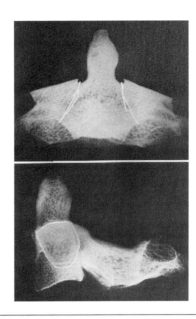

FIGURE 6   Radiograph of an isolated C2 vertebra with wire loops tied around the lateral extensions of the C2 vertebral body. This demonstrates the anatomical basis of the ring of C2 seen on the lateral radiograph.
[From Harris, et al: Low (type III) odontoid fracture: A new radiographic sign. *Radiology* 1984; 153:353–356, with permission.]

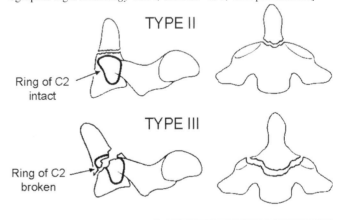

FIGURE 8   The Ring of C2 and Odontoid Fractures.
Type II ("high") fracture through the base of the dens with an intact ring of C2.
Type III ("low") fracture through the superior portion of the body of C2 with a disrupted ring of C2.
[From Rogers LR: *Radiology of Skeletal Trauma.* Churchill-Livingstone, 2002, with permission.]

Patient Outcome

In Patient 2, there is disruption of the "ring of C2" due to a type III odontoid fracture (Figure 9, *arrows*).

Close inspection of the lateral view reveals slight malalignment of the **posterior cervical line**; i.e., the spinolaminar junction of C2 (*asterisk*) is displaced posterior to the posterior cervical line. This is due to anterior displacement of C1, which is a consequence of the slightly displaced odontoid fracture.

There is a small focal bulge in the **prevertebral soft tissues** anterior to the fracture site at the base of the dens (*white arrowheads*). The **predental space** is obscured by the overlapping posterior edge of the mandible (*black arrowhead*).

CT readily demonstrates the fracture through the body of C2 (Figure 10).

The **open mouth view** often does not show the fracture because the fracture line is oblique to the x-ray beam (Figure 1B). (The overlying superior surface of the tongue makes a V-shaped shadow inferior to the base of the dens.)

The patient was observed in the hospital for several days and then discharged home in a hard cervical collar and referred to a treatment program for alcoholism.

Type III Odontoid Fractures

A type III dens fracture is considered "unstable" because of the potential for the dens to displace anteriorly with neck flexion. However, because of the broad fracture surface extending through the body of C2, this injury can usually be managed nonoperatively. It has a good prognosis for healing, unlike type II odontoid fractures which are frequently complicated by nonunion. Displaced fractures are reduced by traction and also generally heal without surgical fixation (Figure 11).

SUGGESTED READING

Harris JH, Burke JT, Ray RD, et al.: Low (type III) odontoid fracture: A new radiographic sign. *Radiology* 1984;153:353–356.

Harris JH, Mirvis SE: *The Radiology of Acute Cervical Spine Trauma*, 3rd ed. Baltimore, Williams and Wilkins, 1996:443–457.

Van Hare RS, Yaron M: The ring of C2 and evaluation of the cross table lateral view of the cervical spine. *Ann Emerg Med* 1992;21:733–735.

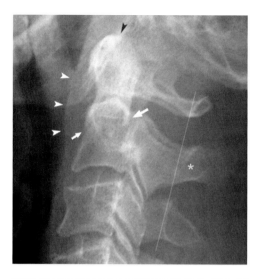

FIGURE 9   Lateral view detail Patient 2.

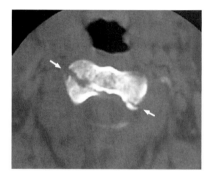

FIGURE 10   CT showing the fracture through the superior portion of the C2 vertebral body.

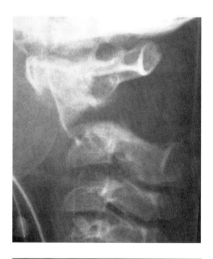

FIGURE 11   A markedly displaced type III odontoid fracture in a 12-year-old girl.

Not all type III odontoid fractures are radiographically subtle.

Cervical Spine: Patient 3

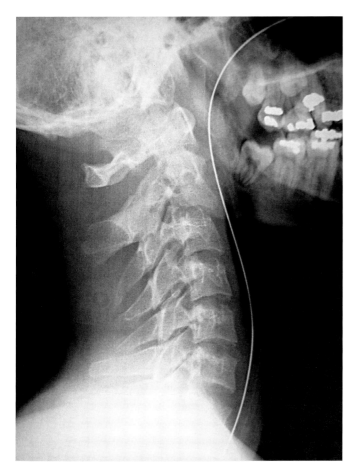

FIGURE 1

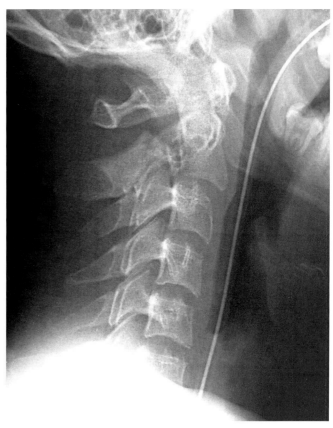

FIGURE 2

A neck injury sustained in a high-speed motor vehicle collision in a young man

A 20-year-old man was returning from a "night on the town" when he drove his car into a garbage truck.

On arrival in the ED, the patient appeared intoxicated. He was hemodynamically stable. He had a forehead contusion. The neurological examination was normal, as was examination of the chest, abdomen and extremities.

His lateral cervical spine radiograph is shown in Figure 1.

• Are there any abnormalities?

The initial lateral view was interpreted as negative for an acute injury. However, the inferior portion of C7 was not seen. In addition, the patient's positioning was rotated; the left and right lateral masses are widely separated.

The patient was maintained in spinal immobilization and the lateral view was repeated with greater traction on the patient's arms (Figure 2).

Although this second view did not show C7, the injury is now more easily seen. The injury, however, was visible on the initial lateral view.

THE IDEAL LESION

The second lateral radiograph more clearly reveals the patient's injury, although the injury was, in fact, visible on the first lateral view.

Although a definite fracture is difficult to detect, there is indirect evidence that a fracture is present, i.e., **malalignment** of the upper cervical spine. The **C2 vertebral body** shows slight anterior displacement (*anterolisthesis*) relative to C3 (*asterisk* in Figures 3 and 4). This displacement is easier to see in the second radiograph (Figure 3).

Slight anterior displacement of the C2 vertebral body relative to C3 may be normal, especially with supine cross-table lateral radiographs in which the neck is slightly flexed. However, a **second radiographic finding** indicates that this C2 anterolisthesis is abnormal.

The spinous process of C2 is displaced slightly posteriorly. This is determined by drawing a line through the C1–C3 spinolaminar junctions: the **posterior cervical line** (PCL) (*lines* in Figures 3, 4, and 5). Normally, the C1, C2, C3 spinolaminar junctions are within 2 mm of a straight line. In this patient, the C2 spinolaminar junction is displaced 3 mm posterior to the PCL (*arrowheads* in Figures 3 and 4). Because the anterior part of C2 is displaced anteriorly, and the posterior part of C2 is displaced posteriorly, the neural arch of C2 must be fractured.

There are subtle signs of the neural arch fractures. In the second radiograph, the superior border of the neural arch is interrupted and has a notched appearance (Figure 3, *arrow*). This is suspicious for a fracture. The first radiograph shows a small indentation along the superior edge of the C2 neural arch (Figure 4, *arrow*).

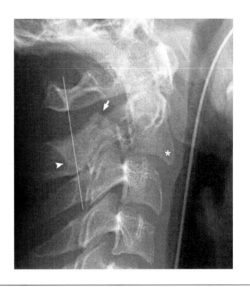

FIGURE 3 Second lateral view (Figure 2).

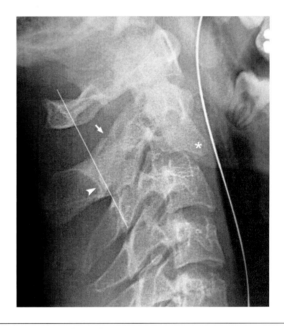

FIGURE 4 First lateral view (Figure 1).

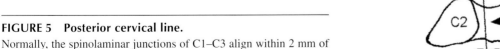

FIGURE 5 Posterior cervical line.

Normally, the spinolaminar junctions of C1–C3 align within 2 mm of a straight line.

With bilateral neural arch fractures (*arrow*), the C2 spinolaminar junction is displaced posterior to the PCL (*arrowhead*). This is due to posterior displacement of the C2 posterior arch fragment as well as anterior displacement of the C2 vertebral body and C1 spinolaminar junction.

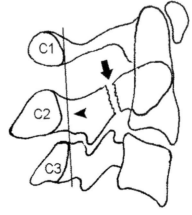

This patient's injury–bilateral neural arch fractures–is known as a **hangman's fracture.** The usual site of fracture is the isthmus or **pars interarticularis,** which is located between the superior and inferior articular facets (Figure 6). This is the weakest part of the C2 neural arch. Alternatively, fractures may occur more anteriorly and extend into the body of C2.

In this patient, the two fractures occur at different levels of the neural arch. They are therefore not overlapping on the lateral view and are not clearly seen on the radiographs.

CT readily demonstrates the bilateral neural arch fractures (Figure 7).

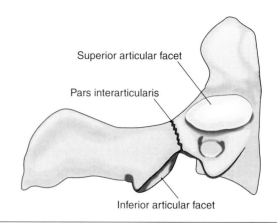

Superior articular facet

Pars interarticularis

Inferior articular facet

FIGURE 6   The pars interarticularis is located between the superior and inferior articular facets.

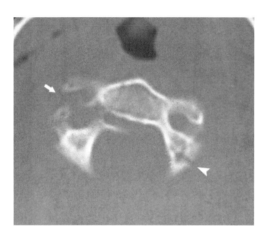
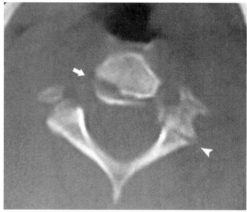

FIGURE 7   CT—Patient 3
There are bilateral fractures through the neural arch of C2.

On the right, the fracture extends into the transverse process and vertebral body (*arrows*). On the left, the fracture is through the pars interarticularis (*arrowheads*).

Hangman's fractures are classified into three types depending on the degree of displacement (Figure 8).

Type I is nondisplaced or minimally displaced (less than 3 mm). This is the most frequent type (65% of cases) and is the most subtle radiographically. Neurological deficits usually do not occur, which contributes to the risk of missing the injury.

In **Type II** fractures (28% of cases), the body of C2 is displaced or angulated with respect to C3.

In **Type III** fractures (7% of cases), the C2–C3 articular facet joints are also disrupted.

When one or both of the fractures involves the posterior portion of the vertebral body rather than the neural arch, the injury is referred to an "**atypical hangman's fracture.**"

Types I and II can usually be managed without operative intervention, whereas Type III injuries often need surgical fixation.

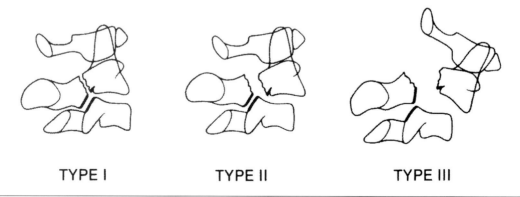

TYPE I   **TYPE II**   **TYPE III**

FIGURE 8   Effendi Classification of Hangman's Fractures.
Type I is minimally displaced. Type II disrupts the C2–C3 intervertebral disk. Type III disrupts the facet joints as well as the intervertebsal disk.
[From Rogers LF: *Radiology of Skeletal Trauma, 3rd ed.* Churchill-Livingstone, 2002, with permission.]

Hangman's Fractures

A typical **mechanism of injury** causing a hangman's fracture is a motor vehicle collision in which the victim's face hits the windshield (Figure 9). **Hyperextension and compression** of the neck causes posterior neural arch fractures. The anterior longitudinal ligament may be torn resulting in anterior slippage (anterolisthesis) of the C2 vertebral body. This vertebral body slippage is the basis for the formal name of a hangman's fracture: **traumatic spondylolisthesis of the axis.**

(*Spondylolisthesis* refers to slippage of one vertebral body relative to the subjacent one at the fibrocartilaginous intervertebral disk. The term *subluxation* should not be used to describe this displacement. The terms subluxation and dislocation refer to displacement of diarthrodial (synovial) joints such as the articular facet joints.)

The **incidence of neurological injury** is low with hangman's fractures, especially types I and II. This is because the spinal canal is widest at C1–C2, and because the fractures through the neural arch tend to enlarge the spinal canal. However, because of the low incidence of fatal spinal cord injury, this fracture would not seen suitable for judicial hangings. In fact, a true hangman's fracture is different from most hangman's fractures that are seen today.

A **judicial hangman's fracture** is produced by a different mechanism of injury. Judicial hangings result in complete, abrupt, and lethal transection of the spinal cord. (A "hungman's fracture" would perhaps be a more accurate term.)

Hangmen did not always produce a hangman's fracture in carrying out their duty. In fact, the hangman's fracture was a relatively recent advance in the "art of hanging." Prior to the late nineteenth century, the hangman's knot was placed in a suboccipital or subauricular position (Figure 10). The spine was often not fractured and the victim died from strangulation and asphyxiation after an often prolonged period of agony. Such strangulation could be inconvenient for judicial hangings because of the relatively long time required to cause death and the occasional non-fatal results. The short distance that the victims dropped also contributed to the prolonged period of strangulation.

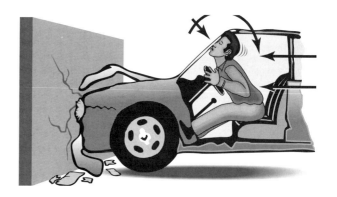

FIGURE 9   The typical mechanism of injury causing hangman's fractures.

Hyperextension and axial compression occur when the head impacts on the windshield. This fractures the posterior skeletal elements of the cervical spine.

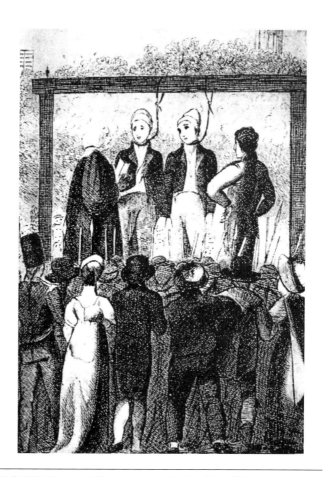

FIGURE 10   A public execution in England, in 1809, of two persons convicted of burglary. The knots are in the subauricular position that causes death by strangulation. In addition, a "short drop" was being used in this double execution.

Public executions were discontinued in the mid-nineteenth century in England.

[From Laurence J: *A History of Capital Punishment.* London, Sampson Low, Marston, 1932.]

In England, during the late nineteenth century, a prison surgeon constructed a device to maintain the hangman's noose in a submental position (Figure 11) (Marshall 1888). In 1913, Fredric Wood-Jones published his study of the injury produced by a submentally placed knot and concluded that this placement yielded the most certain and "humane" results. Hyperextension and forceful *distraction* produce bilateral fractures of the C2 neural arch and cervicocranial separation (Figure 12). The spinal cord is instantly severed causing immediate death. It is therefore the "**ideal lesion**" to be produced by a hanging.

Patient 3 Outcome

The remainder of this patient's trauma evaluation was negative. Neurosurgical evaluation included CT and flexion/extension views, which confirmed the lesion's mechanical stability and the absence of other fractures. The patient was fitted with a halo-vest and referred for further rehabilitation.

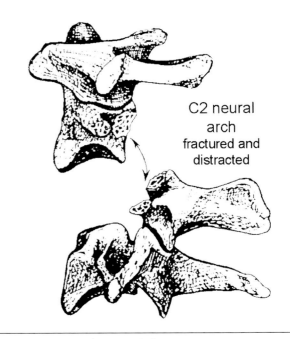

FIGURE 12   A true hangman's fracture.
The "ideal lesion" produced by hanging.

[From Wood-Jones F: The ideal lesion produced by judicial hanging. *Lancet* 1913;1:53.]

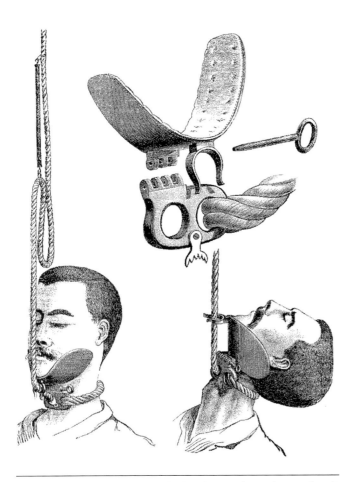

FIGURE 11   A chin trough maintains the rope in a sub-mental position. This assures forceful extension and distraction of the neck, producing a fatal hangman's fracture.

[From Marshall JD: Judicial execution. *Br Med J* 1888;1:179–182.]

'Tis sweet to dance to violins,
When love and life are fair,
But 'tis not sweet with nimble feet
To dance upon the air.

From the Ballad of Reading Goal
Oscar Wilde, 1898

Other Patients with Hangman's Fractures

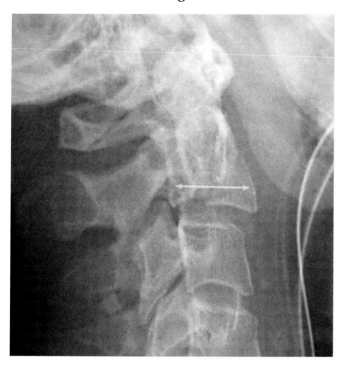

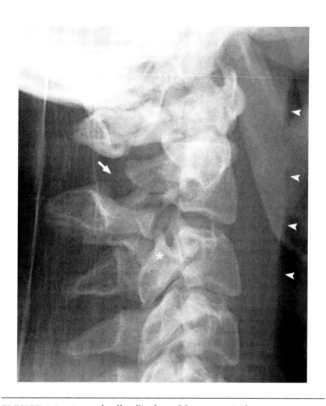

FIGURE 13   An "atypical" hangman's fracture causing a "fat C2" sign.

On one side of the hangman's fracture, there is a vertically oriented fracture through the posterior aspect of the C2 vertebral body. The anterior portion of the vertebral body has displaced anteriorly which causes apparent widening of the C2 vertebral body (*double-headed arrow*).

The **fat C2 sign** is a reliable indicator of a C2 vertebral body fracture. It can also occur with C2 burst fractures, extension teardrop fractures, and type III odontoid fractures that extend low through the body of C2.

FIGURE 14   A markedly displaced hangman's fracture.

Bilateral par interarticularis fractures are easily seen due to displacement of the posterior fragment. The C2–C3 facet joints are disrupted (*asterisk*). There is marked soft tissue swelling (*arrowheads*).

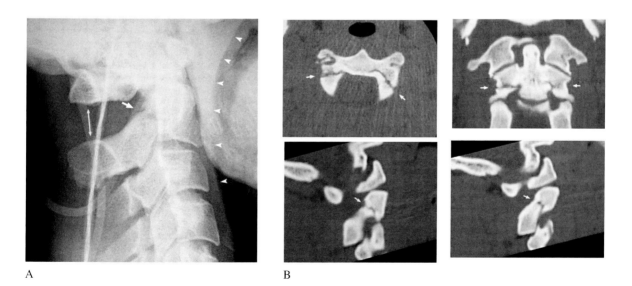

A   B

FIGURE 15   A minimally displaced hangman's fracture—Nearly normal radiographs.

(*A*) There is widening of the C1–C2 interspinous process distance (*double-headed arrow*) and a notch-like defect in the pars interarticularis (*arrow*). There is also soft tissue swelling at and superior to C1 (*arrowheads*).

(*B*) CT axial, coronal, and left and right parasagittal images demonstrate bilateral pars interarticularis fractures (*arrows*).

[Courtesy Peter Gruber, MD, Jacobi Hospital, New York.]

SUGGESTED READING

Clark CR, Benzel EC, Currier BL, et al: *The Cervical Spine,* 4th ed. Lippincott-Raven, The Cervical Spine Research Society Editorial Committee, 2004.

Clark CR, Ducker TB, et al: *The Cervical Spine,* 3rd ed. Lippincott-Raven, The Cervical Spine Research Society Editorial Committee, 1998.

Effendi B, Roy D, Cornish B, et al.: Fractures of the ring of the axis: A classification based on the analysis of 131 cases. *J Bone Joint Surg (Br)* 1981;63:319–327.

Garfin SR, Rothman RH: Traumatic spondylolisthesis of the axis. In Sherk HH (Cervical Spine Research Society Editorial Committee), ed. *The Cervical Spine*, 2nd ed. Lippincott, 1989.

Hammond DN: On the proper method of executing the sentence of death by hanging. *Med Rec NY* 1882;22:426.

James R, Nasmyth-Jones R: The occurrence of cervical fractures in victims of judicial hanging. *Forensic Sci Intern* 1992;54:81–91.

Laurence J: *A History of Capital Punishment.* London: Sampson Low, Marston, 1932.

Marshall JD: Judicial execution. *Br Med J* 1888;1:179–182.

Pellei DD: The fat C2 sign. *Radiology* 2000;217:359–360.

Robertson WGA: Recovery after judicial hanging. *Br Med J* 1935;1:121.

Smoker WRK, Dolan KD: The "fat" C2: A sign of fracture. *AJR* 1987;148:609–614.

Sternbach G, Sumchai AP: Frederic Wood-Jones: The ideal lesion produced by hanging. *J Emerg Med* 1989;7:517–520.

Swichuk LE: Anterior dislocation of C2 in children: Physiologic or pathologic? *Radiology* 1977;122:759–763.
(Initial description of the posterior cervical line. It was first used in children to help distinguish physiologic "pseudosubluxation" of C2 on C3 due to normal ligamentous laxity from traumatic vertebral body slippage.)

van Rijn RR, Kool DR, de Witt Hamer PC, Majoie CB: An abused five-month-old girl: Hangman's fracture or congenital arch defect? *J Emerg Med* 2005;29:61–65.

Wood-Jones F: The ideal lesion produced by judicial hanging. *Lancet* 1913;1:53.

Cervical Spine: Patient 4

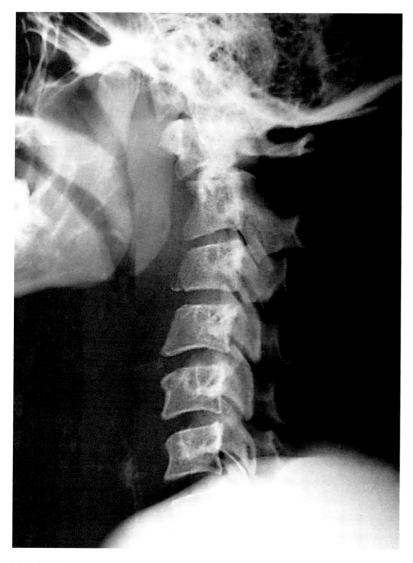

A common clinical scenario causing an axial loading injury to the cervical spine—a dive head-first into a shallow body of water.

[From Galli et al *Emergency Orthopedics: The Spine*. McGraw-Hill, 1989, with permission.]

FIGURE 1

A neck injury in a young man who fell off of a subway platform onto his head

A 37-year-old man lost his balance while standing on a subway platform and fell five feet, head first onto the tracks. He had consumed an alcoholic beverage prior to his fall. Fortunately, a train was not entering the station at the time. He was extricated from the tracks, immobilized, and brought to the ED.

In the ED, the patient was hemodynamically stable. He had a deep, 5-cm scalp laceration, but no other external signs of trauma. He complained of neck pain and a painful burning sensation in his shoulders and upper arms. His neurological examination was remarkable for mild weakness of his hand grasp bilaterally. Lower extremity strength was normal. There was midline tenderness over his cervical spine, but no palpable deformity.

The cervical spine radiograph is shown in Figure 1.

- How would you interpret this radiograph?

DOUBLE TROUBLE

Lateral View—ABCS Approach

The radiograph is technically **inadequate** because the seventh cervical vertebra is not visible (Figure 2). Nonetheless, several significant abnormalities are seen.

The vertebrae are in good **alignment,** although the vertebral column as a whole appears straightened as is common in a supine portable cross-table lateral view of an immobilized trauma victim. In addition, the patient's positioning was slightly rotated causing a lack of superimposition of the articular facets. The "ring of C2" is not clearly seen because of this rotation. The superior portion of the dens is obscured by the overlapping bone of the skull base.

Examination of the **bones** reveals a tiny fragment adjacent to the anterior-inferior corner of **C3** (Figure 2, *arrow*). This represents a **small avulsion fracture** due to traction by the anterior longitudinal ligament during forceful extension of the neck (Figure 3).

Examination of the prevertebral soft tissues reveals marked **soft tissue swelling** that measures 15 mm at C2 and C3 (Figure 2, *arrowheads*).

When one injury is found (e.g., the C3 avulsion fracture), the search for others must continue. This patient, in fact, has two distinct injuries.

The **cervicocranium** appears abnormal (Figure 2). One radiographic landmark in this region is the **predental space**—the space between the dens and the anterior portion of C1 (also known as the *anterior atlanto-dental interval* or AADI). The predental space is normally 3 mm or less (Figure 4). In this patient, the area posterior to the anterior arch of C1 appears "empty." This is because the dens is displaced posteriorly; the predental space is widened, measuring approximately 6 mm (Figures 2 and 5).

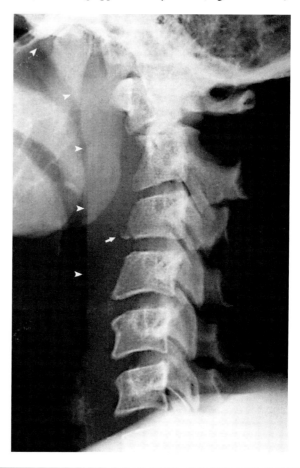

FIGURE 2   Lateral view.

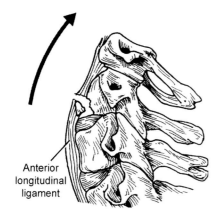

FIGURE 3   **Distractive-extension avulsion fracture**
This is sometimes referred to as a hyperextension "teardrop" fracture.
[From Galli, et al: *Emergency Orthopedics: The Spine*. McGraw-Hill, 1989, with permission.]

Anterior
longitudinal
ligament

The dens is normally held in position against the anterior arch of C1 by the *transverse atlantal ligament* (TAL) (Figures 4 and 6). Widening of the predental space (posterior displacement of the dens) is a sign of TAL disruption. However, TAL rupture is rarely an isolated injury. Most frequently, transverse ligament rupture is associated with a burst fracture of the ring of C1 (Figure 6). This injury was thoroughly described by the neurosurgeon Geoffrey Jefferson in 1920.

The mechanism of injury of a **Jefferson burst fracture** is axial compression. It is usually caused by a fall in which the patient lands head-first, or by a blow to the top of the head. The outward sloping orientation of the atlanto-occipital and atlantoaxial articular surfaces causes the axial loading force to be deflected laterally and split apart the ring of C1 (Figure 7). There are fractures of both the anterior and posterior arches of C1 (Figure 6). The fractures are not usually visible on the lateral radiograph, although occasionally, the posterior arch fracture can be seen (Figure 8).

The incidence of spinal cord injury is low with Jefferson burst fractures. There are three reasons: (1) the spinal canal is widest with respect to the spinal cord at this level, (2) the burst fracture tends to further widen the spinal canal, and (3) spinal cord injuries at this level are usually fatal and the patients do not survive to receive medical attention.

In up to 50% of cases, Jefferson burst fractures are associated with other fractures of the cervicocranium. The most common fractures involve the dens, the C2 posterior arch (hangman's fracture), or C2 vertebral body (Figure 9A).

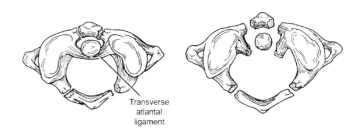

FIGURE 6   Jefferson burst fracture involves the anterior and posterior arches of C1. With a minimally displaced fracture, the transverse ligament is intact. Greater fracture displacement ruptures the transverse ligament.

[From Galli, et al: *Emergency Orthopedics: The Spine*. McGraw-Hill, 1989, with permission.]

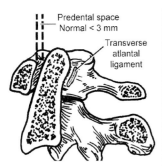 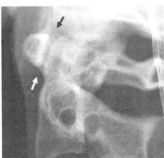

FIGURE 4   Normal predental space.

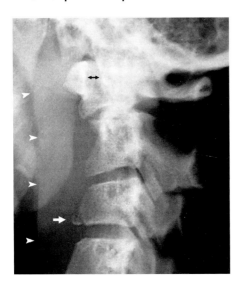

FIGURE 5   Detail of Patient 4's lateral view showing a widened predental space (*double-headed arrow*), C3 avulsion fracture (*arrow*), and soft tissue swelling. (*arrowheads*).

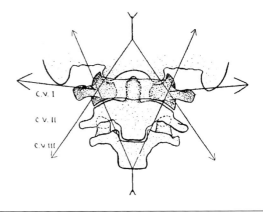

FIGURE 7   Jefferson's depiction of the forces causing a C1 burst fracture. An axial force is applied to the cervicocranium. The oblique orientation of the atlanto-occipital and atlantoaxial articular surfaces causes outward displacement of the C1 lateral masses.

[From Jefferson G: Fracture of the atlas vertebra. *Br J Surg*, Volume 7, 1919. Reprinted with permission. Permission granted by John Wiley & Sons Ltd on behalf of the BJSS Ltd.]

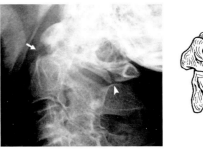 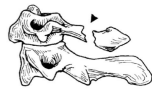

FIGURE 8   C1 posterior arch fracture (*arrowhead*). Confirmation that this is an isolated fracture and not part of a Jefferson burst fracture requires CT. There is also a displaced dens fracture (*arrow*).

[From Galli, et al: *Emergency Orthopedics: The Spine*. McGraw-Hill, 1989, with permission.]

Because a potentially unstable injury was evident on this patient's initial lateral view, the AP and open mouth views were deferred until after the patient's spine was stabilized using Gardner-Wells tongs and traction. On the patient's **open mouth view**, the Jefferson burst fracture is clearly seen (Figure 9). There is lateral displacement of the lateral masses of C1 relative to C2 (*arrowheads*), and asymmetry of the dens between the lateral masses of C1.

CT is excellent at demonstrating C1 fractures. In this patient, there were fractures of both the anterior and posterior arches of C1 (Figure 10, *arrows*). The predental space is widened (*double-headed arrow*), which is indicative of TAL rupture. In this CT myelogram, the spinal cord (*asterisk*) is visible within the relatively large spinal canal, which is one reason that the incidence of cord injury is low with these fractures.

The **management** of a Jefferson burst fracture depends on the **stability of the dens** in relation to C1 and the occiput. This is a function of the integrity of its ligamentous support. The TAL is only one factor. The alar and accessory ligaments also stabilize the dens. The **alar ligaments** extend from the apex of the dens to the base of the occipital condyles (Figure 11). The *accessory ligaments* extend from the lateral masses of C1 to the base of the dens. In most patients, the injury is mechanically stable and treatment can be nonoperative using a rigid halo-vest for immobilization. If the alar ligaments are torn and the dens is completely unstable, C1 and C2 must be surgically fused, even though this will significantly limit mobility of the neck.

The extent of ligamentous disruption can be estimated on the radiographs. On the lateral view, a *predental space* of 3–6 mm implies partial disruption of the transverse ligament; 6–10 mm implies disruption of the transverse ligament, but intact alar and accessory ligaments. Displacement >10 mm signifies complete ligamentous instability. On the *open mouth view*, if the lateral masses of C1 have a combined lateral displacement of 7 mm or more with respect to the lateral masses of C2, there is disruption of the transverse ligament (Figure 12). However, less displacement does not guarantee ligamentous integrity. Treatment decisions are ultimately determined by dynamic studies (flexion/extension views) and/or MRI.

In this patient, the open mouth view showed 10 mm widening of the lateral masses of C1 with respect to C2 and the predental space was 6 mm. This implied rupture of the transverse ligament. Coronal tomographic images of the dens confirmed that there was no concomitant fracture of the dens (Figure 13).

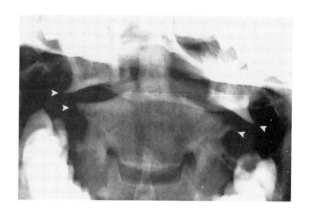

FIGURE 9   Open mouth view—Patient 4.

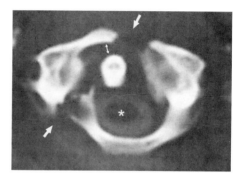

FIGURE 10   CT myelogram—Patient 4.

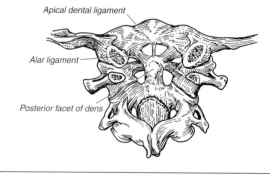

Apical dental ligament

Alar ligament

Posterior facet of dens

FIGURE 11   The alar ligaments viewed from posterior.
In this coronal section, the posterior portions of C1 and the occiput, as well as the TAL have been cut away. The alar ligaments provide secondary support for the dens when the TAL is disrupted.
[From Galli, et al: *Emergency Orthopedics: The Spine.* McGraw-Hill, 1989, with permission.]

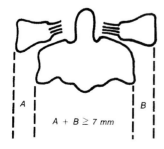

A   B

$A + B \geq 7\ mm$

FIGURE 12 On an open mouth view, displacement of the lateral masses of C1 relative to C2 by 7 mm or more implies that the transverse atlantal ligament is ruptured.

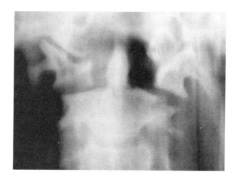

FIGURE 13 Coronal tomography confirms that the dens is not fractured.

Patient Outcome

One hour after the patient's arrival in the ED, his upper extremity paresthesia and weakness worsened. At three hours, the patient had 4/5 weakness of all muscle groups of both arms. This was due to a **central cord syndrome**.

The patient's spinal cord injury was related to the small hyperextension **avulsion fracture at C3**. Forceful extension of the neck causes inward buckling of the ligamentum flavum, which pinches the spinal cord and causes hemorrhage and/or edema within its central portion (Figure 14). The spinal motor and sensory tracts are anatomically arranged such that innervation of the upper extremities is located in the central portions of the spinal cord and lower extremity innervation is located peripherally (Figure 15). Lesions that affect the central portion of the cervical spinal cord therefore cause upper extremity motor and sensory deficits, while sparing the lower extremities.

This patient had two noncontiguous injuries (C1 and C3) due to different mechanisms of injury: *axial compression* caused a C1 burst fracture and *distractive-extension* caused a hyperextension avulsion fracture at C3. It was the second, less dramatic fracture that was responsible for his spinal cord injury.

The patient was treated with high-dose corticosteroids for his spinal cord injury in consultation with the neurosurgery service (although currently there is controversy about this treatment). After one week in the hospital, he recovered strength in his upper extremities. After one month of immobilization in a Halo-vest, flexion/extension views showed no mechanical instability of the cervical spine, and non-operative management was continued.

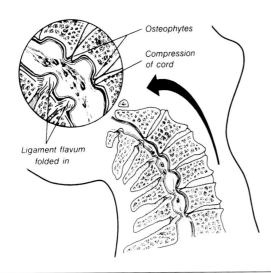

FIGURE 14   Forceful extension of the neck causes inward buckling of the ligamentum flavum which compresses the spinal cord. This results in hemorrhage or edema in the central portion of the spinal cord. Elderly patients are especially prone to this injury because the spinal canal is narrowed by osteophytes.

[From: Galli et al: Emergency Orthopedics: The Spine. McGraw-Hill, 1989. With permission.]

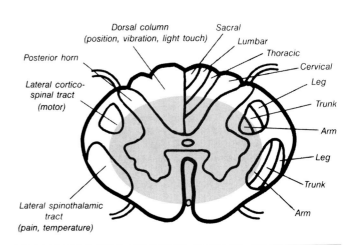

FIGURE 15   Anatomy of the spinal tracts in the cervical spinal cord. The area involved in a central cord syndrome is indicated by *gray shading.*

The tracts innervating the upper extremities are located centrally and are prone to injury during neck extension. The peripheral regions innervating the lower extremities are spared.

SUGGESTED READING

Bracken MB: Steroids for acute spinal cord injury. *Cochrane Database Syst Rev* 2002(3):CD001046.

Dai L, Jia L: Central cord injury complicating acute cervical disc herniation in trauma. *Spine* 2000;25:331–335.

Fehlings MG: Summary statement: The use of methylprednisolone in acute spinal cord injury. *Spine* 2001;26:S55.

Jefferson G: Fracture of the atlas vertebra. Report of four cases and a review of those previously recorded. *Br J Surg* 1920;7:407–422.

Leigh-Smith S, Price R, Summers D: Atlas: Standard diagnostic tests for an unusual fracture. *Emerg Med J* 2005;22:225–226.

Ly JQ: Jefferson fracture. *J Emerg Med* 2002;23:415–416.

Spencer MT, Bazarian JJ: Are corticosteroids effective in traumatic spinal cord injury? *Ann Emerg Med* 2003;41:410–413.

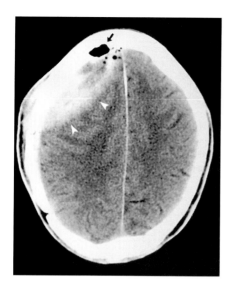

FIGURE 16 Open depressed skull fracture with an epidural hematoma (*arrowheads*) and pneumocephalus (*arrow*).

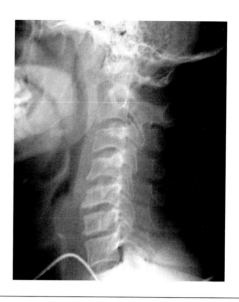

FIGURE 17 Lateral cervical spine view interpreted as negative for acute injury.

PATIENT 4B A 30-year-old construction worker fell from a 10-foot high scaffolding and landed on his head. He had an open depressed skull fracture and epidural hematoma (Figure 16). The lateral cervical spine radiograph was interpreted as negative for an injury (Figure 17). No other serious injuries were evident. The patient was taken immediately to the operating room for evacuation of the hematoma. Spine immobilization, however, was not maintained during the surgical procedure.

Upon awakening from surgery, the patient complained of severe neck pain. Completion of the cervical spine radiographic series revealed a Jefferson burst fracture on the open mouth view (Figure 18). This was confirmed by CT (Figure 19). Fortunately, the patient remained neurologically intact and

suffered no harm despite the delayed diagnosis. Review of the initial lateral view revealed cervicocranial soft tissue swelling (Figure 20, see Patient 1, Figure 5 on p. 376).

The lateral radiograph should not be relied upon to "clear" the cervical spine because it may occasionally miss injuries, particularly of the cervicocranium. Approximately 15% of the patients with cervical spine fractures have normal lateral radiographs and about 4% have a normal three-view series. Cervical spine immobilization must therefore be maintained in patients who have suffered major trauma until the patient can be fully assessed both clinically and radiographically.

In current clinical practice, CT is used as the initial imaging study in patients with severe head injury, and fractures such as this would not be missed.

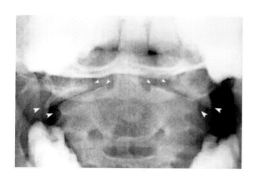

FIGURE 18 Open mouth view shows displacement of the C1 lateral masses characteristic of a Jefferson burst fracture (*arrowheads*).

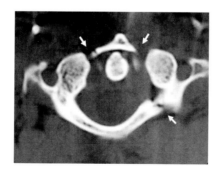

FIGURE 19 CT of C1 demonstrating fractures of the anterior and posterior arches of C1 (*arrows*). The predental space is normal.

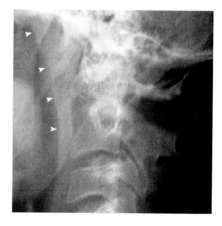

FIGURE 20 Detail of the initial lateral view.

The predental space and posterior arch of C1 are normal, although not well seen due to overlap by the skull base. There is subtle prevertebral soft tissue swelling with loss of the normal concavities superior to C1 and anterior to the dens (*arrowheads*).

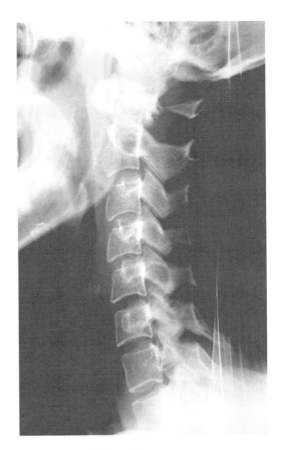

FIGURE 21—Patient 4C

PATIENT 4C   An 18-year-old woman was a rear-seat passenger in a taxicab that stopped short at a traffic light and was "rear-ended" by another car. She was wearing a seat belt. Her head was jolted backward, but there were no other injuries. She was transported to the ED on a long board with spine immobilization.

She complained of mild neck pain and had midline cervical tenderness. Her neurologic examination was normal.

Her lateral cervical spine radiograph is shown (Figure 21).

- Are there any abnormalities?

In this patient, there is a "break" in the posterior arch of C1. However, this is not due to a fracture, but is instead due to a congenital anomaly. There are many developmental anomalies of the cervical spine, and this adds to the difficulties in cervical spine radiograph interpretation. Anomalies of C1 and C2 are common.

This patient has **incomplete ossification of the posterior arch of C1.** The neural arch is completed by a band of fibrous tissue. Lucencies in this region mimic fractures of the posterior arch of C1.

Signs distinguishing this as a congenital anomaly, rather than a fracture, are the well-formed cortical margins that taper smoothly (*arrow*, Figure 22A), the normal width of the predental space, and normal prevertebral soft tissues. In addition, there is compensatory hypertrophy of the anterior arch of C1 (*asterisk*) and a characteristic V-shaped predental space (*arrowhead*). CT confirmed the incomplete arch of C1 (Figure 22B). (CT is not necessary to make this diagnosis.)

In a second patient, the C1 posterior arch defect is due to incomplete ossification of the posterior tubercle (Figure 23).

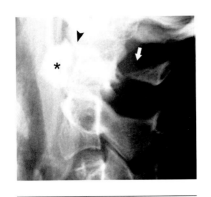

FIGURE 22A

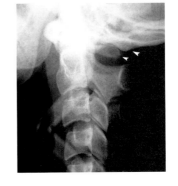

FIGURE 22B

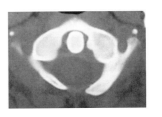

FIGURE 23A   **FIGURE 23B**

Cervical Spine: Patient 5

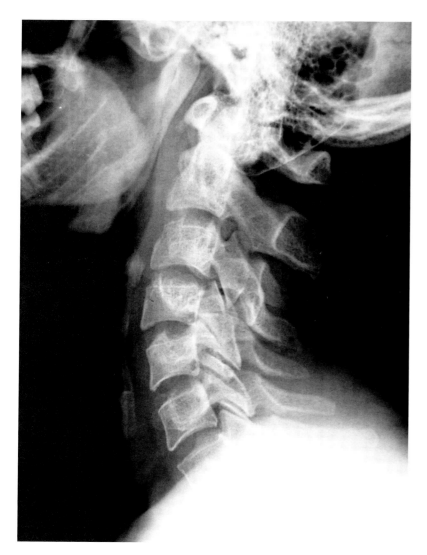
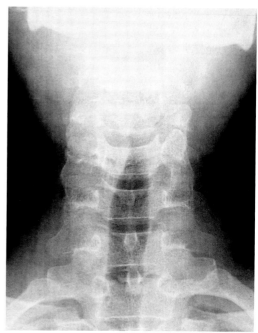
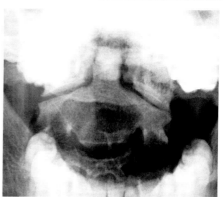

FIGURE 1

Neck pain in a middle-aged man involved in a slow moving motor vehicle collision

A 42-year-old man was the front seat passenger in a car that was struck on the driver's side by another vehicle. Neither car was going at high speed. Damage to the patient's car was limited to the front fender; the windshield was not "spidered." The patient was wearing a seat belt at the time of the collision. He was brought to the ED in full spine immobilization and was triaged to one of the examination rooms.

The patient was awake and alert with no overt signs of trauma. His vital signs were normal. He complained of pain in his neck, lower back, and right wrist. He noted that he had struck his head on the car door and had been "dazed" for a

few seconds, but was uncertain whether he had lost consciousness.

On examination, he had mild midline neck tenderness without deformity. There were good bilateral breath sounds without chest wall tenderness. His abdomen, pelvis, and extremities showed no signs of injury. The neurological examination was normal.

The patient was removed from the "long board" and sent for cervical spine radiography. The radiographs are shown in Figure 1.

- Are there any abnormalities?

BOW TIE

Although **ABCS** (alignment, bone, cartilage, and soft tissues) is a convenient mnemonic device for the interpretation of the lateral cervical spine radiograph, one element seen on the lateral view is not emphasized in this scheme–alignment of the **articular facets** and **lateral masses** of C3–C7.

Each vertebra has two lateral masses and each lateral mass has a superior and inferior articular facet. On the lateral view, each lateral mass has a diamond shape formed by the superior and inferior articular facets and the anterior and posterior cortical surfaces. In a perfectly positioned lateral view, the left and right lateral masses are exactly superimposed. More often, the patient's positioning is slightly rotated and the lateral masses are not exactly superimposed (Figure 2).

In this patient's lateral view (Figure 1), the positioning is slightly rotated and the articular facets do not exactly overlap. However, at C3 there is an abrupt increase in rotation—the two lateral masses of C3 are widely separated. This creates a double-diamond or **bow tie** appearance (Figure 3). **Abrupt rotational malalignment** is characteristic of unilateral facet dislocation.

With **unilateral facet dislocation,** the articular facet of one vertebra has slipped up and over the articular facet of the subjacent vertebra, and the lateral mass has dislocated anteriorly into the subjacent neuroforamina (Figure 4). This is sometimes called "locking" of the facet joint, although a unilateral facet dislocation can be unstable, particularly when the lateral mass is fractured.

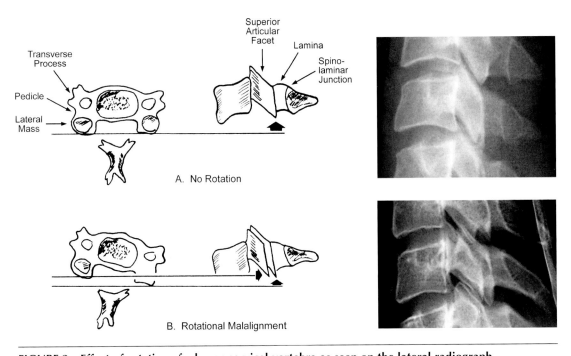

FIGURE 2   **Effect of rotation of a lower cervical vertebra as seen on the lateral radiograph.**

(*A*) Correct alignment (no rotation): the left and right lateral masses are perfectly superimposed on the lateral view.

(*B*) Rotational malalignment: the left and right lateral masses are not superimposed.

[From Gerlock AJ, Kirchner, SG, Heller RM, Kaye JJ: *The Cervical Spine in Trauma, Advanced Exercises in Diagnostic Radiology,* Vol. 7, Saunders, 1978, with permission.]

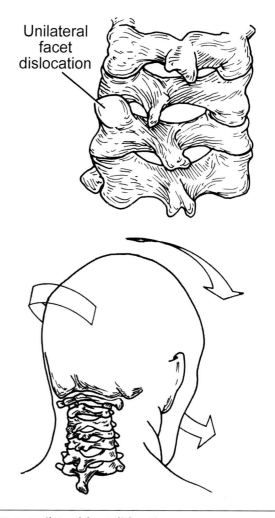

Unilateral
facet
dislocation

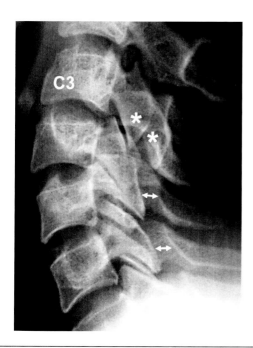

FIGURE 3   Lateral view—Patient 5.

There is abrupt rotational malalignment of the lateral masses at C3.

The lateral masses have a double-diamond or bow tie appearance (*asterisks*). The space between the porterior cortex of the lateral mass and the spinolaminar junction (the "laminar space") is normal at C4 and C5 (*double-headed arrows*) and is obliterated at C3 due to the unilateral facet dislocation.

FIGURE 4   Unilateral facet dislocation.

(*A*) Abrupt rotation causes anterior dislocation of one facet joint while the contralateral facet articulation remains intact.

(*B*) Mechanism of injury is distractive-flexion, which separates the posterior ligamentous structures. A rotational component causes dislocation of the facet joint on one side.

[From Galli et al: *Emergency Orthopedics: The Spine.* McGraw-Hill, 1989, with permission.]

The **mechanism of injury** responsible for unilateral facet dislocation is combined **distractive-flexion,** which separates the posterior elements of the vertebral column, and **rotation,** which directs the injury to one side (Figure 4B).

Unilateral facet dislocation does not usually cause spinal cord injury because the spinal canal is only slightly narrowed. However, displacement of the articular facet into the neuroforamina can cause nerve root injury (in approximately 50% of cases).

The **treatment** of a unilateral facet dislocation can be problematic and various management strategies have been proposed.

Closed reduction with axial traction is successful in one-quarter of cases. If closed reduction fails, open reduction and posterior fixation is recommended. If the dislocation is not reduced and allowed to heal by spontaneous fusion, there is a high incidence of persistent pain and limitation of motion.

Some authors note that closed reduction can be hazardous if there are fracture fragments or disk protrusion into the spinal canal because these can impinge on the spinal cord during traction. Pre-reduction CT and MRI are recommended to identify bone fragments or intervertebral disk herniation in the spinal canal. Open reduction is advised in these cases.

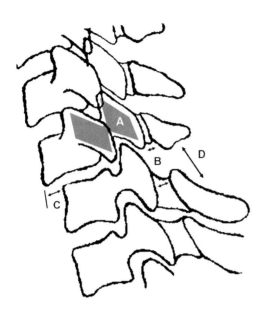

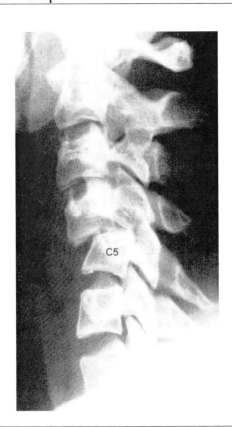

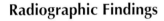

FIGURE 5   Four signs of unilateral facet dislocation.

(*A*) Bow tie: Abrupt rotation causes the articular masses to lie adjacent to one another rather than overlap. Compare to the subjacent vertebrae.

(*B*) Abrupt narrowing of the "laminar space"–space between the posterior cortex of the lateral mass and the spinolaminar junction.

(*C*) Anterior slippage of vertebral body (anterolisthesis) up to 50% of vertebral body width.

(*D*) "Fanning" of the spinous processes.

Radiographic Findings

There are **four radiographic signs of unilateral facet dislocation** (Figure 5). The double-diamond or bow tie is the primary sign, although it can be difficult to see due to overlap with the vertebral body. The most frequent and reliably identified finding is abrupt **narrowing of the "laminar space"**–the space between the posterior cortex of the lateral mass and the spinolaminar junction (Young et al. 1989). The two other signs are due to tearing of the posterior ligaments: anterior slippage of the vertebral body and widening of the space between spinous processes (fanning).

In most instances, unilateral facet dislocation is obvious radiographically (Figure 6). However, the radiographic findings can be subtle in 25–50% of cases (Figure 7).

In Patient 5, a double-diamond is seen at C3 and there is complete loss of the laminar space (Figure 3). However, there is no malalignment of the vertebral bodies, which contributes to the diagnostic difficulty.

FIGURE 6   Unilateral facet dislocation at C4–C5—Obvious.

(*A*) Bow tie configuration of lateral masses at C4.

(*B*) Narrowing of the "laminar space" at C4 and above.

(*C*) Anterior slippage and angulation of C4 vertebral body.

(*D*) Fanning of the spinous processes at C4–C5.

[From Gerlock et al: *The Cervical Spine in Trauma,* Saunders, 1978, with permission.]

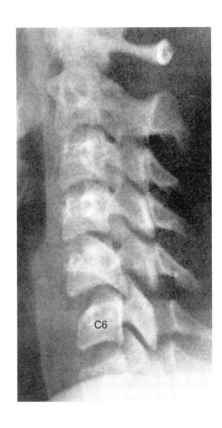

FIGURE 7   Unilateral facet dislocation at C5–C6—Subtle.

(*A*) Bow tie configuration of the lateral masses at C5 and above.

(*B*) Narrowing of the "laminar space" at C5 and above.

(*C*) No vertebral body slippage or spinous process fanning.

[From Harris: *Emerg Radiol* 1994;1:209. Reprinted by permission of the American Society of Emergency Radiology.]

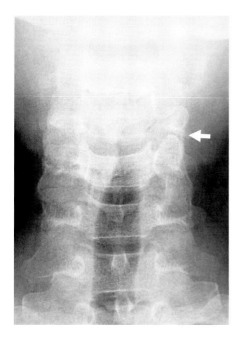

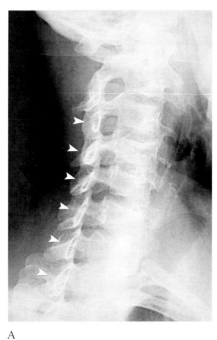

A

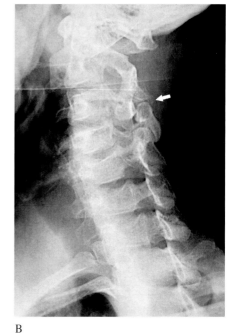

B

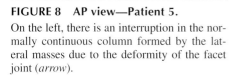

FIGURE 8   AP view—Patient 5.

On the left, there is an interruption in the normally continuous column formed by the lateral masses due to the deformity of the facet joint (*arrow*).

FIGURE 9   Oblique views—Patient 5.

(*A*) Right oblique views shows the normal alignment of the lamina like "shingles on a roof" (*arrowheads*).

(*B*) Left oblique view shows disruption of the laminar orientation at C3–C4 (*arrow*).

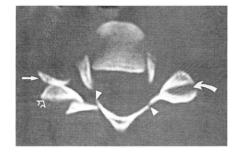

FIGURE 10   CT of unilateral facet dislocation—The reversed hamburger bun sign.

The facet joint on the left is relatively normal and looks like a hamburger on a bun (*curved arrow*). There is slight widening of the joint space due to the injury.

The facet joint on the right is dislocated—the facet of the more superior vertebra (*straight arrow*) lies anterior to the facet of the inferior vertebra (*open arrow*). This looks like a "reversed" hamburger bun. It is also known as a "naked facet."

In addition, there are bilateral laminar fractures (*arrowheads*).

[From Shanmuganathan et al: *AJR* 1994. Reprinted with permission of the American Journal of Roentgenology.]

Additional radiographic views can help confirm a unilateral facet dislocation.

On the **AP view,** the tips of the spinous processes should be aligned in a straight line and be evenly spaced. With a unilateral facet dislocation, the spinous processes at the level of injury may abruptly shift to one side (not seen in this patient). When there is a fracture or deformity of the facet joint, the articular facet surfaces may be visible such that the lateral masses do not form a normal smooth continuous contour (Figure 8).

Oblique views can be helpful in elucidating this injury. On a normal oblique view, the laminae are aligned like the "shingles on a roof." With unilateral facet dislocation, this alignment is disrupted (Figure 9). Oblique views have largely been supplanted by CT.

On **CT,** the articular surfaces of the facets normally face each other and the facet articulation looks like a hamburger bun. With unilateral facet dislocation, the articular facets face outward. This is called a "**naked facet**" or the "**reversed hamburger bun sign**" (Figure 10). In addition, CT can identify fractures of the posterior vertebral arch that are often not visible on the radiographs.

Patient Outcome

This patient's radiographic findings were surprising because, based on his clinical examination, his injuries seemed minor. A CT was done to better define the injury. The unilateral facet dislocation was confirmed, but the articular facets were deformed and hypertrophied, suggesting that this was longstanding (Figure 11). The patient did not recall having had previous trauma, although an injury in early childhood is a likely explanation (Holodny et al. 2002).

Due to the poor outcome associated with unreduced facet dislocation, the benefits of reduction were carefully considered. However, because the patient was asymptomatic, it was decided not to attempt reduction.

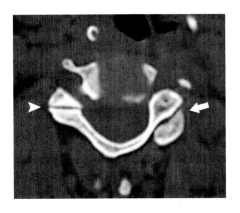
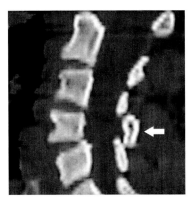

FIGURE 11   CT—Patient 5.

(*A*) Axial image at the C3–C4 facet joints shows a normal facet joint on the right ("hamburger bun") (*arrowhead*), and a dislocated facet on the left ("reversed hamburger bun") (*arrow*). The articular facets have a bulbous deformity because the facet dislocation was chronic.

(*B*) Left parasagittal reformatted image shows posterior displacement of the C4 lamina (*arrow*).

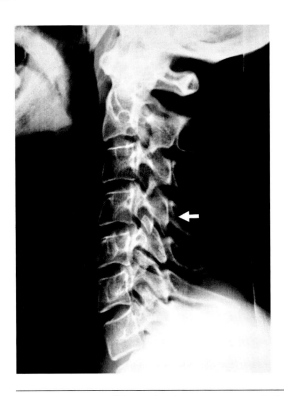
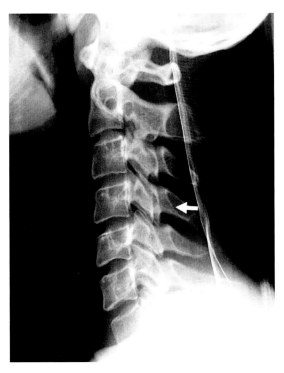

FIGURE 12   Not all bow ties signs represent injuries.

Rotated positioning can mimic a rotational injury such as a unilateral facet dislocation.

(*A*) The initial lateral view shows a bow tie configuration of the lateral masses of C4 (*arrow*). However, each vertebra has a similar bow tie appearance. This is due to rotated positioning of the patient.

(*B*) When the lateral view was repeated with better positioning, the bow ties disappear because the lateral masses are more closely superimposed (*arrow*).

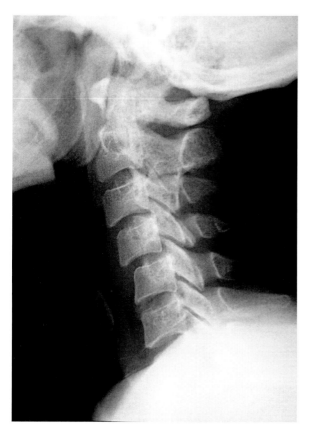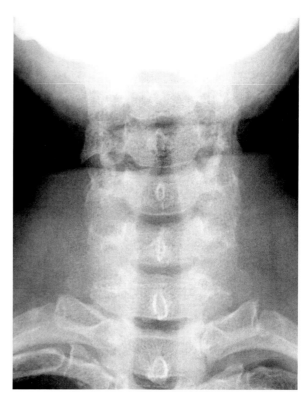

FIGURE 13

PATIENT 5B

A 40-year-old woman had been in a motor vehicle collision one month earlier. She had hit her right shoulder against the passenger side door. She was seen and observed in an ED for several hours. Chest, cervical spine, and shoulder radiographs were interpreted as normal. No serious injuries were diagnosed.

She now sought medical care for persistent right shoulder discomfort and weakness. She was unable to elevate her shoulder and abduct her upper arm.

Shoulder and chest radiographs were normal. Her cervical spine radiographs are shown in Figure 13.

- What is the diagnosis in this patient?

SUGGESTED READING

Daffner SD, Daffner RH: Computed tomography diagnosis of facet dislocations: The "hamburger bun" and "reverse hamburger bun" signs. *J Emerg Med* 2002;23:387–394.

Harris JH: Challenge case. *Emerg Radiol* 1994;1:209–211.

Holodny AI, Sharma V, Rubach E: Long-standing unilateral jumped facets at C3-4 with no apparent history of antecedent trauma. *Emerg Radiol* 2002;9:329–332.

Lingawi SS: The naked facet sign. *Radiology* 2001;219:366–367.

Rhea JT: Rotational injuries of the cervical spine. *Emerg Radiol* 2000;7:149–159.

Shanmuganathan K, Mirvis SE, Levine AM: Rotational injury of cervical facets: CT analysis of fracture patterns with implications for management and neurologic outcome. *AJR* 1994;163:1165–1169.

Young JW, Resnik CS, DeCandido P, Mirvis SE: The laminar space in the diagnosis of rotational flexion injuries of the cervical spine. *AJR* 1989;152:103–107.

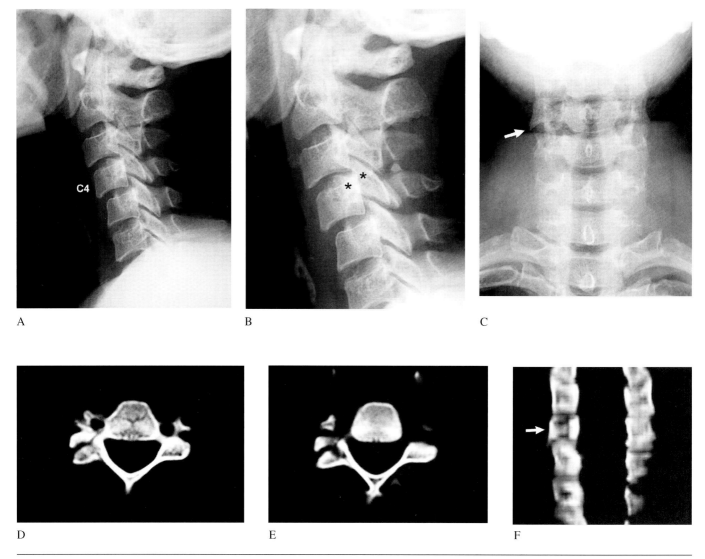

A   B   C

D   E   F

FIGURE 14   An injury with a bow tie sign is not always a unilateral facet dislocation. Patient 5B—Lateral mass fracture.

The lateral cervical spine radiograph shows double-diamonds (bow ties) at C3 and C4 (*A* and *B, asterisks*). There is also slight anterior slippage (anterolisthesis) of C4 on C5.

These findings are due to a fracture and rotational deformity of the right C4 lateral mass. C3 was rotated due to the injury at C4.

On the AP view, there is discontinuity of the right lateral mass column – the C4-C5 facet joint surface is visible (*C, arrow*).The C4 lateral mass is fractured and rotated.

Axial CT and coronal reformatted images confirmed a fracture of the C4 right lateral mass (*D-F*).

The fracture was causing impingement on the right C4 and C5 nerve roots at the C3-C4 and C4-C5 neuroforamina, accounting for the patient's shoulder weakness. A neurosurgery consultant did not feel surgery was indicated due to the long time that elapsed since her injury. She was referred to physical therapy for her C4 and C5 radiculopathies.

The mechanism of injury is compressive-extension with a rotational component. This causes a unilateral posterior element fracture (*G*).

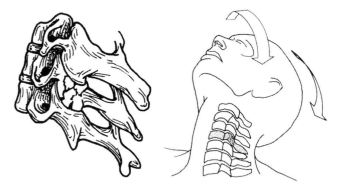

(*G*) A lateral mass fracture is caused by combined compressive extension and rotation (a force opposite to that causing a unilateral facet dislocation, i.e., distractive flexion with rotation).

[From: Galli : et al: *Emergency Orthopedics: The Spine*. McGraw-Hill, 1989, with permission.]

Cervical Spine: Patient 6

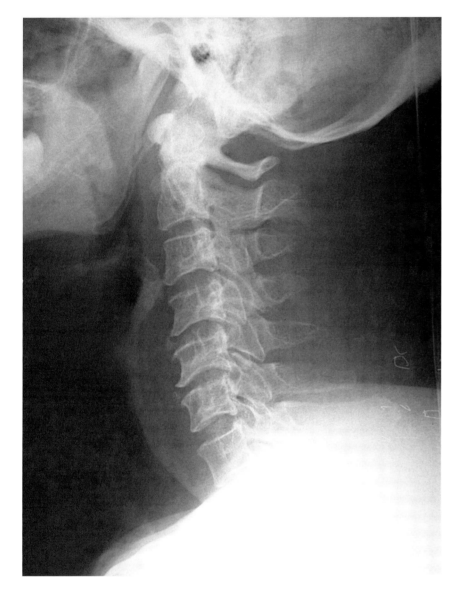

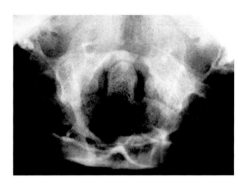

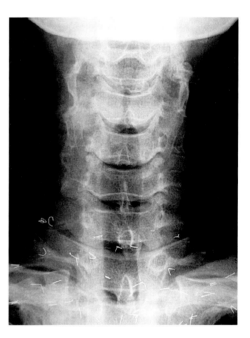

FIGURE 1

Neck pain in a middle-aged man who fell backwards off a ladder the day before coming to the ED

A 54-year-old man presented to the ED with neck, shoulder, and upper back pain. One day earlier, he had fallen six feet from a ladder. He landed feet first, then onto his back. He did not lose consciousness. He was able to get up by himself after the fall and felt that he was "alright." The next day, he decided to see a doctor because of persistent neck and shoulder pain. He was ambulatory on arrival to the ED.

On examination, he appeared healthy and in no apparent distress, resting comfortably on the stretcher. There was tenderness of the posterior neck, upper back, and right trapezius area.

There were no signs of head trauma. He had normal strength, sensation, and reflexes in all four extremities. His neck was then immobilized in a hard plastic cervical collar.

The cervical spine radiographs are shown in Figure 1. Shoulder radiographs were normal. (A Fuchs [submental] view of the dens was obtained rather than an open mouth view.)

- Are there any abnormal findings in these radiographs?

- How would you manage this patient?

DUMB LUCK

The fact that a patient is able to walk into the ED one day after a traumatic event should not dissuade you from considering that he has suffered a serious or unstable cervical spine injury.

In this patient, the **lateral radiograph** is of good technical quality—all seven vertebrae are visible. The patient's positioning is rotated such that the left and right lateral masses are not superimposed (Figure 2). Examination of the **bones** reveals no fracture, although there are chronic **degenerative changes** (**spondylosis**) of C4, C5, and C6—mild loss of vertebral body height, osteophytes, and anterior ligamentous calcification. This is not unexpected in a patient of his age.

The overall **alignment** of the vertebral column appears normal. In patients with degenerative changes, alignment of the *anterior surfaces* of the vertebral bodies is difficult to assess because of vertebral body osteophytes. Alignment can be assessed more accurately using the *posterior surfaces* of the vertebral bodies. In this patient, C5 is displaced 3 mm posteriorly with respect to C6 *(asterisk)*. This is termed **retrolisthesis.**

Malalignment may be due to an acute traumatic injury–a fracture or ligamentous injury. However, minor degrees of malalignment can also occur with nontraumatic conditions such as degenerative spondylosis, ligamentous laxity (common in children), or supine positioning of the patient, especially when the neck is immobilized by a cervical collar. Slight malalignment may be seen in normal individuals.

One often quoted criterion used to assess vertebral stability is that up to 3.5 mm of malalignment (and 11 degree of angulation) can exist between adjacent vertebral bodies without there being **ligamentous instability** (Figure 3). However, this is based on cadaver studies that were undertaken to assist surgeons in assessing spinal stability and planning operative care (White et al. 1975). It should not be used to exclude an injury in ED patients. Ligamentous disruption may be present with lesser degrees of malalignment or even normal alignment. Depending upon the clinical circumstances, further studies such as flexion/extension views or MRI may be needed to detect a nondisplaced or minimally displaced ligamentous injury.

Finally, examination of the **prevertebral soft tissues** reveals a prominent bulge at the level of C5–C6, the same region as the malalignment. Nonetheless, the width of the prevertebral soft tissues is less than 20 mm at this level, which is normal.

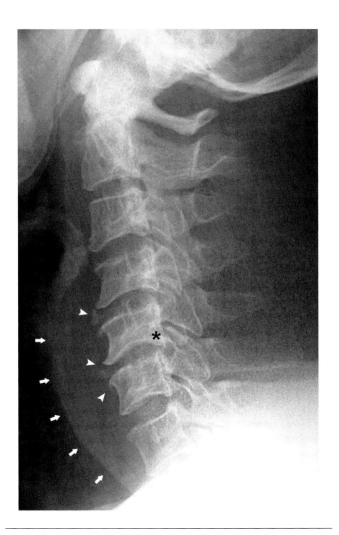

FIGURE 2   Lateral view—Patient 6.

Findings include:

1. Retrolisthesis of C5 *(asterisk)* on C6;
2. Degenerative changes (osteophytes and anterior longitudinal ligament calcification) of the C4, C5, and C6 vertebral bodies *(arrowheads)*;
3. Convexity (budge) in prevertebral soft tissues at C5–C6 and narrowing at C7 *(arrows)*.

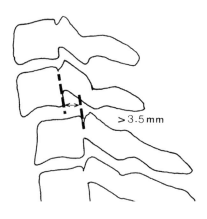

FIGURE 3   Malalignment of up to 3.5 mm can occur in the cervical spine without mechanical instability needing surgical fixation.

Nonetheless, an unstable injury may be present with less malalignment or even normal alignment.

[From Galli: et al: Emergency Orthopedics: The Spine. McGraw-Hill, 1989, with permission.]

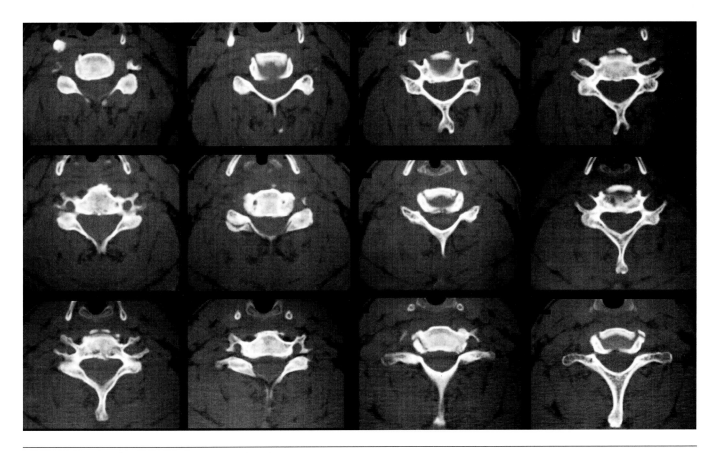

FIGURE 4   CT Patient 6.   C4 to the C6–C7 junction.

This patient had sustained trauma sufficient to injure his cervical spine, even though he was able to walk following the fall. The minor radiographic abnormalities (C5–C6 malalignment and possible soft tissue swelling) were therefore be considered potentially significant and warranting further radiographic evaluation.

A **CT scan** was performed to detect fractures that might not have been visible on the initial radiographs. The CT scan showed only degenerative changes with no fracture (Figure 4).

• What should be done next?

Patient Outcome

Because of the vertebral malalignment, questionable soft tissue swelling, mechanism of injury, and pain on palpation of his neck, **flexion/extension views** were obtained to investigate the possibility of an occult ligamentous injury. This was done at the suggestion of a neurosurgical consultant who advised that after the flexion/extension views were "cleared by radiology," we should send the patient home with a soft foam cervical collar and have him follow up in their clinic in one week.

Surprisingly, on the **flexion view**, there was anterior slippage of C5 with respect to C6, marked "fanning" of the spinous processes, and separation of the facet joints (Figure 5). These findings indicate that the posterior ligaments are completely torn. This is an unstable condition that could lead to spinal cord injury if the patient were to move his neck excessively.

This injury is termed a **hyperflexion sprain.** It is due to a **distractive-flexion** mechanism of injury that tears the posterior spinal ligaments (Figure 6). It is also called **anterior subluxation** because there is often anterior displacement of the articular facet joints.

The patient was hospitalized and treated with surgical fixation using posterior plates and screws (Figure 7).

The following day, the attending radiologist re-read the patient's radiographs. Before examining the flexion/extension views, he noted that the initial lateral view showed only "**chronic degenerative changes** with **no acute injury.**" The key radiographic finding that had been initially interpreted as being suggestive of an injury (vertebral body malalignment) was *not*, in fact, due to an acute injury.

Second, the prevertebral soft tissue thickness is less than 20 mm, which is normal. Furthermore, narrowing of the soft tissues normally occurs at the cervicothoracic junction, although usually not with such a pronounced budge as in this patient (see p. 423) (Harris and Mirvis 1996, pp. 45–48, 185–187).

The correct rationale for ordering flexion/extension views was the patient's significant pain following an injury of sufficient force to cause a cervical injury. In addition, the prevertebral soft tissue bulge is especially prominent and therefore could be considered an equivocal radiographic sign of potential significance. This adds support to the decision to obtain flexion/extension views. MRI would have been an alternative imaging test, although it is not usually readily available in the ED and is costly relative to flexion/extension radiography.

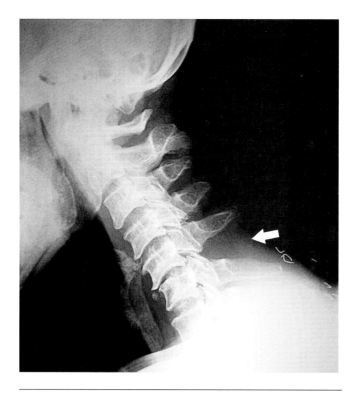

FIGURE 5   Flexion view revealed an unstable injury.
There is fanning of the C5–C6 spinous processes *(arrow)*, anterior subluxation of the facet joints, anterolisthesis of the C5 vertebral body, and narrowing of the anterior aspect of the C5–C6 intervertebral disk.

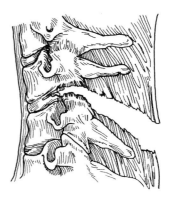

FIGURE 6   Hyperflexion sprain tears the posterior spinal ligaments—the supraspinous and interspinous ligaments, ligamentum flavum, articular facet joint capsules, and posterior longitudinal ligament.

[From Galli: et al: *Emergency Orthopedics: The Spine.* McGraw-Hill, 1989, with permission.]

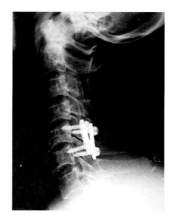
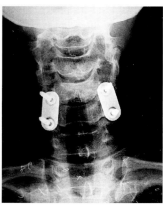

FIGURE 7   Postoperative fixation with posterior plates and screws.

FLEXION/EXTENSION RADIOGRAPHY

This patient represents the rare instance in which flexion/extension radiography revealed an unstable cervical spine injury that would have been missed if flexion/extension views had not been obtained in the ED. It was especially unusual because no fractures were identified on CT.

Flexion/extension radiography is used to detect mechanically unstable ligamentous injuries of the cervical spine. In **surgical practice,** flexion/extension views are used in patients with known cervical spine injuries to assess vertebral stability and aid in planning definitive surgical treatment. Such studies should not be performed in the ED.

The use of flexion/extension views in the ED is controversial. Flexion/extension views are used to diagnose a **nondisplaced isolated ligamentous injury** (no associated fracture) in a patient with normal or equivocal radiographs. Such injuries are rare, although potentially devastating if missed.

In the past, flexion/extension radiographs were ordered fairly frequently in the ED. In Lewis' series (1991), they were ordered in 13% of all cervical spine trauma cases. Brady et al. (1998) surveyed 144 emergency physicians and found that 87% of physicians obtained flexion/extension views for 20% or more of their patients. Such frequent use of flexion/extension radiography made sense before CT of the cervical spine became widely available because it provided an extra measure of assurance that the cervical spine was uninjured. With the widespread use of CT in the ED for patients with equivocal radiographs and those at high-risk for cervical spine injury, flexion/extension radiography is now performed rarely, if at all, in the ED.

Indications for Flexion/Extension Views in ED Patients

There are two circumstances in which flexion/extension views have been advocated for ED patients (Table 1): (1) patients with **severe neck pain** and **normal initial cervical spine radiographs** and (2) patients with **equivocal findings on the initial radiographs** and a clinical presentation compatible with a cervical spine injury, i.e., significant neck pain (Appendix A, Hockberger et al. 2006, Wales, et al.1980, Marion et al. 2000, Hadley et al. 2002, Daffner et al. 2002).

Equivocal findings that are suggestive but not diagnostic of an acute fracture or ligamentous injury include slight vertebral malalignment or isolated prevertebral soft tissue swelling (see p. 419-421). CT of the area in question should be performed prior to flexion/extension radiography to detect any unseen fractures that would preclude ED flexion/extension radiography. When there are **definite radiographic signs** of cervical spine injury, flexion/extension views should *not* be performed in the ED.

With the availability of **multidetector CT** (MDCT), which is able to quickly image the entire cervical spine, CT should be used prior to flexion/extension views both in patients with normal as well as equivocal initial radiographs. However, CT cannot directly detect ligamentous injury. Therefore, if the CT is negative for an acute injury, flexion/extension radiography (or MRI) may still be needed in patients at high-risk of cervical injury. However, the frequency of such injuries is exceedingly low, even among major trauma victims. In one series, there were no unstable ligamentous injuries discovered among 366 obtunded high-risk major trauma patients who had normal MDCT (Hogan et al. 2005).

The distinction between patients with **normal** and **equivocal radiographs** is important. In past studies, 80% of patients referred for flexion/extension views had normal initial radiographs and the frequency of injuries was very low (1%). Patients with equivocal radiographic findings had a higher incidence of injury (14%). However, the criteria for "equivocal" radiographic findings are not clearly defined.

There are **two caveats** to the use of flexion/extension views in the ED. **First,** there is the potential for causing **neurological damage** when an injured spine is moved. Dynamic studies should therefore only be performed in fully alert and cooperative patients under adequate supervision. The motion should be done by the patient and halted if the patient experiences severe pain or neurological symptoms.

Second, muscle spasm in an acutely injured patient can prevent adequate movement of the neck and mask a ligamentous injury (Webb et al. 1976, Herkowitz and Rothman 1984, Lewis et al. 1991, Insko et al. 2002). When neck motion is not adequate, ligamentous injury cannot be definitively excluded. If adequate flexion/extension views cannot be obtained, the patient should be referred for repeat examination in one week, at which time muscle spasm will usually have abated.

TABLE 1

Indications and Contraindications for Flexion/Extension Views in the ED

Indications

  Severe neck pain and normal CSR
  Equivocal or suspicious CSR (slight malalignment)

Contraindications

  Altered mental status
  Unable to cooperate with active motion of neck
  Definite injury on CSR
  Neurological deficit referable to cervical spine injury
  Unable to flex or extend the neck adequately due to muscle spasm
    or pain (relative contraindication)

CSR–cervical spine radiography

What Is the Evidence Regarding the Use of Flexion/Extension Radiography in the ED?

Retrospective Studies

There have been eight retrospective studies to assess the usefulness of flexion/extension views in stable patients with normal or equivocal radiographs. These studies demonstrate a low, but not zero, incidence of occult ligamentous injury. In combining the results of these studies, 1503 patients had flexion/extension radiography, 41 of which revealed an injury (2.7%). Seven of these patients (17%) needed surgical fixation. However, all of these studies antedate the use of MDCT to evaluate patients at high risk for cervical spine injury.

Four of the studies distinguished between patients with normal and equivocal radiographs. A considerably higher incidence of injury was found among patients with equivocal radiographs. Of the 899 patients, with **normal initial radiographs,** 9 had abnormal flexion/extension views (1%), of which 3 needed surgery. Lewis was the only investigator to find significant injuries in patients with *normal* initial radiographs—among 71 patients, 4 had abnormal flexion/extension views (6%), of which 3 needed surgery (4%) (Lewis 1991).

Of the 208 patients with **equivocal radiographs,** 30 had abnormal flexion/extension views (14%). Among the studies that reported treatment, four patients needed surgery and three needed halo-vest immobilization.

The yield of flexion/extension radiography is therefore considerably higher in patients with equivocal initial radiographs. However, most flexion/extension views are performed in patients with normal initial radiographs (approximately 80%). Because the yield is so low in these cases, flexion/extension views could potentially be omitted in such patients.

In a retrospective review of the **NEXUS** cervical spine database of 818 patients with cervical spine injuries, 86 patients (10.5%) had flexion/extension views (Pollack et al. 2001). In patients with *normal* initial radiographs, *no* cases of occult ligamentous injury were disclosed by flexion/extension views. Four patients did have ligamentous injuries disclosed by flexion/extension radiography. However, all four patients had other injuries visible on the initial cervical spine radiographs. The authors conclude that flexion/extension views add little to the evaluation of patients with normal radiographs and are not warranted.

Patients whose initial radiographs were *equivocal* (suggestive, but not diagnostic, of an injury) were *not* analyzed in this study. In fact, 6.5% of injured patients in the NEXUS database had suggestive but nondiagnostic initial radiographs (Mower et al. 2001) and some of these patients may have had their injuries disclosed by flexion/extension views.

Case Reports

Several case reports and small case series have shown that occult isolated ligamentous injuries do occur and, when inadequately diagnosed or treated, can cause progressive mechanical and neurological deterioration. Twenty-four such cases have been reported in six articles (Webb et al. 1976, Evans 1976, Scher 1979, Hershkowitz and Rothman 1984, Fazl et al. 1990, King et al. 2002). None of the patients suffered an abrupt severe neurological injury. Nonetheless, missed cervical spine injuries resulting in spinal cord injury while under medical care do still occur and have been reported in the recent medical **malpractice literature** (Berlin 2003, Papadatos 2005). In these two cases, an unstable hyperflexion strain was missed on initial evaluation due to inadequate clinical and radiographic examination (See Appendix B).

Equivocal Radiographic Findings

The distinction between normal and equivocal radiographic findings is important because patients with equiocal findings have a higher incidence of occult ligamentous injury. However, criteria distinguishing normal from equivocal findings are not clearly defined (Table 2).

Equivocal radiographic findings may be due to traumatic or nontraumatic conditions. **Slight malalignment** can occur with minimally displaced but potentially unstable ligamentous injuries (Harris 2002, Lee et al.1986). Slight malalignment may also be due to chronic **nontraumatic conditions** such as degenerative spondylosis, congenital variants, ligamentous laxity (common in young children), or supine positioning of a patient immobilized in a cervical collar that causes slight flexion of the neck (Table 3) (Harris and Mirvis 1996, pp. 252–261).

The presence of **prevertebral soft tissue swelling,** especially when associated with other equivocal findings, strongly suggests the presence of an acute traumatic injury and merits further study with CT and, if negative, possibly flexion/extension views or MRI.

TABLE 2
Equivocal Radiographic Findings

- Vertebral body malalignment <2 mm
- Vertebral body angulation—slight focal kyphosis
- Intervertebral disk space narrowing
- Slight facet joint malalignment
- Slight widening of the interspinous process distance
- Isolated prevertebral soft tissue swelling

TABLE 3
Nontraumatic Conditions Causing Vertebral Malalignment

Spondylosis—Degenerative changes
  Vertebral body malalignment (spondylolisthesis)

Positioning—Supine, immobilized in cervical collar
  Straightening, malalignment, angulation

Ligamentous laxity in children
  Pseudosubluxation (C2–C3)
  Predental space widening (up to 5 mm)

Types of Isolated Ligamentous Injuries

An understanding of "equivocal" radiographic findings requries knowledge of the various types of isolated ligamentous injuries and the associated radiographic findings. These findings may be similar to those seen with nontraumatic conditions. It should also be noted that the radiographs may be normal despite the presence of an unstable but nondisplaced ligamentous injury.

There are three types of **isolated ligamentous injuries** (i.e., without an associated fracture): hyperflexion sprain, hyperextension sprain, and transverse atlantal ligament tear (Table 4). All can potentially be detected using flexion/extension views. Signs of these injuries should be sought when examining cervical spine radiographs. When there are subtle but definite signs of injury, flexion/extension views should not be performed in the ED. When the radiographic findings are questionable, flexion/extension radiography or MRI can help exclude an acute injury. (CT should be performed first in order to detect unseen fractures.)

TABLE 4
Isolated Ligamentous Injuries

Hyperflexion sprain—Anterior subluxation

Hyperextension sprain

Transverse atlantal ligament tear—Atlanto-axial dissociation

Hyperflexion Sprain

Hyperflexion sprain is the most frequent of the three injuries. It is the most dangerous and the major reason for obtaining flexion/extension views (Figure 5).

The mechanism of injury is **distractive-flexion,** which tears the posterior cervical ligaments. This occurs when the head is thrown forward such as during abrupt deceleration in a motor vehicle collision or by a direct blow to the back of the head (Mower et al. 2001). Hypeflexion sprain is also called "**anterior subluxation**" because anterior displacement of the facet joints and vertebral bodies often occurs with this injury.

The **spectrum of injury** ranges from partial tears of the supraspinous or interspinous ligaments which are mechanically stable, to complete disruption of all the posterior ligaments resulting in gross mechanical instability. When the ligamentous injury is partial, there may be progressive mechanical deterioration of the cervical vertebrae over time. This is referred to as "delayed instability".

When minimally displaced, hyperflexion sprain can have **subtle radiographic findings** or even normal radiographs (Table 5, Figures 8–10). A flexion view may be necessary to disclose the injury. Such injuries are uncommon, but when misdiagnosed, have the potential for causing an abrupt spinal cord injury if there is excessive motion of the neck.

TABLE 5

Radiographic Signs of Hyperflexion Sprain

- Anterior slippage of vertebral body (anterolisthesis)
- Kyphotic angulation between vertebral bodies
- Widening of posterior intervertebral disk space
- Anterior subluxation of facet joints
- Separation (lack of parallelism) of facet joint surfaces
- Increased distance between spinous processes ("fanning")
- Vertebral body wedge compression fracture (when an anterior compressive force accompanies hyperflexion)

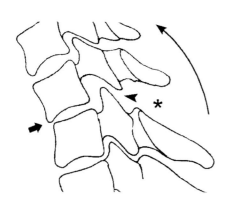

FIGURE 8   Radiographic signs of hyperflexion sprain.

(A) Anterolisthesis and kyphotic angulation of vertebral bodies (*arrow*).

(B) Anterior subluxation and separation (loss of parallelism) of facet joint (*arrowhead*).

(C) Separation ("fanning") of spinous processes (*asterisk*).

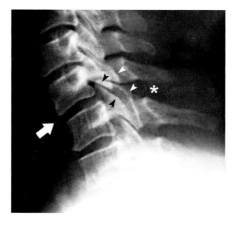

FIGURE 9   Hyperflexion sprain—Subtle signs.

There is vertebral body anterolisthesis (*arrow*), subluxation of the facet joints (*arrowheads*), and widening of interspinous process space (*asterisk*).

[From Schwartz DT, Reisdorff EJ: *Emergency Radiology.* McGraw-Hill, 2000]

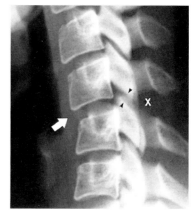

FIGURE 10   Hyperflexion sprain— Subtle signs.

There is slight anterolisthesis and kyphotic angulation at C4 (*arrow*), C4–C5 facet joint subluxation and separation (*arrowheads*), and interlaminar space widening (spinous process fanning) (X).

Hyperextension Sprain

Hyperextension sprain is due to distractive-extension, which tears the anterior longitudinal ligament (Robert et al. 2000). Radiographic findings include widening of the anterior portion of the intervertebral disk space, prevertebral soft tissue swelling, and frequently a small avulsion fracture from the anterior–inferior corner of the vertebral body (Figure 11).

Transverse Atlantal Ligament Rupture

Transverse ligament rupture is usually associated with a Jefferson burst fracture of C1, although *isolated* transverse ligament rupture (without an associated fracture) does occur rarely.

There may be widening of the predental space (Figure 12, see Patient 4 on page 397). However, when there is no displacement of the dens relative to C1, the predental space is normal and injury becomes apparent only during neck flexion.

These injuries have occasionally been reported in children (Pennecot et al. 1984, Fielding et al. 1974).

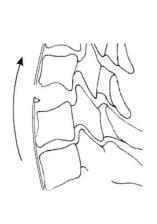 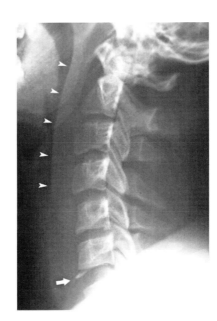

FIGURE 11   Hyperextension sprain.

(*A*) Distractive-extension causes widening of the anterior aspect of the intervertebral disk space and a small avulsion fracture from the inferior endplate of the vertebral body.

(*B*) A 16-year-old boy was in a motor vehicle collision. He had bilateral upper extremity weakness due to a central cord syndrome.

There is widening of the anterior aspect of the C6–C7 intervertebral disk and a small avulsion fracture from the inferior endplate of C6 (*arrow*). Prevertebral soft tissue swelling extends to the cervicocranium (*arrowheads*).

These are definite radiographic signs of injury and flexion/extension views should *not* be performed in the ED. Subsequent MRI and flexion/extension views revealed that the injury was mechanically stable (partial ligamentous tear) and the patient was managed with a hard plastic cervical collar.

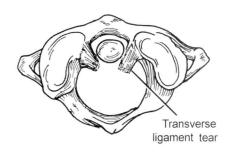

FIGURE 12   Transverse atlantal ligament tear without displacement of the dens.

[From *Galli,* et al: *Emergency Orthopedics: The Spine.* McGraw Hill, 1989, with permission.]

DEGENERATIVE CHANGES OF THE CERVICAL SPINE

Degenerative changes (known as **spondylosis**) are seen in individuals older than 40 years and are common after age 65. These include: vertebral body flattening (platyspondylia), osteophyte formation, ligamentous calcification, and facet joint or intervertebral disk space narrowing (Table 6). The latter two conditions can cause vertebral body malalignment or slippage, which is known as **spondylolisthesis** .

The radiographic finding seen with degenerative spondylosis can have an appearance similar to nondisplaced or minimally displaced fractures or ligamentous injuries. Awareness of these findings can prevent radiograph misinterpretation leading to unnecessary imaging studies. On the other hand, deformities due to degenerative changes can make injuries difficult to detect on radiography. Therefore, additional imaging with CT is often necessary. Furthermore, degenerative changes predispose to skeletal and neurological injury even with relatively minor trauma because they limit flexibility of the cervical spine and cause narrowing of the spinal canal and neuroforamina. For this reason, MDCT of the cervical spine should be obtained in the elderly when there is significant neck pain, even if the mechanism of injury was minor, e.g., a fall from standing.

Spondylolisthesis can occur in either an anterior or posterior direction (Figures 13–15). (The direction of vertebral body slippage is named by displacement of the superior vertebral body.)

When there is degeneration of the intervertebral disk, the disk space is narrowed and, because of the slope of the articular facet surfaces, the superior vertebra slips posteriorly. **Degenerative disk disease** (DDD) thereby causes **retrolisthesis** (Figures 13 and 15A).

Degeneration of the articular facet joints causes joint space narrowing. The superior vertebra is thereby displaced anterior relative to the subjacent one. **Degenerative joint disease** (DJD) thus causes **anterolisthesis** (Figures 14 and 15B).

Both retrolisthesis and anterolisthesis often occur in the same patient. The amount of displacement may be as much as 6 mm (Penning 1989, Lee et al. 1986).

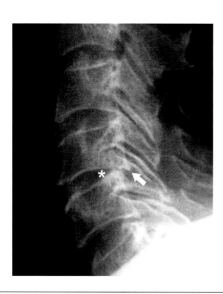

FIGURE 13   Retrolisthesis of C4 (*arrow*) on C5 due to intervertebral disk space narrowing (*asterisk*).

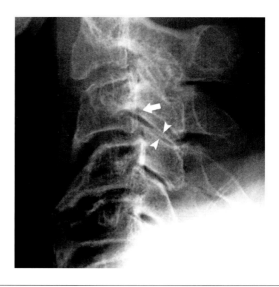

FIGURE 14   Anterolisthesis of C3 (*arrow*) on C4 due to facet joint narrowing (*arrowheads*). There are also marked anterior osteophytes.

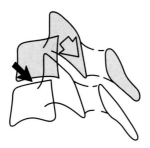

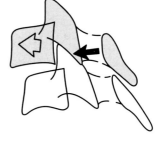

FIGURE 15   Degenerative spondylolisthesis.

Retrolisthesis is due to degenerative disk disease which causes disk space narrowing (*black arrow*). Posterior slippage of the vertebral body occurs due to the oblique orientation of the facet joints (*open arrow*).

Anterolisthesis is caused by degenerative narrowing of the facet joint (degenerative joint disease) (*black arrow*). This causes anterior slippage of the vertebral body (*open arrow*).

Degenerative spondylolisthesis is **mechanically stable** because the intervertebral ligaments are intact. On flexion/extension radiography, there may be some movement between the vertebral bodies, although the amount of movement should be less than 3 mm. In addition, there should be no widening of the interspinous process distance ("fanning" of the spinous processes) and widening (loss of parallelism) of the facet joints during flexion (Figures 9 and 10) (Lee 1986).

The term **subluxation** is sometimes used to describe vertebral body slippage although, strictly speaking, "subluxation" refers only to malalignment of synovial (diarthroidal) joints such as the facet joints. For vertebral body malalignment at the fibrocartilaginous intervertebral disk, the term "**spondylolisthesis**" is preferred. This applies to both nontraumatic conditions and traumatic injuries.

TABLE 6

Degenerative Changes of the Cervical Spine—Spondylosis

1. Vertebral body flattening mimics a wedge compression fracture

2. Osteophytes at the margins of the vertebral bodies obscure anterior vertebral body alignment

3. Anterior longitudinal ligament calcification could be mistaken for an avulsion fracture of the vertebral body endplate

4. Degenerative spondylolisthesis (vertebral body malalignment) could be misinterpreted as traumatic spondylolisthesis
   Anterolisthesis due to facet joint narrowing (DJD)
   Retrolisthesis due to disk space narrowing (DDD)

SOFT TISSUE CHANGES OF THE LOWER CERVICAL SPINE

Prevertebral soft tissue swelling can serve as a radiographic clue to an otherwise occult injury. However, soft tissue swelling of the lower cervical spine is infrequently seen in patients with cervical spine injuries, in contrast to cervicocranial soft tissue swelling, (see Patient 1, Figures 4–7 on pages 376–377). The esophagus is interposed between the tracheal air column and vertebral bodies, and a prevertebral soft tissue thickness of up to 20 mm is normal (see Introduction to Cervical Spine Radiography, Table 2 on page 365). Soft tissue swelling of the lower cervical spine is seen in as few as 5% of spinal injuries (DeBehnke 1984). On the other hand, injuries to the lower cervical spine can cause soft tissue swelling that extends up to the level of C2 and C3, where it is more readily identified (Figure 11).

As with the cervicocranium, alterations in the **contour of the prevertebral soft tissues** of the lower cervical spine may be useful at detecting an injury. However, the criteria for an abnormal contour of the lower cervical soft tissues are less well defined than for the cervicocranium. Normally, there may be a "tucking-in" or narrowing at the cervicothoracic junction (Figure 16) (Harris and Mirvis 1996, pp. 45–48, 185–187).

In **Patient 6,** the soft tissue thickness of the lower cervical prevertebral soft tissues is normal – less than 20 mm (Figure 2). However, there is a prominent soft tissue bulge anterior to C5 and C6 and narrowing at C7. Although this could be interpreted as normal, soft tissue narrowing at C7 is usually less pronounced than in this patient (Figure 16). In addition, anterior vertebral body osteophytes can cause anterior bowing of the soft tissues (Figure 14), although probably not to the extent seen in Patient 6.

It is therefore uncertain whether this patient's soft tissues should be considered normal, abnormal, or equivocal. However, in the setting of significant trauma, this apparent soft tissue swelling merits additional investigation to exclude an acute injury with CT, flexion/extension views, or MRI.

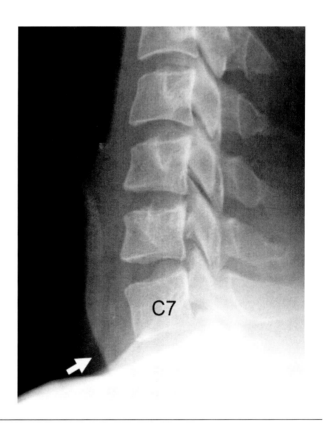

FIGURE 16   Prevertebral soft tissues at the cervicothoracic junction normally "tuck-in" (become narrow) (*arrow*).

FLEXION/EXTENSION RADIOGRAPHY—TECHNIQUE AND INTERPRETATION

Flexion/extension radiography should only be performed on alert and cooperative patients who do not have a definite injury on radiography or CT. The patient may be sitting (preferable) or in a supine position and must be under the direct supervision of a properly instructed clinician or radiology technician. The patient should perform the motion, stopping if severe pain or neurological symptoms develop. The patient first extends their neck, since this is usually the more stable maneuver, and then flexes.

The **safety** of properly performed ED flexion/extension views has been demonstrated in eight retrospective series. Among 1500 cases, only one complication (transient paresthesia) was reported (Ralston et al. 2001).

Criteria for adequate flexion/extension studies are variable. Some authors state that 30 degrees of flexion and extension are required (Marion et al. 2000). Rosen's Textbook of Emergency Medicine suggests that 15 degrees is sufficient to disclose most injuries "aside from minor subluxations" (Hockberger and Kirchenbaum 2002).

Extension can also be judged to be adequate when the spinous processes are nearly touching. Flexion is adequate when the body of the mandible is vertically oriented—perpendicular to the transverse plane (Figure 17). All seven vertebrae must be visible on both the flexion and extension views.

Criteria for abnormal flexion/extension radiography (instability) include >2 mm vertebral body displacement or >11 degree angulation (Knoop et al. 2001, Lewis et al. 1991, White et al. 1975). Other signs of ligamentous injury include: increased separation of the spinous processes ("fanning"), widening of the facet joints (loss of parallelism), widening of the intervertebral disk space, and widening of the predental space.

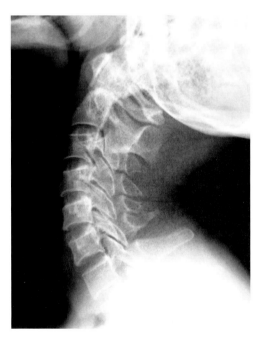
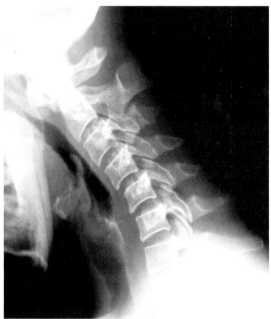

FIGURE 17   Normal flexion/extension views.

With complete extension, the spinous processes are nearly touching. With complete flexion, the body of the mandible is vertically oriented.

Note that with flexion, there may be a slight amount of vertebral body slippage (<2 mm) and angulation, displacement of the facet joints and widening of the interspinous process distances.

OTHER IMAGING MODALITIES FOR PATIENTS WITH SUSPECTED OCCULT LIGAMENTOUS INJURIES

MRI

MRI is highly sensitive at detecting ligamentous injury and can be used as an alternative to flexion/extension radiography to exclude ligamentous injury. However, it is expensive and not readily available in the ED. MRI is most useful in major trauma victims to evaluate ligamentous and neurological injury during hospitalization. MRI directly visualizes edema and hemorrhage within injured ligaments. However, when MRI reveals a nondisplaced ligamentous injury, flexion/extension radiography (or dynamic MRI) may still be needed to distinguish a stable partial ligament tear from a complete unstable ligamentous injury (Benzel et al. 1996, D'Alise et al. 1999, Katzberg et al. 1999, Benedetti et al. 2000, et al. Albrecht 2001).

Helical CT

Helical CT, particularly **multidetector CT** (MDCT) with coronal and sagittal reformatted images is considerably more sensitive at detecting fractures than conventional radiography. Many patients with apparently isolated ligamentous injuries will have fractures or malalignment detected by CT. However, an isolated ligamentous injury (without any fractures or displacement) could theoretically still be missed by CT.

There have been several published series investigating the ability of helical CT with coronal and sagittal reformatted images to exclude cervical spine injury (Hansen et al. Emerg Radiol 2000, Ptak et al. 2001, Diaz et al. 2005, Padaychee 2006, Hogan et al. 2005). These series were primarily in high-risk patients admitted to an inpatient trauma service. They had a 10% incidence of cervical spine injury. Approximately 1–2% of injuries were missed by CT yielding a sensitivity of 98–99% and negative predictive value (NPV) of 99.8%. Some injuries were disclosed by flexion/extension views, including one odontoid fracture (Bolinger 2004). Occasional cases of occult ligamentous injury missed by CT and detected by MRI have been reported (Benedetti et al. 2000).

Hogan et al. (2005) studied thin-section MDCT in obtunded high-risk trauma victims. MRI was performed in 366 patients with normal MDCT scans. Four occult ligamentous injuries were found (NPV of CT was 99%). However none of these injuries were unstable (NPV for unstable injury was 100%). Subtle signs of ligamentous injury were found on retrospective review of two patients' CT scans (slight facet joint widening). Overall, 12 patients (3.3%) had injuries detected by MRI, including 7 spinal cord contusions (NPV of MDCT was 97%).

Although the incidence of spinal injury in patients with a normal MDCT is very low, even among major trauma victims, and the cervical spine can generally be "cleared" on the basis of a normal MDCT, spine immobilization should still be maintained in the ED in patients at greater risk of cervical injury—patients who are obtunded (usually due to major head trauma), and patients with excessive neck pain or signs or symptoms of spine cord injury. Even among these later patients, the incidence of injury is very low when the CT is normal.

Among less severely injured patients, such as those who could potentially be discharged from the ED, an unstable injury would be exceedingly rare when the CT does not disclose an injury. Nonetheless, **Patient 6** represents the unusual circumstance in which CT failed to detect an injury and flexion/extension views were necessary.

ALTERNATIVE STRATEGIES TO ED FLEXION/EXTENSION RADIOGRAPHY

There are several clinical strategies that have been advocated as alternatives to the use of flexion/extension radiography in the ED.

One strategy is to immobilize the patient in a **hard plastic cervical collar** and refer the patient for repeat examination and delayed flexion/extension views in 1 week. At this time, muscle spasm will have abated and adequate studies can be obtained. Cervical immobilization collars that are adequate for patients with potentially unstable cervical spine injuries should be used (*Miami-J* or *Aspen collars*). Other cervical collars that are commonly available in the ED are either not appropriate for long-term use (extrication collars) or provide inadequate immobilization (soft foam collars). This approach is emphasized in the trauma, neurosurgery, and radiology literature (Marion et al. 2000, Hadley et al. 2002, Daffner et al. 2002). In Patient 6, however, who had a highly unstable cervical spine injury, collar immobilization would have been risky unless the immobilization was truly secure.

Some authors do *not* recommend immobilization in a collar because the incidence of injury is so low. They instead recommend instructing the patient to **avoid significant physical activity**, to seek medical attention immediately if there is increasing pain or neurological symptoms, and refer the patient for follow-up in one week (Hockberger and Kirshenbaum 2002, Mower et al. 2001). Such instructions are always prudent when discharging a patient from the ED following neck trauma.

In his review of anterior subluxation injuries, Mower suggests that because the yield of flexion/extension views is so low in patients with *normal* radiographs and because there have been no reported cases of abrupt neurological deterioration in such patients, these patients can be managed without ED flexion/extension radiography. However, in Patient 6 such a strategy would have been dangerous, although (his cervical spine radiographs could be considered equivocal rather than truly normal because of the questionable prevertebral soft tissue swelling).

SUMMARY: What is a Reasonable Approach to ED Patients with Suspected Occult Ligamentous Injuries?

The **traditional approach** to diagnosing occult ligamentous injuries in the ED is to perform **flexion/extension radiography** in patients with **normal** or **equivocal** radiographs who are having excessive pain. However, the yield of flexion/extension radiography is exceedingly low, especially in patients who are otherwise well and could potentially be discharged from the ED.

There are no currently accepted guidelines that address the diagnosis of occult ligamentous injury of the cervical spine, although it is agreed that such injuries, while rare, are potentially devastating. To avoid missing such an injury, the clinician should be alert to this injury, perform a thorough clinical evaluation, and look for subtle radiographic signs suggestive of ligamentous injuries.

With the current widespread use of **MDCT** in patients at **high risk** of cervical spine injury (>5% incidence of injury), the role of ED flexion/extension radiography has been substantially reduced (Figure 18 and Introduction to Cervical Spine Radiology, Appendix on p. 363). Nonetheless, in hospitalized major trauma victims that are obtunded or having substantial neck pain or neurological symptoms, spine immobilization should be maintained in the ED even when the CT is normal because of the small but significant risk of an occult spinal cord or ligamentous injury (see Figure 22 on p. 429) (Hogan et al. 2005).

In centers where MDCT is readily available, only **low-risk patients** undergo **cervical spine radiography.** Such patients can generally be cleared when the radiographs are **normal.**

In patients with **equivocal** radiographs, the incidence of injury is higher. However, "equivocal findings" are not clearly defined. The term encompasses slight malalignment that could be due to a ligamentous injury (such as hyperflexion sprain), findings associated with non-traumatic conditions (such as degenerative spondylosis), and prevertebral soft tissue swelling (Tables 2–6). Whenever an injury may be present, **CT** should be performed. In most instances, CT is able to confirm or exclude an acute injury. However, in rare cases, an occult unstable ligamentous injury may be present when the CT does not reveal an injury, as illustrated by Patient 6.

To avoid missing a radiographically occult injury in the ED, prior to final "clearance" of the cervical spine, the clinician should carefully **reexamine the patient,** looking for **excessive pain** or tenderness or **limited range of motion,** i.e., testing neck rotation as in the Canadian Cervical Spine Rule, as well as flexion and extension (Figure 18).

In most instances, the patient will have an **adequate range of motion** and only **mild or paraspinal tenderness** that can be attributed to muscular strain. The patient can then be confidently cleared of cervical spine injury. However, instructions should always be provided for the patient to return if there is increasing pain or neurological symptoms.

When there is **excessive pain** or **limitation of motion,** there are several management options (Figure 18). One is to simply instruct the patient to **avoid significant physical activity** and to return immediately if there is increased pain or neurological symptoms (Mower et al. 2001). This is sufficient in the vast majority of non-high-risk ED patients whose initial radiographs are *normal.* This is also a reasonable approach when the radiographs show only nontraumatic abnormalities such as degenerative changes or congenital anomalies. Nonetheless, such preexisting conditions can mask injuries as well as predispose to injury, and CT may be needed to exclude a fracture.

Other management options include (1) immobilization in an appropriate hard plastic cervical collar and schedule a follow-up appointment; (2) perform flexion/extension views in the ED; or (3) obtain MRI either in the ED, during a hospital admission, or as an outpatient. If not already obtained, MDCT of the cervical spine should be performed in patients with excessive pain.

As mentioned above, the use of **flexion/extension radiography** in the ED is controversial. Flexion/extension views have a greater role when the radiographs and CT are equivocal, e.g., show minor degrees of malalignment (Daffner et al. 2002). When the patient's neck pain is excessive and the range of motion is limited, flexion/extension views would likely be inadequate and unable to fully exclude an injury. Immobilization in an appropriate cervical collar and referral for follow-up in several days when the pain has abated is a reasonable approach. When neck motion is not limited, flexion/extension views will be adequate, although a ligamentous injury is unlikely to be present. Rarely, ED flexion/extension views will reveal an unstable ligamentous injury, as in Patient 6.

Because these injuries are rare, clinical judgment should be exercised to avoid excessive testing with CT or flexion/extension radiography or excessive management with collar immobilization. On the other hand, since an occult ligamentous injury can have devastating consequences if missed, it is reasonable to investigate a relatively large number of patients to avoid missing one case.

Finally, **common pitfalls** responsible for missed cervical spine injuries should be avoided. These include (1) inadequate radiographs (poor visualization of C7 or the cervicocranium) (2) missed subtle radiographic findings; and (3) performing an inadequate clinical examination, particularly in patients who are difficult to evaluate due to intoxication, altered mentation or other severe injuries (King et al. 2002, Berlin 2003, Papadatos 2005, Appendix B).

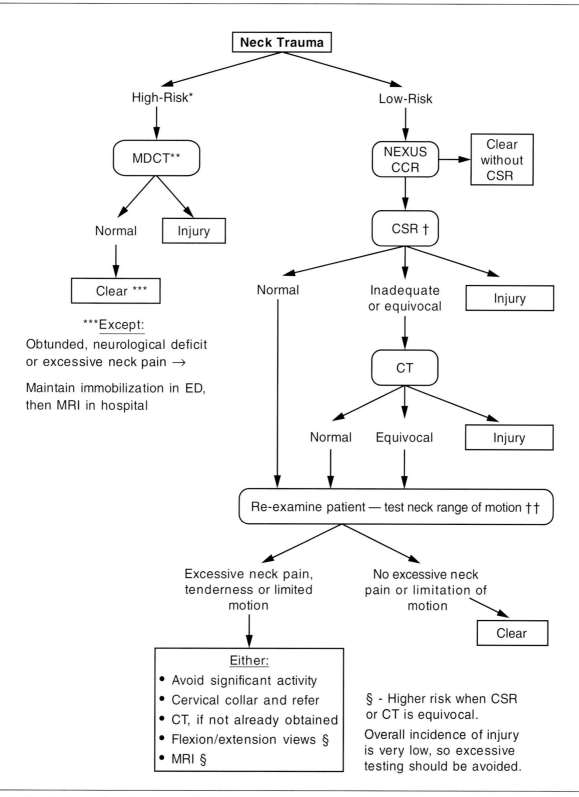

FIGURE 18   Cervical spine imaging strategy in the ED.

* High-risk patients (>5% incidence of cervical spine injury) are selected based on the mechanism of injury and presence of other severe injuries. They are usually undergoing CT of another body region.

   If the patient is hemodynamically unstable and cannot undergo CT, a single cross-table lateral cervical spine view can be obtained to identify obvious injuries that need emergency stabilization.

** CT can also be used as the initial test when head CT is being performed or in the elderly with degenerative spondylosis.

† Low-risk patients undergoing CSR have <1% incidence of cervical spine injury (Hanson 2000). A mild analgesic medication should be administered while the patient is awaiting radiography or CT.

†† After CSR and/or CT, all patients with studies that do not reveal an acute injury should be **carefully reexamined** before final clinical clearance for signs of an occult injury—excessive pain or tenderness, limited range of motion, or neurological signs or symptoms.

MDCT, multidetector CT; NEXUS or CCR (Canadian C-spine rule), clinical decision rules; CSR, cervical spine radiography (three-view series).

Patient 6 Summary

In this patient, flexion/extension views were obtained because the initial radiographs were interpreted as being suggestive of an acute injury. The vertebral body malalignment (retrolisthesis), however, was in fact due to degenerative spondylosis (Figure 19). (Hyperflexion sprain causes anterior, not posterior, vertebral displacement.) Second, the apparent prevertebral soft tissue bulge at the lower cervical spine could be considered suspicious for an acute injury. However, soft tissue swelling is uncommon in the lower cervical spine and the criteria for swelling are not well defined.

The correct rationale for ordering flexion/extension views was that the patient was having considerable pain, had had a fall of sufficient force to cause an unstable cervical injury. In addition, there was questionable soft tissue swelling on radiography. (Neck range of motion was not tested prior to flexion/extension views, which presumably would have revealed substantial pain indicative of a significant injury.) In this case, however, the patient (and his doctors) got *lucky*. (MRI could also have been used to detect the ligamentous injury, but is difficult to obtain in the ED.)

The CT (Figure 2) showed only degenerative changes and was essentially negative for acute injury. This could have been falsely reassuring. However, sagittal and coronal reformatted images were not generated, which might have revealed a ligamentous injury—slight facet joint widening not visible on the axial images.

It is perhaps not entirely coincidental that the traumatic ligamentous disruption occurred at the same level as the degenerative retrolisthesis. Ligamentous injury is more likely to occur at a region of degenerative spondylolisthesis. Weakening of the intervertebral disk and periarticular ligaments, as well as diminished flexibility at that level, account for this vulnerability.

A second possibility is that the disk space narrowing and vertebral malalignment (retrolisthesis) were acute, due to intervertebral disk rupture and herniation. However, the presence of other degenerative changes suggests that the retrolisthesis was chronic. In addition, a preoperative MRI did not reveal an acute intervertebral disk rupture at C5-6.

At the **lower cervical spine,** several **metallic objects** can be seen (Figure 20). Thoracolumbar spine radiographs obtained to evaluate the patient's entire spine revealed similar innumerable metallic densities (Figure 21). These were from acupuncture treatment the patient had received years earlier in Korea. Some practitioners in Asia leave fragments of the acupuncture needles (often gold) embedded under the skin to achieve a more lasting effect. This is known as **Hari acupuncture** (Hollander et al. 1991).

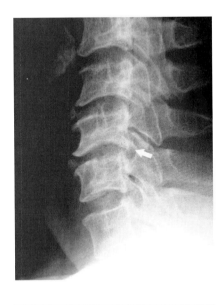

FIGURE 19　Initial lateral view—Patient 6

Degenerative retrolisthesis at C5-6 (*arrow*) due to disk space narrowing and soft tissue swelling at C5-6.

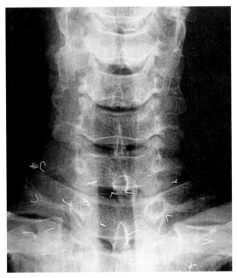

FIGURE 20　AP view of cervical spine.

Numerous residual subcutaneous metallic acupuncture needles in the upper thoracic region.

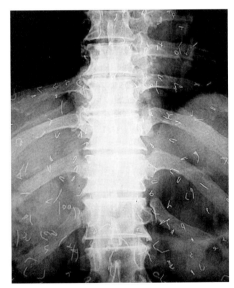

FIGURE 21　Lower thoracic spine.

Innumerable residual acupuncture needles in the subcutaneous tissues of the back.

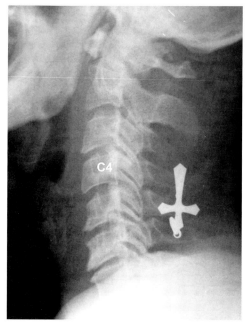

A. Initial lateral view was normal.

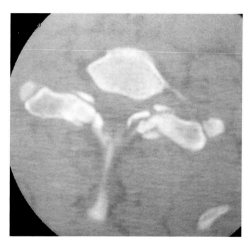

B. CT revealed C7 facet fractures.

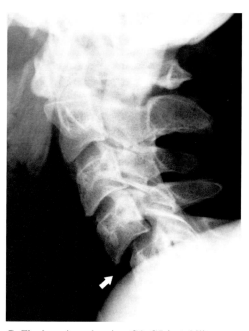

C. Flexion view showing C4–C5 instability.

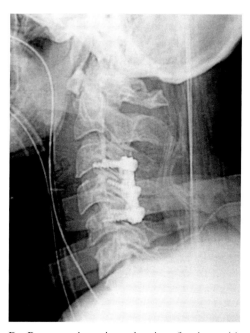

D. Postoperative view showing fixation with posterior plates and screws.

FIGURE 22   Another occult unstable ligamentous injury—Normal radiographs, minor fractures on CT.

A 32-year-old man dove off the stage at a rock concert expecting to be caught by the crowd. Instead, he was dropped to the ground.

On arrival in the ED, he had an incomplete spinal cord injury with 2/5 strength of his left biceps, 0/5 weakness of his right arm and both legs. There was sparing of rectal tone, light touch above C7, and position sense in his legs. Aside from a 4 cm scalp laceration, there were no other injuries.

Initial cervical spine radiograph was negative for an acute injury (A).

Helical CT was performed, which revealed C7 facet fractures (B) and a small nondisplaced fracture of the right inferior articular facet of C5.

Flexion/extension radiography was performed by the neurosurgery service to investigate vertebral stability.

The flexion view revealed an unstable ligamentous injury at C4–C5 (C, arrow). (Alternatively, MRI would have revealed the ligamentous injury, although flexion views might still have been needed to demonstrate instability.)

The patient was treated with posterior stabilization with plates and screws (D). He eventually recovered partial strength of his upper extremities.

Radiography and CT provided no evidence of the severe vertebral instability, although the magnitude of injury was clinically evident in this patient due to his spinal cord injury.

SUGGESTED READING

DeBehnke DJ, Havel CJ: Utility of prevertebral soft tissue measurements in identifying patients with cervical spine fractures. *Ann Emerg Med* 1994;24:1119–1124.

Harris JH: Malalignment: Signs and significance. *Eur J Radiol* 2002;42:92–99.

Harris JH, Mirvis SE: *The Radiology of Acute Cervical Spine Trauma*, 3rd ed. Williams and Wilkins, 1996.

Hoffman JR, Mower WR, Wolfson AB, et al.: Validity of a set of clinical criteria to rule out injury to the cervical spine in patients with blunt trauma. *New Engl J Med* 2000;343:94–99.

Lee C, Woodring JH, Rogers LF, Kim KS: The radiographic distinction of degenerative slippage (spondylolisthesis and retrolisthesis) from traumatic slippage of the cervical spine. *Skel Radiol* 1986;15:439–443.

Mower WR, Clements CM, Hoffman JR: Anterior subluxation of the cervical spine. *Emerg Radiol* 2001a;8:194–199.

Mower WR, Oh JY, Zucker MI, Hoffman JR for NEXUS Group: Occult and secondary injuries missed by plain radiography of the cervical spine in blunt trauma patients. *Emerg Radiol* 2001b;8:200–206.

Penning L: Obtaining and interpreting plain films in cervical spine injury. In Sherk HH, ed. *The Cervical Spine*, 2nd ed. Lippincott, 1989: 106–141.

Touger M, Gennis P, Nathanson N, et al.: Validity of a decision rule to reduce cervical spine radiography in elderly patients with blunt trauma. *Ann Emerg Med* 2002;40:287–293.

Flexion/extension views

Brady WJ, Kini N, Duncan C, Young JS: Flexion-extension cervical spine radiography in blunt trauma: A survey of emergency physicians. *Emerg Radiol* 1998;5:375–380.

Knopp R, Parker J, Tashjian J, Ganz W: Defining radiographic criteria for flexion-extension studies of the cervical spine. *Ann Emerg Med* 2001;38:31–35.

Pollack CV, Hendey GW, Martin DR, Hoffman JR, Mower WR, for the NEXUS Group: Use of flexion-extension radiographs of the cervical spine in blunt trauma. *Ann Emerg Med* 2001;38:8–11.

White AA, Johnson RM, Panjabi MM, Southwick WO: Biomechanical analysis of clinical stability in the cervical spine. *Clin Orthop* 1975;109:85–96.

Retrospective series of flexion/extension views

Brady WJ, Moghtader J, Cutcher D, Exline C, Young J: ED use of flexion-extension cervical spine radiography in the evaluation of blunt trauma. *Am J Emerg Med* 1999;17:504–508.

Dwek JR, Chung CB: Radiography of cervical spine injury in children: Are flexion-extension radiographs useful for acute trauma? *AJR* 2000;174:1617–1619.

Insko EK, Gracias VH, Gupta R, et al.: Utility of flexion and extension radiographs of the cervical spine in the acute evaluation of blunt trauma. *J Trauma* 2002;53:426–429.

Lewis LM, Docherty M, Ruoff BE, et al.: Flexion-extension views in the evaluation of cervical spine injuries. *Ann Emerg Med* 1991;20:117–121.

Myers P, Mimran DDG, Bozeman WP: Adequacy and utility of acute flexion extension x-rays after minor blunt trauma. *Acad Emerg Med* 2003;10:562. Abstract.

Ralston ME, Chung K, Barnes PD, et al.: Role of flexion-extension radiographs in blunt pediatric cervical spine injury. *Acad Emerg Med* 2001;8:237–245.

Wang JC, Hatch JD, Sandhu HS, Delamarter RB: Cervical flexion and extension radiographs in acutely injured patients. *Clin Orthop* 1999;365:111–116.

Woods WA, Brady WJ, Pollock G, Kini N, Young JS: Flexion-extension cervical spine radiography in pediatric blunt trauma. *Emerg Radiol* 1998;5:381–384.

Case reports and case series of occult or missed ligamentous injury of the cervical spine

Berlin L: CT versus radiography for initial evaluation of cervical spine trauma: What is the standard of care? *AJR* 2003;180:911–915.

Evans DK: Anterior cervical subluxation. *J Bone Joint Surg (Br)* 1976;58-B:318–321.

Fazl M, LaFebvre J, Willinsky RA, Gertzbein S: Posttraumatic ligamentous disruption of the cervical spine, an easily overlooked diagnosis: Presentation of three cases. *Neurosurgery* 1990;26:674–678.

Fielding JW, Cochran GVB, Lawsing JF, Hohl M: Tears of the transverse ligament of the atlas. *J Bone Joint Surg (Am)* 1974;56-A:1683–1691.

Herkowitz HN, Rothman RH: Subacute instability of the cervical spine. *Spine* 1984;9:348–357.

King SW, Hosler BK, King MA, Eiselt EW: Missed cervical spine fracture-dislocations: The importance of clinical and radiographic assessment. *J Manipulative Physiol Ther* 2002;25:263–269.

Papadatos A: Missed cervical spine injury yields huge award ($31 million). *Emerg Med News* 2005: 10–12. (*Med Malpract Verdicts Settl Exp* 2004;20[4])

Pennecot GF, Leonard P, Peyrot des Gachins S, et al.: Traumatic ligamentous instability of the cervical spine in children. *J Pediatr Orthop* 1984;4:339–345.

Robert KQ, Ricciardi EJ, Harris BM: Occult ligamentous injury of the cervical spine. *South Med J* 2000;93:974–976.

Scher AT: Anterior cervical subluxation: An unstable position. *AJR* 1979;133:275–280.

Webb JK, Broughton RBK, McSweeney T, Park WM: Hidden flexion injury of the cervical spine. *J Bone Joint Surg (Br)* 1976;58-B:322–327.

Recommended protocols for the use of flexion/extension radiography

Daffner RH, Dalinka MK, Alazraki N, et al.: Suspected cervical spine trauma (ACR Appropriateness Criteria). American College of Radiology, 2002. www.acr.org.

Hadley MN, Walters BC, Grabb PA, et al, for the American Association of Neurological Surgeons/Congress of Neurological Surgeons: Radiographic assessment of the cervical spine in symptomatic trauma patients. *Neurosurgery* 2002;50(3 Suppl):S36–S43.

Hockberger RS, Kaji AH, Newton EJ: In Marx J et al, ed. *Rosen's Emergency Medicine: Concepts and Clinical Practice*, 6th ed. Mosby, 2006.

Hockberger RS, Kirshenbaum KJ: In Marx J et al: *Rosen's Emergency Medicine: Concepts and Clinical Practice*, 5th ed. Mosby, 2002.

Marion D, Domeier R, Dunham CM, et al.: Determination of cervical spine stability in trauma patients (Update of the 1997 EAST cervical spine clearance document), Trauma Practice Guidelines, Chapter 3 update. Eastern Association for the Surgery of Trauma, 2000, www.east.org.

Marion D, Domeier R, Dunham CM, et al.: Practice management guidelines for identifying cervical spine injuries following trauma. Trauma Practice Guidelines, Chapter 3. Eastern Association for the Surgery of Trauma, 1998, www.east.org

Wales LR, Knopp RK, Morishima MS: Recommendations for evaluation of the acutely injured cervical spine: A clinical radiologic algorithm. *Ann Emerg Med* 1980;9:422–428.

Fluoroscopic flexion/extension views in obtunded trauma patients

Anglen J, Metzler M, Bunn P, Griffiths H: Flexion and extension views are not cost-effective in a cervical spine clearance protocol for obtunded trauma patients. *J Trauma* 2002;52:54–59.

Bolinger B et al.: Bedside fluoroscopic flexion and extension cervical spine radiographs for clearance of the cervical spine in comatose trauma patients. *J Trauma* 2004;56:132–136.

Brooks RA, Willett KM: Evaluation of the Oxford protocol for total spinal clearance in the unconscious trauma patient. *J Trauma* 2001;50:862–867.

Davis JW, Kaups KL, Cunningham MA, et al.: Routine evaluation of the cervical spine in head-injured patients with dynamic fluoroscopy: A reappraisal. *J Trauma* 2001;50:1044–1047.

Davis JW, Parks SN, Detlefs CL, et al.: Clearing the cervical spine in obtunded patients: The use of dynamic fluoroscopy. *J Trauma* 1995;39:435–438.

Helical CT in cervical spine trauma

Blackmore CC: Evidence-based imaging evaluation of the cervical spine in trauma. *Neuroimag Clin North Am* 2003;13:283–291.

Brohi K, Healy M, Fotheringham T, et al.: Helical computed tomographic scanning for the evaluation of the cervical spine in the unconscious, intubated trauma patient. *J Trauma* 2005;58:897–901.

Daffner RH: Helical CT of the cervical spine for trauma patients: A time study. *AJR* 2001;177:677–679.

Diaz JJ, Aulino JM, Collier B, et al.: The early work-up for isolated ligamentous injury of the cervical spine: Does computed tomography scan have a role? *J Trauma* 2005;59:897–904.

Hanson JA, Blackmore CC, Man FA, Wilson AJ: Cervical spine injury: Accuracy of helical CT used as a screening technique. *Emerg Radiol* 2000;7:31–35.

Hanson JA, Blackmore CC, Mann FA, Wilson AJ: Cervical spine injury: A clinical decision rule to identify high-risk patients for helical CT screening. *AJR* 2000;174:713–717.

Hogan GJ, Mirvis SE, Shanmuganathan K, Scalea TM: Exclusion of unstable cervical spine injury in obtunded patients with blunt trauma: Is MR imaging needed when multi-detector CT findings are normal? *Radiology* 2005;237:106–113.

Ptak T, Kihiczak D, Lawrason JN, et al.: Screening for cervical spine trauma with helical CT: Experience with 676 cases. *Emerg Radiol* 2001;8:315–319.

MRI in cervical spine trauma

Albrecht RM, Kingsley D, Schermer CR, et al.: Evaluation of cervical spine in intensive care patients following blunt trauma. *World J Surg* 2001;25:1089–1096.

Benedetti PF, Fahr LM, Kuhns LR, Hayman LA: MR imaging findings in spinal ligamentous injury. *AJR* 2000;175:661–665.

Benzel EC, Hart BL, Ball PA, et al.: Magnetic resonance imaging for the evaluation of patients with occult cervical spine injury. *J Neurosurg* 1996;85:824–829.

D'Alise MD, Benzel EC, Hart BL: Magnetic resonance imaging evaluation of the cervical spine in the comatose or obtunded trauma patient. *J Neurosurg* 1999;91(1 Suppl):54–59.

Katzberg RW, Benedetti PF, Drake CM, et al.: Acute cervical spine injuries: Prospective MR imaging assessment at a level 1 trauma center. *Radiology* 1999;213:203–212.

Permanent needle acupuncture

Chiu ES, Austin JHM: Acupuncture needle fragments. *New Engl J Med* 1995;332:304 and 1792–1793.

Gerard PS, Wilick E, Schiano T: Imaging implications in the evaluation of permanent needle acupuncture. *Clin Imaging* 1993;17:36–40.

Hollander JE, Dewitz A, Bowers S: Permanently imbedded subcutaneous acupuncture needles: Radiographic appearance. *Ann Emerg Med* 1991;20:1025–1026.

APPENDIX A: PUBLISHED RECOMMENDATIONS FOR FLEXION–EXTENSION RADIOGRAPHY

Eastern Association for the Surgery of Trauma—2000

Alert and awake patients with neck pain

- Obtain three-view CSR and CT of suspicious areas or areas not well visualized.
- If CSR is normal, obtain flexion/extension views.
- If voluntary painless excursion does not exceed 30 degrees, replace collar and repeat flexion/extension views in 2 weeks.

Marion D, Domeier R, Dunham CM, et al: Determination of cervical spine stability in trauma patients. (Update of the 1997 EAST cervical spine clearance document), Trauma Practice Guidelines, Chapter 3 update. Eastern Association for the Surgery of Trauma, 2000, www.east.org.

Neurosurgery—2002

- **Awake patient** with neck pain and normal CSR
  Discontinue immobilization after

  a. normal adequate flexion/extension views or
  b. normal **MRI** within 48 hours.

- **Obtunded patient** with normal CSR
  Discontinue immobilization after

  a. fluoroscopic flexion/extension views, or
  b. normal **MRI** within 48 hours, or
  c. at discretion of treating physician.

Note: No "physician discretion" is mentioned for clearance of awake patients with normal CSR.

Hadley MN, Walters BC, Grabb PA, et al. Radiographic assessment of the cervical spine in symptomatic trauma patients. *Neurosurgery* 2002;50(3 Suppl):S36–S43.

American College of Radiology Appropriateness Criteria—2002

Flexion/extension views are not helpful except to ensure that minor malalignment in patients with cervical spondylosis are fixed deformities.

Muscle spasm in acutely injured patients usually precludes adequate examination.

Flexion/extension views are best reserved for 7–10 days. If ligamentous instability is suspected, MRI is indicated.

Daffner RH, Dalinka MK, Alazraki N, et al.: *Suspected Cervical Spine Trauma* (ACR Appropriateness Criteria). American College of Radiology, 2002. www.acr.org.

Rosen's Textbook of Emergency Medicine—2002

Indications for ED flexion/extension views

- Normal CSR with severe, persistent neck pain.

- Minor malalignment on CSR.

Minor subluxation may be masked by muscle spasm.

If neck pain is persistent, flexion/extension radiography should be repeated in 1week. If negative, MRI should be obtained to exclude ligamentous injury or disk herniation.

Hockberger RS, Kirshenbaum KJ: Spine in Marx J, et al: *Rosen's Emergency Medicine: Concepts and Clinical Practice*, 5th ed., Mosby, 2002.

APPENDIX B: MISSED CERVICAL SPINE INJURY CASES

Papadatos A: Missed cervical spine injury yields huge award. *Emerg Med News,* 2005, 10–12.

A 41-year-old truck driver was involved in a rollover. He was transported to a trauma center in spine immobilization. He had a scalp hematoma. The emergency physician ordered several radiographic studies, including cervical spine radiographs. The radiology resident interpreted all the radiographs as normal. However, the cervicothoracic junction was not visualized and the radiologist did not request additional studies.

Subsequently, a nurse removed the cervical collar and the patient walked 10 feet and collapsed. The patient sustained an **anterior subluxation** of the cervical spine and a spinal cord injury causing paralysis from the chest down with minimal residual strength in his arms.

The patient and his family sued claiming that when he presented to the ED, he had been complaining of paresthesias in his fingers and, given the mechanism of injury, a correct and timely diagnosis should have been made. The physicians failed to diagnose two small cervical fractures, as well as a ligamentous injury that rendered the spine unstable. He claimed that had the injury been correctly diagnosed and treated, he would not have suffered a spinal cord injury. The verdict was reportedly $31 million. (*Med Malpract Verdicts Settl Exp* 2004;20[4]) (Dallas County [TX] District Court, Case No. 01-1793-E.)

Comment   This patient had a dangerous mechanism of injury but did not have any other significant injuries aside from that of his cervical spine. The radiographs were inadequate by not visualizing the cervicothoracic junction, although the level of injury is not stated in the case report. The injury may have had subtle radiographic findings or not been visible on the radiographs. CT would have been indicated if C7 could not be seen or simply on the basis of the severe mechanism of injury. An anterior subluxation injury is primarily ligamentous, and when nondisplaced, may have minimal or normal radiographic findings. MRI or flexion/extension views may be needed to detect this injury. However, because CT revealed "small" fractures, flexion/extension views were not indicated in the ED. In addition, if the patient had been carefully re-examined after the initial radiographs including assessment of neck mobility, the magnitude of his injury might have been evident.

King et al: Missed cervical spine fracture-dislocations: The importance of clinical and radiographic assessment. *J Manipulative Physiol Ther* 2002;25:263–269.

An elderly man had been discharged from an ED after a motor vehicle collision in which he was the driver of an automobile that was struck on the passenger side by an oncoming car. The initial radiographs showed only disk space narrowing at C5–C6, which was attributed to degenerative changes (Figure 23).

One week later, the patient presented to a chiropractor complaining of severe neck pain and upper extremity weakness. Radiographs revealed complete vertebral dislocation. CT revealed fractures of the posterior elements of C5–C6 and MRI revealed spinal cord compression. Surgical reduction and fixation was performed.

Had CT been obtained initially, the fractures would have been discovered earlier. ED flexion/extension views would also have revealed the injury, but would not have been indicated after CT detected the fractures.

On close inspection of the initial radiograph, the region of C5–C6 is suspicious for a traumatic injury rather than degenerative spondylosis. There was anterolisthesis of C5 without facet joint narrowing, which suggests that the malalignment was due to vertebral fractures and not degenerative changes.

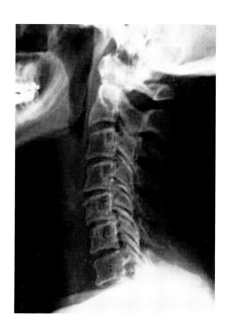
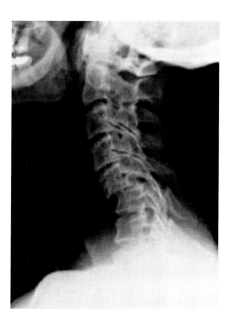

FIGURE 23   A 77-year-old man was injured in a motor vehicle collision.

(*A*) Initial cervical spine radiograph was interpreted as showing degenerative changes at C5–C6. However, on close inspection, there is no facet joint space narrowing that would be expected with degenerative anterolisthesis and the vertebral body was deformed suggesting a fracture.

(*B*) One week later, there is bilateral facet joint dislocation and anterolisthesis of C5 on C6—an anterior subluxation injury.

[From King, et al: *J Manipulative Physiol Ther* 2002;25, with permission.]

APPENDIX B: MISSED CERVICAL SPINE INJURY CASES (CONTINUED)

Berlin L: CT versus radiography for initial evaluation of cervical spine trauma: What is the standard of care? *AJR* 2003;180:911–915.

A 37-year-old man who was driving while intoxicated, lost control of his motor vehicle. The vehicle overturned and he was trapped inside. He was extricated from the vehicle, immobilized and transported to a nearby hospital.

In the ED, the patient was conscious but appeared inebriated. He was thrashing about and needed to be restrained on the stretcher. The patient admitted that he had been drinking but denied that he had lost consciousness or was experiencing pain. Physical examination was otherwise unremarkable, and sensory and motor function of all extremities was normal.

Cervical spine radiographs were obtained including a cross-table lateral view, followed by AP, open-mouth, and two oblique views. The radiologist's interpretation was: "Limited examination because of patient's inability to cooperate for positioning and hold still. No obvious fracture or dislocation is seen."

The patient was admitted to the hospital for observation. On the surgical ward, the patient appeared inebriated, was "unable to follow orders" and was "thrashing around." He was again placed in restraints. The plan was to allow the patient to "sleep it off" during the night. Later that night, the patient reported to a nurse that his arms and legs were "beginning to feel numb" and he was having difficulty moving them. The nurse did not notify the house physician.

The following morning the attending physician examined the patient and found "profound sensory and motor loss" below the patient's neck. A CT scan was obtained which showed fractures of C5-C6 facets on the left and **anterior subluxation** of C5 on C6.

The patient underwent surgery, during which the cervical spine was reduced and a fusion performed. The patient remained permanently paraplegic.

Three months later, the patient filed a malpractice lawsuit against the hospital, emergency physician, hospital physicians, and radiologist. All defendants settled for a total amount of $8 million. The plaintiff's lawyers contended that CT is currently the standard of care.

Comment Although this case was presented as justification for CT as a standard of care, the more substantial deviation from acceptable medical care was that with technically inadequate radiographs, CT should be obtained to better visualize the cervical spine. In addition, the clinical evaluation and treatment were inadequate.

The patient's alcohol intoxication and lack of cooperation with the examination also contributed to the missed injury by making clinical evaluation difficult.

Hyperflexion sprain (anterior subluxation) is a highly unstable injury that may have few if any radiographic abnormalities. This is a third recent case report of a missed predominantly ligamentous injury resulting in spinal cord injury.

INTRODUCTION TO CRANIAL CT

Computed tomography (CT) is the most useful neuroimaging study in emergency medicine practice because it readily detects acute blood collections and intracranial lesions causing mass effect. These are the most important immediate considerations in patients presenting with head trauma, headache, or stroke.

MRI is superior for imaging parenchymal abnormalities and has replaced CT in most *nonemergency* neurodiagnosis. MRI produces images in the sagittal and coronal planes and can better depict the anatomic characteristics of intracranial lesions. In addition, MR images are not degraded by bone artifacts that hamper visualization of the posterior fossa and brainstem on CT (Figure 1).

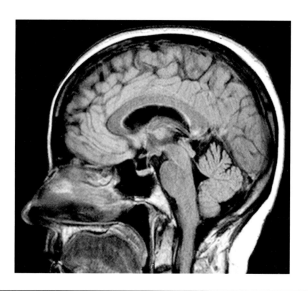

HOW TO READ A HEAD CT

Many intracranial lesions produce CT findings that are easy to identify (Figure 2). A *rudimentary approach* to CT interpretation uses symmetry in comparing the right and left sides of the brain, locates the midline, and notes any midline shift.

However, to detect more subtle abnormalities, as well as to confirm that a CT scan is normal, a methodical approach to CT interpretation is necessary. This depends on knowledge of normal CT anatomy as well as the CT manifestations of various intracranial disorders.

Using a **systematic approach,** each CT slice is examined individually looking for specific anatomical landmarks (Table 1). If a lesion is found, on adjacent CT slices are then examined to determine its extent.

CT interpretation also entails a complementery **targeted approach** in which specific abnormalities related to the patient's clinical presentation are sought, for instance head trauma, headache or an acute focal neurological deficit (Table 2).

FIGURE 1   Midsagittal MRI.

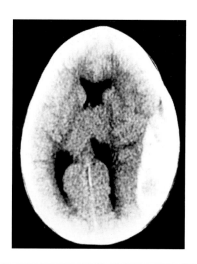

FIGURE 2   A CT that is easy to interpret.
Acute epidural hematoma in an 11-month-old child who fell from the height of a chair.

TABLE 1

Systematic Approach to Head CT Interpretation

Symmetry—Compare left and right sides of the cranium

Midline—Look for midline shift

Cross-sectional anatomy—Review anatomical landmarks for each slice

    Brain tissue—Gray matter, white matter, intracerebral lesions
    CSF spaces—Ventricles, basal cisterns, cortical sulci, and fissures
    Skull and soft tissues—Scalp swelling, fractures, sinuses, orbits

Subdural windows—Look for blood collections adjacent to the skull

Bone windows—Skull, orbits and sinuses, intracranial air

TABLE 2

Targeted Approach to CT Interpretation

Trauma—Blood (extra-axial, intraparenchymal), cerebral edema, fractures, pneumocephalus, scalp swelling, coup, and contra-coup injuries

Headache—Blood in the basilar cisterns (SAH), masses, hydrocephalus, cerebral venous sinuses thrombosis, paranasal sinusitis

Stroke—Examine region of neurological deficit for blood, edema, or masses

CRANIAL CT TECHNIQUE

Head CT slices are oriented obliquely, parallel to the base of the skull, and not in a true axial plane (Figure 3). This reduces the number of slices that are degraded by artifacts caused by the dense bone at the base of the skull (see Figure 10 on p. 440). The effect of this oblique orientation is that on the inferior CT slices, the frontal lobes are anterior, but posteriorly, the cerebellum is seen, rather than the occipital lobes.

Slice thickness is shown as 10 mm through the upper and mid cerebral hemispheres and 5 mm through the lower cerebral hemispheres and brainstem. With current helical CT scanners, all slices are 3 mm to 5 mm thick.

MRI is not degraded by bone artifacts and so the slices are oriented in a true axial plane.

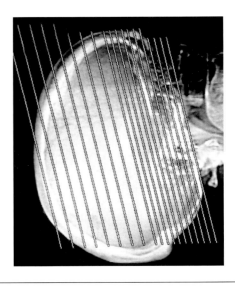

FIGURE 3   Scout topogram showing the oblique orientation of CT slices that parallel the base of the skull.

BRAIN ANATOMY

The principal anatomical landmarks on CT are the cerebral spinal fluid (CSF) spaces of the brain. These include the four ventricles (intracerebral CSF), the extracerebral CSF spaces including the cortical fissures and sulci, and the cisterns at the base of the brain (Figures 4–6).

The two **lateral ventricles** have a C-shape that is formed by the bodies, anterior (frontal) horns, posterior (occipital) horns, and inferior (temporal) horns. The temporal horns are normally slit-like and barely visible; when dilated, they are a sensitive indicator of hydrocephalus.

The **third ventricle** is a slit-like CSF containing space located in the midline between the basal ganglia. The anterior-inferior portion of the third ventricle (the *infundibulum*) tapers like a funnel toward the hypothalamus and pituitary stalk. Posteriorly and inferiorly, the third ventricle drains into the **aqueduct of Sylvius** (cerebral aqueduct) located in the midbrain and then to the **fourth ventricle,** which lies between the cerebellum and pons in the posterior fossa.

The **midbrain** (*mesencephalon*) is the most superior part of the brainstem. In cross section, it has a heart shape (Figure 7). The anterior portion of the midbrain is formed by the *cerebral peduncles*—white matter tracts that carry the main motor innervation of the body, the corticospinal tracts. The posterior portion of the midbrain is the *quadrigeminal plate* with four small nodules—two superior colliculi and two inferior colliculi.

Basilar Cisterns

Relatively large extracerebral CSF spaces are located at base of the cerebral hemispheres and extend around the brainstem and cerebellum (Figure 6). Portions of the basilar cisterns are given

specfic names based on their CT appearance, although they, in fact, form one continuous CSF space.

Superior to the sella turcica is the large **suprasellar cistern.** This contains the *circle of Willis* and is therefore the key region to inspect for signs of aneurysmal subarachnoid hemorrhage (SAH). Inferiorly, the **pre-pontine cistern** lies anterior to the pons. Superiorly, the cisterns surround the midbrain (**perimesencephalic cisterns**). The anterior portion is located between the cerebral peduncles and is known as the **interpeduncular cistern.** The posterior portion is the **quadrigeminal plate cistern.** The quadrigeminal plate cistern extends superiorly over the cerebellum where it is called the **superior cerebellar cistern.**

CSF Circulation

The CSF is formed by the *choroid plexus* located in the lateral ventricles, the third ventricle and, to a small extent, the fourth ventricle. The choroid plexus is often calcified and visible on CT. CSF flows from the lateral ventricles, through the foramina of Monro into the third ventricle and then through the aqueduct of Sylvius into the fourth ventricle. The CSF then drains through perforations in the fourth ventricle (foramina of Magendi and Lushka) into the cisterns at the base of the brain. CSF first enters the *cisterna magna* (cerebellomedullary cistern), then flows inferiorly to bathe the spinal cord, anteriorly into the cisterns at the base of the brain, and superiorly around the cerebral hemispheres. CSF is eventually resorbed into the systemic venous circulation at the arachnoid granulations of the superior sagittal sinus. CSF forms at a fairly brisk rate of 30–60 mL/hr. Obstruction to CSF flow can therefore quickly cause neurological deterioration.

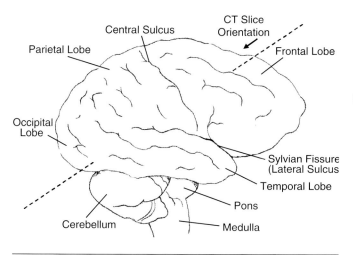

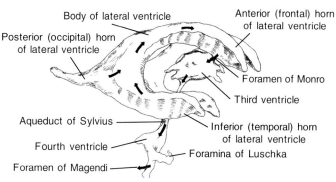

FIGURE 4   Lateral view of the brain.
The Sylvian fissure extends from the surface of the brain over the temporal lobe to the basilar cisterns at the base of the brain.

FIGURE 5   Ventricles of the brain.
Arrows depict the flow of CSF from the lateral ventricles (choroid plexus) to the third and fourth ventricles and out the foramina of Magendie and Luschka to the basilar cisterns.

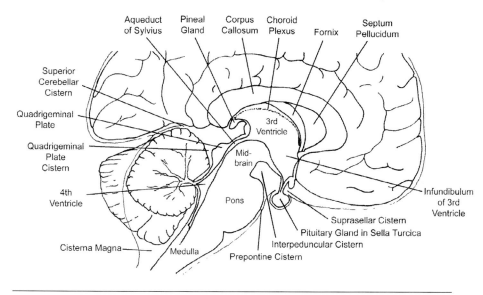

FIGURE 6   Midsagittal section showing the basilar cisterns and brainstem anatomy.

FIGURE 7   Midbrain cross-section.
The cerebral peduncles are anterior and the quadrigeminal plate is posterior.

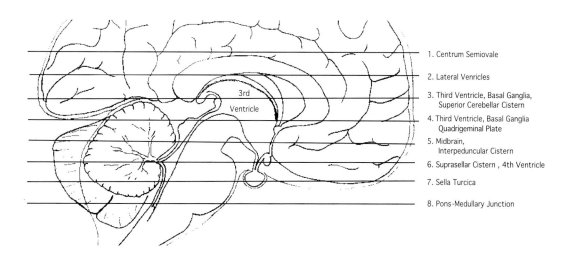

1. Centrum Semiovale

2. Lateral Ventricles

3. Third Ventricle, Basal Ganglia, Superior Cerebellar Cistern

4. Third Ventricle, Basal Ganglia Quadrigeminal Plate

5. Midbrain, Interpeduncular Cistern

6. Suprasellar Cistern , 4th Ventricle

7. Sella Turcica

8. Pons-Medullary Junction

FIGURE 8   CT anatomy—Slice locator.
The slices correspond to the images shown in Figure 9. The slices are oriented obliquely, parallel to the base of the skull.

CT CROSS-SECTIONAL ANATOMY

Each slice has well-defined anatomical landmarks, which should be identified when examining a CT scan (The slice numbering corresponds to that shown in Figures 8 and 9).

Slice 1   The most superior CT slices show the cerebral hemispheres separated by the falx and interhemispheric fissure. Cortical gray and white matter should have a well-defined margin—the *gray/white interface*. On CT, gray matter has slightly higher attenuation (appears lighter) than white matter, which has lower attenuation (appears darker) due to its greater content of fat. The hemispheric subcortical white matter is known as the **centrum semiovale.** The CSF containing cortical *sulci* invaginate between the cortical *gyri*.

Slice 2   The next inferior slice shows the bodies of the **lateral ventricles,** which appear as paired crescent-shaped CSF spaces ("twin bananas").

Slice 3   This slice passes through the middle of the **third ventricle** (a slit-like CSF space in the midline). The **frontal horns** of the lateral ventricles are separated by a membrane, the *septum pellucidum*. The occipital lobes and the occipital horns of the lateral ventricles are located posteriorly and contain the choroid plexus, which is often calcified.

At the posterior margin of the third ventricle is the *pineal gland*, which also is often calcified. Just posterior to the pineal gland is the cisternal space just superior to the cerebellum, the *superior cerebellar cistern.*

The gray matter **basal ganglia** are seen on this and the next slice. The *thalami* lie adjacent to the third ventricle. The heads of the *caudate nuclei* are adjacent to the frontal horns of the lateral ventricles. The more laterally located *lentiform nuclei* are composed of the putamen and globus pallidus. Between the basal ganglia are the V-shaped white matter *internal capsules,* which contain the corticospinal tracts (the main motor innervation of the body).

Slice 4   This slice traverses the lower portion of the third ventricle. The posterior portion of the midbrain—the *quadrigeminal plate* — is seen. The adjacent **quadrigeminal plate cistern** has a crescent shape. This slice has been likened to a "smiley face." The quadrigeminal plate cistern forms the mouth, the third ventricle forms the nose, and the frontal horns form the eyebrows.

Posterior to the quadrigeminal plate cistern is the *cerebellum* that is separated from the occipital lobes by the faint tentorial membrane. The *Sylvian fissure* is also seen on this slice.

Slice 5   This slice traverses though the anterior portion of the **midbrain,** which has a heart-shaped appearance (Figure 7). Between the cerebral peduncles is the small *interpeduncular cistern.* CSF surrounding the midbrain is known as the *perimesencephalic cistern.* The *infundibulum of the third ventricle* is anterior to the interpeduncular cistern. The cerebellum occupies the posterior portion of the slice.

Slice 6   This slice contains the large centrally located **suprasellar cistern,** which is located just superior to the osseus *dorsum sella* (see slice 7). This is also called the "pentagonal cistern" because it has the shape of a five-pointed star. The apex of the star is the *anterior interhemispheric fissure*; the lateral extensions are the medial portion of the *Sylvian fissures*; and the posterior extensions are the *lateral pontine cisterns.*

The **circle of Willis** lies within the suprasellar cistern and is the site of most aneurysmal subarachnoid hemorrhage. The *basilar artery* can be seen just anterior to the pons. The *middle cerebral arteries* are often visible in the lateral extensions of the suprasellar cistern extending into the Sylvian fissures.

The **fourth ventricle** is also seen on this slice. It is located between the pons and cerebellum in the posterior fossa. The temporal lobes contain the **temporal horns of the lateral ventricles,** which normally appear as narrow, barely visible, slits. Enlargement of the temporal horns has a distinctive CT appearance and is a reliable indicator of hydrocephalus (see below).

Slice 7   This slice is through the base of the skull. The **dorsum sella** is a midline bony prominence. The dense *petrous bones* containing the *mastoid air cells*, separate the *posterior fossa* from the middle (temporal) cranial fossae. Streak artifacts emanating from the petrous bones degrade images of the posterior and middle cranial fossae.

The *frontal sinuses* and base of the frontal lobes and anterior cranial fossa are also seen.

Slide 8   This slice traverses the inferior portion of the posterior fossa at the junction of the pons and medulla. Anteriorly, the orbits, ethmoid air cells, and sphenoid sinus are seen.

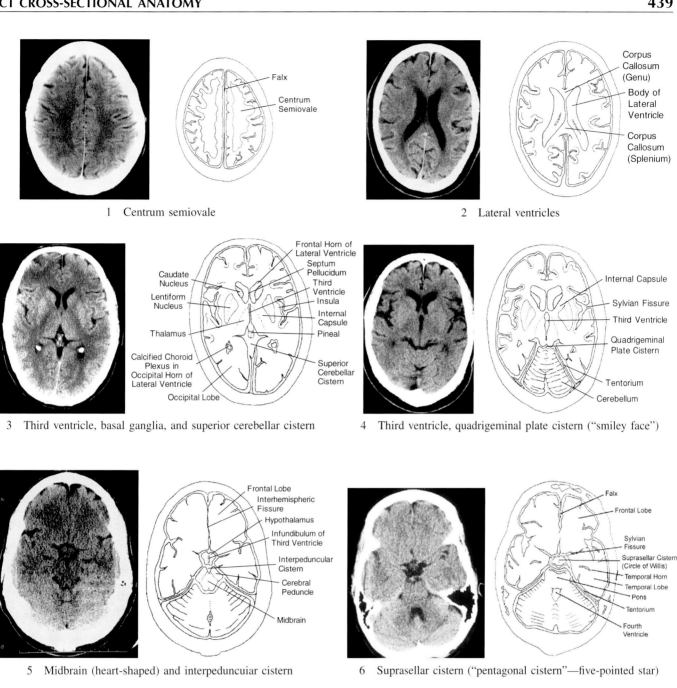

1 Centrum semiovale

2 Lateral ventricles

3 Third ventricle, basal ganglia, and superior cerebellar cistern

4 Third ventricle, quadrigeminal plate cistern ("smiley face")

5 Midbrain (heart-shaped) and interpeduncuiar cistern

6 Suprasellar cistern ("pentagonal cistern"—five-pointed star)

7 Sella turcica

8 Pons-medullary junction

FIGURE 9   Cross-sectional anatomy of eight typical CT slices from the mid-cerebral hemispheres to the lower brainstem.

Head CT Artifacts

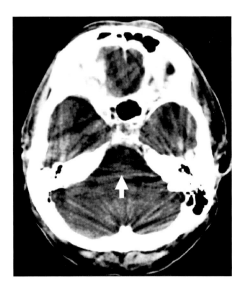

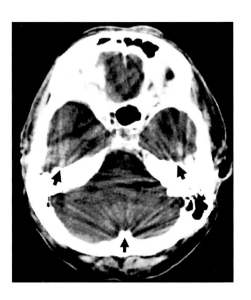

Beam hardening artifact

Loss of image definition occurs in regions adjacent to dense cortical bone. For example, the brainstem is obscured at the level of the petrous portions of the temporal bones (*arrow*).

This is a consequence of "hardening" of the x-ray beam as it passes through cortical bone, i.e., the softer x-rays (lower frequency) are absorbed to a greater extent. The remaining "harder" x-rays are unable to adequately image soft tissues.

Streak artifacts

Alternating dark and light bands radiate from regions of dense cortical bone (*arrows*).

This is due to differences in x-ray beam "hardening" as it passes through regions of dense cortical bone in different directions. The x-ray beam attenuation measurements for a particular location vary depending on the direction of the x-ray beam. This occurs because the extent of x-ray beam hardening varies depending on the amount of cortical bone that it passes through.

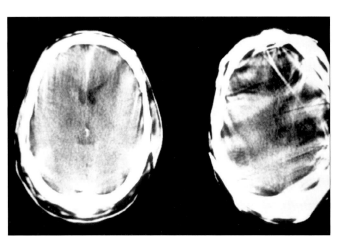

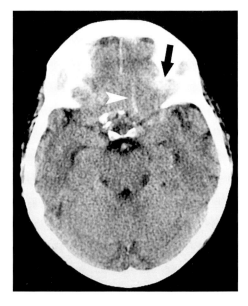

Motion artifact

The head is in different positions as the x-ray source rotates around the patient creating streaks (alternating dark and light bands) and image degradation.

Partial volume artifact

In the region of the skull base, a portion of the CT slice thickness may contain bone (appears white) and portion may contain brain tissue (appears medium gray). The pixel is assigned an intermediate value (an average value) that can mimic blood (appears light gray) (*black arrow*).

A linear streak of traumatic subarachnoid blood is visible at the base of the frontal lobe (*white arrow*). This is not an artifact.

FIGURE 10   Head CT artifacts.

SUGGESTED READING

Barrett JF, Keat N: Artifacts in CT: Recognition and avoidance. *RadioGraphics* 2004;24:1679–1691.

Castillo M: *Neuroradiology Companion: Methods, Guidelines, and Imaging Fundamentals,* 3rd ed. Lippincott Williams & Wilkins, 2005.

Cwinn AA, Grahovac SZ: *Emergency CT Scans of the Head: A Practical Atlas.* Mosby, 1998

Gean AD: *Imaging of Head Trauma.* Raven, 1994.

Greenberg JO: *Neuroimaging: A Companion to Adams and Victor's Principles of Neurology,* 2nd ed. New York: McGraw-Hill, 2000.

Huddle DC, Chaney DB, Glazer M: Emergency imaging of the brain. In: Schwartz DT, Reisdorff EJ, ed. *Emergency Radiology.* New York: McGraw-Hill, 2000.

Kretschmann HJ, Weinrich W: *Cranial Neuroimaging and Clinical Neuroanatomy: Atlas of MR Imaging and Computed Tomography,* 3rd ed. Thieme, 2004.

Latchaw RE, Kucharczyk J, Moseley ME (eds): *Imaging of the Nervous System.* Elsevier-Mosby, 2005.

Lee SH, Rao KCVG, Zimmerman RA: *Cranial MRI and CT,* 4th ed. New York: McGraw-Hill, 1999.

Orrison WW: *Neuroimaging.* Saunders, 2000.

Osborn A, Blaser S, Salzman K: *Diagnostic Imaging: Brain.* Amirsys, 2004.

Ramsey RG: *Neuroradiology,* 3rd ed. Saunders, 1993.

Schnitzlein HN, Murtagh FR: *Imaging Anatomy of the Head and Spine,* 2nd ed. Baltimore: Urban and Schwarzenberg, 1990.

Wolf R: Essentials of neuroimaging. *Radiologic Clin North Am,* 2005.

Zimmerman RA, Gibby WA, Carmody RF (eds): *Neuroimaging: Clinical and Physical Principles.* Springer, 2000.

CT Interpretation Accuracy

Alfaro D, Levitt MA, English DK, Williams V: Accuracy of interpretation of cranial computed tomography scan in an emergency medicine residency program. *Ann Emerg Med* 1995;25:169–174.

Erly WK, Ashdown BC, Lucio RW, et al: Evaluation of emergency CT scans of the head: Is there a community standard? *AJR* 2003;180:1727–1730.

Funaki B, Szymski GX, Rosenblum JD. Significant on-call misses by radiology residents interpreting computed tomographic studies: Perception versus cognition. *Emerg Radiol* 1997;4:290–294. [Four subtle head CT findings missed in 1 year (SDH, SAH, pneumocephalus, temporal contusion.]

Levitt MA, Dawkins R, Williams V, Bullock S: Abbreviated educational session improves cranial computed tomographic scan interpretations by emergency physicians. *Ann Emerg Med* 1997;30:616–626. [A 1-hour course reduced missed major findings from 11% to 3%.]

Perron AD, Huff JS, Ullrich CG, Heafner MD, Kline JA: A multicenter study to improve emergency medicine residents' recognition of intracranial emergencies on computed tomography. *Ann Emerg Med* 1998;32:554–562.

Schriger DL, Kalafut M, Starkemaan S, et al: Cranial computed tomography interpretation in acute stroke: physician accuracy in determining eligibility for thrombolytic therapy. *JAMA* 1998;279:1293–1297.

Head CT: Patient 1

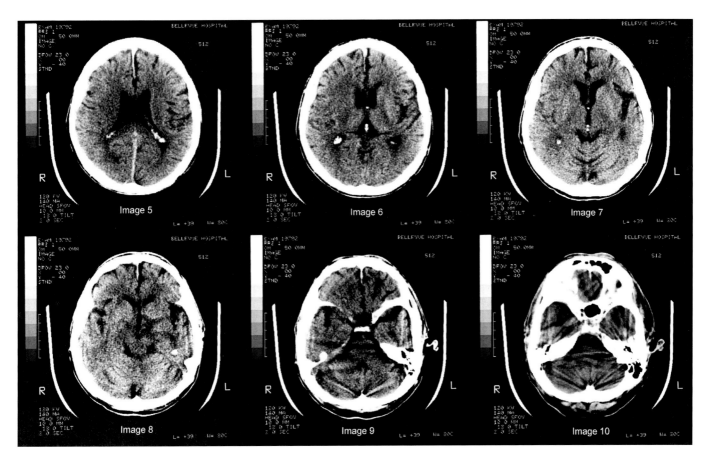

FIGURE 1

Head injury in an elderly man found on the ground outside a bar; head CT was "normal"

A 75-year-old man was found lying on the sidewalk outside a bar. There was a 2-cm laceration on the back of his head. Upon arrival in the ED, he appeared intoxicated. His speech was slurred, but he followed simple commands appropriately. There were no focal neurological deficits. The scalp laceration was cleaned and sutured.

He was given intravenous hydration and thiamine, and was observed for 4 hours in the ED. During this time, his mental status gradually improved. His blood tests were unremarkable aside from an ethanol level of 295 mg/dL. Because of the

patient's age, history of alcoholism, and evident head trauma, a head CT was obtained (Figure 1).

The CT is interpreted as being negative.

After four hours, he was alert and at his "baseline" mental status and wanted to leave.

• Do you agree with the CT interpretation?

A subtle but significant injury was present but difficult to see. Is anything else needed to make the finding more evident?

• How is a CT image created?

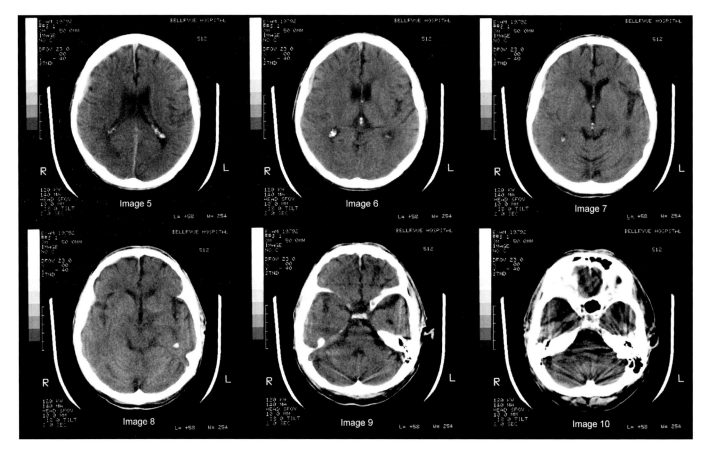

FIGURE 2

CT IN HEAD TRAUMA

To correctly interpret a head CT, it is important to consider whether it has been performed using correct technique and whether all the information needed is being displayed.

The slice orientation should be parallel to the base of the skull and the head should not be tilted. **Head tilt** can cause apparent asymmetry.

In this CT, there is asymmetry of the Sylvian fissures—the fissure appears larger on the left than the right (image 7). This is, in part, due to improper positioning of the patient. The patient's head was slightly tilted and so within each slice, the right side of the brain is shown at a slightly more superior level than the left side. This is confirmed by noting the asymmetry of the petrous bones of the skull base in image 9.

Even accounting for the effect of head tilt, the left Sylvian fissure and adjacent cortical sulci are slightly enlarged compared to the right (images 6 and 7). This was due to mild loss of brain tissue of the left cerebral hemisphere (encephalomalacia), which was likely the result of old trauma or cerebrovascular disease in this elderly patient.

To visualize the significant but subtle acute traumatic abnormality in this patient, additional images are required. As should be routine in cases of head trauma, these images are shown in Figure 2.

• How do these images differ from those shown in Figure 1?

• What do they show?

HOW A CT IMAGE IS CREATED

A CT scan is not a direct radiographic images. It is a mathematically constructed digital picture derived from measurements of a narrow x-ray beam as it passes through the patient in a multitude of different directions (Figures 3 and 4).

CT scanning has two major advantages over conventional radiography. **First,** it provides cross-sectional (tomographic) slices of the body. **Second,** CT can distinguish tissue density differences with far greater sensitivity than can conventional radiography. For example, CT can distinguish CSF and brain tissue and even white and gray matter, which is not possible using conventional radiography.

This discrimination of tissue density differences exceeds that which can be displayed on a single grayscale image. Therefore, every CT slice is displayed as two or three images, each of which shows a different range of tissue densities over the range of radiographic image densities (the grayscale).

The units of radiodensity in CT imaging are named **Hounsfield units** (HU) in honor of Godfrey Hounsfield, one of the inventors of CT scanning (he received the 1979 Nobel Prize for Medicine or Physiology). Water is assigned a value of zero, air a value of −1000 HU, and dense cortical bone a value of +1000 HU (Figure 5).

Brain tissues have a fairly narrow range of density values from approximately +20 to +60 HU. CSF is close to water density (0–10 HU). Acutely clotted blood has higher attenuation (+100 HU or greater). The image display (the "window") for viewing brain tissues is therefore set to best show this range of Hounsfield units.

The CT "window" is defined by two parameters: (1) the **window level** sets the tissue density that is shown as a middle gray and (2) the **window width** sets the range of tissue densities that is distributed over the image's grayscale from white to black. All tissue densities outside the window width will be either white (if the tissue is more radiopaque than the upper limit of the window) or black (if the tissue is more radiolucent). These parameters are analogous to image **brightness** and **contrast** in digital photography.

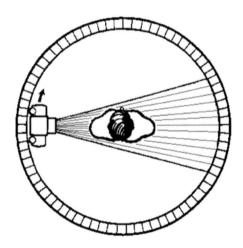

FIGURE 3   Schematic diagram of a CT scanner.

The x-ray source rotates around the patient. The x-rays are measured by detectors on the opposite side of the patient. One revolution is made in 1 second or less.

[From Ballinger PW, Frank ED: *Merrill's Atlas of Radiographic Positions and Radiographic Procedures*, 8th ed. Mosby, 1995, with permission.]

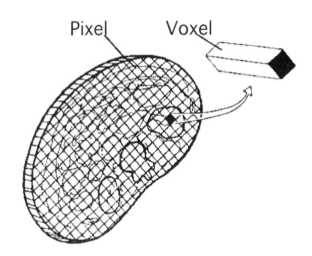

FIGURE 4   After the x-ray data is obtained for the slice, a computer calculates the radiodensity (x-ray beam attenuation) in Hounsfield units (HU) for each picture element (pixel).

The Hounsfield number of the pixel represents the average radiographic density of the tissues located within the volume element (voxel). The thickness of the voxel equals the thickness of the CT slice (3 or 5 mm).

The HU values are displayed a shades of gray on the CT image.

CT imaging in **head trauma** should include three display windows: brain windows, bone windows, and subdural windows (Figure 5).

In **brain windows,** a narrow window width is used to best discriminate the soft tissue details of the brain. The entire grayscale spans only a narrow range of tissue densities (0 to 70-80 HU). The effect is that gray matter (+45 HU) is shown as a different shade of gray than white matter (+30 HU). However, on brain windows, both acute clotted blood and skull appear white and therefore cannot be distinguished (Figure 6A). In addition, both air and CSF (water) appear black. The window level is set at 25–35 HU and the window width is set at 70–80 HU.

For **subdural windows,** the middle gray (window level) remains at (25–35 HU), but the window width is wider (200–250 HU). Brain tissue density differences are not well discriminated and, so the brain appears a more uniform gray. However, substances of greater radiodensity can be differentiated, e.g., bone and acutely clotted blood.

With brain windows, a small subdural hematoma has the same white appearance as the adjacent skull, and can be difficult or impossible to see. On subdural windows, the blood collection appears light gray and is readily distinguished from the adjacent skull (Figure 6).

For **bone windows,** the window level is set at 500–1000 HU and window width at 1000–2000 HU. Bone windows are mainly used to visualize fractures, although they are also useful for detecting pneumocephalus (intracranial air) and fluid within the paranasal sinuses (see subsequent cases).

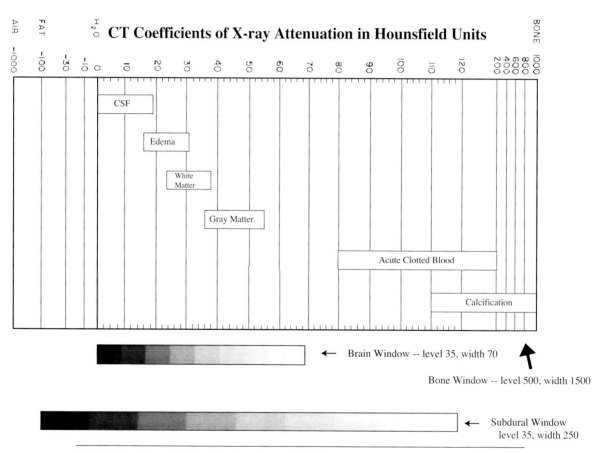

FIGURE 5 Hounsfield unit values in cranial CT.

Tissue attenuation values that are important for brain imaging occupy a narrow range (0–80 HU). These are best displayed using **brain window** settings.

A wider window width (**subdural window**) is needed to detect clotted blood collections (e.g., SDH) located adjacent to the skull.

Osseous structures are visualized using **bone window** settings.

[Adapted from Ramsey RG: *Neuroradiology,* 3rd ed. Saunders, 1993.]

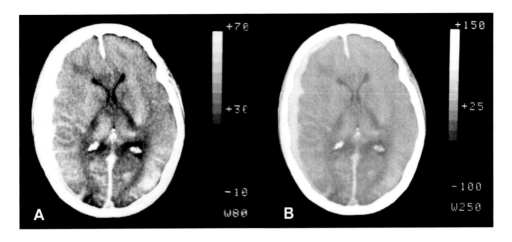

FIGURE 6   Subdural hematoma and subdural windows.

(*A*) On the **brain window** image, the crescent-shaped subdural hematoma has the same white appearance as the skull. (level +30, width 80)

(*B*) On the **subdural window** image, the blood collection is readily distinguished from skull. There is slight midline shift to the left (subfalcine herniation). (level +25, width 250)

Patient Outcome

In Patient 1, there is a small extra-axial blood collection in the right parietal area (Figure 7 and Figures 1 and 2 [images 5, 6, 7]). It has a crescent shape, which suggests that it is a subdural hematoma. There is no mass effect or midline shift.

A small asymptomatic subdural hematoma does not require surgical evacuation. However, the patient needs close observation in the hospital for at least 24, hours, looking for signs of neurological deterioration and expansion of the hematoma.

The initial interpretation of the CT was negative for signs of acute trauma and the patient was discharged from the ED. The "official" reading the next day identified the subdural hematoma. An attempt was made to recall the patient to the ED, but he could not be located.

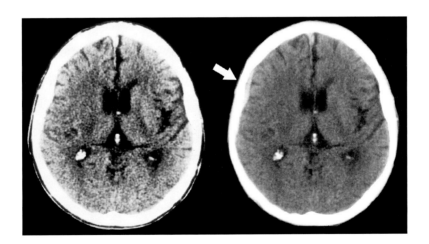

FIGURE 7   Small SDH missed on initial CT interpretation—Patient 1, image 6.

A small SDH is nearly invisible on the **brain window** (*A*). It causes apparent slight thickening of the skull at the right frontoparietal area.

The **subdural window** image (*B*) reveals the subdural blood collection (*arrow*).

The Beatles and the CT scanner

In addition to being cultural icons and responsible for much great music in the 1960s, the Beatles can also be credited with a role in the invention of the CT scanner.

Godfrey Hounsfield was a computer engineer working for British EMI (Electrical and Musical Industries) in the 1950s and 60s. In 1967, he conceived a novel medical imaging technology, adopting a mathematical curiosity to a new method of generating radiographic images.

The mathematical puzzle concerned a square grid of numbers in which each cell of the grid contains an integer. The numbers were then summed along each row, column and diagonal of the grid (Figure 8). The mathematical problem concerned how to calculate the number contained within each cell from the sums of the rows, columns and diagonals. This problem was solved in the early 1900s, more than 50 years before Hounsfield's invention.

Hounsfield's genius was to recognize that this mathematical problem could be applied to measurements of a pencil-thin x-ray beam that was directed through a patient in many different directions. From these measurements, the tissue density at all points in the patient in the plane being scanned could thereby be determined.

In 1967, Hounsfield proposed this novel medical imaging system to British EMI, which had never before manufactured radiologic imaging equipment. The company, awash in cash from the sales of Beatles recordings, agreed to provide the funding – and the rest is history.

The earliest scanners in medical use were known as "EMI scanners," although soon lost out to more established radiologic equipment manufacturers. (EMI did not realize that they had a "hit" as big or bigger than the Beatles). This same concept of computed tomography is now also used in MRI, PET and SPECT (nuclear scintigraphic) scanners.

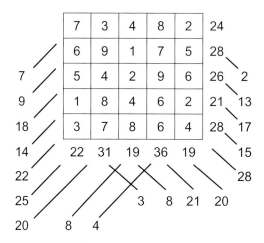

FIGURE 8   Mathematical schema of computed tomography.

In this simplified example, a 5 x 5 grid contains numbers from 1 to 9.

The puzzle is to determine the numbers in each of the cells of the grid from the sum of the integers in each row, column and diagonal. There is insufficient information using only the horizontal and vertical summations to do this calculation, so the diagonal sums are necessary. This is analogous to deriving a topographic image from measurements of x-ray beam attenuation as it passes through the patient in a multitude of different directions.

In CT scanning, the grid size is 256 x 256 and the range of integers is from −1,000 to +1,000. (The original CT scanners used an 80 x 80 grid.)

Current CT scanners use different, more efficient image reconstruction algorithms, one of which was developed by Allan Cormack who shared the Nobel Prize with Hounsfield.

SUGGESTED READING

Friedland GW, Thurber BD: The birth of CT. *AJR* 1996;167: 1365–1370.

Garvey CJ, Hanlon R: Computed tomography in clinical practice. *BMJ* 2002;324:1077–1080.

Hounsfield GN: Computerized transverse axial scanning (tomography) 1. Description of system. *Br J Radiol* 1973;46:1016–1022.

Oransky I: Obituary: Sir Godfrey N. Hounsfield. *Lancet* 2004;364:1032.

Petrik V, Apok V, Brtton JA, et al: Godfrey Hounsfield and the dawn of computed tomography. *Neurosurgery* 2006;58:780–787.

Head CT: Patient 2

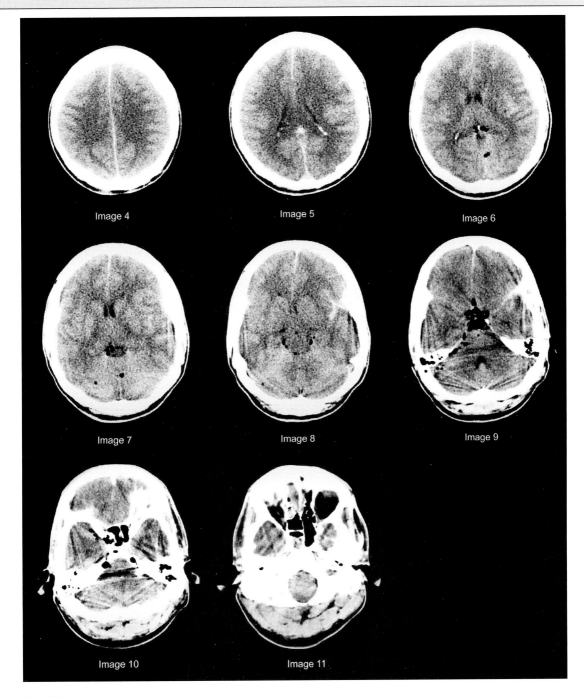

FIGURE 1

Head injury in a young man struck with a bat

During a robbery, a 34-year-old local shopkeeper was hit on the head with a wooden bat and he lost consciousness.

On arrival to the ED, he was awake but oriented only to person.

There were multiple contusions on the right side of his head and blood draining from his nose, but he had no difficulty maintaining his airway. His pupils were equal and he was able to move all four extremities. The initial Glasgow coma scale (GCS) score was 14. His vital signs were normal and, aside from the head injury, there was no other evident trauma. After initial stabilization, a head CT was performed (Figure 1).

- What are the findings on his head CT?
  (There are six abnormalities)

SECONDARY INJURY

The primary goal of emergency CT scanning in a patient with head trauma is rapid identification of a surgically correctable lesion such as large subdural, epidural, or intracerebral hematoma. Clinical outcome can be substantially improved with prompt surgical treatment.

Many patients, however, do not have such lesions despite significant head injury. Lesions that cannot be surgically corrected include nonhemorrhagic cerebral contusions, diffuse axonal injury (DAI), and smaller intracranial hemorrhages. The clinical status of patient with these injuries can range from minor concussion to coma. Patients with these injuries are at risk for delayed development of intracranial hematomas or cerebral edema. These are known as **secondary injuries.**

Although this patient's CT does not show lesions requiring immediate surgical intervention, there are several findings of significant head injury.

On **CT image 5** (Figure 2), the ventricles appear small. Such **slit-like ventricles** are a sign of diffuse cerebral edema due to the traumatic brain injury. Another sign of diffuse cerebral edema is effacement (thinning or obliteration) of the cortical sulci.

On this and the adjacent images (Figure 2 and Figure 1, images 5, 6, and 7), **slight midline shift** to the right can be seen. This is indicative of a mass lesion in the left cranial compartment,

although the lesion itself is nearly impossible to see. However, in the left parietal region, the skull appears slightly thickened (Figure 2).

Blood collections that are adjacent to the skull can be difficult to visualize when the CT images are displayed in standard **brain window** settings (see Patient 1). Therefore, the CT slices must also be displayed at a setting that allows discrimination of a blood collection from the adjacent skull. These are known as a **subdural windows** (or "intermediate" windows). When viewed using brain windows, both clotted blood and the skull appear white (Figure 2), whereas with subdural windows, acutely clotted blood appears as a light shade of gray that is readily distinguishable from bone, which appears white (Figure 3).

It is sometimes difficult to determine whether small hematomas are subdural or epidural. They are therefore simply termed "extra-axial blood collections" (extra-axial means outside of the brain). In addition, this blood collection is *opposite* the site of impact—a **contrecoup injury**. It results from impact of the brain on the skull opposite the site of initial injury. Hemorrhage on the same side as the impact is a **coup injury.** The primary site of impact is often indicated by scalp swelling or a skull fracture.

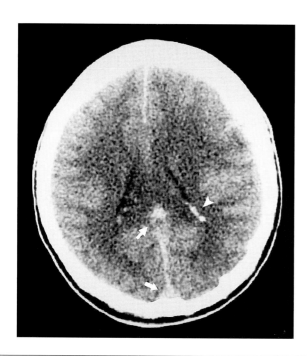

FIGURE 2   Image 5—Brain window.
1. Slit-like ventricles; effacement of cortical sulci.
2. Slight midline shift.
3. Skull appears thick left parietal region.
4. Calcified choroid plexus (*arrowhead*).
5. Normal venous sinuses in posterior falx (*arrows*).

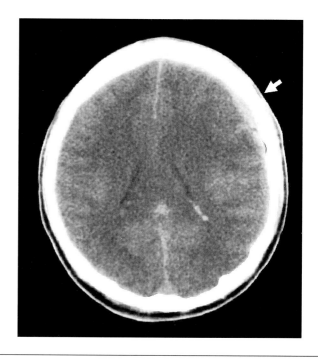

FIGURE 3   Image 5—Subdural window.
Small subdural hematoma (*arrow*).

The next two inferior slices (**CT images 6 and 7**) also show the small extra-axial blood collection (Figures 4 and 5). It is more likely a subdural hematoma (SDH) because it has a crescent shape. In addition, there is no associated skull fracture, and the blood collection is opposite the site of initial impact.

Also seen in images 6 and 7 are white lines extending inward from the cortical surface (Figures 4 and 5). This is blood located within the cortical sulci and represents **traumatic subarachnoid hemorrhage** (SAH). In **image 8,** the subarachnoid blood has a Y-shape owing to its location within the Sylvian fissure

(Figure 6, *arrow*). In **image 7,** a linear white streak that parallels the skull is not in an anatomical location but is instead a **streak artifact** emanating from adjacent dense cortical bone (Figure 5, *arrowhead*).

In **images 6–9,** there are several small black (very low attenuation) regions that are not CSF collections since they are round and have very well-defined margins (like bubbles) (Figures 4–7). These represent air in the cranial cavity—**pneumocephalus.**

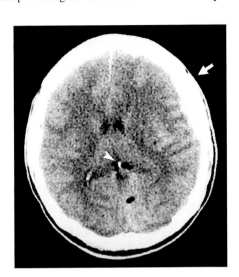

FIGURE 4A   Image 6—Brain window.

1. Slight midline shift.
2. Apparent skull thickening left parietal region (*arrow*).
3. Pineal gland calcified (*arrowhead*)–normal.
4. Pneumocephalus (black bubbles) is easier to visualize using subdural windows (see Figure 4B).

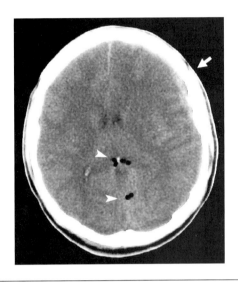

FIGURE 4B   Image 6—Subdural window.

1. Small left parietal SDH and SAH (*arrow*).
2. Pneumocephalus (*arrowheads*) in superior cerebellar cistern (adjacent to pineal gland), and in cortical sulcus of the left occipital lobe adjacent to the posterior interhemispheric fissure.

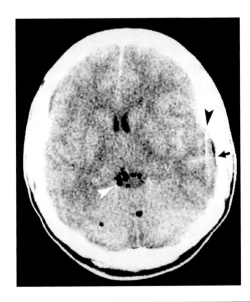

FIGURE 5   Image 7

1. Pneumocephalus in occipital sulci and superior cerebellar cistern (*white arrowhead*).
2. Traumatic SAH (*black arrow*).
3. Streak artifact (*black arrowhead*).

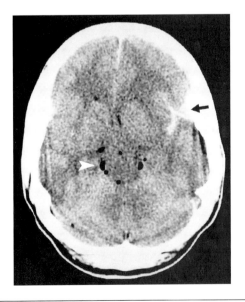

FIGURE 6   Image 8

1. Traumatic SAH in left Sylvian fissure (*black arrow*).
2. Pneumocephalus surrounds the midbrain (*arrowhead*).

In **image 9,** a large collection of air is in the suprasellar cistern ("pentagonal cistern") (Figure 7). Pneumocephalus can be easier to see on subdural windows and *bone windows* because brain tissue and CSF are shown as gray shades, whereas air is black (Figures 4B and 7B). On brain windows, both air and CSF appear black (Figures 4A and 7A).

Pneumocephalus is a sign of an open skull fracture. Air may originate from the outside environment in the case of an open depressed skull fracture. However, in this patient, air at the base of the brain originates from a fracture extending into the adjacent craniofacial sinuses—a **basilar skull fracture.**

The sixth CT finding is an air/fluid level in the **sphenoid sinus** (Figure 8, **CT image 11**). In the setting of head trauma, this fluid is blood due to a fracture (not sinusitis). This finding and pneumocephalus are two indirect signs of a basilar skull fracture. Both the pneumocephalus and sphenoid sinus air/fluid levels are seen better on the bone windows (Figures 7B and 8B). However, the fracture itself is not visible. The fissures and perforations seen at the skull base are neurovascular groves or sutures and not fractures (Table 1).

TABLE 1

Patient 2—Six CT Findings

1. Slit-like ventricles and sulcal effacement (diffuse cerebral edema)

2. Slight midline shift

3. Small subdural hematoma (left parietal)

4. Traumatic subarachnoid hemorrhage

5. Pneumocephalus

6. Sphenoid sinus air/fluid level, mastoid air cell opacified

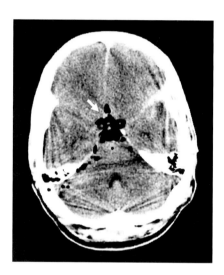

FIGURE 7A   Image 9—Brain window.
1. Pneumocephalus in suprasellar cistern (*arrow*).
2. Streak artifacts (alternating dark and light bands) radiate from the dense bone of the skull base.

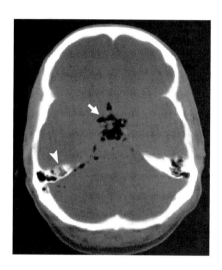

FIGURE 7B   Image 9—Bone window.
1. Pneumocephalus (*arrow*).
2. Fluid (blood) in right mastoid air cells (*arrowhead*).

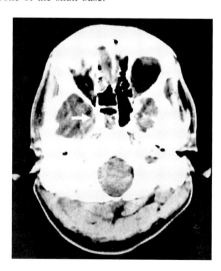

FIGURE 8A   Image 11—Brain window.
1. Air/fluid level in sphenoid sinus (*arrow*).
2. Blood in the right ethmoid air cells.

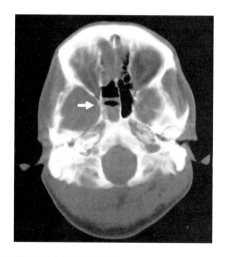

FIGURE 8B   Image 11—Bone window.
Sphenoid sinus air/fluid level (*arrow*).

Fissures in skull base are normal neurovascular groves and perforations, not fractures. The fracture itself is not visible.

A **basilar skull fracture** can involve the anterior, middle, or posterior cranial fossa (Figure 9). Basilar fractures can have two significant clinical **complications**.

First, they can directly damage adjacent vital structures such as the vestibulocochlear, facial, optic, or olfactory nerves. Middle or inner ear structures can also be disrupted. The immediate development of a facial nerve palsy is an indication for emergency surgical decompression, whereas the delayed onset of facial paralysis is caused by edema and managed nonoperatively.

The **second** potential complication of a basilar skull fracture is meningitis. The tightly adherent dura mater is usually torn and the cranial contents are exposed to the adjacent craniofacial sinuses. Prophylactic antibiotics do not prevent the meningitis and may increase the risk of infection with antibiotic-resistant organisms.

The **diagnosis of a basilar skull fracture** can be made on clinical examination: hemotympanum, raccoon eyes, or Battle's sign (the latter two take several hours to develop), as well as CSF rhinorrhea or otorrhea. **In this patient,** hemotympanum was noted during his initial ED evaluation.

Emergency head CT is used in patients with basilar skull fractures to detect associated intracranial injuries, especially hematomas. Standard CT slices (5-mm thick) usually only visualize indirect signs of the fracture. Direct visualization of the fracture requires a thin-section (1.5 mm) dedicated **temporal bone CT** (Figure 10). Such studies are not needed in the emergency department.

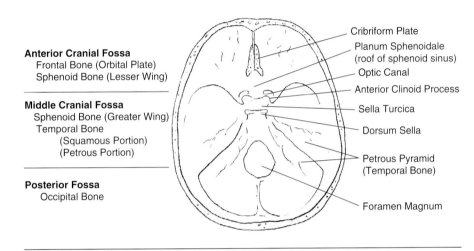

Anterior Cranial Fossa
Frontal Bone (Orbital Plate)
Sphenoid Bone (Lesser Wing)

Middle Cranial Fossa
Sphenoid Bone (Greater Wing)
Temporal Bone
(Squamous Portion)
(Petrous Portion)

Posterior Fossa
Occipital Bone

Cribriform Plate
Planum Sphenoidale
(roof of sphenoid sinus)
Optic Canal
Anterior Clinoid Process
Sella Turcica
Dorsum Sella
Petrous Pyramid
(Temporal Bone)
Foramen Magnum

FIGURE 9 Diagram of the skull base.

Basilar skull fractures can involve the frontal bone (cribriform plate causing CSF rhinorhea and raccoon eyes), middle cranial fossa (sphenoid and temporal bones), or posterior fossa (occipital bone and foramen magnum).

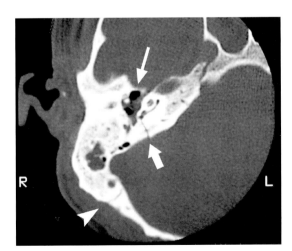

R L

FIGURE 10 Temporal bone CT.

1. Transverse fracture of temporal bone (*arrow*).
2. Normal suture between the temporal and occipital bones (*arrowhead*).
3. Air in internal auditory canal (*long arrow*).

Patient Outcome

The patient was admitted to the Neurosurgical Intensive Care Unit for close monitoring and serial head CT scans. CT done the next day revealed expansion of the left subdural hematoma, a new left temporal contusion, and increased midline shift (Figure 11).

Despite the worsening CT findings, the patient remained clinically stable. He was managed with careful control of blood pressure and intravenous fluids, and did not require endotracheal intubation. His mental status gradually improved over the next several days.

His month-long hospital course was complicated by post-traumatic meningitis. The patient therefore had **two secondary injuries** during his hospital stay: delayed intracranial hemorrhage and meningitis.

Upon discharge, he had mild cognitive deficits and a right sensory-neural hearing loss. He was referred for further rehabilitation.

Delayed Intracranial Hemorrhage

Delayed intracranial hemorrhage is a major concern following head trauma. Patients admitted to the ICU are monitored with serial head CT scans to screen for delayed complications including hemorrhage and worsening cerebral edema. Delayed intracranial hemorrhage is usually seen in patients with severe head injuries (i.e., abnormal mental status and/or abnormal initial CT scans).

Delayed intracranial hemorrhage generally does not occur in patients with minor head trauma who are neurologically normal and have normal CT scans. Such patients can usually be safely discharged from the ED. Nonetheless, Snoey and Levitt (1994) described three cases of delayed subdural hematoma occurring 1–3 months after minor head trauma. All patients had negative initial CT scans. Each patient had several ED visits for persistent headache and each time the headache was attributed to a postconcussive syndrome. Only when neurological deficits developed was a repeat CT scan ordered. In each case, a large SDH was discovered that required surgical drainage.

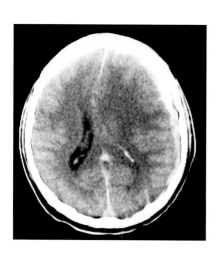
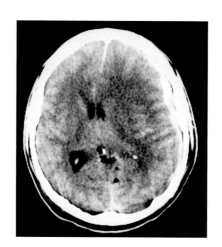
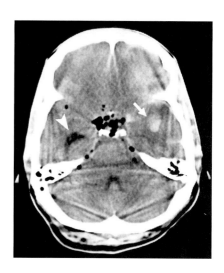
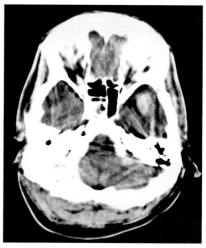

FIGURE 11   Head CT the next day.

Delayed intracranial hemorrhage (secondary injury).

1. Expansion of the left parietal SDH
2. Increasing midline shift
3. Hydrocephalus—dilation of the right lateral ventricle including the temporal horn (*arrowhead*) due to compression of third ventricle that obstructs CSF flow
4. New temporal lobe contusion (*arrow*)

The patient remained clinically stable despite the worsening CT findings.

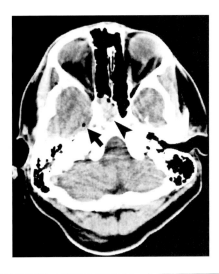

FIGURE 12   Another patient with a basilar skull fracture—Subtle CT signs.

CT findings are (1) a single small air collection in the middle cranial fossa—pneumocephalus (*arrow*) and (2) fluid in the sphenoid sinus (*arrowhead*).

Both findings would be easier to see on bone windows.

A *targeted review* of the CT in patients with clinical signs of a basilar skull fracture (e.g. hemotympanum) incorporates a search for these findings. Such an approach to CT interpretation leads quickly to the pertinent findings.

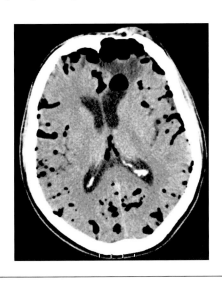
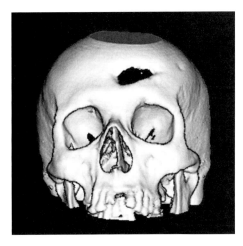

FIGURE 13   Massive pneumocephalus.

A 30-year-old man was struck on his forehead with a peanut butter jar. He presented to the ED with a forehead laceration and mild confusion.

A head CT demonstrated massive pneumocephalus.

On further questioning, the patient stated that he had sustained a gun shot wound to the head several years earlier. There was a residual frontal bone defect as illustrated by a facial bone CT with 3D surface-rendered images.

Surgical evacuation of air and repair of the dural tear were performed.

There is no radiographic evidence of **tension pneumocephalus.** Tension pneumocephalus causes compression of the frontal lobes with concomitant traction on the medial portions of the frontal lobes by the bridging cortical veins. This gives the frontal lobes a bifid peaked appearance, the "Mount Fuji sign" (Michel 2004, Heckmann and Ganslande 2004).

SUGGESTED READING

Heckmann JG, Ganslandt O: The Mount Fuji sign. *N Engl J Med* 2004;350:18.

Michel SJ: The Mount Fuji sign. *Radiology* 2004;232:449–450.

Nageris B, Hansen MC, Lavelle WG, et al: Temporal bone fractures. *Am J Emerg Med* 1995;13:211–214.

Sherman SC, Bokhari F: Massive pneumocephalus after minimal head trauma. *J Emerg Med* 2003;25: 319–320.

Snoey ER, Levitt MA: Delayed diagnosis of subdural hematoma following normal computed tomography scan. *Ann Emerg Med* 1994;23:1127–1131.

How to Read a Head CT in a Patient with Head Trauma

CT interpretation is most efficient when specific findings related to the patient's clinical presentation are sought. In patients with head trauma, **first,** look for large subdural, epidural, or intracerebral hematomas that require emergency surgical treatment.

Second, using a **targeted approach,** review each slice for intra and extra-axial blood collections, midline shift, ventricular compression or enlargement (hydrocephalus), and fractures (Table 1). Examine the brain adjacent to the site of impact (evident by scalp swelling or fracture) for *coup* injures, as well as opposite the site of impact for *contra-coup* injuries. Examine brain, subdural, and bone windows.

Third, search carefully for **easily missed injuries** (Table 2). Although some of these easily missed injuries have been considered "clinically insignificant" by certain investigators, agreement on this point is not universal (Stiell 2000, 2001). Such injuries are associated with a higher incidence of adverse outcome, including delayed intracerebral hemorrhage (Schultz 2002, Atzema 2002). Close observation of the patient, possibly as an in-patient for 24 hours, is warranted. On the other hand, a *normal CT* does not guarantee that delayed bleeding will not occur (Snoey 1994).

TABLE 1

Targeted Approach to Head CT Interpretation in Patients with Head Trauma

Examine each slice for:

1. **Extra-axial blood**—SDH, EDH, traumatic SAH (Figures 1–4)

2. **Intraparenchymal blood**—Hemorrhagic contusion and hematoma (Figure 5)

3. **Midline shift**—May be greater than the width of a SDH due to underlying cerebral edema (Figure 3)

4. **Ventricles:**
   Compressed (unilateral or bilateral)—Mass effect of hematoma or cerebral edema (Figure 6)
   Enlarged (usually asymmetrical)—Obstruction to CSF flow (hydrocephalus)
      (see Introduction to Head CT, Figure 2, page 435, and Patient 2, Figure 11, page 454)

5. **Scalp swelling**—Indicates site of impact to the head (Figure 2)

6. **Fractures**—Examine bone windows and "scout" lateral skull view (Figures 2B, 9, and 10)

7. **Pneumocephalus** (intracranial air)—A sign of open skull fracture (seen best on bone windows) (see Patient 2, pages 451–452, 455)

8. **Craniofacial sinuses**—Blood or air/fluid level; examine bone windows (Figures 2B, 9, and 10)

TABLE 2

Easily Missed Injuries—Head Trauma

1. **Small SDH**—Difficult to see adjacent to skull; use subdural windows (see Patients 1 and 2, pages 447 and 450).

2. **Interhemispheric or tentorial SDH**—Blood adjacent to falx or tentorium causes increased attenuation (whiteness) (Figure 7). Falx calcification can mimic blood. Subdural windows can help distinguish blood from calcification.

3. **Blood at base of frontal or temporal cranial fossae**—Difficult to distinguish from "partial volume artifact" caused by adjacent bone of the skull base (Figure 8).

4. **Diffuse axonal injury**—"Slit-like" ventricles due to diffuse cerebral edema; petechial hemorrhages at the gray/white interface. Indicative of severe brain injury (Figure 6 and Patient 2, Figure 2, page 450).

5. **Linear skull fracture** or **depressed skull fracture**—Difficult to see if in axial plane; use "scout" lateral skull film (Figures 9 and 10).

6. **Pneumocephalus**—A sign of an open skull fracture (best seen using bone windows) (Figure 10E and Patient 2, page 452).

7. **Basilar skull fracture**—Pneumocephalus; fluid in sphenoid sinus or mastoid air cells; fracture is not usually seen directly (see Patient 2).

8. **Isodense SDH** (subacute, 1 week old)—Blood collection is same attenuation as brain tissue; see midline shift and absence of cortical sulci.

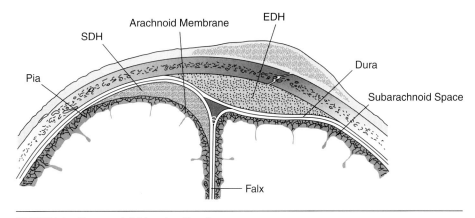

FIGURE 1   Extra-axial blood collections.

The *dura* is composed of an inner (meningeal) and an outer (periosteal) layer (Figure 1). These two layers split to form the dural venous sinuses (S). The dura is firmly attached to the skull at the cranial sutures: the *coronal suture* between the frontal bone and parietal bones, and the *lambdoidal suture* between the parietal bones and the occipital bone.

The *arachnoid membrane* is loosely adherent to the inner layer of the dura. The subarachnoid space invaginates into the cortical sulci on the surface of the brain.

Subdural hematoma (SDH) collects in the virtual space between the dura and loosely attached arachnoid membrane. It usually has a **crescent shape** lying between the skull and cerebral convexities (Figure 3). The SDH does not cross the falx or tentorium; it may follow the contour of and lie adjacent to the falx or tentorium (Figure 7). Subdural blood does not extend into the cortical sulci. Hemorrhage originates from torn *bridging veins* that drain the cerebral cortex, traverse the subdural and subarachnoid spaces, and enter the superior sagittal sinus (S).

Epidural hematoma (EDH) is located between the dura and the skull. The EDH tends to have a **lenticular shape** (biconvex) because of the firm attachment of the dura to the skull, particularly at the cranial sutures. It occasionally crosses the midline, and it is usually associated with an overlying skull fracture, which tears a meningeal artery. Parietal EDH are most common, but frontal and occipital EDH can occur (Figure 2).

Traumatic subarachnoid hemorrhage (SAH) collects within the subarachnoid space under the arachnoid membrane and invaginates into the cortical sulci and fissures (Figure 4).

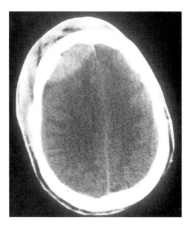
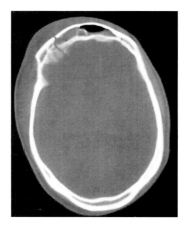

FIGURE 2   Epidural hematoma.

Typical lenticular (biconvex) shape. Although most epidural hematomas are temporo-parietal, frontal and occipital EDH do occur. In this case, there is an associated frontal skull fracture, fluid (blood) in the frontal sinus, and considerable overlying soft tissue swelling.

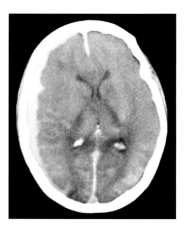

FIGURE 3   Subdural hematoma.

Crescent shape due to blood overlying the cerebral convexity.

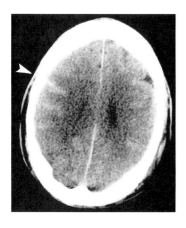
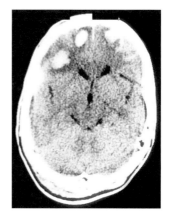

FIGURE 4   Traumatic SAH.

Blood invaginates into the cortical sulci (*arrowhead*).

FIGURE 5   Intracerebral hematomas.

Hemorrhagic contusions (intra-axial blood) involving the frontal lobes.

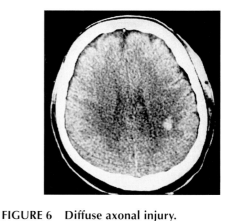

FIGURE 6   Diffuse axonal injury.

Slit-like lateral ventricles due to diffuse cerebral edema. A small (petechial) hemorrhage is caused by shear forces at the gray/white interface when the brain is subjected to a forceful impact.

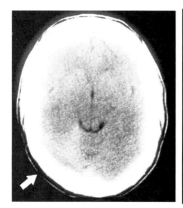
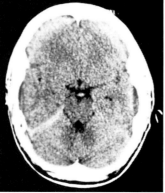

FIGURE 7   Tentorial SDH.

The right side of the tentorial membrane has a higher attenuation due to overlying blood (*arrow*). This is sometimes called "pseudoenhancement" because it mimics the increased attenuation that normally occurs with intravenous contrast administration. True enhancement, however, is symmetrical.

A repeat CT scan the next day showed a more well-defined tentorial opacity.

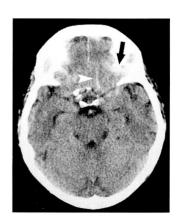

FIGURE 8   Traumatic SAH

At base of the frontal cranial fossa (*arrowhead*).

Partial volume artifact due to the skull base mimics blood (*black arrow*). Blood can be distinguished from the bone of the skull base by its appearance (linear if SAH; rounded if a contusion) and its extension to the next superior CT slice.

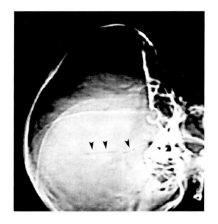
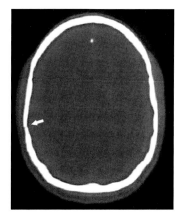

FIGURE 9   Linear skull fracture.

A vertically oriented linear skull fracture is visible on the lateral scout skull topogram (*arrowheads*) and the bone window image (*arrow*).

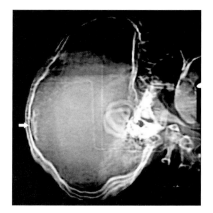
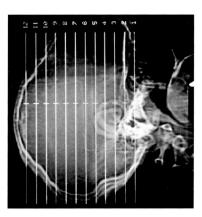
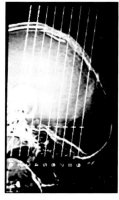

A   Scout laterd skull radiograph   B   Axial CT slice orientation   D   Coronal CT slice orientation

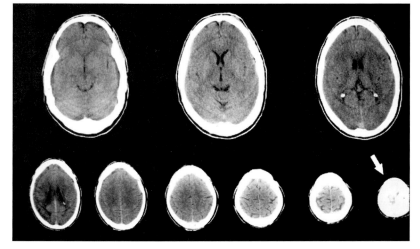
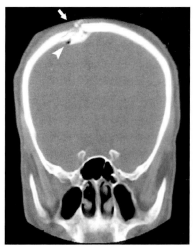

C   Axial CT   E   Coronal CT

FIGURE 10   Depressed skull fracture.

A depressed skull fracture at the most superior aspect of the skull is more easily seen on the scout lateral skull topogram (*arrows* in *A* and *B*) than on the axial CT images (C, *arrow*) because the fracture is in the plane of the CT slices.

A coronal CT readily shows the fracture (*D* and *E*). A small collection of air (pneumocephalus) is adjacent to the fracture, i.e., an "open" skull fracture (*arrowhead* in *E*).

This patient had bilateral leg weakness. Although bilateral lower extremity weakness is usually due to a spinal cord injury, in this patient it was caused by bilateral parafalcine cerebral contusions at the motor cortex that innervates the lower extremities.

SUGGESTED READING

Cooper PR, Golfinos JG, eds. *Head Injury,* 4th ed. New York: McGraw-Hill, 2000.

Cwinn AA, Grahovac SZ: *Emergency CT Scans of the Head: A Practical Atlas.* Mosby, 1998.

Gean AD: *Imaging of Head Trauma.* Raven, 1994.

Go JL, Zee CS, eds. Imaging of head trauma. *Neuroimag Clin North Am* 2002;12:165–343.

Hammoud DA, Wasserman BA: Diffuse axonal injuries: Pathophysiology and imaging. *Neuroimag Clin North Am* 2002;12:205–216.

Huddle DC, Chaney DB, Glazer M: Emergency imaging of the brain. In Schwartz DT, Reisdorff EJ, eds. *Emergency Radiology.* New York: McGraw-Hill, 2000.

Johnson PL, Eckard DA, Chason DP, et al: Imaging of acquired cerebral herniations. *Neuroimag Clin North Am* 2002;12:217–228.

Stallmeyer MJB, Morales RE, Flanders AE: Imaging of traumatic neurovascular injury. *Radiol Clin North Am* 2006;44:13–39.

Swartz KR, Fee DB, Dempsey RJ: Blossoming traumatic epidural hematoma. *J Emerg Med* 2003;25:451–452.

Young RJ, Destian S: Imaging of traumatic intracranial hemorrhage. *Neuroimag Clin North Am* 2002;12:189–204.

Subtle Signs of Cranial Trauma

Atzema C, Mower WR, Hoffman JR, et al: Defining "clinically unimportant" CT findings in patients with blunt head trauma (abstract). *Acad Emerg Med* 2002;9:451. [From NEXUS II, 11 of 82 pts. (11%) had poor outcome, all of whom had abnormal mental status or coagulopathy.]

Doezema D, King JN, Tandberg D, et al: Magnetic resonance imaging in minor head trauma. *Ann Emerg Med* 1991;20:1281–1284.

Erly WK, Ashdown BC, Lucio RW, et al: Evaluation of emergency CT scans of the head: Is there a community standard? *AJR* 2003;180:1727–1730.

Funaki B, Szymski GX, Rosenblum JD. Significant on-call misses by radiology residents interpreting computed tomographic studies: Perception versus cognition. *Emerg Radiol* 1997;4:290–294. [Four subtle head CT findings missed in one year (SDH, SAH, pneumocephalus, temporal contusion).]

Schultz J, Atzema C, Mower W, Hoffman J: Isolated cerebral contusion and limited subarachnoid hemorrhage on head CT scanning for minor blunt head trauma is clinically important (abstract). *Acad Emerg Med* 2002;9:411. [From NEXUS II: 29 of 47 pts. (62%) with "minor" CT abnormalities had serious adverse outcomes.]

Snoey ER, Levitt MA: Delayed diagnosis of subdural hematoma following normal computed tomography scan. *Ann Emerg Med* 1994;23:1127–1131.

Stiell I, Lesiuk H, Vandemheen K, et al: Obtaining consensus for the definition of "clinically important" brain injury in the CCC study (abstract). *Acad Emerg Med* 2000;7:572. [Although the "majority" of physicians felt that these findings were "clinically insignificant," nearly 50% were not in agreement, especially the emergency physicians surveyed.]

Head Trauma Imaging Clinical Decision Rules

Haydel MJ, Preston CA, Mills TJ, et al: Indications for computed tomography in patients with minor head trauma. *New Engl J Med* 2000;343:100–105.

Hollander JE, Go S, Lowery DW, et al: Interrater reliability of criteria used in assessing blunt head injury patients for intracranial injuries. *Acad Emerg Med* 2003;10:830–835.

Masters SJ, et al: Skull x-ray examinations after head trauma: Recommendations of a multidisciplinary panel and validation study. *N Engl J Med* 1987; 316:84–91.

Miller EC, Derlet RW, Kinser D: Minor head trauma: Is computed tomography always necessary? *Ann Emerg Med* 1996;27:290–294.

Mower WR, Hoffman JR, Herbert M, et al: Developing a clinical decision instrument to rule out intracranial injuries in patients with minor head trauma: Methodology of the NEXUS II investigation. *Ann Emerg Med* 2002;40:505–514.

Stiell IG, Wells G, Vandemheen K, et al: The Canadian CT Head Rule for patients with minor head trauma. *Lancet* 2001;357:1392–1396.

Sun BC, Hoffman JR, Mower WR: Evaluation of a modified prediction instrument to identify significant pediatric intracranial injury after blunt head trauma. *Ann Emerg Med* 2007;49:325–332; 333–334.

Head CT: Patient 4

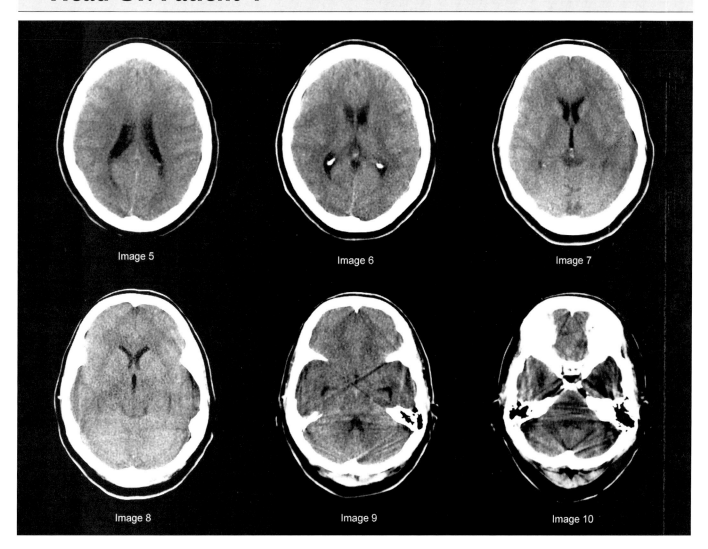

Image 5

Image 6

Image 7

Image 8

Image 9

Image 10

FIGURE 1

An occipital headache and vomiting in a middle-aged woman; head CT was "normal"

A 42-year-old woman presented to the ED with headache and posterior neck pain of one and a half hour's duration. The onset of the headache was sudden and was accompanied by one episode of vomiting.

She had seen a physician two days earlier for neck pain and was told she had a "pinched nerve."

On examination, she was an overweight female in mild distress due to her headache. The patient was fully alert and oriented with no focal neurological deficits. She resisted full flexion of her neck.

A noncontrast head CT was obtained and interpreted as normal (Figure 1).

- What should be done next?

The next day, the official CT reading diagnosed subarachnoid hemorrhage.

- What are the CT findings of subarachnoid hemorrhage on this CT?

HOW BAD IS A HEADACHE

Because the patient's headache had characteristics suspicious for subarachnoid hemorrhage (SAH)—sudden onset, association with vomiting, and mild nuchal rigidity—and because CT can occasionally miss SAH, a lumbar puncture was performed in the ED. The spinal fluid was blood tinged and, after centrifugation, the supernatant fluid had xanthochromia. She was admitted to the hospital for further evaluation of SAH.

Subarachnoid hemorrhage is a potentially life-threatening cause of headache. In 85% of cases, SAH is due to leakage or rupture of an aneurysm at the base of the brain (circle of Willis). The patient classically presents with an abrupt onset of severe headache ("thunder-clap"), which may be accompanied by an altered level of consciousness, seizure, or focal neurological deficits. When there is a large hemorrhage, the gravity of illness is obvious both clinically and on CT.

When a lesser quantity of blood leaks from the aneurysm, the patient may present solely with headache. The clinical and CT findings can be subtle and the diagnosis can potentially be missed. Such misdiagnosis can have devastating consequences when the patient later suffers a massive hemorrhage causing permanent neurological disability or death.

In up to 50% of cases, a small bleed causing a "sentinel" or "warning" headache precedes a large hemorrhage by hours, days, or weeks. Half of these patients may have sought medical attention and may have been misdiagnosed, i.e., up to 25% of SAH are missed on initial presentation (Kowalski 2004, Mayer 1996). Patients with such small bleeds benefit most from prompt diagnosis and treatment because they are neurologically intact at the time of initial presentation and a subsequent major hemorrhage can be prevented.

SAH should therefore always be considered in patients presenting to the ED with headache. Clinical features that are important to consider include the rapidity of onset, severity, and similarities or differences relative to prior headaches. The headache of SAH is typically abrupt in onset or rapidly progresses to maximal intensity over seconds or minutes. It is often associated with nausea, vomiting, and neck stiffness. However, there have not been any prospective studies to determine the clinical features of sentinel headache or to develop criteria that can guide clinical assessment of the likelihood of SAH, although such studies are in progress (Perry 2002, 2003 and 2005).

Noncontrast CT is the imaging study of choice to diagnose SAH. However, the CT findings of a small SAH can be subtle and, in some patients, CT may fail to show signs of SAH. This is particularly true if more than 12–24 hours has elapsed since the onset of headache (CT sensitivity is then as low as 80%). However, a CT scan will occasionally be normal even if performed within 12 hours of headache onset. CT sensitivity is as high as 98% under optimal circumstances, but is more realistically in the range of 95-96%. (van der wee 1995, Perry 2004, Morgenstern 1998, Edlow and Wyer 2000, Schwartz 2002).

Because the consequences of missing a sentinel headache SAH can be so devastating, patients with a normal CT in whom *SAH is suspected* should have a lumbar puncture (LP) to examine the cerebral spinal fluid (CSF) for evidence of hemorrhage (ACEP 1996, Edlow and Caplan 2000). However, clinical criteria defining when SAH should be suspected and when it can be deemed improbable have not been established (Coats 2006, Perry 2006, Pines 2006).

The second noteworthy observation made in the studies of missed SAH is that the most common diagnostic error is not obtaining a CT scan (approximately 75% of cases). In about 15% of cases, CT or LP results are misinterpreted, and in 10% or fewer cases, LP is not performed when the CT is negative (Kowalski 2004, Mayer 1996). Unfortunately, the clinical characteristics of the patients with missed SAH were not investigated, which would be useful information for practicing clinicians. However, it can be concluded that an increased awareness of SAH presenting solely with headache, as well as liberal use of CT is such cases, would avoid many missed cases of SAH.

Finally, in addition to SAH, **other serious causes of headache** must be considered including meningitis, tumors, intracranial hematomas, cerebral venous sinus thrombosis, sinusitis, toxin exposure (e.g., carbon monoxide), and vasculitis (e.g., temporal arthritis).

WHAT ARE THE CT SIGNS OF SUBARACHNOID HEMORRHAGE?

Aneurysmal SAH occurs in the subarachnoid spaces at the base of the brain where the circle of Willis is located. On CT, blood in the basilar cisterns has greater x-ray attenuation (appears whiter) than brain tissue, whereas normal CSF has lower attenuation (appears darker). Because many of the CT findings of SAH involve midline structures, identification of an abnormality cannot rely on comparison of the two sides of the brain. Accurate CT interpretation therefore requires a clear understanding of CT neuroanatomy.

The primary site of SAH is the **suprasellar cistern**—the location of the circle of Willis. The suprasellar cistern is also known as the "pentagonal cistern" because it is shaped like a five-pointed star. From there, blood may spread to the anterior interhemispheric fissure, the Sylvian fissures and then to the cortical sulci on the surface of the cerebral hemispheres (Figures 2–5).

SAH is also often seen on the next superior slice that passes through the **midbrain** (*mesencephalon*). In cross section, the midbrain has a heart-shaped appearance. The "lobes" of the heart are the *cerebral peduncles* and in between the cerebral peduncles is the **interpeduncular cistern**. With a larger bleed, the **perimesencephalic cisterns** are filled with blood, which outlines the entire midbrain (Figure 6).

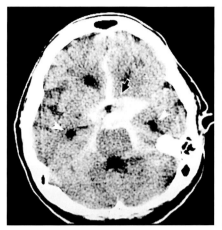

A. SAH in suprasellar cistern

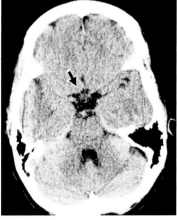

B. Normal suprasellar cistern

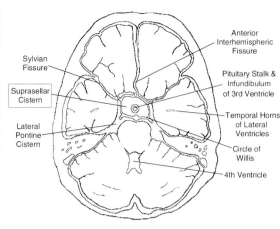

C. Suprasellar cistern anatomy

FIGURE 2   Suprasellar cistern—SAH and normal anatomy.

(*A*) Massive SAH fills the *suprasellar cistern* ("pentagonal cistern") (*black arrow*). Blood extends anteriorly to the anterior interhemispheric fissure, laterally to the left Sylvian fissure, and posteriorly to the lateral pontine cisterns.

In the center of the blood-filled suprasellar cistern is the distended, CSF-containing *infundibulum* of the third ventricle within the pituitary stalk (black). The temporal horns of the lateral ventricles are dilated (*arrowheads*). These findings are indicative of *hydrocephalus*.

(*B*) Normal suprasellar cistern (*arrow*) containing CSF. The temporal horns of the lateral ventricles are barely visible.

(*C*) CT anatomy at the level of the suprasellar cistern (see A–A in Figure 3). (The pituitary stalk is not normally visible).

FIGURE 3   Mid-sagittal section showing orientation of CT slices through the basal cisterns.

(Anatomy described from anterior to posterior.)

(A–A) Frontal lobes, **suprasellar cistern** with pituitary stalk (contains the inferior extent of the infundibulum of 3rd ventricle), pons, fourth ventricle, and cerebellum.

(B–B) Frontal lobes, infundibulum of 3rd ventricle, **interpeduncular cistern,** midbrain, and cerebellum.

FIGURE   4   (left) Contrast CT showing normal vascular enhancement of the major arteries of the circle of Willis (anterior, middle and posterior cerebral arteries) located in the suprasellar cistern.

FIGURE   5   (right) A   "giant" aneurysm (>10mm) at the origin of the left middle cerebral artery (patient shown in Figure 2A).

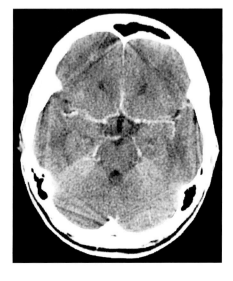

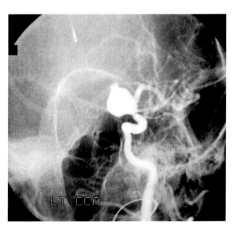

In a **sentinel leak SAH**, only a small quantity of blood enters the CSF and the CT signs of SAH can be subtle (Table 1). SAH may be limited to the anterior interhemispheric fissure, Sylvian fissure, interpeduncular cistern, or prepontine cistern (see Patient 4C below). In some cases, a small amount of blood mixes with CSF and appears *isodense* (gray) rather than white. The presence of SAH can then be inferred only by the absence of CSF (dark) where it should normally be located, i.e., the basilar cisterns are not visible.

To identify SAH on CT, one should first locate the *dorsum sella*, a bony prominence in the midline at the base of the skull (Figure 1, image, 10), and then examine the next superior slice for blood in the basilar cisterns (image 9).

Hydrocephalus

SAH can cause acute hydrocephalus. Blood in the subarachnoid space impedes the flow of CSF in the basilar cisterns and around the cerebral hemispheres, and interfere with CSF resorption as the superior sagittal sinus. This causes **communicating hydrocephalus**, in which all the four ventricles become dilated. Acute communicating hydrocephalus can also be caused by meningitis. Communicating hydrocephalus may also be a chronic finding in patients who have had prior intracranial disorders. Even though hydrocephalus itself is not diagnostic of SAH, it may be the most visible CT sign of SAH.

Although the bodies of the lateral ventricles are enlarged with hydrocephalus, there are no reliable measurements to assess such enlargement. However, a distinctive CT feature of hydrocephalus is dilation of the **temporal horns** of the lateral ventricles. The temporal horns are normally barely visible (Figure 2B). When distended, they have a comma shape or "mustachioed" appearance—the "**Juan Valdez sign**" (Figures 6A, 7A, 8A, and 9).

A second characteristic sign of hydrocephalus is the dilation of the third ventricle, particularly the **infundibulum** (Figure 3). The third ventricle appears rounded rather than slit-like, and the infundibulum that extends towards the pituitary stalk appears as a distinct black circle (containing CSF) that is surrounded by blood (white) in the suprasellar cistern (Figures 2A and 8A).

Intraventricular blood

In some patients, blood in the basilar cisterns refluxes into the ventricles, initially the **fourth ventricle,** then the third and even the lateral ventricles (Figure 8A). This occurs because the slight

TABLE 1

CT Signs of SAH

Blood in the basilar cisterns
    Suprasellar cistern
    Interpeduncular cistern
    Sylvian fissure
    Anterior interhemispheric fissure
    Prepontine cistern
Isodense basilar cisterns
Hydrocephalus
    Temporal horns of lateral ventricles
    Infundibulum of third ventricle
Reflux of blood into fourth ventricle

pressure gradient that normally exists between the fourth ventricle and basilar cisterns is reversed when there is blood in the subarachnoid space.

If a blood clot forms within the ventricles, intraventricular CSF flow can be obstructed, resulting in **noncommunicating hydrocephalus** (obstructive hydrocephalus). Emergency insertion of a ventriculostomy drain might be necessary to prevent transtentorial herniation in such patients (usually massive SAH).

Patient Outcome

In Patient 4, a small amount of subarachnoid blood is present on the CT slice at the level of the midbrain— CT image 9. A small white spot is seen in the **interpeduncular cistern** where there is normally dark CSF (Figure 7). (Note that all slices are 10-mm thick and so the suprasellar cistern is not seen on a single slice.)

Although this patient did not appear to be in acute distress due to her headache, clues to its serious nature were the sudden onset, awakening her from sleep, and the mild nuchal rigidity.

A cerebral angiogram was performed, which showed an irregular narrowing of the supraclinoid internal carotid artery and middle cerebral artery possibly due to spasm or thrombosis of an aneurysm. The patient remained stable. A head CT performed one week later showed complete resolution of the hemorrhage.

An aneurysm is not identified in 15% of patients with SAH. Patients with limited perimesencephalic hemorrhage and negative angiograms have a low risk of rebleeding. The bleeding site is presumably venous or capillary (nonaneurysmal) (Rinkel 1990).

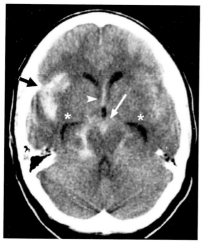

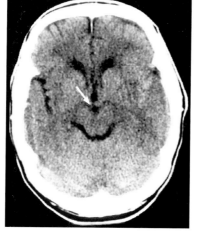

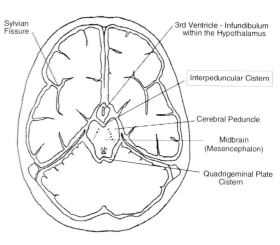

A. SAH in perimesencephalic cisterns   B. Normal interpeduncular cistern   C. Midbrain anatomy

FIGURE 6   Perimesencephalic cisterns and midbrain—SAH and normal anatomy.

(*A*) SAH in the perimesencephalic cisterns surrounding the "heart-shaped" midbrain.

The interpeduncular cistern is filled with blood (*white arrow*). Blood also extends into the *anterior interhemispheric fissure* (*white arrowhead*) and the right *Sylvian fissure* (*black arrow*).

Hydrocephalus causes distension of the *infundibulum of the third ventricle* (black area just anterior to the interpeduncular cistern), and the *temporal horns* of the lateral ventricles (*asterisks*).

(*B*) Normal CT showing the **interpeduncular cistern** containing CSF (*white arrow*).

(*C*) CT anatomy at the level of the midbrain (See B–B in Figure 3).

FIGURE 7   Patient 4—Subtle SAH.

(*A*) **Image 9**—There is minimal SAH in interpeduncular cistern (*arrow*). Just anterior to the interpeduncular cistern is the infundibulum of the third ventricle containing CSF (black) (*open arrowhead*).

Hydrocephalus causes distension of the temporal horns of the lateral ventricles (*arrowheads*).

(*B*) **Image 7**—"Not every white spot in the midline is blood." A normal calcified pineal gland (*arrow*) is located posterior to the third ventricle.

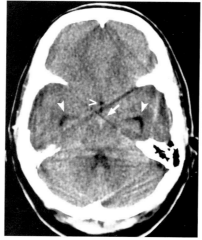

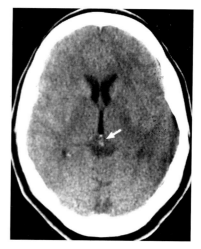

A. Patient 4—CT Image 9   B. Patient 4—CT Image 7

FIGURE 8   Moderate SAH.

(*A*) Blood fills the **suprasellar cistern** (*arrow*) and extends anteriorly and laterally.

Hydrocephalus is present. The infundibulum of the third ventricle is distended (a round black region in the center of the blood-filled suprasellar cistern). The temporal horns of the lateral ventricles are also distended–the "Juan Valdez sign".

Blood has refluxed into the **fourth ventricle** (*arrowhead*). This should not be misinterpreted as a calcified choroid plexus.

(*B*) Right internal carotid angiogram reveals a 4 mm × 8 mm aneurysm at the junction between the middle cerebral artery and posterior communicating artery (*arrow*).

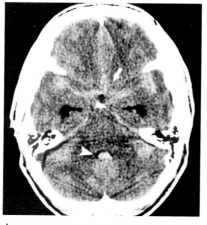

A

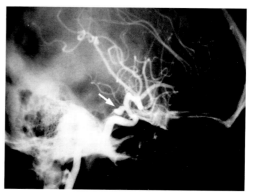

B

Two Additional Patients with SAH whose CT Scans were Initially Interpreted as Normal

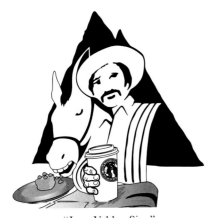

"Juan Valdez Sign"
Mustachioed appearance of the dilated temporal horns of the lateral ventricles.

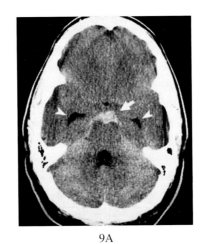

9A

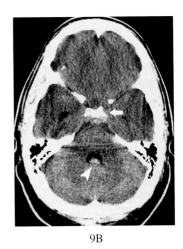

9B

PATIENT 4B A 54-year-old man presented with headache of one day duration. The CT was initially interpreted as negative for SAH. However, a significant quantity of blood is present anterior to the midbrain (Figure 9A, *arrow*). This blood was misinterpreted as bone extending up from the dorsum sella (Figure 9B, *arrow*).

In addition, blood is present in the fourth ventricle (Figure 9B, *arrowhead*). There is mild hydrocephalus—dilated temporal horns of the lateral ventricles, the "Juan Valdez" sign (Figure 9A, *arrowheads*).

After four attempts at lumbar puncture, blood-tinged spinal fluid was obtained. There were 15,000 red cells in the first tube and 10,000 in the fourth. The supernatant fluid was clear and colorless, without xanthochromia. The blood in the CSF was felt to be traumatic. The patient felt better and was discharged home.

The official CT report identified the SAH and the patient was recalled for hospitalization. No aneurysm was found on angiography (nonaneurysmal perimesencephalic SAH).

Three factors contributed to the diagnostic error in this case. First, even though there was a decrement in the CSF red cell count between the first and fourth tubes, the CSF was "persistently bloody" and therefore suggestive of SAH. Second, xanthochromia was assessed by the laboratory by visual inspection and the reliability of this method is questionable. In addition, the absence of xanthochromia does not exclude SAH. Third, accurate CT interpretation and identification of SAH would have avoided the problem of distinguishing between a traumatic tap and SAH by making CSF examination unnecessary.

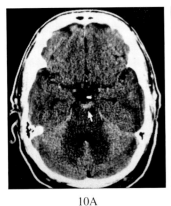

10A

10B

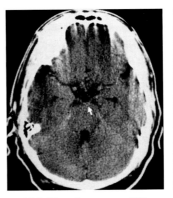

10C Next day, repeat CT

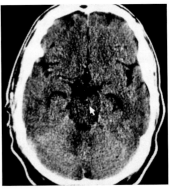

10D Next day, repeat CT

PATIENT 4C A 58-year-old man presented with intermittent headaches for 4 days. He vomited once on the day of presentation to the ED.

The CT was initially interpreted as negative. The patient felt well. He was discharged home and was referred to a neurologist.

The official CT interpretation the next day noted blood in the prepontine cistern (Figure 10A, *arrow*) and interpeduncular cistern

(Figure 10B, *arrow*). There is mild hydrocephalus with distention of the temporal horns of the lateral ventricles.

The patient was recalled to the ED the next day. A repeat CT showed resolution of the prepontine and interpeduncular blood (Figures 10C and D, *arrows*). MRI confirmed the presence of subacute blood in the prepontine cistern. Cerebral angiography did not show an aneurysm.

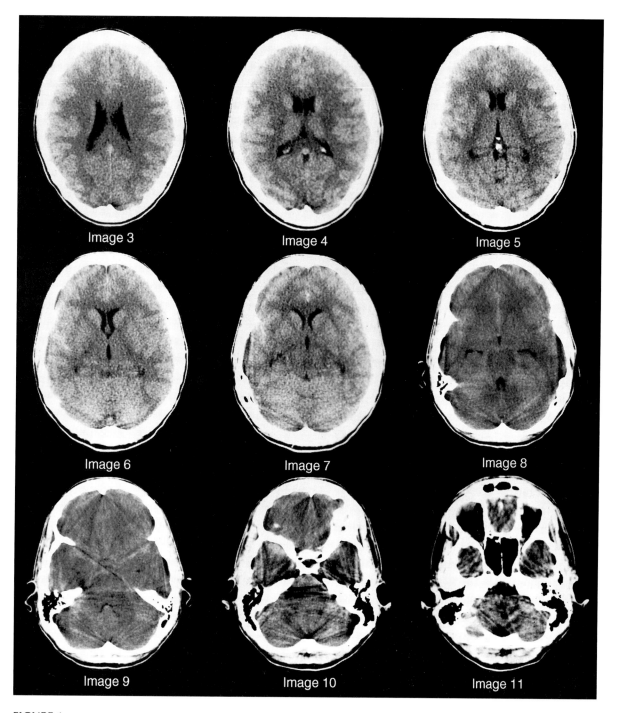

Image 3   Image 4   Image 5

Image 6   Image 7   Image 8

Image 9   Image 10   Image 11

FIGURE 1

PATIENT 4D A 30-year-old elementary school teacher presented with a frontal headache and photophobia.

She had a history of "migraine" headaches for 1 year, but had not seen a doctor for this. For the past 2 days, she had a persistent headache. The headache became worse that morning. She described it as "pulsating." It began in the right frontal region, then spread to the right side of the head, and then became diffuse. She vomited once. She had a history of panic attacks for which she was taking paroxetine.

A head CT was performed and was interpreted as normal. The patient was discharged on analgesic medications.

The following day the CT was read by the attending radiologist as showing SAH. The patient was recalled to the hospital.

• Which signs of SAH are present on the CT scan?

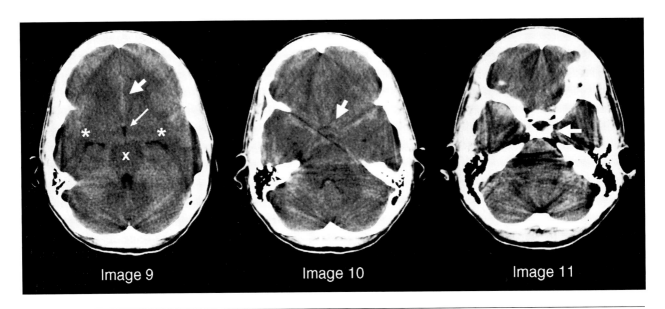

Image 9   Image 10   Image 11

FIGURE 12   Patient 3D—Isodense subarachnoid blood in the suprasellar cistern.

HOW TO READ A HEAD CT IN A PATIENT SUSPECTED OF HAVING SAH

First, look for blood in the basilar cisterns. Then, examine the ventricles for signs of hydrocephalus or intraventricular blood.

1. Locate the **basilar cisterns** by identifying the **dorsum sella,** a bony prominence in the midline at the base of the skull (*arrow*, **image 11**). Then examine the next superior slice for evidence of blood in the basilar cisterns (**image 10**).

   The **suprasellar cistern** in located in the center of **image 10** (just superior to the dorsum sella in image 11). Normally, the suprasellar cistern is filled with CSF (dark) and looks like a five-pointed star (pentagonal cistern) (see Figure 2B).

   In this patient, the suprasellar cistern is barely visible because it is filled with a mixture of blood and CSF that is attenuating to brain (*arrow*). Blood that is slightly hyperattenuating (white) is seen extending laterally into the Sylvian fissures and lateral pontine cisterns, although this is partly obscured by streak artifacts emanating from thick ridges of the skull is base.

   In the next superior slice (**image 9**), the heart-shaped midbrain (**X**) is surrounded by slightly hyperattenvating blood in the perimesencephalic cisterns rather than normally hypoattenuating (dark) CSF (see Figures 6 and 7A). Blood in the anterior interhemispheric fissure appears white (*large arrow*), which lies just anterior to the CSF-filled (dark) infundibulum of the third ventricle (*long arrow*).

2. **Hydrocephalus** is often seen in patients with SAH. Dilation of the temporal horns of the lateral ventricles and the third ventricle, particularly the infundibulum are most readily recognized. In this patient, the temporal horns are slightly dilated (*asterisks*) having a mustachioed appearance ("Juan Valdez sign").

3. Look for **intraventricular blood**, particularly in the fourth ventricle, for evidence of blood that has refluxed from the subarachnoid spaces (see Figures 8A and 9B).

Patient Outcome

When the patient returned to the ED, she was alert and oriented and complained of a persistent headache. There was slight nuchal rigidity and minimal (1 mm) anisocoria (right > left). A repeat head CT showed disappearance of the SAH.

A cerebral angiogram revealed a 3 mm by 7 mm aneurysm of the right posterior communicating artery (possibly accounting for the slight dilatation of the patient's right pupil). The patient underwent aneurysm surgery and made an uneventful recovery.

WHY IS IT IMPORTANT TO DETECT SUBTLE SIGNS OF SAH ON CT?

Although it could be argued that accurate CT interpretation is of secondary importance because patients with normal CT scans will undergo a lumbar puncture, identification of subtle signs of SAH is important for **three reasons.**

First, in some patients LP is *not* performed when the CT is normal—as many as 40–50% of patients in current series (Perry 2002 and 2005, Schofield 2004, Morgenstern 1998). In these cases, CT misinterpretation would lead to misdiagnosis of SAH. In one recent series, misinterpretation of CT accounted for 11% of missed SAH (Mayer 1996). In another series, CT (or LP) misinterpretation accounted for 16% of missed cases (Kowalski 2004). (Failure to perform CT was the most common reason SAH was missed—in 73% of cases, and failure to perform LP when the CT was normal accounted for 7% of missed cases.)

Second, even when patients do routinely undergo LP when the CT is normal, interpretation of LP results can be problematic when there is a "traumatic tap." Traumatic taps occur in 15% of LPs (Shah 2002 abstract), and blood due to a traumatic LP can be difficult or impossible to distinguish from SAH. Accurate CT interpretation will reduce the number of times that LP is needed to diagnose SAH and the attendant difficulties interpreting traumatic spinal taps (Schwartz 2002).

Various criteria have been proposed to differentiate blood due to a **traumatic tap** from SAH, but none are well-established or foolproof (Shah 2002). For example, Van der Wee uses the presence of xanthochromia measured *spectrophotometrically* and mandates that the LP be performed at least 12 hours after symptom onset to allow for development of xanthochromia. Although logical, this strategy is impractical in emergency practice. Furthermore, *visual inspection* in used in nearly all hospitals to assess xanthochromia, even though it is less sensitive than spectrophotometry. Morgenstern's criteria for SAH are an RBC count of more than 1,000 cells/mm^3 with a decrement of less than 25% from the first and to the last tubes, *and* the presence of xanthochromia by visual inspection. Morgenstern and others have found that spectrophotometric measurement of xanthochromia gave occasional false-positive results (Graves 2004, Perry 2005 abstract).

In their review, Edlow and Caplan (2000) state that LP should *not* be delayed 12 hours in patients with suspected SAH and that "patients with persistently bloody CSF without xanthochromia should undergo vascular imaging when the level of clinical suspicion of SAH is high." Although these are reasonable conclusions given the available evidence, the terms "persistently bloody" and "high clinical suspicion" are not precisely defined.

The problem of misinterpreting a traumatic tap is significant for two reasons. First, if there is a concurrent traumatic tap and SAH, the bloody CSF could be mistakenly attributed solely to trauma (since there is a decrement in RBC count) and the diagnosis of SAH would be erroneously excluded (see Patient 3B). Second, if bloody CSF is mistakenly interpreted as due to SAH rather than a traumatic tap, the patient will require one or more cerebral angiograms to search for a cerebral aneurysm—an invasive procedure with potential morbidity. Noninvasive imaging studies such as magnetic resonance angiography and CT angiography cannot reliably exclude aneurysms smaller than 5 mm (Ellegala 2005, Jayaraman 2004). Although infrequent, such errors could become comparatively common when patients at very low risk of SAH are undergoing LP (Pines 2006).

Third, accurate CT interpretation is important to reliably detect other serious disorders that cause headache such as intracranial masses or hematomas, arteriovenous malformations, sphenoid sinusitis, and cerebral venous sinus thrombosis.

SUGGESTED READING

Coats TJ, Lofthagen R: Diagnosis of subarachnoid haemorrhage following a negative computed tomography for acute headache: A Bayesian analysis. *Europ J Emerg Med* 2006;13:80-83.

Davenport R: Acute headache in the Emergency Department. *J Neurol Neurosurg Psychiatry* 2002; 72 (suppl II): ii33–37.

Edlow JA: Diagnosis of subarachnoid hemorrhage in the emergency department. *Emerg Med Clin North Am* 2003;21:73–87.

Edlow J, Caplan L: Pitfalls in the diagnosis of subarachnoid hemorrhage. *New Engl J Med* 2000;342:29–36.

Van Gijn J, Kerr RS, Rinkel GJ: Subarachnoid hacmorrhage. *Lancet* 2007;369(9558):306–318.

Van Gijn J, Rinkel GJ. Subarachnoid haemorrhage: Diagnosis, causes and management. *Brain* 2001;124: 249–278.

CT for SAH
Adams HP, Kassell NF, Torner JC, Sahs AL: CT and clinical correlations in recent aneurysmal subarachnoid hemorrhage: A preliminary report of the Cooperative Aneurysm Study. *Neurology* 1983; 33:981-988.

Boesiger BM, Shiber JR: Subarachnoid hemorrhage diagnosis by computed tomography and lumbar puncture: Are fifth generation CT scanners better at identifying subarachnoid hemorrhage? *J Emerg Med* 2005; 29:23-27. (100% sensitive, but only 5 cases of SAH included; meaninglessly wide confidence intervals).

Edlow JA, Wyer PC: How good is a negative cranial computed topographic scan result in excluding subarachnoid hemorrhage? *Ann Emerg Med* 2000;36:507–516.

Given CA, Burdette JH, Elster AD, Williams DW: Pseudo-subarachnoid hemorrhage: a potential imaging pitfall associated with diffuse cerebral edema. *AJNR* 2003; 24: 254–256.

Hoffman JR: Computed tomography for subarachnoid hemorrhage: What should we make of the evidence. *Ann Emerg Med* 2001;37;345-349.

Prosser RL, Edlow JA, Wyer PC. Feedback: Computed tomography for subarachnoid hemorrhage. *Ann Emerg Med* 2001;37:679-685.

O'Neill J, McLaggan S, Gibson R: Acute headache and subarachnoid haemorrhage: A retrospective review of CT and lumbar puncture findings. *Scott Med J* 2005;50:151-153.

Morgenstern LB, Luna-Gonzales H, Huber JC, et al: Worst headache and subarachnoid hemorrhage: Prospective, modern computed tomography and spinal fluid analysis. *Ann Emerg Med* 1998; 32: 297–304.

Perry JJ, Stiell IG, Wells GA, et al: The sensitivity of computed tomography for the diagnosis of subarachnoid hemorrhage in ED patients with acute headache (abstract). *Acad Emerg Med* 2004;11: 435–436.

Sames, TA, Storrow AB, Finkelstein JA, et al: Sensitivity of new-generation computed tomography in subarachnoid hemorrhage. *Acad Emerg Med* 1996;3:16-20.

Schwartz DT: Computed tomography and lumbar puncture for diagnosis of subarachnoid hemorrhage: The importance of accurate interpretation. *Ann Emerg Med* 2002;39:190–192.

Sidman R, Connolly E, Lemke T: Subarachnoid hemorrhage diagnosis: lumbar puncture is still needed when the computed tomography scan is normal. *Acad Emerg Med* 1996;3:827-31.

Singal BM: A tap in time? (editorial) *Acad Emerg Med* 1996;3:823.

Van der Wee N, Rinkel GJE, Hasan D, van Gijn J: Detection of subarachnoid hemorrhage on early CT: is lumbar puncture still needed after a negative scan ? *J Neurol Neurosurg Psychiatr* 1995;58: 357–359.

Clinical criteria for SAH

American College of Emergency Physicians. Clinical policy on the initial approach to adolescents and adults presenting to the emergency department with a chief complaint of headache. *Ann Emerg Med* 1996;27:821–44.

American College of Emergency Physicians. Clinical policy: Critical issues in the evaluation and management of patients presenting to the emergency department with acute headache. *Ann Emerg Med* 2002;39:108-122.

Leblanc R: The minor leak preceding subarachnoid hemorrhage. *J Neurosurg* 1987;66:35-39.

Linn FH, Rinkel GJ, Algra A, et al: The notion of "warning leaks" in subarachnoid haemorrhage: are such patients in fact admitted with a rebleed? *J Neurol Neurosurg Psychiatry* 2000;68:332-6.

Linn FH, Rinkel GJ, Algra A, et al: Headache characteristics in subarachnoid haemorrhage and benign thunderclap headache. *J Neurol Neurosurg Psychiatry* 1998;65:791-3.

Linn FH, Wijdicks EF: Causes and management of thunderclap headache: a comprehensive review. *Neurologist.* 2002;8:279-89.

Linn FH, Wijdicks EF, van der Graaf Y, et al: Prospective study of sentinel headaches in aneurysmal subarachnoid hemorrhage. *Lancet* 1994; 344:590-593. 12 of 103 patients with sudden severe headache had SAH.

Perry JJ, Stiell IG, Wells GA, et al: Clinical decision rule for emergency department patients with acute headache (abstract). *Acad Emerg Med* 2002; 9: 360–361.

Perry JJ, Stiell IG, Wells GA, et al: The value of history in the diagnosis of subarachnoid hemorrhage for emergency department patients with acute headache (abstract). *Acad Emerg Med* 2003;10:553.

Perry JJ, Stiell IG, Wells GA: Attitudes and judgment of emergency physicians in the management of patients with acute headache. *Acad Emerg Med* 2005;12:33–37.

Perry JJ, Stiell IG, Wells GA, et al: A clinical decision rule to safely rule out subarachnoid hemorrhage in acute headache patients in the emergency department (abstract). *Acad Emerg Med* 2006;13:S9.

Perry JJ, Stiell IG, Wells GA, et al: Interobserver agreement in the assessment of headache patients with possible subarachnoid hemorrhage (abstract). *Acad Emerg Med* 2006;13:s138.

Perry JJ, Stiell IG, Wells GA, et al: Arrival in the emergency department by ambulance for headache: a marker of high risk for subarachnoid hemorrhage (abstract). *Acad Emerg Med* 2006;13:s138-s139.

Misdiagnosis of SAH

Kowalski RG, Claassen J, Kreiter KT, et al: Initial misdiagnosis and outcome after subarachnoid hemorrhage. *JAMA* 2004;291: 866–869.

Mayer PL, Awad IA, Todor R, et al: Misdiagnosis of symptomatic cerebral aneurysm: Prevalence and correlation with outcome at four institutions. *Stroke* 1996;27:1558–1563.

Papadatos A: Expert witness: Headache with upper respiratory symptoms. *Emerg Med News,* Feb. 2005, pp. 30, 35.

Seymour JJ, Moscati RM, Jehle DV: Response of headaches to non-narcotic analgesics resulting in missed intracranial hemorrhage. *Am J Emerg Med* 1995;13:43-45. (3 cases; all has severe headache and other worrisome symptoms)

LP and CSF examination for SAH

Foot C, Merfield E: Suspected subarachnoid haemorrhage with a negative CT head scan: What next? *Emergency Medicine (Australasia)* 2000;12:212–217.

Graves P, Sidman R: Xanthochromia is not pathognomonic for subarachnoid hemorrhage. *Acad Emerg Med* 2004;11:131–135.

Perry JJ, Sivilotti M, Stiell IG, et al. Should spectrophotometry be used to diagnose xanthochromia in the cerebrospinal fluid of alert patients suspected of having subarachnoid hemorrhage? *Acad Emerg Med* 2005;12(5):s173.

Pines JM: A cost-utility analysis for evaluating low-risk suspected subarachnoid hemorrhage: Is lumbar puncture always needed? (abstract) *Acad Emerg Med* 2006;13:S17-S18

Pines JM, Szyld D: Risk tolerance for the exclusion of potentially life-threatening diseases in the ED. *Am J Emerg Med* 2007;25:540-544.

Schofield MLA, Lorenz E, Hodgson TJ, Yates S, Griffiths PD: How well do we investigate patients with suspected subarachnoid hemorrhage? The continuing need for cerebrospinal investigations. *Post Grad Med* 2004;80:27–30.

Shah KH, Edlow JA: Distinguishing traumatic lumbar puncture from true subarachnoid hemorrhage. J Emerg Med 2002; 23:68-73.

Shah KH, Richard KM, Nicholas S, Edlow JA: Incidence of traumatic lumbar puncture. *Acad Emerg Med* 2002;9:410.

Aneurysm diagnosis

Ellegala DB, Day AL: Ruptured cerebral aneurysms. *N Engl J Med* 2005;352: 121–124.

Jayaraman MV, Mayo-Smith WW, Tung GA, et al: Detection of intracranial aneurysms: Multi-detector row CT angiography compared with DSA. *Radiology* 2004;230;510–518. (CT sensitivity only 90%).

Tomandl BF, Kostner NC, Schempershofe M, et al: CT angiography of intracranial aneurysms: A focus on postprocessing. *RadioGraphics* 2004;24:637-655.

Nonaneurysmal SAH

Rinkel GJE, Wijdicks EFM, Vermeulen M, et al: Outcome in perimesencephalic (nonaneurysmal) subarachnoid hemorrhage: a follow-up study in 37 patients. *Neurology* 1990;40:1130–1132.

Van Gijn J, van Dongen KJ, Vermeulen M, Hijdra A: Perimesencephalic hemorrhage: a nonaneurysmanl and benign from of subarachnoid hemorrhage. *Neurology* 1985;35:493–497.

Head CT: Patient 5

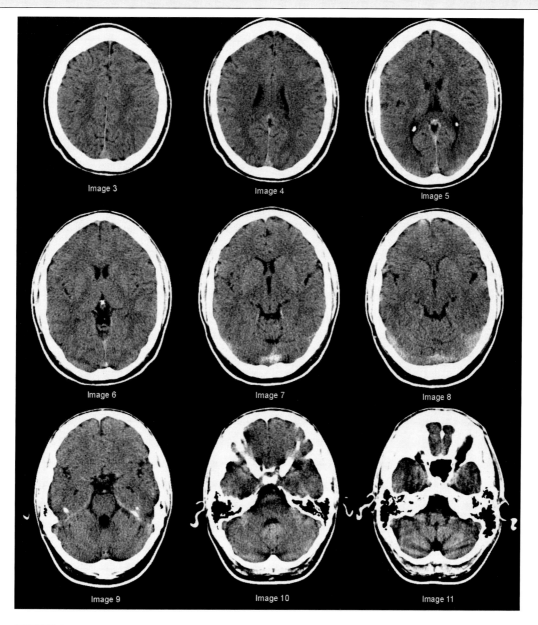

Image 3   Image 4   Image 5
Image 6   Image 7   Image 8
Image 9   Image 10   Image 11

FIGURE 1

Persistent headache for five days in a young man

A 24-year-old man presented with a persistent headache of 5 day's duration. It had increased in severity several hours before coming to the ED. The headache was relatively constant and had intermittent exacerbations. It was bitemporal, but worse on the right than left. At the time of his initial evaluation, the pain was rated 5/10 in severity. He had taken 800 mg of ibuprofen with partial relief.

There was no associated fever, sinus congestion, neck stiffness, or visual or focal neurological symptoms. There was no family history of migraine or other headache disorder. The patient had begun his third year of law school 3 weeks earlier.

He had no significant past medical history. He had not recently traveled outside of New York City and had no history of head trauma.

His physical examination was essentially normal, including vital signs, head, neck, and neurological examinations. There was no nuchal rigidity.

A head CT was obtained (Figure 1).

- Are there any abnormalities?

(Had an LP been performed, the CSF cell count and chemistries would have been normal.)

CEREBRAL DVT

Examination of a head CT in a patient with headache begins by looking for symmetry and midline shift. Next, the basilar cisterns are examined for evidence of SAH. Ventricular size and shape are assessed; ventricular enlargement may be a sign of hydrocephalus. Finally, several serious disorders can produce other, sometimes subtle, CT findings should be sought.

On this patient's head CT, there is no midline shift, mass effect, or asymmetry. The basilar cisterns and ventricles are normal. On image 7 (Figure 2A), there is a small hyperattenuating region (white) in the posterior midline. This represents clotted blood. However, rather than being an extra-axial hematoma, it represents clotted blood within a cerebral venous sinus. It is located at the confluence of the superior sagittal sinus and transverse sinuses (the *torcula*) (Figure 3). On image 8 (Figure 2B), there is diffuse hyperattenuation in the region of the transverse sinuses. These findings are due to cerebral venous sinus thrombosis.

The **clinical presentation** of **cerebral venous sinus thrombosis (CVST)** can range from isolated headache to stroke and seizure. Strokes and seizures are due to venous hemorrhagic infarction. However, the greatest diagnostic difficulty occurs in patients who present solely with headache. The **headache** is typically severe and persistent, although it may have an abrupt onset mimicking SAH ("thunderclap"). Many, but not all, patients have risk factors for venous thrombosis—a hypercoagulable state (e.g., familial thrombophilia, postpartum, lupus anticoagulant), local trauma, or infection (e.g., mastoiditis) (Bousser and Ferro 2007).

Noncontrast CT may show a hyperattenuating (thrombosed) venous sinus such as the superior sagittal sinus, transverse sinus, or straight sinus. In one series, noncontrast CT showed a **hyperattenuating venous sinus** (also referred to as "hyperdense" venous sinus) in 60% of patients with CVST who presented solely with headache (Cumurciuc 2005). However, in a number of recently published case reports, noncontrast CT did show hyperattenuating venous sinuses (Barrett 2005, Khandelwal 2004). Noncontrast CT can therefore play an important role in the diagnosis of CSVT when hyperdense venous sinuses are seen in a patient with headache (Figure 2).

One difficulty in using non-contrast CT for the diagnosis of CVST is that in some normal individuals, the cerebral venous sinuses are mildly hyperattenuating and asymmetrical (Figure 4). Nonetheless, in a patient with headache, hyperattenuating venous sinuses should prompt investigation for CVST. Finally, a normal CT does not exclude CVST and the diagnosis should be pursued with additional imaging whenever CVST is suspected (e.g., the patient has risk factors for CVST).

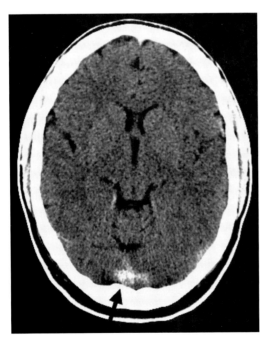

A. CT Image 7

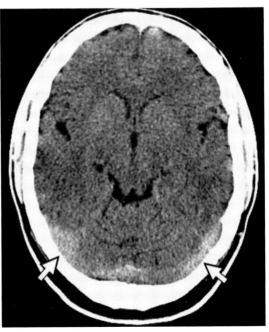

B. CT Image 8

FIGURE 2   Patient 5—Noncontrast CT images 7 and 8
Noncontrast CT shows a hyperattenuating (thrombosed) superior sagittal sinus (*arrow*, A) and slightly hyperattenuating transverse sinuses (*arrows*, B).

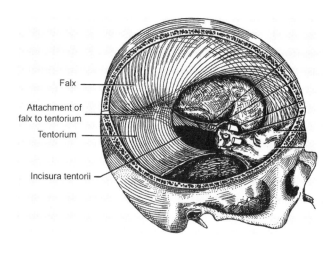

3A. Falx and tentorium—location within the skull

3B. Cerebral venous sinuses in relation to falx and tentorium

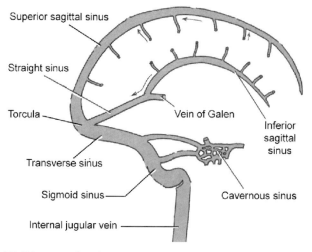

3C. Diagram of major cerebral venous sinuses (the transverse sinus, sigmoid sinus and internal jugular vein are bilateral)

3D. Base of skull showing location of cerebral venous sinuses

FIGURE 3   Anatomy of the cerebral venous sinuses.

[From Pansky B: *Review of Gross Anatomy*, 6th ed. McGraw-Hill, 1996, with permission.]

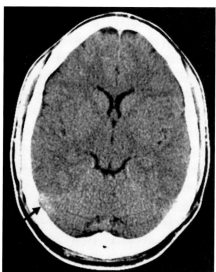

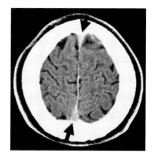

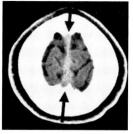

B and C. Normal superior sagittal sinus (*arrows*)

FIGURE 4   Normal cerebral venous sinuses.

In some individuals, the cerebral venous sinuses are normally mildly hyperattenuating (*arrows*). This contributes to the difficulty in discriminating the noncontrast CT signs of cerebral venous sinus thrombosis. Nonetheless, in a patient with headache, hyperattenuating venous sinuses should prompt an investigation for cerebral venous sinus thrombosis.

(*A*) The transverse sinus is located in the regions where the tentorium inserts on the occipital region of the skull (*arrow*).

(*B* and *C*) The superior sagittal sinus is seen on the most superior CT slices (*arrows*).

A. Normal transverse sinus with slightly increased attenuation

Definitive diagnosis of CVST is made using contrast CT or MRI. **Contrast CT** shows a filling defect in a venous sinus—the "empty delta sign" (Figure 5 and 6). A specialized contrast CT protocol, **CT venography,** has higher sensitivity at detecting CVST and is easier to interpret. Timing of the scan is optimized for maximal venous sinus enhancement after the contrast bolus and thin sections (1 to 1.5 mm) are acquired. Sagittal and coronal reformated images can be made from these data. This is best accomplished using a multidetector CT scanner.

Standard **MRI** sequences (T1-weighted and T2-weighted) can miss venous sinus thrombosis, and so **MR venography** should be obtained. These are displayed as three-dimensional (3D) images (Figure 7). Both CT and MR venography are highly accurate for the diagnosis of CVST, and represent improvements over standard contrast CT or MRI. However, large studies of these new technologies have yet to be performed (Khandelwal et at. 2006, Smith and Hourihan 2006, Leach et al. 2006, Rodallec et al. 2006, Brousser and Ferro 2007).

If a **lumbar puncture** is performed in a patient with headache who has CVST, there may be an *isolated elevated opening pressure* (no other CSF abnormality). Opening pressure should therefore be measured when performing LP on a patient with headache. Intracranial hypertension is due to diminished CSF resorption in the superior sagittal sinus. It occurs when there is extensive superior sagittal sinus thrombosis.

The finding of an isolated elevated opening pressure is also seen in **idiopathic intracranial hypertension** (formerly known as *pseudotumor cerebri* or *benign intracranial hypertension*). Therefore, cerebral venous sinus thrombosis (could be termed "pseudo-pseudotumor cerebri") must be excluded before making a definite diagnosis of idiopathic intracranial hypertension (Khandelwal 2004). Both disorders are often, although not always, associated with papilledema. Treatment and potential complications, however, differ substantially.

Treatment of CVST consists of anticoagulation. This is true even in patients who have developed hemorrhagic infarction

(see Patient 5B) (Williams 2004). Although CVST had been considered a rare disorder with poor prognosis, recent investigations have revealed that it is more common than previously believed and, when properly treated, can have a better outcome.

CVST should be suspected in patients with headache who have risk factors for cerebral thrombosis (hypercoagulability), in patients with headache and papilledema, when LP reveals an elevated opening pressure but otherwise normal CSF, or with hyperattenuating cerebral venous sinuses on noncontrast CT.

Patient Outcome

In this patient, the CT finding of a hyperattenuating venous sinus was recognized, although the radiologist noted that this might be a normal finding (Figure 5). To confirm the diagnosis, a contrast CT was performed using thin-section technique with an intravenous contrast bolus timed to maximize cerebral venous sinus opacification. The axial images demonstrated the "empty delta sign" (Figure 6A).

Sagittal and coronal reformatted images clearly demonstrate the extent of thrombosis. In this patient, thrombosis was limited to the confluence of the superior sagittal sinus and transverse sinuses and the posterior portion of the superior sagittal sinus (Figure 6B and C). Further confirmation of the diagnosis was obtained using MRI with MRV sequences displayed as 3-D reformatted images (Figure 7).

The patient was started on heparin anticoagulation and discharged from the hospital several days later on oral coumadin. Investigation for a hypercoagulable predisposition revealed *methylene tetrahydrofolate reductase deficiency*, a familial disorder causing hyperhomocysteinemia (usually mild) that is associated with accelerated atherosclerosis and recurrent arterial and venous thromboses (Welch 1998).

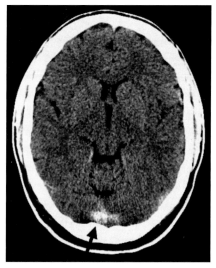

5A. Noncontrast CT, image 7

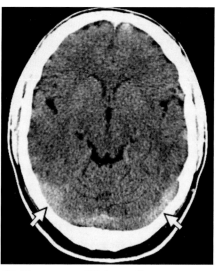

5B. Noncontrast CT, image 8

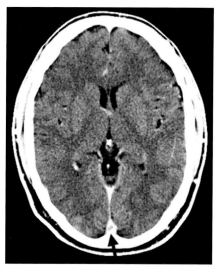

6A. Contrast CT

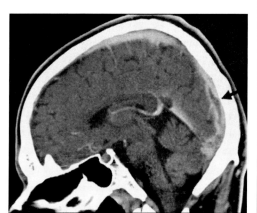

6B. Contrast CT—Mid-sagittal section

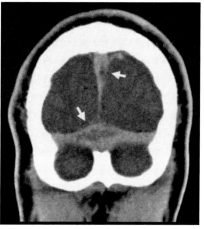

6C. Contrast CT—Coronal section (posterior slice)

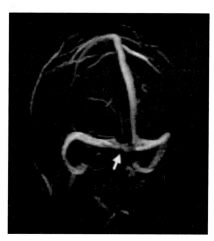

7. MRV 3D image (left-posterior view)

Cerebral venous sinus thrombosis—Patient 5.

FIGURE 5   Noncontrast CT shows a hyperattenuating (thrombosed) superior sagittal sinus (*arrow, A*) and slightly hyperattenuating transverse sinuses (*arrows, B*).

FIGURE 6   (*A*) Contrast CT reveals a "filling defect" (thrombus) within the superior sagittal sinus —the **"empty delta sign"** (*arrow*).

FIGURE 6   (B and C) Sagittal and coronal reformatted MDCT images demonstrate thrombosis at the confluence of the superior sagittal sinus and transverse sinuses (*arrows*).

FIGURE 7   MR venography 3D image (posterior view) shows thrombosis of the transverse sinus near its confluence with the superior sagittal sinus (*arrow*).

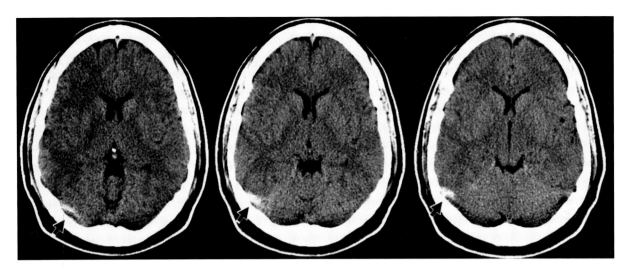

FIGURE 8   Patient 4B—Initial noncontrast CT showing hyperattenuation of the right transverse sinus (*arrows*).

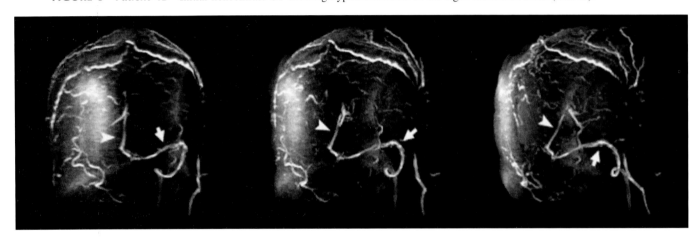

FIGURE 9   MR venography shows an absence of signal (thrombosis) of the superior sagittal, right transverse and sigmoid sinuses, and internal jugular vein. Signal is present only in the straight sinus (*arrowheads*), left transverse and sigmoid sinuses (*arrows*) and left internal jugular vein. The scalp veins are distended due to increased transosseous collateral blood flow.

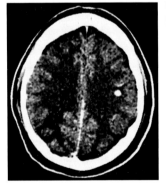 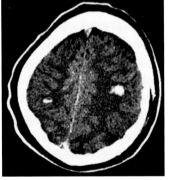

FIGURE 10   Noncontrast CT on days 2 and 3 showing subcortical white matter hemorrhage due to venous infarction.

PATIENT 5B   A 28-year-old man presented with a persistent headache of 3 week's duration that increased on the day of admission. The physical examination was normal.

Head CT showed hyperattenuation in the region of the right transverse sinus (Figure 8). However, this was interpreted as a "normal variant." LP revealed 25 red blood cells without xanthochromia, which was interpreted as a traumatic tap. CSF protein and glucose were normal. Opening pressure was not measured.

MRI/MRV obtained the next day revealed extensive thrombosis of the superior sagittal sinus and right transverse and sigmoid sinuses (Figure 9). Shortly after the MRI, the patient had a generalized seizure and developed a right hemiparesis and aphasia. A head CT then revealed several small parenchymal hemorrhages in the subcortical white matter (Figure 10). MRI showed corresponding areas of infarction with hemorrhage consistent with venous infarction.

The patient was treated with anticoagulant and anticonvulsant medications. His aphasia eventually resolved and the strength of his right arm and leg improved. No conditions predisposing to thrombosis were found on further testing.

SUGGESTED READING

Clinical Features

Agostoni E: Headache in cerebral venous thrombosis. *Neurol Sci* 2004;25 Suppl 3:S206–S210.

Allroggen H, Abbott RJ: Cerebral venous sinus thrombosis. *Postgrad Med J* 2000;76:12–15.

Barrett J, Alves E: Postpartum cerebral venous sinus thrombosis after dural puncture and epidural blood patch. *J Emerg Med* 2005;283:41–342.

Beeson MS, JA Vesco, Reilly BA, Little KJ: Dural sinus thrombosis. *Am J Emerg Med* 2002;20:568–569.

Bousser MG: Cerebral venous thrombosis: Diagnosis and management. *J Neurol* 2000;247:252–258.

Bousser MG, Ferro JM: Cerebral venous thrombosis: An update. *Lancet Neurology* 2007;6:162–170.

Bretatau G: Cerebral venous thrombosis: 3-year clinical outcome in 55 consecutive patients. *J Neurol* 2003;250:29–35.

Cumurciuc R, Crassard I, Sarov M, Valade D, Bousser MG. Headache as the only neurological sign of cerebral venous thrombosis: a series of 17 cases. *J Neurol Neurosurg Psychiatry* 2005;76:1084–1087.

de Bruijn S, de Haan RJ, Stam J: Clinical features and prognostic factors of cerebral venous sinus thrombosis in a prospective series of 59 patients. *J Neurol Neurosurg Psychiatry* 2001;70:105–108.

de Bruijn SF, Stam J, Kappelle LJ. Thunderclap headache as first symptom of cerebral venous sinus thrombosis. *Lancet* 1996;348: 1623–1625.

Diener HC: Cerebral venous thrombosis: Headache is enough. *J Neurol Neurosurg Psychiatry* 2005;76:1043.

Ferro JM, Canhao P, Stam J, Bousser MG, Barinagarrementeria F: Prognosis of cerebral vein and dural sinus thrombosis: Results of the International Study on Cerebral Vein and Dural Sinus Thrombosis (ISCVT). *Stroke* 2004;35:664–670. www.ISCVT.com

Kimber J: Cerebral venous sinus thrombosis. *QJM* 2002;95:137–142.

Masuhr F, Mehraein S, Einhaupl K: Cerebral venous and sinus thrombosis. *J Neurol* 2004;251:11–23

Quattrone A, Bono F, Oliveri RL, et al: Cerebral venous thrombosis and isolated intracranial hypertension without papilledema in CDH (chronic daily headache). *Neurology* 2001;57:31–36.

Stam J: Thrombosis of the cerebral veins and sinuses. *New Engl J Med* 2005;352:1791–1798.

van Gijn J: Cerebral venous thrombosis: Pathogenesis, presentation and prognosis. *J R Soc Med* 2000;93:230–233.

Williams DT, Sue MW, Gabriel EA, Liu AK: Cerebral venous thrombosis: Hemorrhagic stroke requiring acute heparin anticoagulation. *J Emerg Med* 2004;27:295–297.

Hoffman JR: Correspondence. *J Emerg Med* 2006;31:111–113.

Idiopathic intracranial hypertension (pseudo-tumor cerebri)

Biousse V, Ameri A, Bousser M. Isolated intracranial hypertension as the only sign of cerebral venous thrombosis. *Neurology* 1999;53: 1537–1542.

Evans RW, Dulli D: Pseudo-pseudotumor cerebri. *Headache* 2001;41:416–418.

Higgins JN, Gillard JH, Owler BK, Harkness K, Pickard JD. MR venography in idiopathic intracranial hypertension: unappreciated and misunderstood. *J Neurol Neurosurg Psychiatry* 2004;75: 621–625.

Khandelwal S, Miller CD: Distinguishing dural sinus thrombosis from benign intracranial hypertension. *Emerg Med J* 2004;21:245–247.

Leker R, Steiner I: Features of dural sinus thrombosis simulating pseudotumor cerebri. *Eur J Neurol* 1999;6:601–604.

Imaging in CVST

Cwinn AA, Grahovac SZ: *Emergency CT Scans of the Head*. Mosby, 1998, pp. 81–83 and 181–184.

Fink JN, McAuley DL: Mastoid air sinus abnormalities associated with lateral venous sinus thrombosis: Cause or consequence? *Stroke* 2002;33:290–292.

Khandelwal N, Agarwal A, Kochhar R, et al: Comparison of CT venography with MR venography in cerebral sinovenous thrombosis. *AJR* 2006;187:1637–1643.

Leach JL, Fortuna RB, Jones BV, Gaskill-Shipley MF: Imaging of cerebral venous thrombosis: Current techniques, spectrum of findings and diagnostic pitfalls. *RadioGraphics* 2006;26:S19–S43.

Lee EJY: The empty delta sign. *Radiology* 2002;224 788–789.

Lee SK, ter Brugge K: Cerebral vein thrombosis in adults: The role of imaging in evaluation and management. *Neuroimag Clin North Am* 2003;13:139–152.

Provenzale JM: CT and MR imaging and nontraumatic neurologic emergencies. *AJR* 2000;174::289–299.

Provenzale JM: Nontraumatic neurologic emergencies: Imaging findings and diagnostic pitfalls. *Radiographics* 1999;19:1323–1331.

Rodallec MH, Krainik A, Feydy A, et al: Cerebral venous thrombosis and multidetector CT angiography: Tips and tricks. *RadioGraphics* 2006;26:S5–S18.

Smith R, Hourihan MD: Investigating suspected cerebral venous thrombosis. *BMJ* 2007;334:794–795.

Teasdale E: Cerebral venous thrombosis: Making the most of imaging. *J R Soc Med* 2000;93:234–237.

D-dimer in CVST

Crassard I, Soria C, Tzourio C, et al: A negative D-Dimer assay does not rule out cerebral venous thrombosis: A series of 73 patients. *Stroke* 2005;36:1716–1719.

Lalive PH, de Moerloose P, Lovblad K, Sarasin FP, Mermillod B, Sztajzel R: Is measurement of D-dimer useful in the diagnosis of cerebral venous thrombosis? *Neurology* 2003;61:1057–60.

Tardy B, Tardy-Poncet B, Viallon A, et al. D-Dimer levels in patients with suspected acute cerebral venous thrombosis. *Am J Med* 2002;113:238–241. (Sensitivity 100%.)

Methylene tetrahydrofolate reductase deficiency

Welch GN, Loscalzo J: Homocysteine and atherothrombosis. *N Engl J Med* 1998;338:1042–1050.

How to Read a Head CT in a Patient with Headache

In addition to reviewing each CT slice for its anatomical landmarks, an organized search should be made for signs of various disorders that can cause headache. These include (1) aneurysmal SAH, (2) an intracranial mass such as a tumor, abscess, or hematoma (intracerebral or subdural), (3) arteriovenous malformation (AVM), (4) cerebral venous sinus thrombosis, or (5) sinusitis (Table 1).

First, compare the left and right cerebral hemispheres for **symmetry** and look for **midline shift** indicative of an intracranial mass.

Second, examine the **basilar cisterns** for evidence of **SAH**.

Third, examine the **ventricles**. Ventricular enlargement may represent obstructive (noncommunicating) hydrocephalus due to a mass causing obstruction to CSF flow. Enlargement of all the four ventricles (communicating hydrocephalus) is associated with SAH and meningitis or may be a chronic condition. Small ventricles may be seen in idiopathic intracranial hypertension (pseudotumor cerebri) or diffuse cerebral edema.

Fourth, examine the **brain parenchyma** for anatomical distortion or altered attenuation indicative of a mass lesion, bleed or vascular malformation.

Fifth, examine the major **cerebral venous sinuses**, particularly the superior sagittal sinus and transverse sinuses, for increased attenuation (hyperdensity) indicative of thrombosis. The superior sagittal sinus is seen in the midline where the falx attaches to the skull in the superior CT slices and in the occipital region. The transverse sinuses are visible where the tentorium attaches to the occipital region of the skull.

Sixth, the paranasal **sinuses**, in particular the sphenoid sinus and ethmoid air cells should be examined for signs of sinusitis, i.e., filling with fluid. Sinus aeration is more easily assessed on bone windows.

Finally, a careful search should be made for disorders that can have subtle **CT findings that are easily missed.** These include SAH (CT is occasionally entirely normal), an intracerebral mass or AVM (causing only subtle parenchymal irregularity), an isodense SDH (particularly if bilateral and not causing midline shift), and cerebral venous sinus thrombosis.

TABLE 1

What to Look for on a Head CT in a Patient with Headache

1. **Symmetry and midline shift**—Compare left and right sides of cranium.

2. **SAH**—Blood in the basilar cisterns; look at the CT slice just superior to the dorsum sella

3. **Ventricles enlarged**—Obstructive hydrocephalus (mass lesion causing ventricular obstruction); Communicating hydrocephalus (SAH or meningitis)
   Ventricles small (or normal)—Idiopathic intracranial hypertension (pseudotumor cerebri)

4. **Brain parenchymal distortion**—Masses, edema, hemorrhage, vascular malformation

5. **Cerebral venous sinuses**—Hyperattenuating in cerebral venous sinus thrombosis

6. **Sinusitis**—Fluid or air/fluid levels in sphenoid, ethmoid, or frontal sinuses (use bone windows)

DIAGNOSTIC TESTING IN PATIENTS WITH HEADACHE

The initial diagnostic test in the evaluation of ED patients with headache is generally a **noncontrast CT.** Other tests may be needed when the CT is normal depending on the diagnostic considerations (Table 2).

Lumbar puncture is needed to detect **meningitis** or **SAH** (when the CT is normal). Opening pressure should be measured because an isolated elevated **opening pressure** (no other CSF abnormality) may be a sign of either *idiopathic intracranial hypertension* ("pseudotumor cerebri") or *cerebral venous sinus thrombosis* (CVST) CT is not needed prior to LP in selected patients suspected of having meningitis (see Patient 7).

Several disorders causing headache can be missed on noncontrast CT and require **contrast CT** or **MRI** for diagnosis. These include: (1) a small nonhemorrhagic AVM; (2) cerebral venous sinus thrombosis; (3) carotid or vertebral artery dissection; and (4) a small CNS tumor or abscess not causing mass effect (Purdy and Kirby 2004). Depending on the clinical circumstances, these further investigations can be done during the ED visit, upon hospitalization, or as an outpatient.

Finally, **medical causes** of headache must also be considered, including toxins (e.g., carbon monoxide poisoning) and vasculitis (e.g., temporal arteritis).

TABLE 2

Diagnostic Testing in Patients with Headache

Diagnostic Test	Suspected Diagnosis
Noncontrast CT	SAH (if CT normal, then LP), hematoma (ICH, SDH), mass (tumor or abscess) AVM, CVST, sphenoid sinusitis
LP	Meningitis (CT before LP if an intracranial mass is suspected) SAH (if CT normal) Idiopathic intracranial hypertension and CVST (elevated opening pressure)
Contrast CT or MRI	Small tumor or abscess, AVM, CVST (CTV or MRV) Cervicocranial artery dissection (CTA or MRA)
Other tests	Carbon monoxide poisoning (carboxyhemoglobin level) Temporal arteritis (ESR, temporal artery biopsy)

ICH, intracranial hematoma; SDH, subdural hematoma; AVM, arteriovenous malformation; CVST, cerebral venous sinus thrombosis; CTA, CT angiography; MRA, magnetic resonance angiography; MRV, magnetic resonance venography; ESR, erythrocyte sedimentation rate CTV, CT venography.

Examples of various head CT findings in patients with headache are shown in the following figures:

midline shift and mass effect (Figure 1);

SAH (Patient 4 on page 461);

ventricular enlargement due to obstructive hydrocephalus (Figure 3) or communicating hydrocephalus Patient 7, Figure 4, page 489);

small ventricles in idiopathic intracranial hypertension (Figure 2);

brain parenchymal distortion due to an AVM (Figures 5–7);

hyperattenuating cerebral venous sinuses (Patient 5 on page 471); and

paranasal sinus disease.

The need for contrast CT or MRI in patients with normal or nearly normal noncontrast CT scans is illustrated for:

AVM (Figures 5–7);

cerebral venous sinus thrombosis (Patient 5, Figures 6–9 pages 475–476),

and parenchymal tumors (Figure 9).

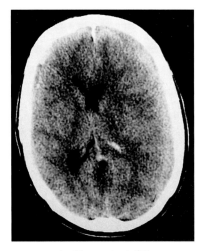
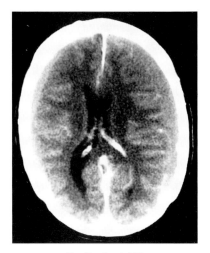

A. Noncontrast CT   B. Contrast CT

FIGURE 1   Isodense (subacute) subdural hematoma (SDH).

An isodense SDH in a 76-year-old man who complained of headache. The patient had, at baseline, mild cognitive deficits, but there was no change in his mental status. He had no history of head trauma. On examination, there were no focal neurological deficits.

(*A*) **Non-contrast CT** showed a moderate amount of midline shift to the right. The cortical sulci and gyri do not extend to the inner surface of the skull—characteristic of an isodense SDH. The

clotted blood in a SDH lyses over 7 to 14 days becoming isoattenuating relative to brain tissue, i.e., a subacute SDH.

(*B*) **Contrast CT** revealed the margins of the isodense SDH on the left and a smaller isodense SDH on the right. Contrast is visible in the pial blood vessels on the cortical surface. Intravenous contrast improves visualization of an isodense SDH, but is not always necessary to make this diagnosis.

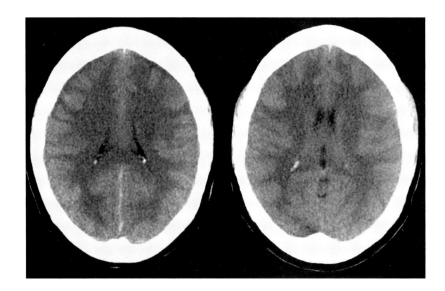

FIGURE 2   Idiopathic intracranial hypertension (Pseudotumor cerebri).

A 25-year-old woman presented to the ED with a headache of 7 day's duration. She was overweight, but her physical examination was otherwise normal. Funduscopic examination revealed papilledema (obscured optic disk margins without hemorrhage). Her visual acuity was normal.

A noncontrast CT was obtained to exclude an intracranial mass causing headache and papilledema.

The CT was noteworthy for small ventricles, which may be seen with idiopathic intracranial hypertension. However, the diagnostic utility of this finding has been questioned because in a young adult, small ventricles are a normal finding.

Lumbar puncture opening pressure was 35 cm water.

The patient was hospitalized for further neurological evaluation. She was treated with analgesic medications and a weight-reduction diet was prescribed.

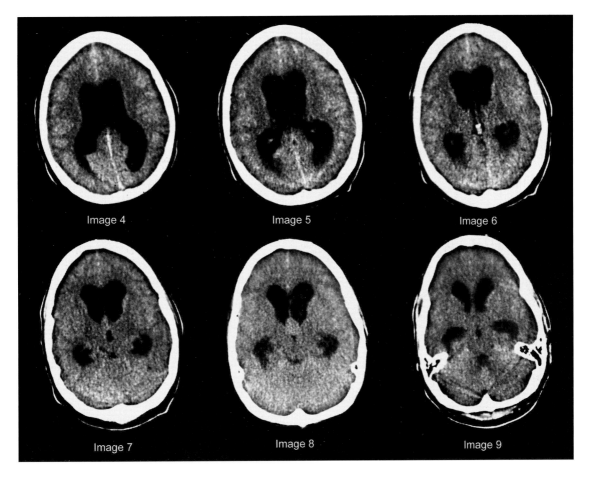

Image 4 Image 5 Image 6

Image 7 Image 8 Image 9

FIGURE 3

PATIENT 6A

A 21-year-old man developed severe headache shortly after awakening. He collapsed soon after his arrival at work. In the ED, he was confused and lethargic.

An emergency head CT was performed to "rule-out bleed" (Figure 3).

- What was the cause of this patient's severe headache and collapse?

The ventricles are markedly dilated (Figure 3) including the bodies of the lateral ventricles (images 4 and 5), the frontal and occipital horns (image 6), and the temporal horns (images 8 and 9). The superior portion of the third ventricle anterior to the calcified pineal gland is also dilated (image 6). This ventricular enlargement represents hydrocephalus.

The fourth ventricle, within the posterior fossa, is, however, normal in size (image 9). This is therefore obstructive (noncommunicating) hydrocephalus.

The cause of obstruction is seen on image 8 (Figure 4). There is a mass lesion within the third ventricle (*asterisk*), which is obstructing the foramina of Monro. (*Arrows* = dilated temporal horns)

The mass is a *colloid cyst of the third ventricle*. Other third ventricular tumors that can cause obstructive hydrocephalus include ependymomas and suprasellar tumors.

An emergency ventriculostomy drain was inserted. The colloid cyst was subsequently drained and excised.

Third ventricular tumors can present with sudden collapse due to acute hydrocephalus, or with intermittent headaches that worsen with the head tilted forward and are relieved when lying supine. The later presentation is due to a ball-valve pressure phenomenon. Sinusitis can cause a similar positional headache.

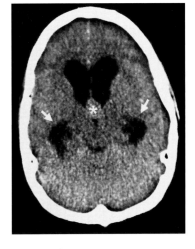

FIGURE 4

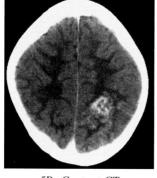

5A. Noncontrast CT   5B. Contrast CT

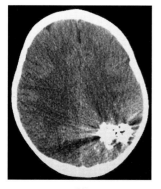

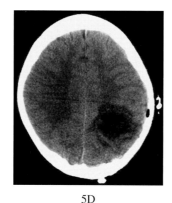

5C   5D

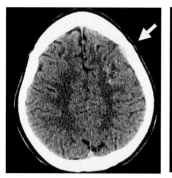

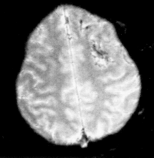

6A. Noncontrast CT   6B. MRI—T2-weighted

ARTERIOVENOUS MALFORMATIONS

CT signs of AVM can be subtle when there is no associated hemorrhage. Contrast CT or MRI may be needed for diagnosis.

FIGURE 5   A 9-year-old boy presented with headache of several day's duration.

(*A*) Noncontrast CT showed a subtle parenchymal irregularity in the left occipital lobe. This was seen on only one slice (*arrows*).

The CT was initially interpreted as negative. The following day, the patient was recalled to the ED.

(*B*) Contrast CT shows the AVM.

(*C*) Therapeutic embolization of the AVM.

(*D*) Later resection of the AVM.

FIGURE 6   An 18-year-old woman presented with new onset of focal seizure involving the right arm.

(*A*) Noncontrast CT showed parenchymal irregularity and slight calcification due to an AVM (*arrow*).

(*B*) MRI showed the AVM as a "signal void" (black) in the left fronto-parietal region.

FIGURE 7   A 28-year-old woman presented with progressive headache of one day's duration.

She had had headaches for the past 4 months, which were diagnosed as "migraine." The current headache was more persistent and accompanied by lethargy.

(*A*) Noncontrast CT demonstrated intraventricular hemorrhage. The AVM is not clearly seen.

(*B*) Contrast CT revealed enhancement of the left frontal AVM (*arrow*).

(*C*) Left internal carotid artery angiogram demonstrated an anterior cerebral artery AVM (lateral and frontal views).

She was treated with embolization and resection of a portion of the left frontal lobe.

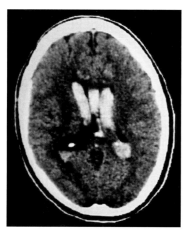

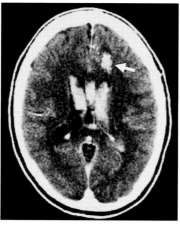

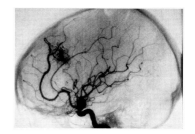

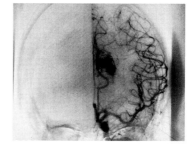

7A. Noncontrast CT   7B. Contrast CT   7C

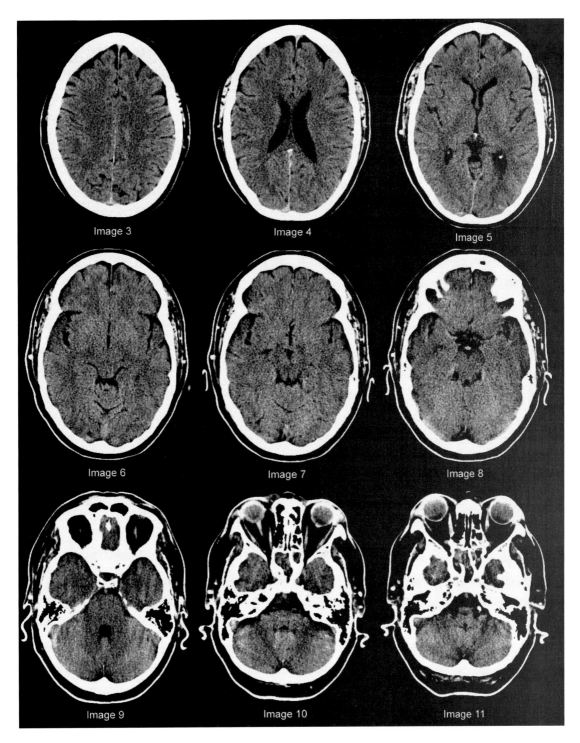

Image 3   Image 4   Image 5

Image 6   Image 7   Image 8

Image 9   Image 10   Image 11

FIGURE 8

PATIENT 6B

A 55-year-old woman presented with a persistent headache of one week's duration. Her physical examination was normal.

On CT (Figure 8), the cerebral hemispheres and other cranial structures are symmetrical and there is no midline shift. There is no blood in the suprasellar cistern (image 8) or interpeduncular cistern (image 7).

The ventricles are normal in size. There are no brain parenchymal lesions. The transverse cerebral venous sinuses (image 8) and superior sagittal sinus (images 3 and 4) are not hyperattenuating.

- What abnormality is present? (for answer see Figure 10)

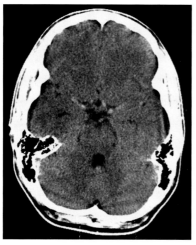

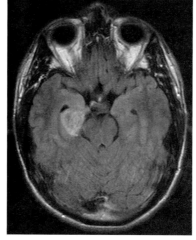

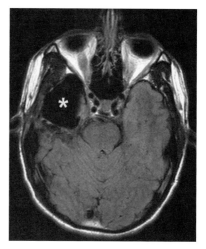

A Noncontrast CT   B MRI with gadolinium   C Postoperative MRI

FIGURE 9   Noncontrast CT may be entirely normal in a patient with a parenchymal brain tumor.

A 28-year-old man fainted at work. The episode was not observed, but he seemed to regain consciousness gradually according to the coworkers that heard him fall. In the ED, he was fully alert and had a normal neurological examination. Because of the suspicion of a seizure, noncontrast CT was obtained which was normal (*A*).

He was hospitalized and a gadolinium-enhanced MRI showed a focal lesion in the right medial temporal lobe consistent with a primary CNS neoplasm (*B*). Surgical resection revealed an anaplastic astrocytoma (*C*).

Small tumors that are not visible on CT would more likely present with a seizure or focal neurological symptoms than with a headache alone. A tumor causing a headache would be expected to be large enough to be seen on a noncontrast CT due to its mass effect. Nonetheless, small tumors causing headache that are not visible on noncontrast CT and require MRI for diagnosis have been reported (Purdy and Kirby 2004).

DIAGNOSTIC TESTING IN ED PATIENTS WITH HEADACHE

Head CT is indicated in patients with headache when any of the disorders listed in Table 2 are suspected (SAH, intracranial masses, CVST, sphenoid sinusitis). Although this simple statement is correct, it is not especially helpful in ED patients. Headache is a nonspecific symptom and there are few characteristics that can reliably distinguish between uncommon but potentially serious causes of headache (such as SAH, CVST) and more common benign causes of headache (migraine, tension, or cluster headache). Often, the only distinguishing feature of a serious condition is that the headache is of new onset or has changed from prior headaches (ACEP 1996). A low threshold should be maintained for ordering CT in ED patients with a new or unusual headache.

Diagnostic testing is needed for patients with severe or persistent headache. Other features that suggest the need for head CT include headache that is of abrupt onset, unusual in quality, or associated with vomiting or focal neurological symptoms. An abrupt onset ("thunder clap") headache suggests SAH, although only a minority of ED patients with thunder clap headache have SAH (10–15%). Furthermore, patients with SAH may occasionally present without an immediate-onset severe headache. Findings on physical examination that indicate a need for CT include neck stiffness, papilledema, an altered level of consciousness, and any focal neurological signs. Relief of headache with analgesic medications does not reliably exclude a serious cause of headache, especially when other dangerous features are present.

Patients at higher risk of having a serious cause of headache include the elderly, young children, immunocompromised patients and those with cancer known to metastasize to the brain.

Patients who may not need CT in the ED due to a headache's likely benign etiology include patients with a relatively mild headache, patients who experience prompt and complete relief with analgesic medications, headache of short duration, and headache without dangerous features (vomiting, neck stiffness, altered mentation, papilledema, or focal neurological signs such as cranial nerve deficits). Patients with a headache typical of their chronic headache syndrome also generally do not require CT. A patient with a likely benign cause of headache should be treated symptomatically, referred for follow-up examination, and instructed to return to the ED if symptoms worsen or persist.

The need for additional testing also depends on the suspected diagnoses. **LP** is indicated in patients of having suspected meningitis (CT should be performed first if a mass lesion might be present, or when SAH is suspected and the CT is normal). LP measurement of opening pressure is important in patients with suspected idiopathic intracranial hypertension and possibly CVST.

Contrast CT or MRI is indicated in patients suspected of having a nonhemorrhagic AVM (look for subtle parenchymal irregularities on the noncontrast CT, Figure 5A), CVST (see Patient 5), or when an intracranial mass is suspected clinically or on the noncontrast CT (Figure 9) (Evans 2004, Purdy and Kirby 2004).

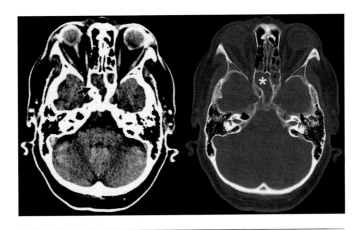

FIGURE 10   Patient 6B (image 10)—Sphenoid sinusitis.

In patients with headache, the inferior CT slices should be examined for signs of sinusitis. In Patient 6B, opacification of the sphenoid and ethmoid sinuses is seen in CT image 10 (Figure 10A, *arrow*) and image 11. Fluid in the sinuses is more easily seen on bone windows (Figure 10B, *asterisk*).

Patients with **sphenoid sinusitis** may present with a persistent, poorly localized headache, or a headache localized to the vertex of the head. They may not have sinus tenderness, sinus congestion, or fever. Serious complications can occur including orbital cellulitis, cavernous sinus thrombosis, and meningitis.

A patient with sphenoid sinusitis who appears well and is otherwise healthy, can be treated with oral antibiotics and prompt follow up. Hospitalization and intravenous antibiotics are warranted in patients who are ill-appearing or immunocompromised. Lumbar puncture should be performed if meningitis is suspected.

SUGGESTED READING

American College of Emergency Physicians. Clinical policy on the initial approach to adolescents and adults presenting to the emergency department with a chief complaint of headache. *Ann Emerg Med* 1996;27:821–844.

American College of Emergency Physicians. Clinical policy: Critical issues in the evaluation and management of patients presenting to the emergency department with acute headache. *Ann Emerg Med* 2002;39:108–122.

Detsky ME, McDonald DR, Baerlocher MO, et al: Does this patient with headache have a migraine or need neuroimaging? *JAMA* 2006;296:1274–1283.

Evans RW, ed.: Secondary headache disorders. *Neurol Clin* 2004;22(1):xi–xii.

Gladstone JP, Dodick DW: From hemicrania lunaris to hemicrania continua: An overview of the revised international classification of headache disorders. *Headache: J Head Face Pain* 2004; 44:692–705.

Headache Classification Subcommittee of the International Headache Society. The Internaitonal Classification of Headache Disorders, 2nd edition. *Cephalalgia* 2004;24(Suppl. 1):1–160.

Kaniecki R: Headache assessment and management. *JAMA* 2003; 289:1430–1433.

Purdy RA, Kirby S: Headaches and brain tumors. *Neurol Clin* 2004; 22:39–53.

Rothrock JF: Headaches due to vascular disorders. Neurol Clin 2004; 22:21–37.

Idiopathic Intracranial Hypertension
Friedman DI, Jacobson DM: Diagnostic criteria for idiopathic intracranial hypertension. *Neurology* 2002;59:1492–1495.

Friedman DI: Pseudotumor cerebri. *Neurol Clin North Am* 2004; 22:99–131.

Jacobson DM, Karanjia PN, Olson KA, et al: Computed tomography ventricular size has no predictive value in diagnosing pseudotumor cerebri. *Neurology* 1990;40:1454–1455.

Colloid Cyst of the Third Ventricle
Ferrera PC, Kass LE: Third ventricle colloid cyst. *Am J Emerg Med* 1997;15:145–147.

McDonald JA: Colloid cyst of the third ventricle and sudden death. *Ann Emerg Med* 1982;11:365–367.

Opeskin K, Anderson RM, Lee KA: Colloid cyst of the third ventricle as a cause of acute neurological deterioration and sudden death. *J Paediatr Child Health* 1993;29:476–477.

Read EJ: Colloid cyst of the third ventricle. *Ann Emerg Med* 1990;19:1060–1062.

Weisz RR, Fazal M: Colloid cyst of the third ventricle: A neurological emergency. *Ann Emerg Med* 1983;12:783–785.

Sphenoid Sinusitis
Goldman GE, Fontanarosa PB, Anderson JM: Isolated sphenoid sinusitis. *Am J Emerg Med* 1993;11:235–238.

Nordeman L, Lucid EJ: Sphenoid sinusitis: a cause of debilitating headache. *J Emerg Med* 1990;8:557–559.

Head CT: Patient 7

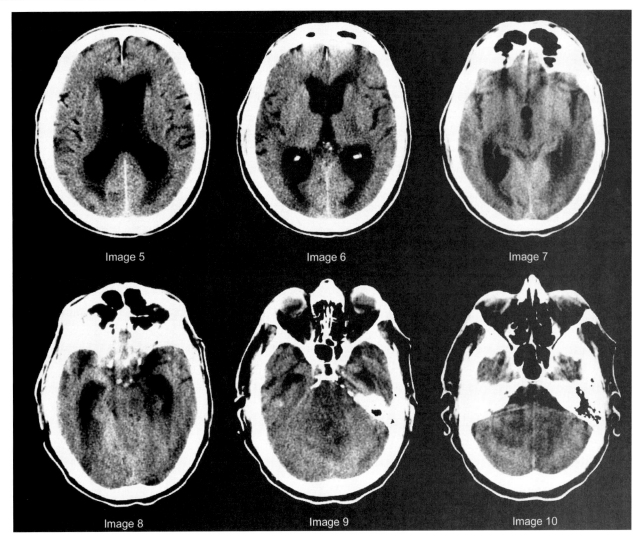

Image 5   Image 6   Image 7

Image 8   Image 9   Image 10

FIGURE 1

Lethargy and fever in an elderly man; head CT was performed prior to LP

A 79-year-old man presented to the ED with weakness, anorexia, and lethargy of two day's duration. His next door neighbor called for an ambulance.

In the ED, he complained of a mild headache, but did not have abdominal pain, vomiting, diarrhea, cough, or urinary symptoms.

On examination, he was an elderly man who was lethargic and oriented only to person and place. His verbal responses and responses to simple commands were slow. His vital signs were normal aside from a temperature of 100.9°F (rectal).

His pupils were equal and reactive and extraocular motion was normal. Funduscopic examination was limited by cataracts. His neck was supple. His heart, lung, and abdominal

examinations were normal. Neurological examination revealed normal strength, sensation, and reflexes in all extremities.

Given the patient's low-grade fever without an identified source, slowed mentation and complaint of headache, meningitis was a diagnostic consideration. Because his fundi could not be visualized, a noncontrast head CT was performed prior to lumbar puncture (Figure 1).

There is no midline shift or mass effect.

- Is it safe to perform a lumbar puncture?

NB. Because the CT slice orientation was not parallel to the skull base, the anterior portions of the lower slices (8–10) extend into the orbits.

REMEMBER THE FOURTH VENTRICLE

Intracranial lesions causing mass effect are important to identify prior to performing a lumbar puncture (LP) in patients suspected of having meningitis because they increase the risk of post-LP herniation. The risk of herniation is greatest when a mass causes unequal pressure between intracranial compartments.

Although contrast CT is better than noncontrast at detecting intracerebral masses such as tumors and abscesses, a lesion that is causing significant mass effect can usually be detected on a noncontrast scan. Therefore, noncontrast CT is generally felt to be an acceptable means of excluding an intracranial mass prior to LP.

In this patient's CT, there is no evident distortion of brain parenchyma and no midline shift. However, a sizable intracranial mass is present. Had the patient undergone lumbar puncture, fatal herniation would have been the likely outcome.

This patient's CT is notable for **ventricular enlargement** (Figure 2). Ventricular enlargement is an expected finding in elderly patients and is usually due to cerebral **atrophy** (loss of brain tissue). Atrophy is also termed *ex-vacuo hydrocephalus*.

Ventricular enlargement may also be caused by excess CSF within the ventricles, which is known as **hydrocephalus.** Hydrocephalus may due to obstruction to CSF flow, diminished CSF resorption or, rarely, increased CSF production (e.g., a choroid plexus tumor).

Cerebral atrophy can be distinguished from hydrocephalus on CT by comparing the relative enlargement of the ventricles and cortical sulci. With atrophy, the cortical sulci are enlarged, whereas with hydrocephalus, the cortical sulci are normal in size or small (effaced, meaning "thinned") (Figure 3).

Hydrocephalus is classified as either *communicating* or *non-communicating* ("obstructive") depending on whether or not there is a lesion within the ventricular system that is obstructing the flow of CSF (Table 1).

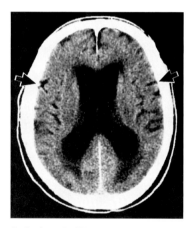
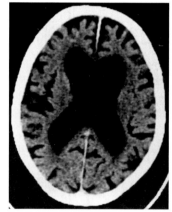
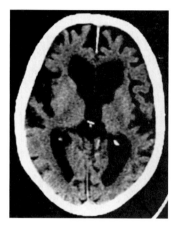

2. Patient 7–CT Image 5   3A. Atrophy   3B. Atrophy

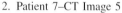

Ventricular enlargement

FIGURE 2   Hydrocephalus—Image 5 of Patient 7 shows dilated lateral ventricles. The cortical sulci are not enlarged (*arrows*). This patient's ventricular enlargement is therefore due to hydrocephalus, not cerebral atrophy.

FIGURE 3   Cerebral atrophy—CT of another patient showing diffuse cortical atrophy. There is ventricular enlargement as well as enlargement of the cortical sulci due to volume loss of the cortical gyri.

TABLE 1

Classification of Hydrocephalus

Communicating hydrocephalus

    Extraventricular obstructive hydrocephalus (EVOH)

    Dilation of all four ventricles

    An acute or chronic sequela of, most often, SAH or meningitis

Non-communicating ("obstructive") hydrocephalus

    Intraventricular obstructive hydrocephalus (IVOH)

    Dilation of ventricles proximal to obstructing lesion; distal ventricles are normal sized

    Obstructing lesion either intraventricular or extrinsic (compressing ventricular system)

Ex-vacuo hydrocephalus—Diffuse cortical atrophy

    Dilation of ventricles and enlargement of cortical sulci

Non-communicating hydrocephalus is also known as *obstructive hydrocephalus* or, more precisely, *intraventricular obstructive hydrocephalus* (IVOH) because there is a blockage of CSF flow within the ventricular system. The ventricles proximal to the obstruction are dilated, whereas the ventricles distal to the obstruction are normal in size.

Obstruction to CSF flow usually occurs at one of the narrow segments of the ventricular system—the foramena of Monro, the third ventricle, the aqueduct of Sylvius or the fourth ventricle. The obstruction may be due to a lesion within the ventricular system or a extraventricular mass causing extrinsic compression of the ventricular system. Because patients with obstructive hydrocephalus can deteriorate rapidly due to herniation, emergency ventricular decompression with a ventriculostomy drain is often necessary (Patient 6A, p.481).

Communicating hydrocephalus is caused by obstruction to CSF flow outside of the ventricles (in the basilar cisterns or around the cerebral convexities) or by diminished CSF resorption at the arachnoid villi in the superior sagittal sinus. It is also known as *extraventricular obstructive hydrocephalus* (EVOH). In communicating hydrocephalus, there is uniform dilation of the entire ventricular system, including the fourth ventricle.

Communicating hydrocephalus may be acute or chronic. **Acute communicating hydrocephalus** is usually caused by infection (meningitis) or blood within the CSF (subarachnoid hemorrhage). The inflammatory exudate or blood within the subarachnoid spaces impedes extraventricular flow of CSF (Figure 4 and Patient 4, Figures 2-12 on pages 463–468).

Chronic communicating hydrocephalus is often a residual finding of prior subarachnoid hemorrhage, meningitis, or other CNS disorder. Chronic communicating hydrocephalus can be asymptomatic, cause chronic headaches, or be associated with *normal pressure hydrocephalus* in elderly patients (dementia, ataxia, and urinary incontinence). Because there is no pressure differential between intracranial compartments, communicating hydrocephalus is not considered a contraindication to lumbar puncture (Figure 5).

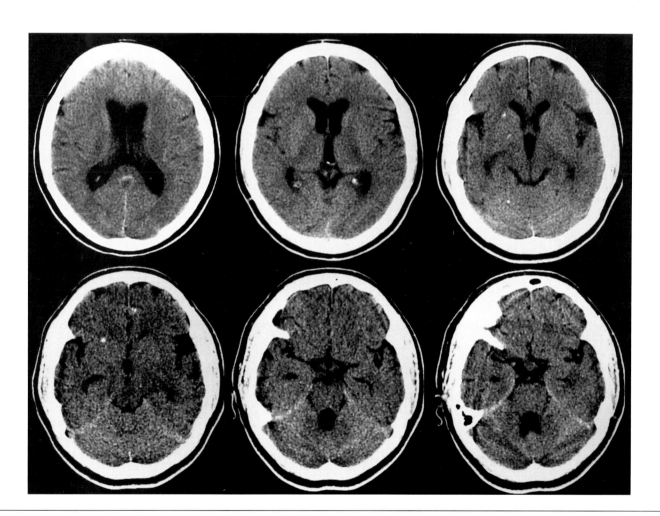

FIGURE 4   Communicating hydrocephalus due to meningitis.

A 40-year-old Hispanic woman presented with persistent headache of five day's duration. She had previously been healthy. Physical examination was normal aside from *papilledema*.

CT revealed *communicating hydrocephalus* with dilated lateral, third, and fourth ventricles. In addition, several punctate calcifications are

seen in the cerebral hemispheres indicative of **neurocysticercosis** (upper right and lower left CT slices). Lumbar puncture revealed 70 leukocytes/mm^3 with lymphocyte predominance. CSF serology titers were positive for cysticercosis.

The patient was treated with albendazole and her headaches resolved.

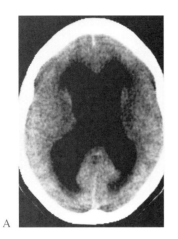
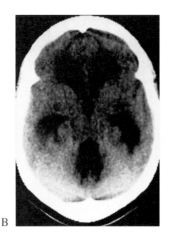
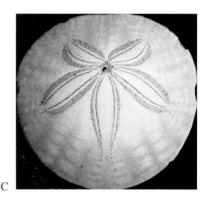

FIGURE 5   Chronic communicating hydrocephalus.

(*A*) The lateral ventricles are markedly enlarged and the cortical sulci are completely effaced.

(*B*) The fourth ventricle (posterior) is dilated, which confirms that this is communicating hydrocephalus. The frontal horns and temporal horns of the lateral ventricles and the third ventricle (central round structure) are dilated.

(*C*) The appearance of image B has been likened to that of a **sand dollar** (an invertebrate shell found on the beach).

This is severe chronic communicating hydrocephalus in a patient who had had meningitis many years earlier.

Patient Outcome

In Patient 7, the **lateral ventricles** are markedly enlarged; however, there is no enlargement of the cortical sulci as would be expected with cerebral atrophy. The **third ventricle** is also enlarged and has a rounded appearance (Figure 6).

Most importantly, the **fourth ventricle** is not seen in its usual location within the posterior fossa between the pons and cerebellum (Figures 7 and 8). This patient, therefore, has **noncommunicating (obstructive) hydrocephalus.**

In this case, the ventricular obstruction is due to extrinsic compression of the fourth ventricle by a posterior fossa mass. However, the obstructing mass lesion is not visible because it is isodense (isoattenuating) relative to brain tissue. The only evidence of the mass is obliteration of the fourth ventricle.

Fortunately, patient's the obstructive hydrocephalus was recognized and a lumbar puncture was not performed. Herniation would otherwise have been the likely outcome. Instead, a **contrast CT** was performed, which revealed a large ring-enhancing lesion in the posterior fossa (Figure 9). A ventriculostomy drain was inserted to reduce the intracranial pressure and avert herniation (Figure 10A).

The next day, the patient underwent craniotomy and excision of the lesion (Figure 10B). The lesion proved to be an **abscess**.

When his medical records were reviewed, it was discovered that he had presented to the ED two weeks earlier and antibiotics had been prescribed for otitis media. It is not known whether he took the medication, but otitis media with mastoiditis was the likely cause of his brain abscess. The patient made a good postoperative recovery.

When examining all head CT scans, be sure to **look for the fourth ventricle**—this is especially important when the fourth ventricle cannot be seen.

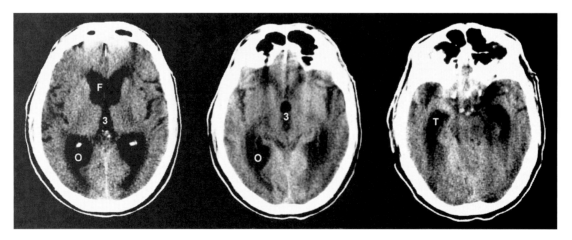

FIGURE 6   Patient 7—Images 6–8
Noncontrast CT showing marked enlargement of the frontal horns (F), occipital horns (O) and temporal horns (T) of the lateral ventricles, and the third ventricle (3).

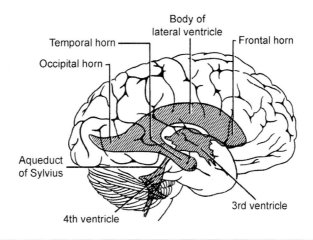

FIGURE 7   Ventricles of the brain.

The fourth ventricle is located in the posterior fossa between the pons and cerebellum.

[From Pansky, *Review of Gross Anatomy,* 6th ed., McGraw-Hill, 1996.]

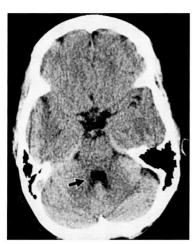

A. **Normal fourth ventricle**

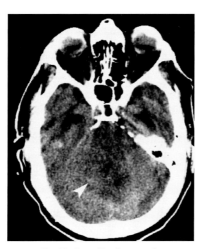

B. **Patient 7—Image 9**

FIGURE 8.   The fourth ventricle.

(*A*) In another patient, the fourth ventricle has a normal size and location in the posterior fossa (*arrow*).

(*B*) Image 9 shows obliteration of the fourth ventricle (*arrowhead*).

(The CT slice orientation is suboptimal and extends anteriorly into the orbits.)

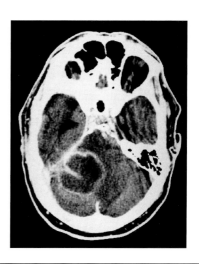

FIGURE 9   Patient 7—Contrast CT.

A ring-enhancing lesion in the posterior fossa compresses the fourth ventricle.

FIGURE 10   Patient 7—Outcome.

(*A*) Emergency insertion of a ventriculostomy drain into the right lateral ventricle to avert the impending herniation.

(*B*) Postoperative CT showing excision and drainage of brain abscess.

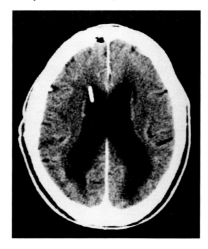

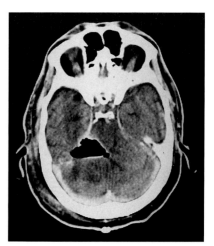

A

B

WHAT CT FINDINGS PROHIBIT PERFORMING A LUMBAR PUNCTURE?

There are four principal CT findings indicative of unequal pressure between the three intracranial compartments (the right and left supratentorial compartments, and the posterior fossa). These are: 1) midline shift, 2) obstructive hydrocephalus, 3) compression of the basilar cisterns, and 4) compression of the fourth ventricle (Table 2). These signs of mass effect can usually be detected on a noncontrast CT (Figures 11–13). The associated intracranial mass may or may not be visible.

Masses in the **posterior fossa** are notoriously difficult to detect on CT. Displacement or compression of the fourth ventricle may be the only sign of a posterior fossa mass. However, because the posterior fossa is relatively small, any mass, even without deforming the fourth ventricle, poses a risk of herniation. One author therefore advocates performing a contrast CT (or MRI) prior to LP when a posterior fossa mass is suspected, i.e., abnormal cerebellar or brainstem findings on clinical examination, recent otitis media, or history of posterior fossa tumor (Gower et al. 1987).

In the presence of certain other CT finding, the safety of performing an LP is likely but not definite. These findings include: (1) a supratentorial lesion that is not causing midline shift or mass effect, and (2) communicating hydrocephalus.

With **communicating hydrocephalus**, pressures between intracranial compartments are equal and LP is felt to be safe. However, herniation has occurred in patients with meningitis who had "normal" CT scans. These patients may have had communicating hydrocephalus and elevated intracranial pressure. Therefore, following LP, such patients should be closely monitored for signs of neurological deterioration. Lumbar puncture using a small caliber needle (22 gauge) and removal of a limited quantity of CSF (3–4 mL) may be advisable.

TABLE 2

What to Look for on a Head CT before Performing LP

CT signs of unequal pressure between intracranial compartments are contraindications to LP

1. Midline shift—Subfalcine herniation

   Unequal pressure between left and right supratentorial compartments
   Also, look for intracerebral masses not causing midline shift

2. Noncommunicating (obstructive) hydrocephalus—Intraventricular obstruction to CSF flow

   Enlargement of ventricles proximal to an obstructing lesion and normal-sized ventricles distal to the obstruction(particularly the fourth ventricle)

3. Basilar cisterns compressed—Elevated pressure at the tentorial notch (midbrain compression)

   Lateral ventricles and third ventricle may be small due to diffuse cerebral edema, or enlarged due to obstructive hydrocephalus. Midline shift may or may not be present.

4. Posterior fossa mass—Displacement or compression of the fourth ventricle

   A mass can be difficult to detect; contrast CT may be necessary

---

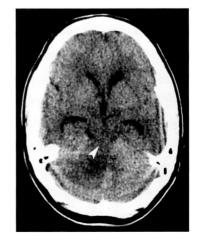

FIGURE 11   The quadrigeminal plate cistern is compressed (*arrowhead*) by a posterior fossa mass.

In addition, the temporal horns are dilated and the fourth ventricle is compressed

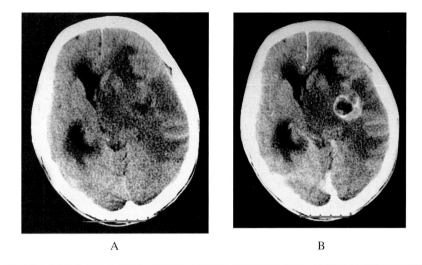

A   B

FIGURE 12 Herniation can occur following lumbar puncture.

A 30-year-old man with AIDS was admitted to the hospital for an altered level of consciousness and fever. He was lethargic but had "no focal neurological deficits" and reportedly no papilledema. A head CT could not be obtained promptly and so LP was performed. Thirty minutes later, he had a respiratory arrest and was intubated.

A noncontrast CT revealed a left cerebral mass causing ventricular compression and midline shift (*A*). Contrast CT revealed a ring-enhancing lesion with surrounding cerebral edema consistent with CNS toxoplasmosis (*B*). The patient expired 24 hours later.

This patient clearly should not have had an LP without first obtaining a head CT. A much safer strategy would have been to administer antibiotics effective against meningitis because of the delay in performing a head CT and LP.

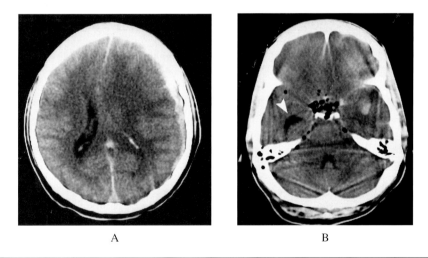

A   B

FIGURE 13 Obstructive hydrocephalus as a consequence of head trauma.

(*A*) Midline shift (subfalcine herniation) due to a subdural hematoma compresses left lateral ventricle. The third ventricle is also compressed, which obstructs the flow of CSF. The right lateral ventricle is dilated.

(*B*) Dilation of temporal horn of the right lateral ventricle (*arrow*) is indicative of hydrocephalus. The fourth ventricle is normal in size.

Such patients must be closely observed for signs of transtentorial herniation.

INDICATIONS FOR CT PRIOR TO LP IN PATIENTS WITH SUSPECTED MENINGITIS

Because of the potential risk of herniation following lumbar puncture, clinical signs of an intracerebral mass causing increased intracranial pressure must be sought before performing a lumbar puncture. If any of these findings are present, CT should be obtained prior to LP (Table 3).

CT is readily available in the ED and, although rare, herniation following LP can be fatal. Therefore, some practitioners nearly always obtain CT prior to LP. However, the presence of an intracranial mass is uncommon in patients suspected of having meningitis, particularly if there are no suggestive clinical signs, and routine use of CT prior to LP is therefore questionable. Unnecessary CT scans add to the cost of medical care, and frequently delay administration of antibiotics, which may worsen outcome in patients with bacterial meningitis. When CT is being obtained prior to LP in patients with suspected meningitis, empiric antibiotic therapy should be administered before performing CT and LP.

Clinical findings suggestive of an intracranial mass include focal neurological deficits and papilledema (or absence of spontaneous venous pulsations) on funduscopic examination (Table 3). Patients with an altered level of consciousness are at higher risk of harboring an intracranial mass because they are more difficult to examine for focal neurological deficits. Furthermore, altered mental status itself may be an early sign of brainstem compression. Finally, patients with medical conditions that are associated with intracranial masses should have CT before LP. These include immunosuppression (e.g., AIDS) and a history of prior intracranial mass lesion (Hasbun et al. 2001, Gopal et al. 1999, Linden 2000, Archer 1993, Gower et al. 1987).

TABLE 3

Indications for CT Scanning Prior to LP in Patients Suspected of having Meningitis

1. Focal neurological deficits—Focal signs or symptoms

2. Altered level of consciousness—GCS score <14

3. Papilledema

4. Risk factors for intracranial mass lesion

   AIDS, immunosuppressive therapy, known malignancy with propensity for intracranial metastasis, history of intracranial mass lesion, recent otitis media or paranasal sinus infection, recent head trauma or neurosurgical procedure

5. Seizure within 1 week

6. Severe headache and vomiting—a sign of increased intracranial pressure

7. Age ≥ 60 years (Hasbun et al. 2001)

8. Other disorders that require CT for diagnosis are suspected : SAH, intracranial hemorrhage, brain abscess

Administration of antibiotics must not be delayed while awaiting CT and LP.

There are few prospective data regarding the sensitivity of these clinical signs for excluding an intracranial mass prior to LP and the frequency of mass lesions.

Hasbun (2001) studied 301 adult patients with suspected meningitis. Meningitis was diagnosed in 83 (28%) of the patients. CT was performed prior to LP in 235 patients (78%), i.e., 22% of patients had LP without CT. Fifty-six of the patients (24%) had abnormal CT scans, eleven of whom (5%) had mass effect (severe in 3 and mild or moderate in 8). Only four patients (2%) had CT findings that prohibited LP The frequency of contraindications to LP was thus very low, although the frequency of abnormal CT scans was fairly high (24%).

Hasbun identified five clinical features that were associated with a CNS mass on CT. In the absence of all five features, CT could potentially be omitted. The five features were:

1. focal neurological deficits;

2. altered level of consciousness (Glasgow Coma Scale [GCS] score <14 or inability to answer two questions or follow two commands);

3. underlying diseases that can cause cerebral mass lesions (immunocompromize, history of CNS disease);

4. seizure within the past week; and

5. Age ≥ 60 years.

Papilledema was not found to be useful because it was present in only one patient.

Ninety-six of the 235 patients (41%) had none of the five high-risk features and could potentially forgo CT prior to LP. However, three of these 96 patients had abnormal CT scans and one had mild mass effect. Nonetheless, all three of these patients did undergo LP and none had untoward consequences. The *negative predictive value* of Hasbun's criteria was high: 97% for any CT abnormality and 99% for mass effect (93 of 96 patients had normal CT scans).

However, because the number of patients with significant CT abnormalities was so low, providing their results only as "negative predicative value" overstates the accuracy of the decision criteria. In fact, the *sensitivity* of these criteria was only moderate. To exclude *any* CT abnormality, the decision criteria had 95% sensitivity, i.e., 3 out of 56 cases with abnormal CT were missed by the decision criteria. For a CT finding of mass effect, sensitivity was only 91%; 1 of 11 cases was missed (lower 95% confidence interval of sensitivity was 75%). However, in this case the mass effect was mild and LP was performed without an adverse outcome. Unfortunately, the clinical features of the one patient whose CT showed mass effect despite the absence of risk factors was not described. This might have elucidated an additionally clinically useful risk factor. In addition, although LP was not harmful, the CT findings were likely relevant to patient care.

Nonetheless, this study does support the use of clinical criteria in deciding to omit CT prior to LP in patients suspected of having meningitis. None of the four patients with CT findings that prohibited LP would have been missed (although the number of such patients was small).

Summary

Two prospective studies (Hasbun and Gopal) suggest that the likelihood of a mass lesion is very low in patients suspected of having meningitis, and their results, in concert with good clinical judgment, allow omission of CT before LP in selected patients. However, these studies were small, the number of patients with masses was low, and there has been no prospective validation of the results. The study results, therefore, do not prove when CT can be omitted. Whenever LP is planned but the clinician is concerned about another disorder that could be detected by CT, it should be obtained first, especially when CT is readily available. When CT cannot be quickly obtained and interpreted, empirical antibiotics should be administered prior to CT and LP.

Because information about bacterial sensitivity to antibiotics could be compromised if antibiotics have been administered, LP should be performed as expeditiously as possible, even when CT is being performed first.

Many patients with bacterial meningitis – typically elderly adults with fever, nuchal rigidity, and depressed levels of consciousness (present in 88% of cases) – have clinical features that indicate a need for CT before LP, e.g., advanced age (per Hasbun) and altered mental status. In these cases, the diagnostic evaluation must be expedited and the administration of antibiotics must not be delayed.

On the other hand, a patient who may not need CT before LP is typically a young otherwise healthy adult who is alert, has a normal neurological examination including a normal mental status, no papilledema, no risk factors for a CNS mass such as HIV infection, and a clinical presentation compatible with meningitis (headache fever, and some degree of neck stiffness). The absence of fever may cast sufficient doubt on the diagnosis to prompt ordering CT before LP (Linden 2000). Other disorders that depend on CT for diagnosis must not be considerations such as SAH, intracerebral hemorrhage, brain abscess or tumor.

Young children and infants generally do not undergo CT before LP. This is because of the increased risk of radiation exposure in young children and because the chance of there being a CNS mass in the absence of suggestive clinical findings is exceedingly low.

SUGGESTED READING

Meningitis Diagnosis

Attia J, Hatala R, Cook DJ, Wong JG: Does this adult patient have meningitis? *JAMA* 1999;282:175–181. (Correspondence: *JAMA* 2000;283:1004.)

van de Beek D, de Gans J, Tunkel AR, et al: Community-acquired bacterial meningitis in adults. *N Engl J Med* 2006;354:44–53.

CT before LP in Patients with Suspected Meningitis

Abrahamian FM, Moran GJ, Talan DA, Gupta M, et al: Community-acquired bacterial meningitis (correspondence). *N Engl J Med* 2006; 354:1429–1432.

Gopal AK, Whitehouse JD, Simel DL, Corey GR: Cranial computed tomography before lumbar puncture: A prospective clinical evaluation. *Arch Intern Med* 1999;159:2681–2685.

Gower DJ, Baker AL, Bell WO, Ball MR: Contraindications to lumbar puncture as defined by computed cranial tomography. *J Neurol Neurosurg Psychiatry* 1987;50:1071–1074.

Hasbun R, Abrahams J, Jekel J, Quagliarello VJ: Computed tomography of the head before lumbar puncture in adults with suspected meningitis. *N Engl J Med* 2001;345:1727–1733.

Johnson PL, Eckard DA, et al.: Imaging of acquired cerebral herniations. *Neuroimag Clin North Am* 2002;12:217–228.

Linden CH: Cranial computed tomography before lumbar puncture. *Arch Intern Med* 2000;160:2868–2870.

Steigbigel NH: Computed tomography of the head before a lumbar puncture in suspected meningitis—Is it helpful? *N Engl J Med* 2001;345:1768–1770. (Editorial)

Tattevin P, Bruneel F, Regnier B, et al.: Cranial CT before lumbar puncture in suspected meningitis. *N Engl J Med* 2002;346:1248–51. (Letters)

van Crevel H, Hijdra A, de Gans J: Lumbar puncture and the risk of herniation: When should we first perform CT? *J Neurol* 2002;249:129–137.

Dangers of LP

Addy DP: When not to do a lumbar puncture. *Arch Dis Childhood* 1987;62:873–875.

Baker ND, Kharazi H, Laurent L, et al.: The efficacy of routine head CT prior to lumbar puncture in the emergency department. *J Emerg Med* 1994;12:597–601.

Pfister HW, Feiden W, Einhaupl KM: Spectrum of complications during bacterial meningitis in adults. *Arch Neurol* 1993;50:575–581.

Rennick G, Shann F, de Campo J: Cerebral herniation during bacterial meningitis in children. *BMJ* 1993;306:953–955.

Richards PG, Towu-Aghantse E: Dangers of lumbar puncture. *BMJ* 1986;292:605–606. (Correspondence 827–828.)

Zisfein J, Tuchman AJ: Risks of lumbar puncture in the presence of intracranial mass lesions. *Mt Sinai J Med* 1987;55:283–287.

Head CT: Patient 8

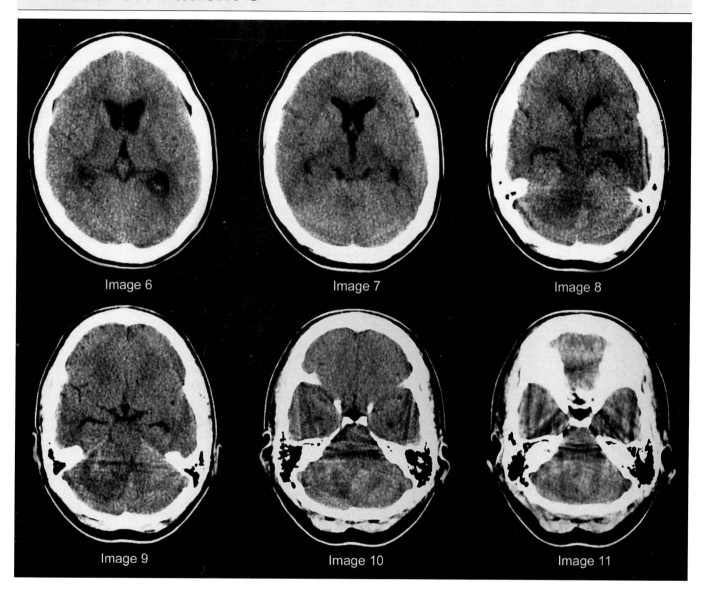

FIGURE 1

Headache, unilateral hearing loss and blurred vision in a young woman

A 29-year-old woman presented with blurred vision of 2 week's duration. She had consulted an optometrist to have her eyeglass prescription checked and was told that she should visit a doctor.

She had a six-month history of intermittent headaches and diminished hearing on the right. She had been to a doctor on two prior occasions for the headache and was prescribed a mild analgesic with some relief. She had mentioned the hearing loss to the doctor, but no further work up was done.

On examination, she was a healthy appearing woman in no distress. There was markedly diminished hearing on the right.

The Weber test localized to the left. Pupillary response and extraocular motion were intact, with slight rotary nystagmus in all directions. There was diminished sensation on the right side of the face. The right corneal reflex was diminished. The gag reflex was also diminished on the right. The tongue was midline. Visual acuity with corrective lenses was 20/25 right eye, 20/30 left eye. Funduscopic examination revealed bilateral papilledema and no hemorrhages.

- What is this patient's diagnosis?

  Her head CT is shown in Figure 1.

CONTRAST ENHANCEMENT

The clinical presentation of this patient is classic for an **acoustic schwannoma** (formerly called acoustic neuroma) or other cerebello-pontine angle tumor. Unfortunately, diagnosis of this disease is occasionally delayed because of its gradual onset and a failure to appreciate the significance of unilateral hearing loss. In this patient, the tumor had grown to a large size causing obstructive hydrocephalus and papilledema.

Tumors (and abscesses) can often be detected on **noncontrast CT** because the lesions are hypo- or hyperattenuating (appear darker or lighter) relative to normal brain tissue. In addition, surrounding edema and mass effect distorts other anatomical structures. Lesions in the posterior fossa are, however, often difficult to detect by CT. This is because adjacent thick cortical bone creates beam-hardening artifacts, which diminish the ability of CT to visualize anatomical detail and to detect slight differences in tissue density (Figure 1, images 10 and 11).

In this patient, the right side of the cerebellum has slightly lower attenuation (appears darker) than the left (Figure 1, images 8 and 9). More importantly, the fourth ventricle is compressed and displaced toward the left, which indicates that the tumor is on the right and compressing the cerebellum and brainstem. In addition, the temporal horns of the lateral ventricles and the third ventricle are mildly enlarged—indicative of hydrocephalus (Figure 2).

After the administration of intravenous contrast, the tumor becomes obvious on CT (Figure 3).

Contrast enhancement is seen in a number of intracranial structures (Table 1, Figure 4). Enhancement occurs in intracerebral lesions (tumors and abscesses) that promote neovascularization with abnormal blood vessels that do not have an intact blood–brain barrier. The enhancement may be homogeneous or, more commonly, ring-like when the central area has diminished vascularity or is necrotic (Figure 4D).

Large and small intracranial blood vessels, both normal and abnormal also exhibit enhancement on a contrast CT (Figures 4A–C).

Finally, intracranial structures that do not have a blood–brain barrier take up contrast. This includes the falx and tentorium (Figure 4B and 4C). Similarly, extra-axial tumors do not have a blood–brain barrier and therefore readily take up contrast, including meningomas and cranial nerve tumors such as acoustic schwannomas (Figure 3). These tumors have a characteristic appearance—dense homogeneous enhancement with well-defined margins.

Acoustic schwannomas are occasionally evident on a noncontrast CT when they cause erosion of the petrous bone. However, small tumors are often only visible on MRI (Figure 5).

Patient Outcome

In this patient, the tumor could not be entirely resected because of its large size. After surgery, the patient had a partial right facial palsy and a sixth nerve palsy causing diplopia.

TABLE 1
_____

Intracranial Structures that Exhibit Contrast Enhancement

1. Vascular structures

    Normal: Major cerebral arteries (Circle of Willis), venous sinuses, and pial vessels on
    surface of cerebral cortex

    Abnormal: AVM, large aneurysms

2. Structures outside the blood–brain barrier

    Dura: Falx, tentorium

    Extra-axial tumors: Meningioma, cranial nerve tumor (homogeneous enhancement)

3. Intracerebral lesions whose vascular supply does not have an intact blood–brain barrier

    Tumors, Abscesses
    Enhancement typically often has a ring-like pattern—the surface of the lesion being is
    well vascularized and the central region poorly vascularized, necrotic or cystic.

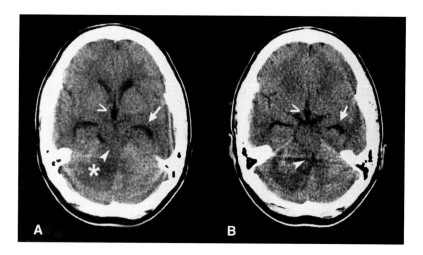

FIGURE 2   Noncontrast CT—Images 8 and 9.

A hypoattenuating mass in the posterior fossa (*asterisk*) compresses the quadrigeminal plate cistern (*arrowhead* in A) and the fourth ventricle (*arrowhead* in B).

There is mild hydrocephalus with dilation of the temporal horns of the lateral ventricles—the "Juan Valdez sign" (*arrows*) and the infundibulum of the third ventricle (*open arrowheads*).

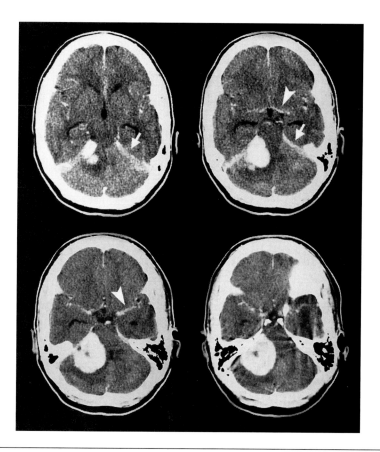

FIGURE 3   Contrast CT.

Homogeneous enhancement is characteristic of an extra-axial tumor such as an acoustic schwannoma or meningioma that does not have a blood-brain barrier. In this patient, the tumor is compressing the brainstem and displacing the fourth ventricle towards the left.

Contrast is seen within larger cerebral blood vessels of the circle of Willis (*arrowheads*). Enhancement of the falx and tentorium is normal (*arrows*).

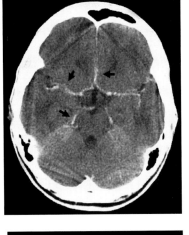

(A) Normal blood vessels.
Major cerebral arteries at the base of the brain—the anterior, middle, and posterior cerebral arteries of the circle of Willis (*arrows*).

(B) Abnormal blood vessel.
Large ophthalmic artery aneurysm (*arrow*).
Enhancement of tentorium is normal (*arrowheads*).

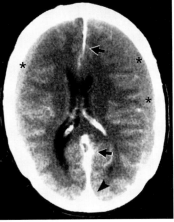

(C) Enhancement of pial vessels on the surface of the brain aids visualization of bilateral isodense subdural hematomas (*asterisks*).
Enhancement of the falx (*arrows*) and superior sagittal sinus (*arrowhead*) is normal.

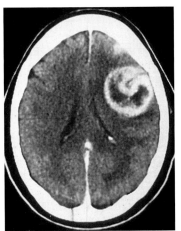

(D) Ring enhancement—Glioblastoma.
Enhancement occurs on the surface of the lesion that is perfused by blood vessels without an intact blood–brain barrier. The central region has diminished vascularity or is necrotic and therefore does not enhance.
The patient presented with a new-onset focal seizure.

FIGURE 4   Intracranial structures that exhibit contrast enhancement.
Structures that enhance include normal and abnormal blood vessels (A, B, C), intracranial structures that do not have a blood–brain barrier such as the falx, tentorium, and extra-axial tumors (B, C), and intracerebral tumors perfused by blood vessels that lack a blood–brain barrier (D).

Other examples of the role of contrast enhancement in the diagnosis of intracranial disorders include cerebral venous sinus thrombosis (Patient 5, Figure 6 on page 475), AVM (Chapter VI-6, Figures 5 and 7 on page 482), and brain abscess (Patient 7, Figures 8 and 9 on page 491).

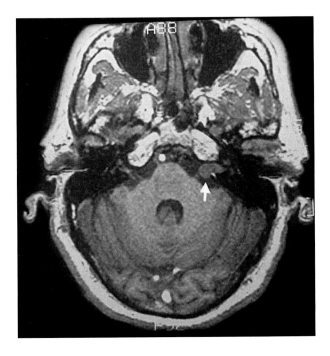

FIGURE 5   MRI of another patient showing a small acoustic schwannoma (*arrow*). This lesion would be impossible to detect by CT.
The patient presented with left-sided hearing loss, tinnitus, and slight unsteadiness with tandem gait.

Head CT: Patient 9

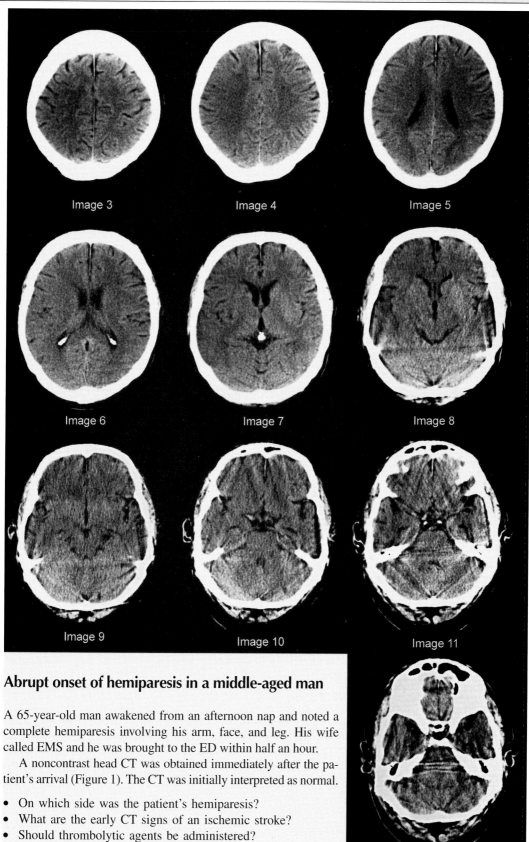

Image 3   Image 4   Image 5

Image 6   Image 7   Image 8

Image 9   Image 10   Image 11

FIGURE 1

Abrupt onset of hemiparesis in a middle-aged man

A 65-year-old man awakened from an afternoon nap and noted a complete hemiparesis involving his arm, face, and leg. His wife called EMS and he was brought to the ED within half an hour.

A noncontrast head CT was obtained immediately after the patient's arrival (Figure 1). The CT was initially interpreted as normal.

- On which side was the patient's hemiparesis?
- What are the early CT signs of an ischemic stroke?
- Should thrombolytic agents be administered?

BRAIN ATTACK

The principal role of CT in patients with a stroke is to exclude intracranial hemorrhage (10–15% of strokes) or other lesions such as a tumor, abscess, or SDH, which could be the cause of the patient's neurological deficit. CT has a limited ability to detect acute ischemic changes within 12–24 hours of onset, although subtle signs of early ischemia can be detected in a substantial proportion of patients, even within 3 hours of stroke onset. After 24 hours, CT is better able to detect an ischemic stroke because there is more pronounced cerebral edema.

With the advent of thrombolytic therapy for patients that present within 3 hours of stroke onset, CT plays two additional roles in emergency patient care. First, and foremost, CT detects hemorrhage, which is an absolute contraindication to thrombolytic therapy. Second, a large area of *early ischemic change* is considered by some clinicians to be a contraindication to the use of thrombolytic therapy because it is associated with an increased risk of hemorrhage. A third potential role of imaging would be to confirm the diagnosis of an acute ischemic stroke, although CT has a limited ability to do this.

CT Signs of Ischemic Stroke

There are **three stages** in the evolution of an ischemic stroke as depicted on CT.

Acute ischemic changes occur within 24 hours and may be visible within three hours of the onset of stroke. These early ischemic changes are due to *cytotoxic edema* that accumulates intracellularly. **Subacute** changes occur after 24 hours, peak in 3 to 5 days, and gradually subside over 1 to 4 weeks. They are due to *vasogenic edema* from leaky capillaries causing interstitial edema. **Chronic** changes evolve over 3 to 6 weeks, and eventually become permanent (Figures 2 and 3, and Table 1).

In an **earlier nomenclature,** early ischemic changes were not recognized and the first CT signs identified were those developing after 24 hours. These were termed "acute" (but are now termed "subacute"). When early ischemic changes were later recognized, they were termed "**hyperacute**" (i.e., occurring within 24 hours and now termed "acute"). This older terminology sometimes appears in radiologists' reports (e.g., the changes seen within the first 24 hours are referred to as "hyperacute").

Ischemic changes are localized to the territory of the involved vessel (Figure 4). Eighty percent of ischemic strokes involve the **middle cerebral artery** (MCA).

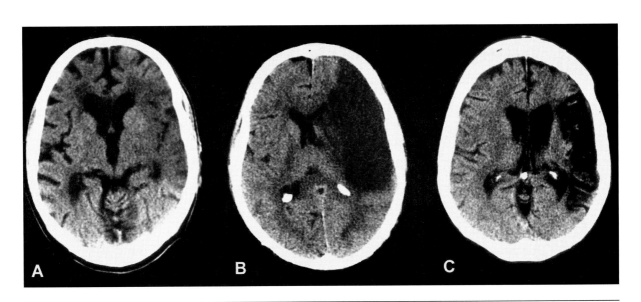

FIGURE 2   Evolution of a large left MCA stroke.

(*A*)   **Acute** (<24 hours)—**Cytotoxic edema** causes slightly decreased attenuation, loss of the normal gray/white interface, and effacement of the cortical sulci (slight mass effect).

(*B*)   **Subacute** (2–7 days)—**Vasogenic edema** in a well-demarcated wedge-shaped region of low attenuation. Considerable mass effect causes midline shift.

(*C*)   **Chronic** (months to years)—Infarct has very low attenuation (similar to CSF); diminished volume causes expansion of the adjacent lateral ventricle ("negative mass effect").

[From Schwartz DT, Reisdorff EJ: *Emergency Radiology.* McGraw-Hill, 2000.]

Acute Ischemic Changes The earliest anatomical change in ischemic brain tissue is **cytotoxic edema.** Ischemic cells are unable to maintain fluid homeostasis, resulting in intracellular edema (Figure 3A). Recent evidence suggests that such brain tissue is, for the most part, irreversibly ischemic, although a zone of potentially salvageable tissue may surround the irreversibly ischemic tissue. This reversibly ischemic tissue is referred to as the "ischemic penumbra" (Von Kummer 2005).

There are **three CT signs of cytotoxic edema** (Table 1, Figure 2A).

The principal CT finding is **loss of the normal differentiation between gray and white matter.** Cytotoxic edema predominantly affects gray matter, making it appear to have a similar attenuation to white matter. Second, there is mass effect, although it is minimal because the edema is limited to the intracellular space. Slight mass effect produces **effacement of the cortical sulci** (i.e., thining). Third, intracellular fluid accumulation causes **slight hypoattenuation** of the cerebral parenchyma (appears slightly darker).

Two subtle CT findings are due to loss of the normal gray/white matter differentiation. Loss of definition of the cortical gray matter in the region of the insula at the base of the Sylvian fissure is the "**insular ribbon sign.**" This is an early sign of an MCA infarction (Figure 6A). Loss of definition of the lentiform nucleus results in the "**disappearing basal ganglion sign**" (see Figure 9 below) (Saenz 2005).

Visualization of the gray/white interface can be improved using a very narrow window width, known as a "**stroke window**"—window width of 10 HU (Figure 6B) (Srinivasan et al. 2006).

Occasionally, a hyperdense thrombus is visible in the proximal portion of the MCA. This is known as the "**MCA sign**" (Figure 5).

Early CT signs of ischemia are often subtle, but usually identifiable, especially when a large vascular territory is involved. When the early ischemic changes involve one-third or less of the MCA territory, they are difficult to identify with certainty, even among experienced neuroradiologists.

Although early ischemic changes were formerly believed to be visible on CT only after 6 or more hours had elapsed from stroke onset, they can, in many cases, be seen within 3 hours. In the NINDS trial, 31% of patients with CT performed within 3 hours of the onset of stroke had early ischemic changes when the CT scans were carefully reviewed (Patel et al. 2001).

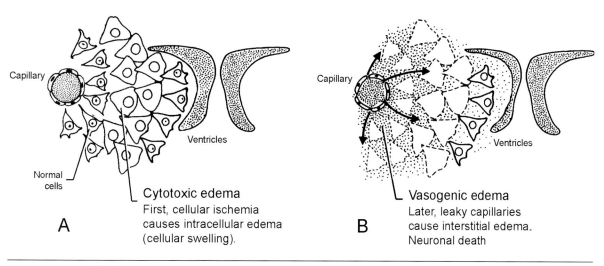

FIGURE 3 **Pathologic changes in ischemic stroke.**

(A) Acute (early) ischemic changes.

In the initial hours, there is cellular ischemia resulting in intracellular edema (**cytotoxic edema**) involving both gray and white matter.

(*B*) Subacute ischemic changes.

After 24 hours, capillary leak results in interstitial edema (**vasogenic edema**) causing greater mass effect (ventricular compression, midline shift).

[From Bradley WG: Magnetic resonance imaging of the central nervous system. *Neurol Res* 1984:6;91–106, with permission.]

Subacute Infarction   After 24 hours, capillary results in accumulation of edema in the interstitial spaces of the brain (Figures 2B and 3B). Edema due to capillary leakage is known as **vasogenic edema.** In the setting of an ischemic stroke, vasogenic edema involves both gray and white matter. The margins of the ischemic area are well-defined (Figures 2B and 4). Mass effect may be considerable and the risk of herniation is greatest at this stage.

Late Subacute Infarction   In some patients, after one week, as the edema subsides, there may be reperfusion of the infarcted brain tissue. The reperfused tissues can have attenuation similar to normal brain tissue and the CT at this stage may appear nearly normal. This transient appearance is called "fogging." In the older terminology, this stage was called "subacute infarction."

In some patients, reperfusion occurs predominantly at the cortical surface of the infarcted tissue. In these cases, the cortical surface has increased attenuation and the gray/white interface appears accentuated (Figure 7A). This can mimic the edema that surrounds a tumor or abscess (*peritumoral edema*). However, with peritumoral edema there is considerable mass effect, whereas with a late subacute stroke, there is minimal or no mass effect. This appearance may persist into the chronic stage.

When the distinction between late subacute stroke and a tumor is uncertain, intravenous contrast can be administered. Blood vessels in the reperfused areas of a stroke do not have an intact blood–brain barrier and the reperfused tissues therefore take up contrast. With cortical reperfusion, contrast enhancement has a "gyral pattern" (Figure 7B), which is distinct from the ring-enhancement pattern of a tumor or abscess.

Chronic Infarction   After 4 weeks, there is cellular resorption in the area of infarction, which develops an attenuation similar to CSF (Figure 2C). Loss of brain tissue causes compensatory enlargement of adjacent ventricles. This is referred to as "negative mass effect."

In cases, the cortical gray matter retains its normal attenuation and there is an accentuated gray/white interface. However, with an old stroke there is considerable volume loss which distinguishes it from peritumoral edema. Chronic strokes do not exhibit contrast enhancement, in contradistinction to late subacute strokes.

TABLE 1

CT Stages of Stroke

Acute—Onset to 24 hours (formerly termed "hyperacute")

    Cytotoxic edema—"early ischemic changes"

        Loss of gray/white matter differentiation
            Insular ribbon sign
            Disappearing basal ganglia sign (lentiform nucleus)
        Effacement of cortical sulci—slight mass effect
        Subtle low attenuation (especially of gray matter)

    Middle cerebral artery sign—thrombosis (hyperattenuating)

    Normal CT in 20–50% of patients

Subacute—24 hours to 7 days (formerly termed "acute")

    Vasogenic edema—Leaky capillaries

    Well-demarkated wedge-shaped area of low attenuation involving both gray and white matter
    Increasing edema causes marked mass effect, maximal at 3–5 days—risk of herniation

Chronic—3 weeks to years

    Resorption of infarcted brain tissue—attenuation similar to CSF
    Volume loss—ex-vacuo dilatation of the ventricle ("negative mass effect")
    In some cases, there is reperfusion at the cortical surface, which appears as an accentuated
    gray/white interface (Figure 7).

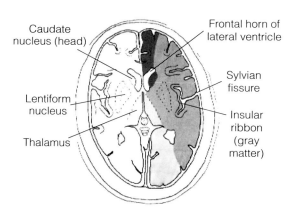

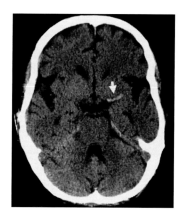

FIGURE 4   Vascular territories at the level of the basal ganglia.
Dark gray–anterior cerebral artery (ACA). Middle gray–Middle cerebral artery (MCA). Light gray–posterior cerebral artery (PCA).

FIGURE 5   MCA sign.
Hyperattenuating (thrombosed) left middle cerebral artery (*arrow*) in a patient with an acute stroke.

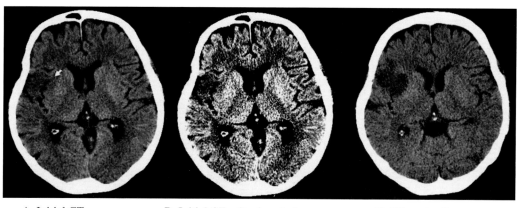

A. Initial CT   B. Initial CT—Stroke window   C. CT on day 2

FIGURE 6   Insular ribbon sign.

A 77-year-old woman presented to the ED three and a half hours after the onset of left arm weakness and dysarthria.

(*A*)   The initial CT shows loss of the normal gray/white differentiation in the anterior portion of the insula (*arrow*) and in the adjacent frontal cortex. The finding is subtle on the brain window. (Compare this to the normal gray/white interface of the opposite cerebral hemisphere.)

(*B*)   **Stroke window**—Using a very narrow window width (10 HU), the gray/white matter interface and the insular ribbon sign are more conspicuous.

(*C*)   The next day, the area of infarction was obvious.

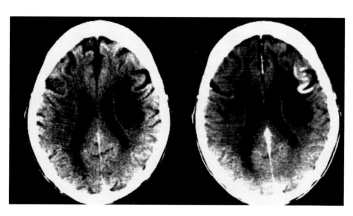

FIGURE 7   Cortical reperfusion—Late subacute infarction (2–4 weeks)

(*A*) Noncontrast CT shows an area of subcortical hypoattenuation. The reperfused cortical surface has an attenuation similar to normal gray matter. This causes an *accentuated gray/white interface*. Mild volume loss causes enlarged cortical sulci.

(*B*) Contrast CT shows enhancement of the superficial area of neovascularization in a **"gyral" pattern.**

[From Cwinn AA, Grahovac SZ: *Emergency CT Scans of the Head: A Practical Atlas.* Mosby, 1998, with permission.]

Patient Outcome

This patient presented with a complete left hemiparesis involving the face, arm, and leg due to a large right MCA territory infarction. The time of onset could not be accurately determined since the stroke was first noted when the patient awakened from a nap. Because the patient had last been seen more than 3 hours earlier, thrombolytic agents were not administered.

In addition, the stroke was severe and the initial CT showed extensive early ischemic changes involving the entire right MCA territory. Both factors augur a poor prognosis and some guidelines caution against using thrombolytic agents in such cases (see Appendix).

On images 4–6 of the patient's initial CT, there is slight hypoattenuation of the cerebral parenchyma, loss of normal the grey/white matter differentiation, and effacement of the cortical sulci (Figure 8).

On the slice that passes through the basal ganglia, there is hypoattenuation of the lentiform nucleus, in addition to the cortical ischemic changes (Figure 9). On image 10, the right MCA is hyperdense indicative of aproximal MCA thrombosis as the cause of the patient's stroke (Figure 10).

The following day, the patient deteriorated further. He was intubated and an emergency head CT revealed marked cerebral edema causing subfalcine and transtentorial herniation (Figure 11). The neurosurgery service was consulted regarding performing a decompressive craniectomy or hemicraniectomy in an heroic attempt to relieve the herniation. The neurosurgeons declined to undertake the procedure because of the patient's age and poor prognosis (Gupta et al. 2004). The patient expired the next day.

This has been termed a "malignant MCA stroke" owing to its grave prognosis.

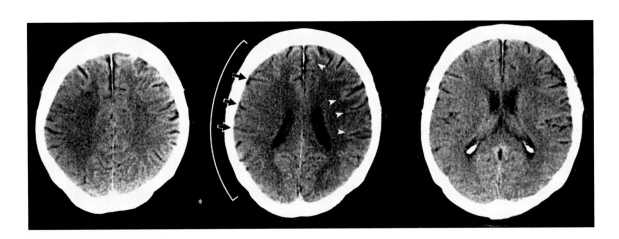

FIGURE 8   Initial CT (images 4-6) showing extensive early ischemic change in the right MCA territory

On the left cerebral hemisphere, the cortical gray–white differentiation is normal (*white arrowheads*).

On the right, there is loss of the gray–white differentiation over the entire right MCA territory (*curved white line*). The entire right MCA territory is slightly hypoattenuating, particularly the cortical gray matter. There is slight mass effect causing effacement (thinning) of the cortical sulci (*black arrows*).

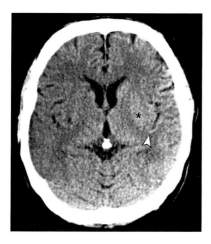

FIGURE 9   Initial CT—Image 7.

There is loss of the normal cortical gray/white differentiation over the entire right MCA territory.

The right lentiform nucleus is not visible—**disappearing basal ganglion sign**. The left lentiform nucleus (*asterisk*) and insular ribbon (gray matter stripe) (*arrowhead*) are normal.

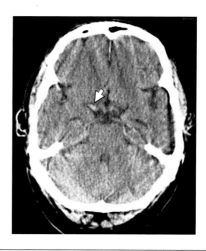

FIGURE 10   Initial CT—Image 10—MCA sign.

The right MCA is hyperattenuating (thrombosed) at the level of the suprasellar cistern (*white arrow*).

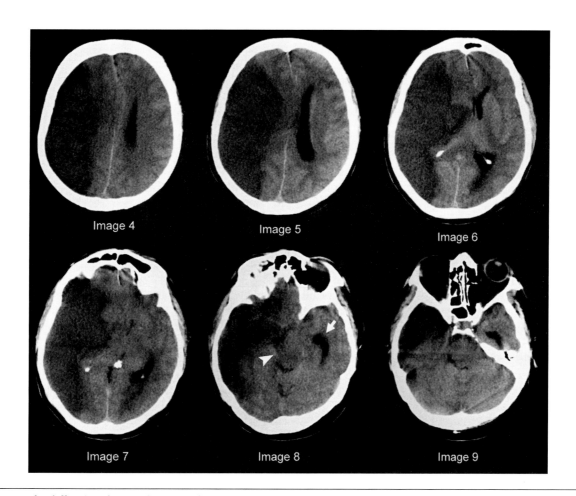

FIGURE 11   CT the following day—Subacute infarction and herniation, a "Malignant" MCA stroke.

There is marked cerebral edema involving the entire right MCA territory. Mass effect causes compression of the right lateral ventricle, midline shift (subfalcine herniation), and uncal (transtentorial) herniation compressing the midbrain and perimesencephalic cistern (*white arrowhead*).

Obstructive hydrocephalus due to compression of the third ventricle causes dilation of the temporal horn of the left lateral ventricle (*white arrow*).

THROMBOLYTIC THERAPY AND EARLY ISCHEMIC CHANGES

Although a hemorrhagic stroke is an absolute contraindication to thrombolytic therapy (Figure 12), early ischemic changes on CT have also been considered a contraindication to thrombolytic therapy when they involve more than one-third of the MCA territory. The NINDS trial found that patients with early ischemic changes involving >1/3 of the MCA territory did poorly and some clinical guidelines have excluded these patients from thrombolytic therapy (AAN 1996, AHA 2007) (see Appendix).

However, re-analysis of the NINDS trial data revealed that although patients with early ischemic changes tended to have poorer outcomes, they still appeared to benefit from, or at least were not harmed by, thrombolytic therapy (Patel et al. 2001). Nonetheless, the NINDS trial did not have sufficient statistical power to detect differences in subgroups of patients, e.g., those with early ischemic changes on CT (Ingall et al. 2004). This issue remains controversial.

In the European ECASS trial, the pilot study (ECASS I) found that patients with early ischemic changes involving more than one-third of the MCA territory had a higher incidence of intracranial hemorrhage and were therefore excluded from receiving thrombolytic therapy in the placebo-controlled randomized trial (ECASS II). The ECASS trial also differed from the NINDS trial in that patients were treated with recombinant tissue plasminogen activator (rt-PA) up to 6 hours after onset of symptoms, whereas in the NINDS trial, only patients who presented within three hours of stroke onset were treated. The ECASS trial did not find a benefit for thrombolytic therapy.

The ability of non-neuroradiologists to identify subtle CT findings of stroke has been a matter of concern. In a study by Schriger et at (1998), hemorrhages were missed in 18% of readings, even though these are absolute contraindications to thrombolytic therapy. Acute infarctions were missed even more frequently. Early infarctions (cytotoxic edema) were missed in over 50% of cases. This casts doubt on the ability of primary care givers to accurately determine the presence of contraindications to thrombolytic therapy on CT. Better education in recognizing signs of stroke on CT could improve these results.

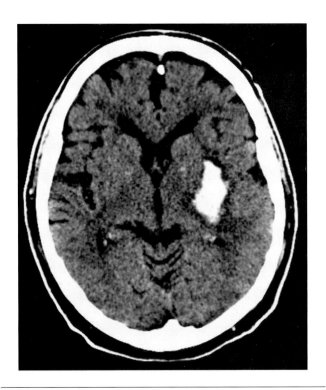

FIGURE 12   Acute hemorrhagic stroke.
The patient presented less than three hours after onset of a right hemiparesis. The CT showed a large basal ganglion bleed.

APPENDIX:

RECOMMENDATIONS FOR THROMBOLYTIC TREATMENT IN ACUTE ISCHEMIC STROKE

Intravenous rt-PA is the recommended treatment within three hours of onset of ischemic stroke. Intravenous rt-PA is not recommended when the time of onset of stroke cannot be ascertained reliably. This includes persons whose strokes are recognized upon awakening.

The diagnosis of stroke must be established by a physician who has expertise in making this diagnosis. A physician who is expert in reading CT scans of the brain must assess the imaging study.

If the CT demonstrates early changes of a recent major infarction, such as sulcal effacement, mass effect, edema, or possible hemorrhage, thrombolytic therapy should be avoided (AAN 1996).*

Thrombolytic therapy is not recommended for persons who have one of the following reasons for exclusion from the NINDS study (1995):

A. Another stroke or any serious head injury in the previous 3 months
B. Prior intracranial hemorrhage
C. Neurological signs that are improving rapidly
D. Isolated mild neurological deficits
    such as ataxia alone, sensory loss alone,
    dysarthria alone, or minimal weakness
E. Seizure at the onset of stroke
F. Major surgery within the preceding 14 days
G. Gastrointestinal or urinary bleeding within the preceding 21 days
H. Recent myocardial infarction
I. Pretreatment systolic blood pressure >185 or diastolic >110
J. Blood glucose <50 or >400
K. Current use of oral anticoagulants or a PT >15 seconds (INR >1.7)
L. Use of heparin in the previous 48 hours and a prolonged PTT
M. Platelet count <100,000

Caution is advised before giving intravenous rt-PA to persons with severe stroke (NIH Stroke Scale >22) (e.g., complete right hemiparesis with aphasia, visual field loss, gaze deviation, and sensory loss = 25) (AAN 1996). *

Because the use of thrombolytic drugs carries the risk of major bleeding, the risks and potential benefits of rt-PA should be discussed whenever possible with the patient and family before treatment is initiated.

From: Quality Standards Subcommittee of the American Academy of Neurology (AAN): Practice advisory: Thrombolytic therapy for acute ischemic stroke: Summary statement. *Neurology* 1996;47:935–839.

See also: Adams HP, del Zoppo G, Alberts MJ, et al: Guidelines for the early management of adults with ischemic stroke: A guideline stroke: A guideline from the American Heart Association/ American Stroke Association Stroke Council. Stroke 2007;38:1655–1711

---

*Although the risk of intracranial hemorrhage and poor outcome was greater in patients with severe stroke or early ischemic changes on CT, the overall benefit of rt-PA included patients with severe stoke and early ischemic changes on CT. There is no evidence to support withholding rt-PA in such patients, although the NINDS trial did not have sufficient statistical power to detect differences between subgroups of patients, e.g. those with early ischemic changes on CT and those with severe stroke (Ingall 2004).

Four factors were associated with an increased risk of intracranial hemorrhage, especially when two or more were present: age >70 years, baseline NIH Stroke Scale >20, serum glucose > 300 mg/dL, and edema or mass effect on the initial CT scan. However, there was no statistically significant evidence that the risk of rt-PA outweighed the benefit.

SUGGESTED READING

Cwinn AA, Grahovac SZ: *Emergency CT Scans of the Head: A Practical Atlas.* Mosby, 1998.

Huddle D, Chaney D, Glazer M: Emergency imaging of the brain. In: Schwartz DT, Reisdorff EJ, eds. *Emergency Radiology.* McGraw-Hill, 2000.

Latchaw RE, Kucharczyk J, Moseley ME (eds): *Imaging of the Nervous System.* Elsevier-Mosby, 2005.

Lee SH, Rao KCVG, Zimmerman RA: *Cranial MRI and CT,* 4th ed. McGraw-Hill, 1999.

van der Worp HB, van Gijn J: Acute ischemic stroke. *New Engl J Med* 2007;357:572–579

CT Signs of Stroke

Burdette JH, Elster AD: Cerebral infarction diagnosis by computerized tomography: Analysis and evaluation of findings-How far have we really come? *AJR* 2006;186:611–612.

Kalafut MA, Schriger DL, Saver JL, Starkman S: Detection of early CT signs of >1/3 middle cerebral artery infarctions: Inter-rater reliability and sensitivity of CT interpretation by physicians involved in acute stroke care. *Stroke* 2000;31:1667–1671.

Moulin T, Cattin F, Crepin-Leblond T, et al.: Early CT signs in acute middle cerebral artery infarction: predictive value for subsequent infarct locations and outcome. *Neurology* 1996;47:366–375.

Schriger DL, Kalafut M, Starkman S, et al.: Cranial computed tomography interpretation in acute stroke: physician accuracy in determining eligibility for thrombolytic therapy. *JAMA* 1998;279: 1293–1297.

Srinivasan A, Goyal M, Al Azri F, Lum C: Imaging of acute stroke. *RadioGraphics* 2006;26:S75–S95.

Von Kummer R: Computed tomography. In: Latchaw RE, Kucharczyk J, Moseley ME, eds. *Imaging of the Nervous System.* Elsevier-Mosby, 2005, pp. 199–213.

Wardlaw JM, Farrall AJ, Perry D, et al for the Acute Cerebral CT Evaluation of Stroke Study (ACCESS) Study Group: Factors influencing the detection of early CT signs of cerebral ischemia: An internet-based, international multiobserver study. *Stroke* 2007;38:1250–1256.

Wardlaw JM, Mielke O: Early signs of brain infarction at CT: Observer reliability and outcome after thrombolytic treatment. *Radiology* 2005;235:444–453.

Weingarten K: Computed tomography of cerebral infarction. *Neuroimaging Clin North Am* 1992;2:409–419.

Thrombolytic Therapy for Acute Stroke

Adams HP, del Zoppo G, Alberts MJ, et al: Guidelines for the early management of adults with ischemic stroke: A guideline from the American Heart Association/ American Stroke Association Stroke Council. *Stroke* 2007;38:1655–1711.

Hacke W, Kaste M, Fieschi C, et al. for the Second European-Australasian Acute Stroke Study Investigators: Randomised double-blind placebo-controlled trial of thrombolytic therapy with intravenous alteplase in acute ischemic stroke (ECASS II). *Lancet* 1998;352:1245–1251.

Hacke W, Kaste M, Fieschi C, et al.: Intravenous thrombolysis with recombinant tissue plasminogen activator for acute hemispheric stroke: the European Cooperative Acute Stroke Study (ECASS I). *JAMA* 1995;274:1017–1025.

Ingall TJ, O'Fallon WM, Asplund K, Goldfrank LR, et al.: Findings from the reanalysis of the NINDS tissue plasminogen activator for acute ischemic stroke treatment trial. *Stroke* 2004;35: 2418–2424.

Kwiatkowski TG, Libman RB, Frankel M, et al.: Effects of tissue plasminogen activator for acute ischemic stroke at one year. *N Engl J Med* 1999;340:1781–1787.

Marler JR, Tilley BC, Lu M, et al.: Early stroke treatment associated with better outcome: The NINDS rt-PA Stroke Study. *Neurology* 2000;55:1649–1655.

NINDS rt-PA Stroke Study Group: Tissue plasminogen activator for acute ischemic stroke. *N Engl J Med* 1995;333:1581–1587.

Quality Standards Subcommittee of the American Academy of Neurology (AAN): Practice advisory: thrombolytic therapy for acute ischemic stroke: summary statement. *Neurology* 1996;47: 935–839.

The ATLANTIS, ECASS, and NINDS rt-PA Study Group Investigators: Association of outcome with early stroke treatment: Pooled analysis of ATLANTIS, ECASS, and NINDS rt-PA stroke trials. *Lancet* 2004;363:768–774.

Early Ischemic Changes and Thrombolytic therapy

Davis SM, Donnan GA: CT screening for thrombolysis: Uncertainties remain. *Stroke* 2003;34:822–823.

Lyden P: Early major ischemic changes on computed tomography should not preclude use of tissue plasminogen activator. *Stroke* 2003;34:821–822.

Patel SC, Levine SR, Tilley BC, et al for the NINDS and rt-PA *Stroke* Study Group: Lack of clinical significance of early ischemic changes on computed tomography in acute stroke. *JAMA* 2001;286:2830–2838. Correspondence: *JAMA* 2002;287:2361–2362.

von Kummer R: Early major ischemic changes on computed tomography should preclude use of tissue plasminogen activator. *Stroke* 2003;34:82–821.

Thrombolytic therapy - Controversy

ACEP Board of Directors. Use of Intravenous tPA for the Management of Acute Stroke in the Emergency Department. http://www.acep.org/webportal/PracticeResources/PolicyStatements/pracmgt/UseofIntravenoustPAforAcuteStroke.htm

Caplan LR: Treatment of acute stroke: Still struggling. *JAMA* 2004;292 1883–1885.

Hoffman JR: Annals supplement on the American Heart Association proceedings, *Ann Emerg Med* 2001;38: 605

Lyden PD, Lees KR, Davis SM: Alteplase for acute stroke revisited: the first 10 years. *Lancet Neurology* 2006; 5: 722–724.

Mann J: Truths about the NINDS study: Setting the record straight. West *J Med* 2002; 176: 192–194.

Silbergleit R, Scott PA: Thrombolysis for acute stroke: The incontrovertible, the controvertible and the uncertain. *Acad Emerg Med* 2005;12:348–351.

Trotter G: Why were the benefits of tPA exaggerated? *West J Med* 2002: 176: 194–198.

Wardlaw JM, Lindley RI, Lewis S: Thrombolysis for acute ischemic stroke: Still a treatment for the few by the few. *West J Med* 2002; 176: 198–199.

Hemicraniectomy for Herniation Due to Stroke

Gupta R, Connolly ES, Mayer S, Elkind MSV: Hemicraniectomy for massive middle cerebral artery territory infarction: A systematic review. *Stroke* 2004;35:539–543.

Vahedi K, Hofmeijer J, Juettler E, et al: Early decompressive surgery in malignant infarction of the middle cerebral artery: A pooled analysis of three randomised controlled trials. *Lancet Neurol* 2007: 6:215–222.

Head CT: Patient 10

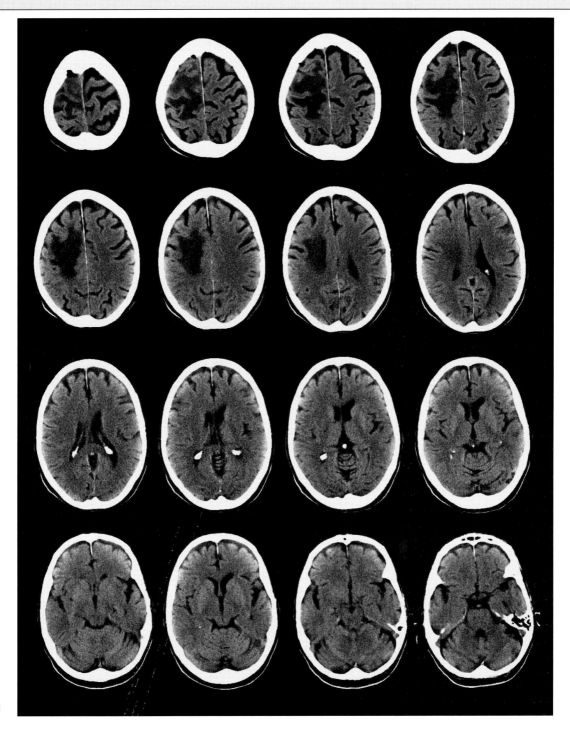

FIGURE 1

Left-sided weakness that began six days earlier in an elderly woman

An 84-year-old woman was admitted to another hospital 4 days earlier for weakness of her left arm and leg that had begun 2 days prior to that admission. A head CT was performed and she was diagnosed as having a stroke. Her family became concerned that "nothing was being done." They signed her out of that hospital and transported her to the ED.

The CT obtained in the ED is shown in Figure 1.

- What was the patient's likely diagnosis?
- What other tests are needed to confirm the diagnosis?

NOT A STROKE

Although this patient presented with a focal neurological deficit and the CT showed cerebral edema in the corresponding region of the right cerebral hemisphere, the patient's disorder was *not* an ischemic stroke. The subcortical white mater has a very low attenuation, while the gray matter is relatively normal in appearance. There is an **accentuation of the gray/white matter interface,** as opposed to the loss of the gray/white interface seen with an acute ischemic stroke (cytotoxic edema) (Figure 2, and see also Patient 9).

In addition, there is considerable **mass effect** due to the cerebral edema, although its effect is moderated by the patient's underlying age-related cerebral atrophy. The cortical sulci are effaced in comparison to the wide cortical sulci and atrophic gyri of the opposite cerebral hemisphere. The right lateral ventricle is compressed, although there is no midline shift (Figure 2).

This is the typical appearance of cerebral edema associated with tumors and abscesses and is known as **peritumoral vasogenic edema.** Tumor angiogenesis promotes the formation of immature blood vessels with abnormal permeability that leak edema into the surrounding interstitial tissues (Figure 3). The edema spreads extensively along white matter tracts, but does not enter the gray matter due to the tight junctions between the cells of the cortical gray matter. The interstitial spaces can accommodate a considerable amount of fluid, which causes pronounced mass effect and hypoattenuation in contrast to cytotoxic edema, which accumulates intracellularly.

The blood vessels that supply the tumor or abscess do not have an intact blood–brain barrier. Therefore the underlying lesion will enhance following the administration of intravenous contrast material. Enhancement is often limited to the periphery of the lesion whereas the central region is avascular or necrotic—**ring enhancement** (Figure 4).

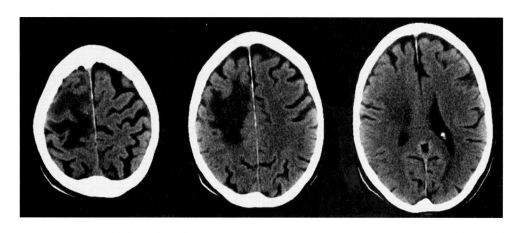

FIGURE 2   Patient 10—Noncontrast CT.

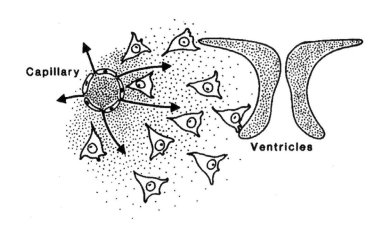

FIGURE 3   Pathogenesis of vasogenic edema.
Leaky capillaries cause increased fluid in the extracellular (interstitial) space.
Edema surrounding a tumor or abscess is confined to white matter.
[From Bradley WG: Magnetic resonance imaging of the central nervous system. *Neurol Res* 1984;6:91–106, with permission.]

Peritumoral edema must be distinguished from edema due to a stroke because the treatment of a tumor or abscess differs substantially from that of a stroke. In addition, corticosteroids can effectively reduce mass effect due to peritumoral edema and can, at least temporarily, avert progression to irreversible herniation.

The CT appearance of peritumoral edema and a stroke differ substantially (Table 1). With an **acute stroke** (cytotoxic edema), there is minimal mass effect and obliteration of the normal gray/white differentiation, whereas with **peritumoral edema,** there is considerable mass effect and accentuation of the gray/white interface (see Patient 9, Figure 3 on page ●). A **subacute stroke** (>24 hours) also produces marked mass effect due to leaky capillaries (vasogenic edema), although it involves both gray and white matter because of the antecedent cellular ischemia and infarction.

A **chronic or late subacute stroke with cortical reperfusion** can mimic peritumoral edema because both have accentuation of the gray–white interface (see Patient 9, Figure 7 on page ●). However, with an old stroke there is volume loss, whereas with a tumor there is mass effect due to vasogenic edema. If the diagnosis is uncertain, a contrast CT or MRI can be used to differentiate these two disorders. A subacute infarction with cortical reperfusion exhibits a *gyral* pattern of enhancement, whereas with tumors or abscesses, the mass lesion itself will enhance (Figure 4B, and Patient 9, Figure 7B). Chronic stokes do not show contrast enhancement.

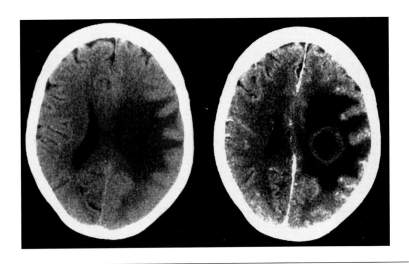

FIGURE 4   **Vasogenic (peritumoral) edema due to a glioma.**

(A) **Noncontrast scan** showing low attenuation edema confined to the white matter. This results in *accentuation* of the gray/white interface. Mass effect is considerable and completely obliterates the lateral ventricle.

(B) **Contrast scan** reveals a ring-like pattern of enhancement of the tumor.

Enhancement of the surface of the tumor is due to neovascularization by immature vessels without an intact blood-brain barrier. The central portion of the tumor is avascular and nonenhancing.

[From Schwartz DT, Reisdorff EJ: Emergency Radiology. McGraw-Hill, 2000.]

TABLE 1

Comparison of Cytotoxic and Peritumoral Vasogenic Edema

	CYTOTOXIC EDEMA	PERITUMORAL EDEMA
Pathology	Cellular ischemia causes neuronal swelling—intracellular edema	Capillary leak causes fluid accumulation in interstitial spaces
Gray/white interface	Diminished—edema involves gray and white matter	Accentuated—edema limited to white matter
Attenuation	Slightly decreased	Markedly decreased
Mass effect	Slight—effacement of cortical sulci	Considerable

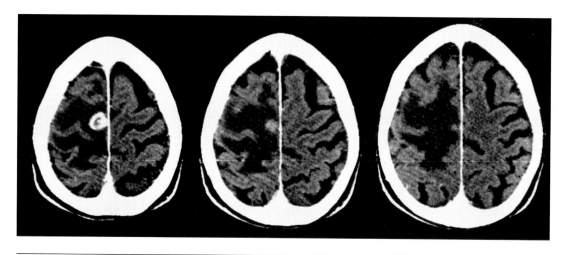

FIGURE 5   Patient 10—Contrast CT.
A ring-enhancing lesion is seen in the superior parietal region. There is extensives urrounding vasogenic edema.

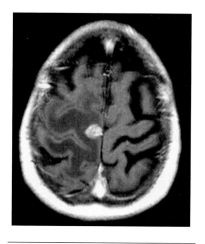

FIGURE 6   T1-weighted MRI.
Following administration of gadolinium-based contrast, the lesion and surrounding edema are visible.

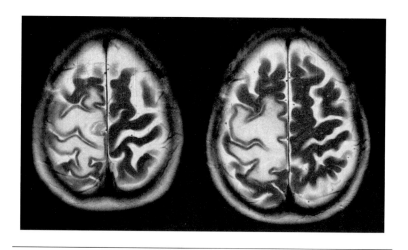

FIGURE 7   T2-weighted MRI.
Extensive vasogenic edema limited to the subcortical white matter has a high signal intensity (appears white). CSF also has high signal intensity and is seen filling the cortical sulci.

Patient Outcome

In this patient, the cerebral edema was correctly recognized as being due to an intracerebral mass rather than an evolving infarction. Contrast CT and MRI revealed a ring-enhancing lesion within the area of vasogenic edema (Figures 5–7). Further evaluation determined that the mass was a metastasis from a primary lung tumor. The patient was treated with dexamethasone and cranial radiation therapy.

Fitzpatrick reported two similar cases of patients with cerebral abscesses that were misdiagnosed as ischemic strokes. In both cases, diagnostic and treatment delay resulted in neurological deterioration. Noncontrast CT findings were characteristic of a mass rather than an infarction with accentuation of the gray/white interface and mass effect. The author advocates obtaining contrast CT in such cases, although misinterpretation of the noncontrast CT contributed to the diagnostic error.

The clinical characteristics of each patient were also not typical for an ischemic stroke. In one, the patient presented with a seizure and Todd's paralysis that gradually resolved. The second patient presented with an acute neurological deficit accompanied by a low-grade fever and altered mental status. The focal neurological deficits improved in both patients and they were discharged from the hospital after a brief admission. Each patient returned 2–3 weeks later after experiencing significant neurological deterioration. Marked mass effect caused transtentorial herniation in both cases.

Fitzpatrick MO, Gan P: Contrast enhanced computed tomography in the early diagnosis of cerebral abscess. *BMJ* 1999;319:239–240.

Head CT: Patient 11

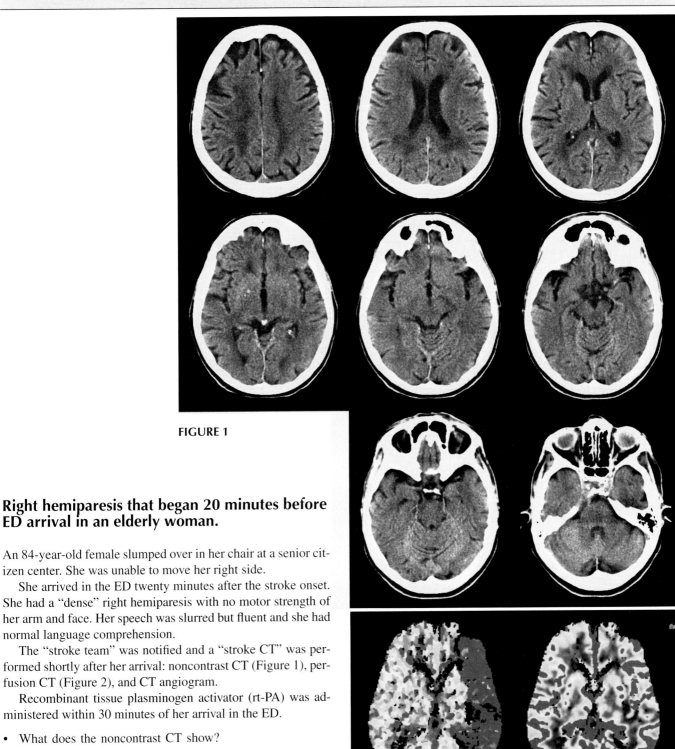

FIGURE 1

Right hemiparesis that began 20 minutes before ED arrival in an elderly woman.

An 84-year-old female slumped over in her chair at a senior citizen center. She was unable to move her right side.

She arrived in the ED twenty minutes after the stroke onset. She had a "dense" right hemiparesis with no motor strength of her arm and face. Her speech was slurred but fluent and she had normal language comprehension.

The "stroke team" was notified and a "stroke CT" was performed shortly after her arrival: noncontrast CT (Figure 1), perfusion CT (Figure 2), and CT angiogram.

Recombinant tissue plasminogen activator (rt-PA) was administered within 30 minutes of her arrival in the ED.

- What does the noncontrast CT show?

- What does the perfusion CT suggest about the potential benefit of thrombolytic therapy?

A. Time-to-peak   B. Cerebral blood volume

FIGURE 2   Perfusion CT
(same level as CT slice in upper right corner of Figure 1)

ADVANCED IMAGING MODALITIES IN STROKE

Several new CT and MR imaging modalities have been developed that could potentially improve acute stroke management (Table 1). The role of these tests include: (1) accurate early identification of an acute ischemic stroke; (2) distinguishing potentially salvageable ischemic brain tissue from irreversible ischemia (the ischemic penumbra); and (3) visualization of the vascular lesion responsible for the ischemic event. The benefits of these imaging modalities have yet to be proven in large clinical trials and their use remains experimental.

Early diagnosis of stroke can be made using diffusion-weighted MRI, perfusion CT and CT angiographic source images. Distinguishing potentially salvageable from irreversibly ischemic brain tissue can be accomplished using perfusion CT or perfusion-weighted MRI (Figure 2). Vascular lesions are demonstrated using CT angiography or MR angiography.

These imaging techniques may, in the future, help select patients for thrombolytic therapy. For example, early imaging confirmation of stroke would positively identify patients having an acute ischemic event and distinguish disorders that can occasionally mimic stroke such as a seizure or complicated migraine, for which thrombolytic therapy is not indicated.

More importantly, distinguishing patients with potentially salvageable brain tissue (an "**ischemic penumbra**") could identify those patients most likely to benefit from thrombolytic therapy, treat patients with unknown time of stroke onset, and possibly extend the therapeutic time limit beyond 3 hours in selected patients who have reversible ischemia (Figure 4).

Identification of an occlusive vascular lesion could also potentially guide stroke therapy. Patients that have discrete occlusion of a major cerebral vessel may benefit most from thrombolytic therapy. Intra-arterial administration of thrombolytics or mechanical clot removal using catheter angiography may be beneficial in patients presenting later than 3 hours if a large and accessible thrombus is identified. CT angiography can also identify an atherosclerotic lesion of the carotid artery as the source of an embolic stroke or total carotid occlusion (Thomas et al 2006).

CT is readily available in most emergency departments. Advances in CT scanner technology, particularly multidetector CT (MDCT), have enabled development of *perfusion CT* and *CT angiography* that use a contrast bolus to assess regional cerebral perfusion and vascular anatomy.

Specialized MR imaging sequences, particularly *diffusion-weighted MRI* and *perfusion-weighted MRI*, have also shown promise in early stroke diagnosis. *Gradient-echo MRI* is able to identify a hemorrhagic stroke with a sensitivity equal to noncontrast CT, allowing MRI to be used as the sole imaging modality in acute stroke. However, in most institutions, MRI is less readily available on an emergency basis.

TABLE 1

Advanced Imaging in Ischemic Stroke

Objective	Imaging Modality
Early diagnosis of stroke	Diffusion-weighted MRI, perfusion CT, CT angiographic source images
Distinguish potentially salvageable brain tissue from irreversibly ischemic tissue	Perfusion CT, perfusion-weighted MRI
Identify vascular lesion	CT angiography, MR angiography

Diffusion-Weighted MRI

Although MRI is generally more sensitive at detecting intracerebral lesions than noncontrast CT, standard MRI sequences (T1-weighted and T2-weighted) are insensitive at detecting early cerebral ischemia (<3–12 hours), i.e., cytotoxic (intracellular) edema. **Diffusion-weighted MRI** (DWI) can reliably detect early ischemic changes based on the different diffusion characteristics of intracellular and extracellular (interstitial) water. With early ischemic changes, intracellular edema (cytotoxic edema) is detected as an abnormal diffusion-weighted imaging signal (Figure 3).

DWI abnormalities are analogous to "acute ischemic changes" seen on noncontrast CT, although the imaging appearance is considerably more conspicuous.

The sensitivity of diffusion-weighted MRI for detecting an early ischemic stroke is 70 to 80% as compared to 30 to 50%

sensitivity of noncontrast CT (Mullins 2002). On the other hand, standard MRI, particularly fluid-sensitive imaging sequences such as T2-weighted and FLAIR (fluid-attenuated inversion recovery), is highly sensitive at detecting interstitial (vasogenic) edema, i.e., subacute stroke. The advantage of FLAIR over T2-weighted imaging is that with FLAIR, CSF has low signal intensity (appears dark) so that superficial cortical lesions are more easily detected (see Patient 10, Figure 7 on page 514).

Brain tissue exhibiting early ischemic changes (cytotoxic edema) is felt to be largely *irreversibly ischemic* and would therefore not benefit from thrombolytic therapy. However, adjacent cerebral tissue may be salvageable, i.e., the "ischemic penumbra".

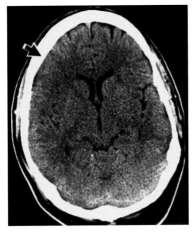 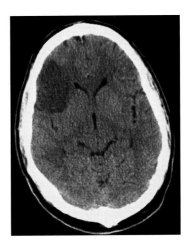

A. **Initial noncontrast CT**
Subtle loss of the gray/white interface in the right frontal region (*arrow*) representing early ischemic change—cytotoxic edema

E. **Noncontrast CT obtained 2 days later**
There is an evolving (i.e., subacute) infarct

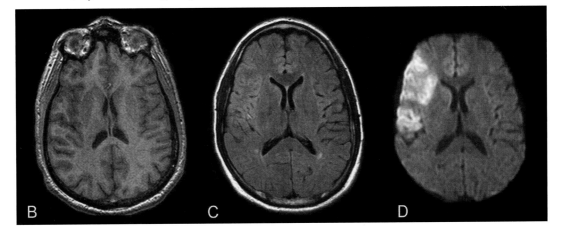

MRI performed within 1 hour of patient's arrival
B and C. T1-weighted and FLAIR images are nearly normal.
D. Diffusion-weighted MRI (DWI) shows early ischemia—cytotoxic edema.

FIGURE 3   Acute stroke confirmed by diffusion-weighted MRI.
A 39-year-old man presented with a left facial weakness that began 3 hours earlier after smoking crack cocaine. He also complained of left arm "tingling," but had a normal examination. A stat noncontrast CT was obtained that was interpreted as normal (A).

MRI was obtained to confirm that the facial palsy was a stroke

and not a peripheral seventh cranial nerve palsy. Due to the delay in presentation, thrombolytic agents were not administered.

The patient's facial paresis improved, but did not entirely resolve. Infarction was presumably due to vasospasm because no carotid artery lesion or cardiac source of embolism was found.

Perfusion CT

Perfusion CT is useful in the early diagnosis of ischemic stroke and is especially promising in distinguishing potentially salvageable brain tissue from irreversibly ischemic tissue – the "ischemic penumbra." Surrounding a "core" of irreversibly ischemic tissue is a zone of reversible ischemia that could potentially benefit from reperfusion therapy – the *ischemic penumbra* (Figure 4).

Penumbra Imaging   Tissue in the ischemic penumbra is not functioning (exhibits a neurological deficit) but is potentially salvageable because the severity and duration of ischemia has not yet caused irreversible injury. Cerebral perfusion is diminished but maintained at a level that permits neuronal recovery if perfusion is re-established.

In reversibly ischemic brain tissue, *cerebrovascular autoregulation* is preserved, i.e., cerebral arterioles dilate in response to ischemia. This maintains perfusion via collateral vessels. For example, if there is occlusion of the middle cerebral artery (MCA), perfusion at the periphery of the ischemic zone may be preserved by flow from vessels supplied by the anterior and posterior cerebral arteries (ACA and PCA) (Figure 4). However, perfusion to

this region is slightly delayed. This characteristic delay in perfusion is detected by perfusion imaging. When the tissue becomes irreversibly ischemic (the "ischemic core"), cerebrovascular autoregulation is lost and collateral perfusion is not maintained.

Perfusion imaging entails administration of a bolus of intravenous contrast. Normal tissues show prompt enhancement due to the appearance of contrast in the cerebral blood vessels. Reversibly ischemic tissues show a delay in the appearance of intravascular contrast because perfusion is via collateral vessels, but the total quantity of contrast delivered is maintained. Irreversibly ischemic tissue receives little or no contrast (Figure 5).

Perfusion CT – Technique   A rapid bolus of intravenous contrast is administered and repetitive CT images (one image per second) are obtained through one or two CT slices the level of the basal ganglia for the duration of the contrast bolus (30–40 seconds). These images show progressive opacification and then wash-out of the cerebral tissues (Figures 6D and 7C). The contrast material appears within the vasculature of the cerebral hemispheres; there is no enhancement of brain parenchyma itself (Tomandl 2003, Srinivasan 2006).

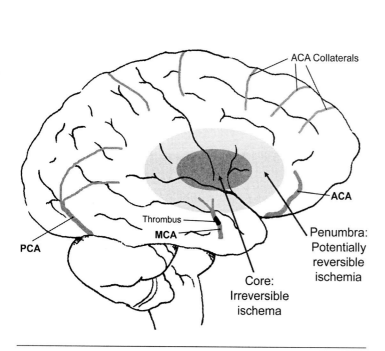

FIGURE 4   Acute stroke—Core and penumbra.

A core of irreversible ishemia is surrounded by a penumbra of reversibly ischemic (potentially salvageable) tissue.

Thrombotic occlusion of the middle cerebral artery (MCA) interrupts blood supply to the region of ischemia. Collateral flow from branches of the anterior and posterior cerebral arteries (ACA and PCA) maintains some perfusion at the periphery of the stroke so long as cerebrovascular autoregulation is intact.

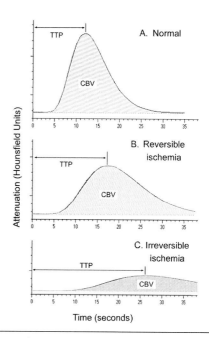

FIGURE 5   Time-Attenuation Curves.

Time-attenuation curves show the progressive opacification of brain tissue following a bolus of intravenous contrast.

(A) Normal timing of opacification = normal time-to-peak (TTP), and normal quantity of opacification – area under the time attenuation curve = normal cerebral blood volume (CBV).

(B) Potentially reversible ischemia – Opacification is delayed (increased TTP), but the total quantity of opacification is maintained (normal CBV).

(C) Irreversibly ischemic tissue – Opacification is very delayed and diminished.

Measurements are made of the timing and quantity of contrast opacification for each pixel of the CT slice. For each pixel, a plot is made of the opacification (attenuation in Hounsfield Units) over time—a **time-attenuation curve** (Figure 5). The rapidity of contrast opacification is expressed as the *time-to-peak* opacification (TTP) or *mean transit time* of the contrast bolus (MTT). The total quantity of opacification of the pixel over the duration of the contrast bolus (the area under the curve) represents the local *cerebral blood volume* (CBV). A third parameter, the local *cerebral blood flow* (CBF), is the CBV divided by MTT.

From these data, color-coded tomographic images (**perfusion maps**) are made for TTP, CBV, and CBF (Figures 6E-F and 7D-E). (The perfusion maps are shown here as shades of gray rather than colored).

Perfusion Maps As mentioned, the initial effect of arterial occlusion is delayed blood flow to the affected region of the brain. The blood arrives via collateral vessels in tissues with intact cerebrovascular autoregulation. On perfusion CT, this appears as a region of increased time-to-peak contrast opacification (TTP) (Figure 6E). However, the total quantity of contrast being delivered to this region of the brain is preserved, i.e., the cerebral blood volume (CBV) remains normal or nearly normal (Figure 6F). This characterizes *potentially salvageable* ischemic brain tissue – the **ischemic penumbra** (Figure 5B).

As ischemia persists or because of poor collateral circulation, the ability of the cerebral vasculature to maintain perfusion by reflex vasodilation is lost, and local cerebral blood flow and blood volume diminishes. On perfusion CT, there is diminished contrast opacification (decreased CBV) in addition to markedly delayed or absent opacification (increased TTP) (Figure 6D-E). This characterizes a region of *irreversible ischemia* – the **ischemic core** (Figure 5C). Irreversibly ischemic tissue is destined to undergo infarction, even if reperfusion occurs. The development of irreversible ischemia depends on the duration of ischemia, the severity of the vascular occlusion, and the abundance of collateral blood vessel.

Perfusion CT can thereby be used to assess the presence and extent of an ischemic penumbra. Tissue in the ischemic penumbra could theoretically benefit from reperfusion following the administration of a thrombolytic agent.

There are as yet no trials ongoing for perfusion CT. Cases have been reported demonstrating that perfusion CT can be successfully used to select patients for thrombolytic therapy when the time of stroke onset is unknown, either because it occurred during sleep, or because the patient had aphasia and could not communicate the time of stroke onset (Hellier 2006).

Early Stroke Diagnosis Perfusion CT also can serve to quickly confirm the diagnosis of an ischemic stroke. The perfusion images that show a region of poor perfusion (non-enhancement) confirms that the neurological deficit is due to a stroke and not a stroke mimic such as a seizure, complicated migraine or peripheral nerve disorder.

In a similar fashion, the **CT cerebral angiogram source images** can be used to demonstrate a region of non-perfusion (no contrast enhancement). This represents the ischemic core and can be used to confirm the diagnosis of ischemic stroke (Camargo 2007). An advantage of CTA is that the entire brain is imaged, not only one or two slices as in perfusion CT. The perfusion CT with perfusion maps are, however, needed to detect an ischemic penumbra.

Perfusion-weighted MRI

Perfusion-weighted MRI (PWI) is analogous to perfusion CT. Following an intravenous bolus of gadolinium-based contrast material, an image of the entire brain is obtained. A region of delayed perfusion (increased TTP), but normal diffusion on DWI – **perfusion/diffusion (PWI/DWI) mismatch** – defines an area of potentially reversible ischemia – anischemic penumbra. Regions of diffusion-weighted signal abnormality (cytotoxic edema) are irreversibly ischemic – the ischemic core.

The disadvantages of PWI relative to perfusion CT are that MRI scanners are not usually available on an emergency basis and the image acquisition time is greater for MRI than CT. One advantage of MRI is that it can provide perfusion imaging of the entire brain, and is not limited to one or two slices as is perfusion CT.

Studies are ongoing that use perfusion MRI to select patients for reperfusion therapy beyond the current three-hour time limit for rt-PA as defined by the NINDS trial (Albers 2006, Furlan 2006, Hacke 2005, Kohrmann 2006, Ribo 2005, Tomalla 2006).

Perfusion imaging and thrombolysis

Perfusion imaging (CT or MRI) could theoretically refine the selection of patients for thrombolytic therapy by identifying those with potentially salvageable ischemic brain tissue (Gonzalez 2006).

Patients with areas of delayed but maintained perfusion (increased TTP with preserved CBV on perfusion CT or a perfusion/diffusion mismatch on MRI) may be more likely to benefit from thrombolytic therapy (Figure 6). In addition, the currently accepted three-hour time limit could potentially be extended in such patients using intravent or intra-arterial thrombolysis or mechanical clot retrieval used instead. Perfusion imaging could also be used when the time of stroke onset is unknown (e.g., the patient awoke with a neurological deficit) to detect a region of reversible ischemia that could be treated with a thrombolytic agent. Finally, perfusion imaging might be able to identify patients with solely irreversible ischemia who, despite being within the three-hour time limit, would not benefit from rt-PA (e.g., due to poor collateral circulation).

Nonetheless, the role of these imaging modalities remains experimental and the use of thrombolytic therapy in acute stroke should adhere to the indications and contraindications established by the NINDS trial (see Patient 9, Appendix on page 509).

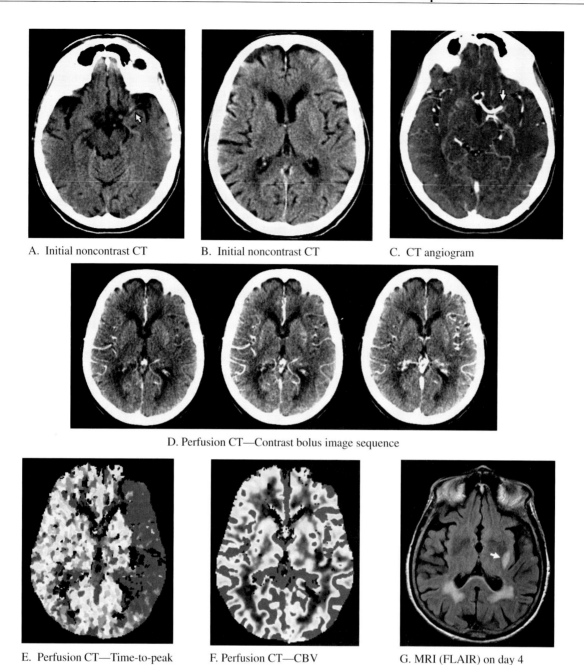

A. Initial noncontrast CT   B. Initial noncontrast CT   C. CT angiogram

D. Perfusion CT—Contrast bolus image sequence

E. Perfusion CT—Time-to-peak   F. Perfusion CT—CBV   G. MRI (FLAIR) on day 4

FIGURE 6   Patient 11 Outcome—Stroke reversal following administration of rt-PA.

(*A* and *B*) **Noncontrast head CT**—Normal aside from a hyperattenuating (thrombosed) left MCA (*arrow*).

(*C*) **CT angiography**—Complete occlusion of the proximal left MCA (*arrow*).

(*D*) **Perfusion CT (base images)**—Right MCA territory begins to opacify and reaches peak opacification before the left side. Opacification of the left MCA territory is delayed, but there is a nearly normal quantity of opacification over the entire duration of the contrast bolus. This indicates that cerebral blood volume is preserved by intact cerebrovascular autoregulation. (Only 3 of approximately 40 images are shown.)

(*E* and *F*) **Perfusion CT (perfusion maps)**—Delayed perfusion (increased time-to-peak–**TTP**) in a large area of the left MCA territory (dark gray), but only a small central area of slightly decreased cerebral blood volume (**CBV**). This is indicative of a large area of potentially salvageable ischemic brain tissue ("ischemic penumbra").

In Patient 11, recombinant tissue plasminogen activator (rt-PA) was administered within 30 minutes of her arrival. The right hemiparesis resolved within one hour upon completion of the rt-PA infusion. (It is also possible that recanalization would have occurred spontaneously without the administration of rt-PA.)

Three days later, **MRI** (*G*) revealed a small area of infarction limited to the left insula and external capsule (*arrow*).

(NB. The likely explanation for the patient's lack of aphasia on presentation despite her left brain ischemia was that she was left-handed and her language center was in the right cerebral hemisphere.)

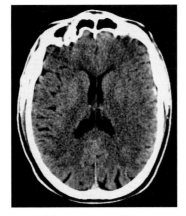

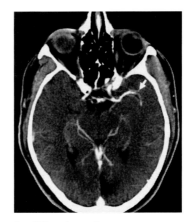

A. Initial noncontrast CT   B. CT angiography

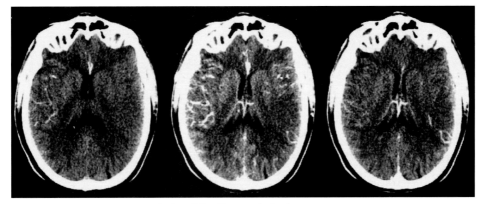

C. Perfusion CT—Contrast bolus image sequence

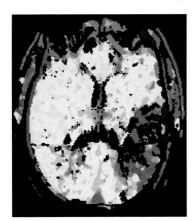

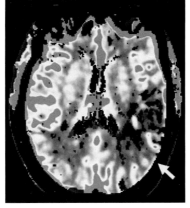

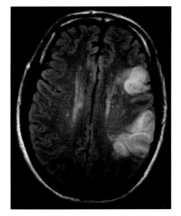

D. Perfusion CT—TTP   E. Perfusion CT—CBV   F. MRI (FLAIR) on day 3

FIGURE 7   Perfusion CT showing predominantly irreversible ischemia.

A 67-year-old attorney presented three and a half hours after the onset of right hemiparesis and aphasia.

(*A*) **Noncontrast CT**—Slight effacement of the cortical sulci in the left posterior MCA territory without loss of the gray/white interface.

(*B*) **CT angiography**—Narrowing of the left MCA (*arrow*) without complete thrombosis.

(*C*) **Perfusion CT (base images)**—Early opacification of the right cerebral hemisphere but delayed and nearly absent opacification of the posterior left MCA territory.

(*D* and *E*) **Perfusion CT (perfusion maps)**—Delayed time-to-peak (TTP) and diminished cerebral blood volume (CBV) in the posterior left MCA territory indicative of irreversible ischemia.

Because of the severity of the patient's neurological deficit and his arrival just after the 3-hour time limit for intravenous thrombolytic therapy, intra-arterial thrombolytics were administered via a left internal carotid artery catheter. However, the defect on the TTP map appeared only slightly larger than on the CBV map (*arrow*), suggesting only a small area of potentially salvageable tissue—a small ischemic penumbra.

There was some improvement in the patient's neurological deficit. Subsequent **MRI** (*F*) showed evolution of the infarction involving roughly the entire area of ischemia seen on the perfusion CT, i.e. little or no reduction in area of infarct.

SUGGESTED READING

Gonzalez RG: Imaging-guided acute ischemic stroke therapy: From "time is brain" to "physiology is brain". *AJNR* 2006;27:728–735.

Muir KW, Buchan A, von KR, et al: Imaging of acute stroke. *Lancet Neurol* 2006;5:755–768.

Mullins ME: Modern emergent stroke imaging: Pearls, protocols, and pitfalls. *Radiol Clin North Am* 2006;44:41–62.

Provenzale JM, Jahan R, Naidich TP, Fox AJ: Assessment of the patient with hyperacute stroke: Imaging and therapy. *Radiology* 2003; 229:347–359.

Srinivasan A, Goyal M, Al Azri F, Lum C: State-of-the-art: Imaging of acute stroke. *RadioGraphics* 2006;26:S75–S95.

Tomandl BF, Klotz E, Handschu R, et al: Comprehensive imaging of ischemic stroke with multisection CT. *RadioGraphics* 2003;23:565–592.

Thomas SH, Schwamm LH, Lev MH: Case records of the Massachusetts General Hospital. Case 16-2006. A 72-year-old woman admitted to the emergency department because of a sudden change in mental status. *N Engl J Med* 2006;354:2263–2271.

Vo KD, Lin W, Lee JM: Evidence based neuroimaging in acute ischemic stroke. *Neuroimag Clin North Am* 2003;13:167–183.

Perfusion CT

Eastwood JD, Lev MH, Provenzale JM: Perfusion CT with iodinated contrast material. *AJR* 2003;180:3–12.

Hellier KD, Hampton JL, Guadagno JV, et al: Perfusion CT helps decision making for thrombolysis when there is no clear time of onset. *J Neurol Neurosurg Psychiatr* 2006;77:417–419.

Hoeffner EG, Case I, Jain R, et al: Cerebral perfusion CT: Technique and clinical applications. *Radiology* 2004;231:632–644.

Hunter GJ, Hamberg LM: Computed tomography perfusion, in Latchaw RE, Kucharczyk J, Moseley ME (eds): Imaging of the Nervous System. *Elsevier-Mosby*, 2005, pp. 273–280.

Klosta SP, Nabavi DG, Gaus C, et al: Acute stroke assessment with CT: Do we need multimodal evaluation? *Radiology* 2004;233:79–86.

Muir KW, Halbert HM, Baird TA, et al: Visual evaluation of perfusion computed tomography in acute stroke accurately estimates infarct volume and tissue viability. *J Neurol Neurosurg Psychiatry* 2006; 77:334–339.

Shetty SK, Lev MH: CT perfusion in acute stroke. *Neuroimag Clin North Am* 2005;15:481–501

Wintermark M, Flanders AE, Velthuis B, et al: Perfusion-CT assessment of infarct core and penumbra: receiver operating characteristic curve analysis in 130 patients suspected of acute hemispheric stroke. *Stroke* 2006;37:979–985.

CT Angiography

Camargo ECS, Furie KL, Singhal AB, et al: Acute brain infarct: Detection and delineation with CT angiographic source images versus nonenhanced CT scans. *Radiology* 2007;244:541–548.

Sanelli PC, Mifsud MJ, Zelenko N, Heier LA: CT angiography in the evaluation of cerebrovascular diseases. *AJR* 2005;184:305–312.

Schaefer PW, Roccatagliata L, Ledezma C, et al: First-pass quantitative CT perfusion identifies thresholds for salvageable penumbra in acute stroke patients treated with intra-arterial therapy. *AJNR* 2006; 27:20–25.

Schramm P, Schellinger PD, Klotz E, et al: Comparison of perfusion computed tomography and computed tomography angiography source images with perfusion-weighted imaging and diffusion-weighted imaging in patients with acute stroke of less than 6 hours duration. *Stroke* 2004;35:1652–1658.

MRI

Davis DP, Robertson T, Imbesi SG: Diffusion-weighted magnetic resonance imaging versus computed tomography in the diagnosis of acute ischemic stroke. *J Emerg Med* 2006;31:269–277.

Lascola CD, Provenzale JM: Magnetic resonance imaging of cerebral ischemia, in Latchaw RE, Kucharczyk J, Moseley ME (eds): Imaging of the Nervous System. *Elsevier-Mosby*, 2005, pp. 215–226.

Makkat S, Vandevenne JE, Verswijvel G, et al: Signs of acute stroke seen on fluid-attenuated inversion recovery (FLAIR) MRI. *AJR* 2002;179:237–243.

Moseley ME, Bammer R: Diffusion-Weighted Magnetic Resonance Imaging, in Latchaw RE, Kucharczyk J, Moseley ME (eds): Imaging of the Nervous System. *Elsevier-Mosby*, 2005, pp. 227–236.

Mullins ME, Schaefer PW, Sorensen AG, et al: CT and conventional and diffusion-weighted MR imaging in acute stroke: Study in 691 patients at presentation to the emergency department. *Radiology* 2002;224:353–360.

MR Perfusion Imaging

Albers GW, Thijs VN, Wechsler L, et al. Magnetic resonance imaging profiles predict clinical response to early reperfusion: The Diffusion and Perfusion Imaging Evaluation for Understanding Stroke Evolution (DEFUSE) study. *Ann Neurol.* 2006;2560:508–517.

Bammer R, Moselely ME: Perfusion Magnetic Resonance and the Perfusion/Diffusion Mismatch, in Latchaw RE, Kucharczyk J, Moseley ME (eds): Imaging of the Nervous System. *Elsevier-Mosby*, 2005, pp. 303–313.

Butcher KS, Parsons M, MacGregor L, et al: Refining the perfusion-diffusion mismatch hypothesis. *Stroke* 2005;36:1153–1159.

Furlan AJ, Eyding D, Albers GW, et al. Dose escalation of desmoteplase for acute ischemic stroke (DEDAS): evidence of safety and efficacy 3 to 9 hours after stroke onset. *Stroke.* 2006;37:1227–1231.

Hacke W, Albers G, Al-Rawi Y, et al: The Desmoteplase in Acute Ischemic Stroke Trial (DIAS): a phase II MRI-based 9-hour window acute stroke thrombolysis trial with intravenous desmoteplase. *Stroke* 2005;36:66–73.

Kohrmann M, Juttler E, Fiebach JB, et al: MRI versus CT-based thrombolysis treatment within and beyond the 3 h time window after stroke onset: a cohort study. *Lancet Neurology* 2006;5:661–667

Lev MH, Koroshetz WJ, Schwamm LH, et al: CT or MRI for imaging patients with acute stroke: Visualization of "tissue at risk"? *Stroke* 2002;33:2736–2737.

Ribo M, Molina CA, Rovira A, et al. Safety and efficacy of intravenous tissue plasminogen activator stroke treatment in the 3 to 6-hour window using multimodal transcranial Doppler/MRI selection protocol. *Stroke* 2005;36:602–606

Schwab M, Fitzek C, Witte OW, Isenmann S: Extending the potential of perfusion imaging with MRI to prevent major stroke. *Lancet Neurol* 2007;6:102–104.

Seitz RJ, Meisel S, Weller P, et al: Initial ischemic event: Perfusion-weighted MR imaging and apparent diffusion coefficient for stroke evolution. *Radiology* 2005;237:1020–1028.

Thomalla G, Schwark C, Sobesky J, et al: Outcome and symptomatic bleeding complications of intravenous thrombolysis within 6 hours in MRI-selected stroke patients: Comparison of a German multicenter study with the pooled data of ATLANTIS, ECASS, and NINDS tPA Trials. *Stroke* 2006;37:852–85

INTRODUCTION TO FACIAL RADIOLOGY

Because the radiographic anatomy of the facial skeleton is complex, attempting to identify a fracture simply by looking for discontinuity or deformity of the facial bones is inefficient and may fail to identify the pertinent findings. Facial fractures are best detected by looking for specific injury patterns (tripod fracture, blow-out fracture, isolated zygomatic arch fracture, or LeFort fracture).

Fracture patterns are best understood by considering the main structural elements of the facial skeleton (Figure 1).

When to Order Facial Radiographs

Does every patient with a "black eye" need an imaging study? There are no clinical decision rules to guide the ordering of facial radiographs.

Many facial fractures can be diagnosed clinically, and signs of specific injuries serve as a guide to ordering facial imaging. Such clinical findings include: palpable deformity of the orbital rim or zygomatic arch (can be masked by soft tissue swelling), malar flattening, periorbital subcutaneous emphysema, infraorbital anesthesia, restriction of ocular motion (especially upward gaze), dental malocclusion, mobility of the maxilla (LeFort fractures), enophthalmus, proptosis, sagging of the lateral canthus, and telecanthus (widening of the intercanthal distance). However, patients with nondisplaced fractures may only have nonspecific clinical findings such as swelling or ecchymosis. Radiography is therefore indicated even without definite signs of a fracture. On the other hand, in patients with massive facial injuries that have a dramatic clinical appearance, the serious associated injuries must be given priority over radiography—namely, airway, intracranial, ocular, and cervical injuries.

In institutions where it is available on an emergency basis, **Multidetector CT** (MDCT) has supplanted facial radiography. Nonetheless, the anatomical landmarks and patterns of facial injury remain the same.

Structural Anatomy

The facial skeleton consists of three horizontal and three vertical supportive struts (Figure 1). Most facial fractures are oriented perpendicular to these supportive struts.

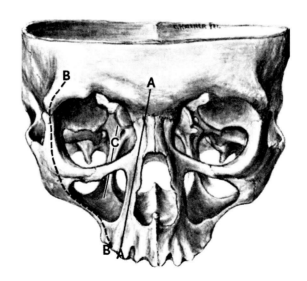

FIGURE 1   **Supportive struts of the facial skeleton.**

Three vertical struts: (A) nasal strut, (B) lateral orbital rim and lateral wall of the maxillary sinus, and (C) pterygoid plate (posterior).

Three horizontal struts: frontal bone (roof of the orbit), zygomatic arch and inferior orbital rim, and hard palate (maxilla).

The walls of the maxillary sinus and orbital floor are cut away in this illustration.

[From: Harris, et al: An approach to mid-face fractures. *Crit Rev Diagn Imaging* 1984;21:105–132. Copyright CRC Press, Boca Raton, FL.]

Facial Radiography

There are several standard radiographic views of the facial skeleton. These views are usually grouped into two radiographic series—a *facial series* and an *orbital series*.

The **facial series** includes a Waters view, a Caldwell view, a lateral view, and a submental-vertical view (bucket-handle view). The **orbital series** includes a Waters view, a Caldwell view, and two oblique orbital views.

The **Waters view** is the most important view and by itself is probably a sufficient screening radiograph for patients with facial injuries. Some authors suggest that only a Waters view be obtained, followed by a CT scan if any sign of injury is detected. When facial radiography is used as the initial imaging test, there is generally no need to obtain a CT scan in the ED because CT is not required to determine initial management. When MDCT is readily available, it can serve as the initial imaging study.

Waters view (Occipito-mental):   A PA projection with the face tilted upward about 40 degrees so that the petrous bones are projected inferior to the maxillary sinuses (Figures 2A and B). The maxillary sinuses are seen without overlapping shadows (Figure 3). The patient should be sitting or standing *upright* and the x-ray beam directed horizontally so that air/fluid level within the maxillary sinus can be seen (see Figure 8 on p. 527).

Caldwell view (Occipito-frontal):   A PA projection with the face tilted downwards about 15 degrees providing a view of the frontal sinuses, superior orbital rim, and ethmoid air cells (Figures 2C and 4).

Submental vertical view: The neck is hyperextended and the x-ray beam is directed from the inferior aspect of the chin to the top of the head (Figures 2D and 5). When underpenetrated ("**bucket-handle view**"), the zygomatic arches are projected free of overlap from the rest of the facial skeleton. When overpenetrated, the sphenoid sinus and maxillary sinuses are visible (**basal view**), although this is not useful for the assessment of facial trauma.

Lateral view: The anterior and posterior walls of the frontal sinus and the pterygoid plates (important for the diagnosis of LeFort fractures) are seen on this view. Due to overlap, most of the remaining facial structures are difficult to interpret (Figure 6).

Oblique orbital views: These views have a limited role in the trauma setting. Both the ipsilateral and contralateral lateral orbital rims (frontozygomatic sutures) are seen (Figure 7).

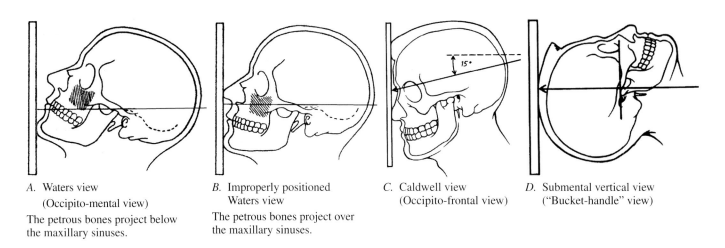

A. Waters view
     (Occipito-mental view)

The petrous bones project below the maxillary sinuses.

B. Improperly positioned
     Waters view

The petrous bones project over the maxillary sinuses.

C. Caldwell view
     (Occipito-frontal view)

D. Submental vertical view
     ("Bucket-handle" view)

FIGURE 2   Positioning for facial radiographs.

[A and B from Ballinger PW: *Merrill's Atlas of Radiographic Positions and Radiologic Procedures*, 8th ed. Mosby, 1995.
C and D from Schubert MJ: *Essentials of Medical Imaging Series: Patient Positioning*. McGraw-Hill, 1999.]

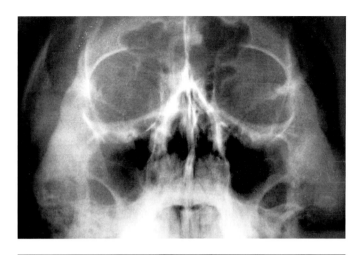

FIGURE 3A   Waters view.

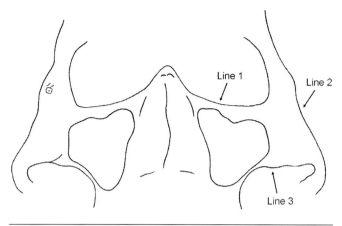

FIGURE 3B   Dolan's lines—Elephant's head in profile.

Aide to interpreting the Waters view

1. Nasion, inferior orbital rim, and lateral orbital rim (medial surface) (= elephant's ear)
2. Lateral orbital rim (= elephant's forehead) and zygomatic arch (lateral surface)
3. Zygomatic arch (medial surface) (= elephant's trunk) and lateral wall of the maxillary sinus (= elephant's chin)

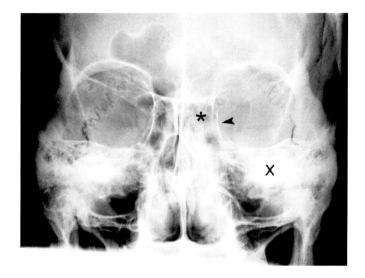

FIGURE 4   Caldwell view.

Medial orbital wall (*arrowhead*) and ethmoid air cells (*asterisk*).

Orbital floor is obscured by overlying petrous bones (X).

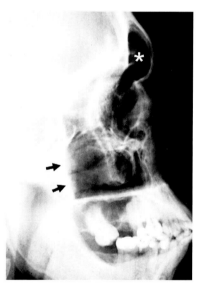

FIGURE 6   Lateral view.

Pterygoid *plates* (*arrows*).

Frontal sinus (*asterisk*).

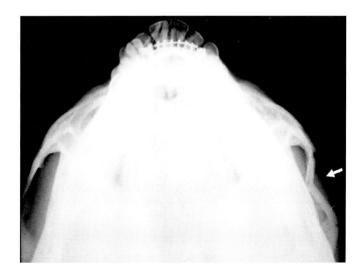

FIGURE 5   Submental-vertical view—Bucket-handle view.

Isolated depressed fracture of left zygomatic arch (*arrow*)

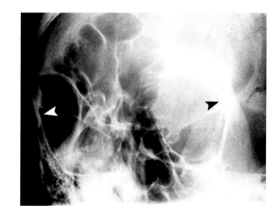

FIGURE 7   Oblique orbital view.

Lateral orbital rims (*arrowheads*).

HOW TO READ FACIAL RADIOGRAPHS

An **ABCS approach** can be tailored to facial radiography. Some factors are of great importance (e.g., soft tissue signs of injury), whereas others play a negligible role (e.g., cartilage, meaning joint spaces) (Table 1). Attempting to delineate every bone contour looking for a break or deformity is time consuming and potentially misleading. Instead, it is more efficient to focus on specific skeletal contours that are important for the diagnosis of facial fractures.

The first step is to judge the **adequacy** of the radiographs. The frontal views should not be rotated and in the Waters view, the petrous bones should project inferior to the maxillary sinuses.

Soft tissue signs of injury are important in identifying facial fractures. These include diffuse opacification due to overlying soft tissue swelling (a nonspecific finding), opacification of the maxillary sinus or ethmoid air cells, and air within the orbit (orbital emphysema). A Waters view should be performed with the patient in an upright position so that fluid (blood) in the maxillary sinus will form a distinctive and easily identified air/fluid level (Figure 8).

Next, the **bones** of the face are examined. **Dolan's lines** are the three principal skeletal contours on the Waters view. These three lines form an **elephant's head** in profile (Figure 3B).

In a complementary **targeted approach** to radiograph interpretation, specific injury patterns are sought. These include "blow-out" fractures of the orbital floor or medial orbital wall, tripod fractures (zygomaticomaxillary complex fractures—ZMC fractures), isolated zygomatic arch fractures (Figure 5), and Le Fort bilateral midface fractures.

TABLE 1

How to Read Facial Radiographs

Waters view (Figure 3)

    Adequacy
        Petrous bones projected inferior to the maxillary sinuses
        No rotation

    Soft tissue signs—often more conspicuous than bony abnormalities
        Periorbital soft tissue swelling (nonspecific)
        Maxillary sinus air/fluid level or opacification (Figure 8)
        Orbital emphysema

    Bones
        Dolan's lines (3)—Elephant's head in profile (Figure 3B)
            Lateral orbital rim (elephant's forehead)
            Inferior orbital rim (elephant's ear)
            Zygomatic arch (elephant's trunk)
            Lateral wall of the maxillary sinus (elephant's chin)
        Nasal septum (midline)

Caldwell view (Figure 4)
        Frontal sinuses and superior orbital rim
        Medial orbital wall (fracture)
        Ethmoid air cells (opacification due to blood)
        Lateral wall of the maxillary sinus (inferior portion)

SMV view—Zygomatic arch fracture (Figure 5)
        The zygomatic arch forms part of a rigid bony ring with the facial skeleton— when only a single zygomatic arch fracture is seen, there must be a fracture elsewhere, such as a tripod fracture

Lateral view (Figure 6)
        Pterygoid plates (LeFort fractures)
        Anterior and posterior walls of the frontal sinus

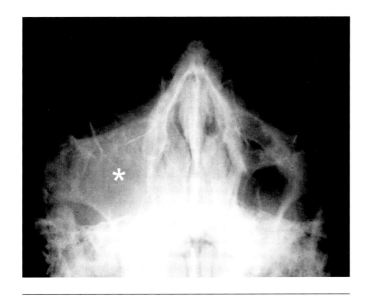

FIGURE 8A   Supine Waters view.
Opacification of right maxillary sinus (*asterisk*) may be due either to overlying soft tissue swelling or fluid in the sinus.

Computed Tomography

Axial Images   Thin sections (1–3 mm) oriented in a true transverse plane (Figures 9A and B). (Head CT slices which are in an oblique plane that is parallel to the base of the skull.)

Coronal Images   The neck is hyperextended and the slices are perpendicular to the axial images (Figures 9C and D). (The cervical spine must be "cleared" before obtaining this view.) The patient should be in a prone position, if possible, so that blood in the maxillary sinus collects inferiorly and orbital floor frac-

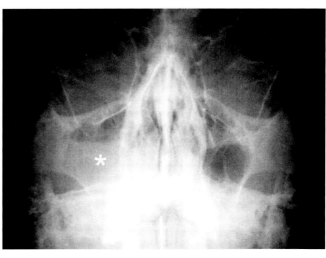

FIGURE 8B   Upright Waters view.
Right maxillary sinus air/fluid level (*asterisk*) confirms that opacification is due to blood in sinus and not overlying soft tissue swelling. The patient had an orbital floor fracture.

tures are more easily seen. Coronal images are needed to detect orbital floor fractures. MDCT is able to generate reformatted coronal sections directly from the axial image data set.

Three-Dimentional Images   Surface-rendered (shaded-surface display) or volumetric images provide easily interpreted views of fracture conformation and displacement. Surface-rendered images do not provide information about fracture extension below the surface, for which two-dimensional images are still needed (Figure 10).

FIGURE 9

A. Axial CT
— Slice orientation.

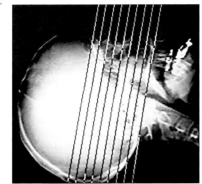

C. Coronal CT
—Slice orientation
with prone positioning.

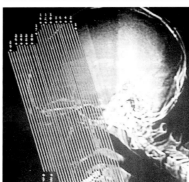

B. **Axial CT.**
Fractures of the right zygomatic arch (*arrow*) and anterior and lateral walls of the maxillary sinus (*arrowheads*).

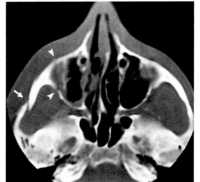

D. **Coronal CT.**
Right maxillary sinus air/fluid level (*asterisk*).

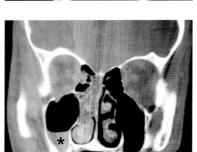

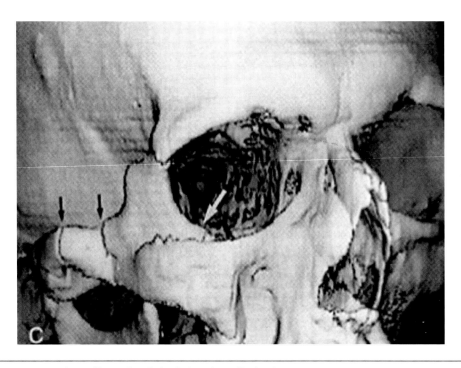

FIGURE 10   Three-dimensional shaded surface display image.
Fractures of the zygomatic arch and inferior orbital rim (*arrows*).
[Rhea JT: Helical CT and three-dimensional CT of facial and orbital injury. *Radiol Clin North Am* 1999;
37: 489–513, with permission.]

SUGGESTED READING

Flores C, Schwartz DT: Facial Radiology. In: Schwartz DT, Reisdorff EJ: *Emergency Radiology.* New York: McGraw-Hill, 2000.

Harris JH, Harris WH: *The Radiology of Emergency Medicine*, 4th ed. Williams and Wilkins, 2000:49–136.

Rogers LF: *Radiology of Skeletal Trauma,* 3rd ed. New York: Churchill Livingstone, 2002.

DelBalso AM: *Maxillofacial Imaging.* WB Saunders, 1990:35–127.

Pearl WS: Facial imaging in an urban emergency department. *Am J Emerg Med* 1999;17:235–237.

Rhea JT: Helical CT and three-dimensional CT of facial and orbital injury. *Radiol Clin North Am* 1999;37:489–513.

Sun JK, LeMay DR: Imaging of facial trauma. *Neuroimag Clin North Am* 2002;12:295–309.

Turner BG, Rhea JT, Thrall JH, Small AB, Novelline RA: Trends in the use of CT and radiography in the evaluation of facial trauma, 1992–2002: Implications for current costs. *AJR* 2004;183:751–754.

Rosenthal E, Quint DJ, Johns M, Peterson B, Hoeffner E: Diagnostic maxillofacial coronal images reformatted from helically acquired thin-section axial CT data. *AJR* 2000;175:1177–1181.

Reuben AD, Watt-Smith SR, Dobson D, Golding SJ: A comparative study of evaluation of radiographs, CT and 3D reformatted CT in facial trauma. *Br J Radiol* 2005;78:198–201.

Goh SH, Low BY: Radiologic screening for midfacial fractures: A single 30-degree occipitomental view is enough. *J Trauma* 2002;52: 688–692.

Pogrel MA, Podlesh SW, Goldman KE: Efficacy of a single occipitomental radiograph to screen for midfacial fractures. *J Oral Maxillofac Surg* 2000;58:24–26.

Altreuter RW: Facial form and function: Films versus physical examination. *Ann Emerg Med* 1986;15:240–244. Discusses when to order facial radiographs.

Facial Radiology: Patient 1

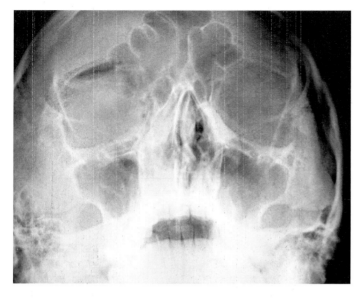

FIGURE 1A   Patient 1A—Waters view.

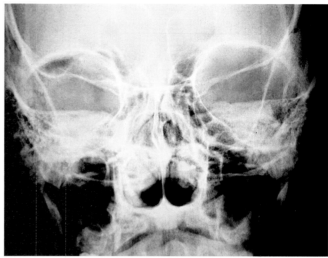

FIGURE 1B   Patient 1A—Caldwell view.

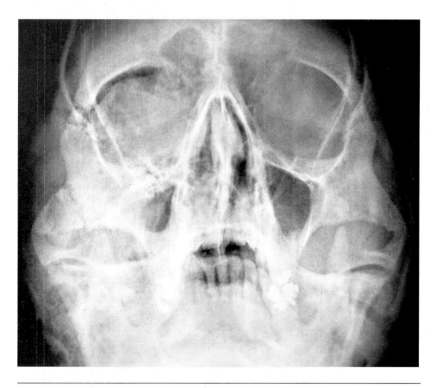

FIGURE 2   Patient 1B—Waters view.

Two patients with black eyes after being punched to the face

Two patients with "black eyes" sustained in altercations (one black eye each). In both patients, the globe was intact. Visual acuity and extra-ocular movements were normal.

• What are the radiographic findings in these patients? (Figures 1 and 2)

ORBITAL EMPHYSEMA

In both of these patients, air is seen within the orbit—orbital emphysema. It appears as a radiolucent (dark) area in the superior portion of the right orbit just below the superior orbital rim (Figures 1 and 2). This is caused by a fracture through one of the walls of the orbit into an adjacent air-filled sinus. The fracture is either through the orbital floor into the maxillary sinus, or the medial orbital wall (lamina papyracea) into the ethmoid air cells. Orbital emphysema is one of the findings of a "blowout" fracture, although it is not unique to that fracture.

A **"blow-out" fracture** occurs when the anterior orbit sustains an impact by an object of larger diameter than the orbit itself, e.g., a baseball or a fist. The blow causes increased intraorbital pressure fracturing its weakest part (the orbital floor or medial orbital wall) and not the globe itself (Figure 3). However, given this mechanism of injury, there is a high incidence of ocular injury (hyphema, vitreous hemorrhage, retinal detach-

ment). An alternative mechanism of injury is a blow to the inferior orbital rim that causes buckling and a fracture of the orbital floor.

Radiographic signs of a blow-out fracture include **soft tissue changes**, which are frequently more easily seen than the fracture itself (Table 1). These soft tissue signs include overlying soft tissue swelling, a maxillary sinus opacification or air/fluid level, and orbital emphysema.

Occasionally, the **orbital floor fracture** can be directly visualized. On the Waters view, when the projection is optimal, the *orbital floor* appears as a thin white line that appears disrupted or displaced if the actual fracture fragments are seen (Figure 4). The *inferior orbital rim* appears as a grayish line superior to the orbital floor and is intact in blowout fractures.

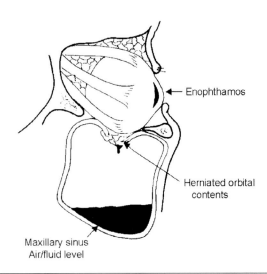

FIGURE 3   Blowout fracture of the orbital floor.

The fracture can cause entrapment of the inferior rectus muscle and injury to the infraorbital nerve.

[From Scaletta TA, Schaider JJ: *Emergent Management of Trauma*, McGraw-Hill, 1996, with permission.]

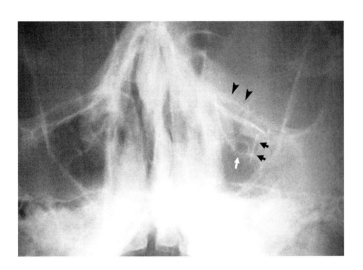

FIGURE 4   Orbital floor fracture.

In another patient, the bright line of a depressed (vertically oriented) orbital floor fragment is visible (*black arrows*).

The margin of the inferior orbital rim is a gray edge (*arrowheads*) projecting superior to the sharp line of the orbital floor. The foramen for the infraorbital nerve is seen near the orbital floor (*white arrow*).

TABLE 1

Radiographic Signs of a Blow-Out Fracture

Waters view

    Overlying soft tissue swelling (nonspecific, occurs with and without fractures)

    Orbital emphysema (especially medial orbital wall fractures)

    Maxillary sinus opacification or air/fluid level (upright Waters view)

    Herniation of orbital contents into the roof of maxillary sinus ("tear-drop" sign)

    Orbital floor (fine white line) is obliterated, widened, displaced downward (trap-door sign)

        or fragmented and seen as a bright white line within maxillary sinus;

        inferior orbital rim and lateral wall of maxillary sinus are intact

Caldwell view

    Fracture or obliteration of medial orbital wall (lamina papyracea)

    Opacification of ethmoid air cells (filled with blood)

Patient 1A

This patient has a **blow-out fracture.** The most obvious radiographic finding is orbital emphysema. On the **Caldwell view**, there is opacification of the ethmoid air cells (Figure 5). This is due to a medial orbital wall fracture, which occurs in 25–50% of blow-out fractures.

On the **Waters view,** there is a second white line paralleling the orbital floor, which is suspicious for a fracture (Figure 6, *black arrow*). However, there is no air/fluid level in the right maxillary sinus, which is usually present in orbital floor fractures. CT confirmed a slightly displaced orbital floor fracture (Figure 7).

The difficulties in directly visualizing an orbital fracture are illustrated on this patient's Waters view. The inferior orbital rim is seen as a grayish band located superiorly to the fine white line of the orbital floor. In this patient, there seems to be a radiolucent break in the inferior orbital rim on the right side (injured side) (Figure 6, *arrowhead*). However, the radiolucent shadow extends beyond the orbital rim. A similar gap is seen on the left (*arrow head*). This pseudofracture is caused by overlying soft tissues of the nose. A rounded gap in the inferior orbital rim is the foramen for the infraorbital nerve (*white arrows*).

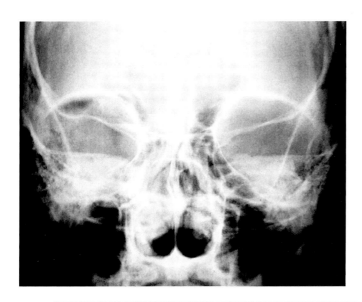
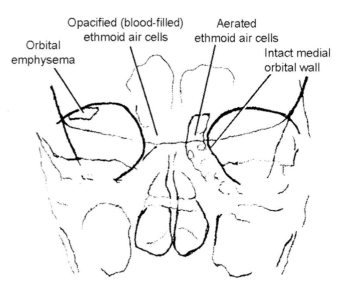

FIGURE 5   Caldwell view—Blow-out fracture—Patient 1A.

There is orbital emphysema and opacification of the ethmoid air cells on the right due to a medial orbital wall blow-out fracture. The fracture itself is not visible, although the medial orbital wall appears slightly widened compared to the normal left side.

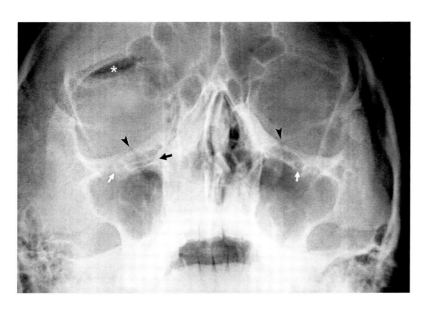

FIGURE 6   Waters view—Blow-out fracture—Patient 1A.

Orbital emphysema (*asterisk*) is a sign of an orbital wall fracture. The fracture is not clearly visible. A double line of the right orbital floor may be due to a depressed orbital floor fracture (*black arrow*).

A radiolucent line extending through each inferior orbital rim is due to the margin of overlying soft tissues and is not a fracture (*arrowheads*). The foramina for the infraorbital nerves perforate the inferior orbital rims (*white arrows*).

Management of Blow-Out Fractures

A blow-out fracture can be managed as an outpatient when there is no entrapment of the inferior rectus muscle (impeding upward gaze), enopthalmus, or ocular injury. The patient should be instructed not to blow his or her nose, which would introduce air, and possibly bacteria, from the sinuses into the orbit. Many authors recommend prophylactic antibiotics to reduce the risk of an orbital infection although its benefit is unproven.

Orbital emphysema is usually of little clinical consequence. However, when a ball-valve mechanism exists, air can become trapped within the orbit causing a progressive increase in intra-orbital pressure. Vision is impaired due to compression and vascular compromise of the optic nerve, an ophthalmologic emergency treated by lateral canthotomy (Jordan et al. 1988).

When the blow-out fracture has caused entrapment of the inferior rectus muscle, the need for and timing of surgical correction is controversial. Some surgeons feel the patient should have elective surgery only if entrapment does not resolve over 10 to 14 days after orbital edema has subsided. Others suggest surgery when more than 50% of the orbital floor is involved.

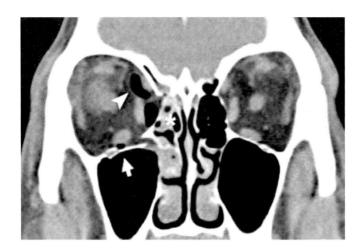 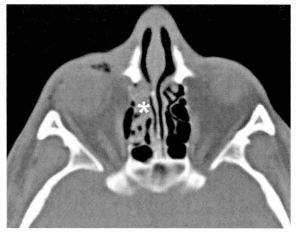

FIGURE 7   CT Blow-out fracture—Patient 1A.

(A) Coronal image shows a medial orbital wall fracture, opacification of the ethmoid air cells (*asterisk*), orbital emphysema (*arrowhead*), and a minimally displaced orbital floor fracture (*arrow*).

(B) Axial image shows opacification of the ethmoid air cells (*asterisk*) due to a medial orbital wall fracture.

Patient 1B

This patient also has orbital emphysema, but does not have a blow-out fracture. In addition to orbital emphysema and an air/fluid level in the maxillary sinus, there are fractures through the inferior orbital rim, zygomatic arch, and lateral orbital rim (often a fronto-zygomatic suture diastasis) (Figure 8A and B). These fractures can be identified on the Waters view by tracing **Dolan's lines,** which form the contours of an elephant's head in profile (Figure 8C).

This fracture of the **zygomaticomaxillary complex** (ZMC) is commonly known as a "**tripod fracture**" (Table 2 and Figure 9). The fourth component of a tripod fracture is a fracture through the lateral wall of the maxillary sinus (not seen on the Waters view in this patient). The anatomy of a tripod fracture is depicted by CT (axial and coronal images) (Figure 10).

A ZMC fracture (tripod fracture) is caused by a direct blow to the malar area ("cheek bone"). The fractures cross the supportive struts of the facial skeleton (see Introduction to Facial Radiology, Figure 1, page 523), and the malar bone is separated from the facial skeleton. Nondisplaced fractures can be managed nonoperatively, whereas displaced fractures require surgical reduction and fixation with mini-plates and screws (Figure 11).

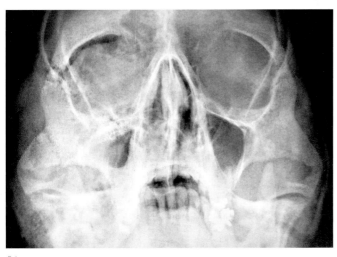

8A

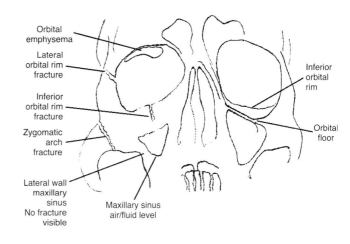

8B

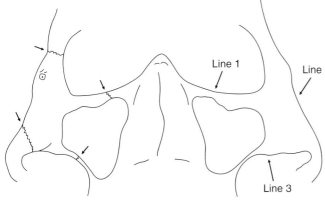

8C. Dolan's lines—Elephant's head in profile.

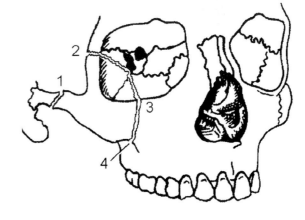

FIGURE 8   Waters view—Tripod fracture—Patient 1B.

Soft tissue signs of an injury include orbital emphysema and a maxillary sinus air/fluid level (*A* and *B*). Examination of the Waters view for fractures entails tracing **Dolan's lines** (*C*), which are normal on the left side of the face. On the right, there are fractures of the zygomatic arch, inferior orbital rim, and frontozygomatic suture diastasis.

FIGURE 9   Zygomatico-maxillary complex fracture —Tripod fracture.

1, Zygomatic arch fracture; 2, lateral orbital rim fracture; 3, inferior orbital rim fracture; 4, lateral wall of maxillary sinus fracture.

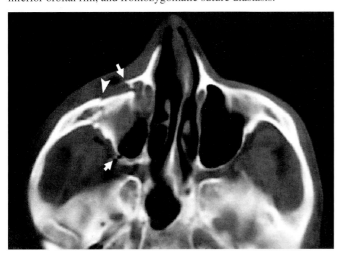

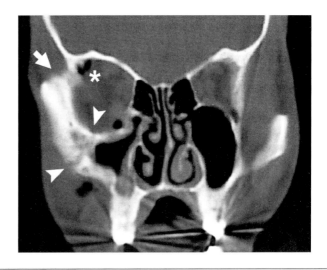

FIGURE 10   CT—Tripod fracture—Patient 1B.

(*A*)   Axial CT at level of zygomatic arch shows fractures through anterior portion of zygomatic arch (*arrowhead*), and the anterior and lateral walls of maxillary sinus (*arrows*).

(*B*)   Coronal CT shows fractures of orbital floor and lateral wall of maxillary sinus (*arrowheads*). There is no fracture evident of the lateral orbital rim in this image (*arrow*). Orbital emphysema is present (*asterisk*).

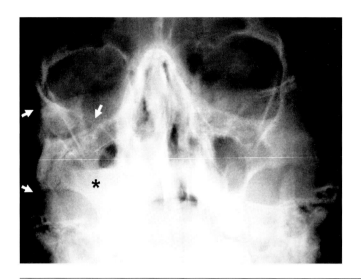 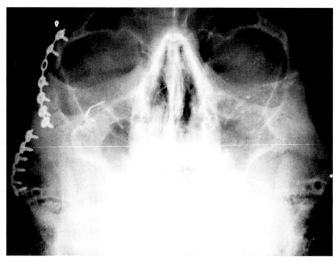

FIGURE 11   Markedly displaced tripod fracture.

(*A*) There are comminuted fractures of the lateral orbital rim, inferior orbital rim, and zygomatic arch (*arrows*). A maxillary sinus air/fluid level is present (*asterisk*).

(*B*) Postoperative view showing reduction and fixation with miniplates and screws.

TABLE 2

Radiographic Signs of a Tripod (ZMC) Fracture

Waters view—Examine Dolan's lines (elephant head in profile)

    Zygomatic arch fracture (single break—confirm on "bucket-handle" view)

    Frontozygomatic suture diastasis or lateral orbital rim fracture

    Inferior orbital rim and orbital floor fracture

    Lateral wall of maxillary sinus fracture

Soft tissue signs

    Maxillary sinus air/fluid level or opacification

    Orbital emphysema

SUGGESTED READING

Brady SM, McMann MA, Mazzoli RA, et al:. The diagnosis and management of orbital blowout fractures: Update 2001. *Am J Emerg Med* 2001;19:147–154.

Isenhour JL, Colucciello SA: Maxillofacial trauma. In: Ferrera PC, Colucciello SA, Marx JA, Verdile VP, Gibbs MA, eds. *Trauma Management: An Emergency Medicine Approach.* Mosby; 2001:185–186.

O'Hare TH: Blow-out fractures: A review. *J Emerg Med* 1991;9: 253–263.

Jordan DR, White GL, Anderson RL, Thiese SM: Orbital emphysema: A potentially blinding complication following orbital fractures. *Ann Emerg Med* 1988;17:853–855.

Sanerov B, Viccellio P: Fractures of the medial orbital wall. *Ann Emerg Med* 1988;17:973–976.

Rumboldt Z, Smith JK, Castillo M: Triple blowout fracture of the orbit. *Emerg Radiol* 2001;8:341–343.

Lee HJ, Jilani M, Frohman L, Baker S: CT of orbital trauma. *Emerg Radiol* 2004;10:168–172.

Facial Radiology: Patient 2

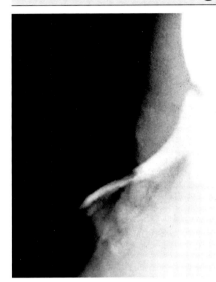

A. Right lateral nasal view.

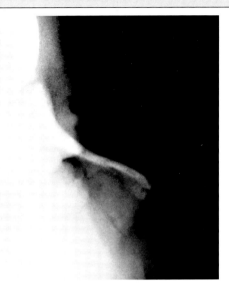

B. Left lateral nasal view.

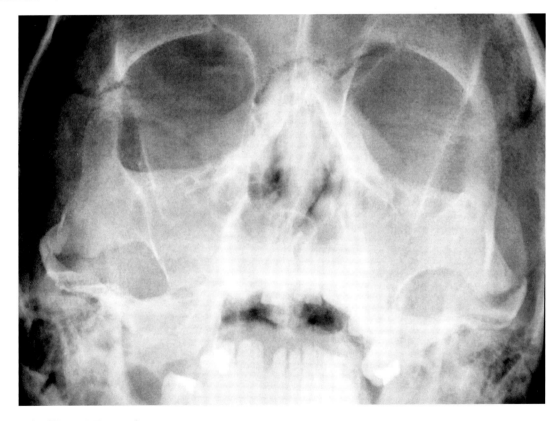

FIGURE 1 *C.* Waters view

A nasal laceration sustained by an elderly man who was in a car that stopped short

A 70-year-old man was the rear seat passenger in a taxi cab that suddenly stopped short. He was thrown forward and hit the bridge of his nose on the divider between the front and rear seats. He did not lose consciousness and had no other injuries.

In the ED, a 2-cm laceration across the bridge of his nose was cleaned and sutured. He was sent for nasal bone radiographs. The nasal series is shown in Figure 1.

- What injury is present?

NOT JUST A BROKEN NOSE

A nasal radiographic series consists of left and right lateral views of the nasal bones and a Waters view (Figure 1). Nasal radiographs are generally not needed in ED patients with nasal trauma because finding a nasal bone fracture does not alter initial management. Displaced nasal factures may need operative reduction, although this is not done at the time of injury because displacement is difficult to assess when there is overlying soft tissue swelling. In some instances, nasal trauma involves more extensive injury.

On Patient 2's nasal radiographs, a fracture is present, although it is superior to the nasal bones (Figure 1). On the Waters view, a fracture through the nasion is visible (Figure 2, *arrow*).

A nasion fracture may be a component of a **nasoethmoid orbital fracture** (NEO fracture). A NEO fracture is a comminuted fracture of the nasion extending into the adjacent portions of the frontal bone, maxilla and orbits (Figure 3). The mechanism of injury is a direct blow to this region, as was sustained by this patient.

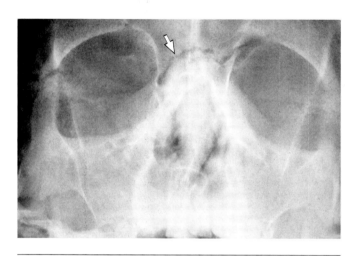

FIGURE 2   Patient 2—Waters view.
Nasion fracture (*arrow*).

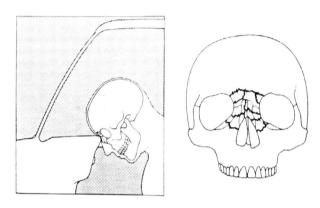

FIGURE 3   Nasoethmoid orbital fracture—NEO fracture.

[From DelBalso AM: *Maxillofacial Imaging.* WB Saunders, 1990, with permission.]

Further examination of the **Waters view** discloses several additional injuries (Figure 4).

First, looking for soft tissue signs of an injury reveals opacification of both maxillary sinuses (*asterisks*). **Second**, tracing the key midface skeletal contours (Dolan's lines) reveals, on the right, a fracture of the lateral orbital rim (*arrow*) and, on the left, a fracture of the zygomatic arch (*arrowhead*).

These findings are associated with tripod fractures. However, interpreting these injuries as "bilateral tripod fractures" would be incorrect. Bilateral midface fractures are the hallmark of a complex of fractures that were first described by René Le Fort in 1901. He experimentally produced these injuries in cadavers.

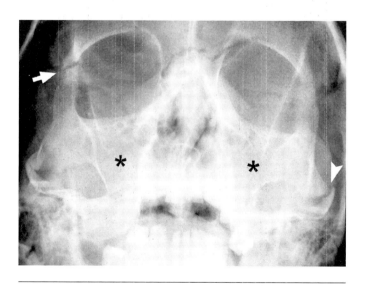

FIGURE 4   Waters view—Patient 2
(See text for explanation)

Le Fort described three types of bilateral midface fractures (Figure 5). The fractures traverse the supportive struts of the facial skeleton (Introduction to Facial Radiology, Figure 1, page 523).

Le Fort 3 extends from the nasion through the lateral orbital rims and zygomatic arches. It is also known as *craniofacial separation*. **Le Fort 2** extends from the nasion through the inferior orbital rims and lateral walls of the maxillary sinuses. Owing to its shape, it is also called a *pyramidal fracture*. **Le Fort 1** does not involve the nasion, but crosses horizontally through the maxillary sinuses just superior to the hard palate. Le Fort injuries often occur in combination, particularly Le Fort 2 and 3 (Table 1).

All three Le Fort fractures extend through to the posterior vertical supportive struts of the facial skeleton—the **pterygoid plates** (Figure 6). This fracture is seen on the lateral view (Figure 7). Indeed, prior to the widespread use of CT for facial fractures, detecting a pterygoid plate fracture was the principal role of the lateral facial view.

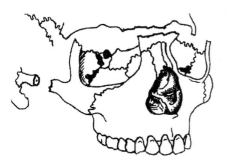 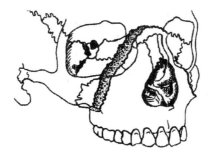 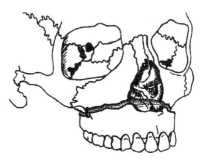

Le Fort 3 – Cranio-facial separation   Le Fort 2 – Pyramidal fracture   Le Fort 1

FIGURE 5   Le Fort fractures.

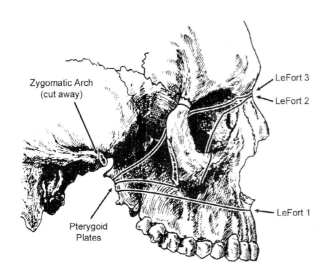

FIGURE 6   Lateral view of Le Fort fractures.
All three types extend through the pterygoid plates.
[Modified from Pansky, *Review of Gross Anatomy*, 6th ed., McGraw. Hill, 1996.]

TABLE 1

Radiographic Signs of Le Fort Fractures

Bilateral midface fractures crossing the facial struts

Waters view:

Bilateral maxillary sinus air/fluid levels or opacification

Le Fort 3

Nasion
Lateral orbital rim
Zygomatic arch

Le Fort 2

Nasion
Inferior orbital rim and orbital floor
Lateral wall of maxillary sinus

Le Fort 1

Nasal septum
Medial walls of maxillary sinus
Lateral walls of maxillary sinus

Lateral view:

Pterygoid plate fractures

Patient Outcome

This patient's Waters view showed a Le Fort 3 injury. By the time the patient returned from the radiology department, he had bilateral periorbital ecchymosis, and the severity of his injury was more evident.

A common impression of Le Fort fractures is that the patient has extensive facial swelling and deformity (i.e., facial flattening known as a "pancake facies"). However, the clinical presentation can be more subtle, as in this patient. All patients with facial trauma should therefore be examined for mobility of the maxilla, the hallmark of a Le Fort injury. The upper teeth are grasped and gently tested for abnormal mobility. The examiner's second hand stabilizes the patient's face and palpates for motion along the lines of Le Fort injures. When this patient was reexamined, mobility of the maxilla was noted.

The patient was admitted to the hospital. A complete facial radiographic series confirmed the fractures seen on the Waters view. The lateral view disclosed characteristic pterygoid plate fractures (Figure 7). Preoperative CT demonstrated combined Le Fort 3 and 2 injuries (Figure 8). The patient was treated with mini-plate and screw fixation (Figure 9).

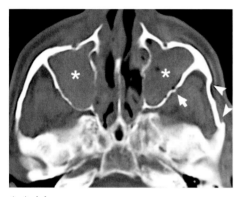 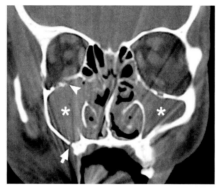 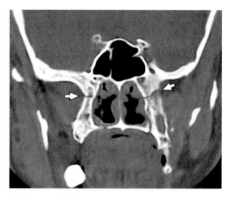

A. Axial   *B.* Coronal CT   *C.* Coronal CT

FIGURE 8   CT showing bilateral maxillary sinus opacification (*asterisks* in *A* and *B*), left zygomatic arch fractures (*arrowheads* in *A*), fracture of the lateral wall of the maxillary sinus (*arrow* in *A* and *B*), orbital floor fracture (*arrowhead* in *B*), and pterygoid plate fractures on the posterior coronal image (*arrows* in *C*).

Fractures of the zygomatic arch and lateral orbital rim are characteristic of Le Fort 3 injuries.

Fractures of the orbital floor and lateral wall of the maxillary sinus are characteristic of Le Fort 2 injuries.

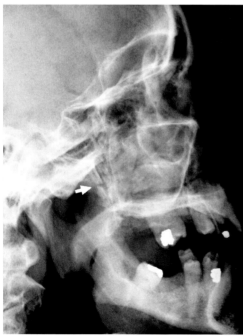

FIGURE 7   Lateral view.
Pterygoid plate fracture (*arrow*).

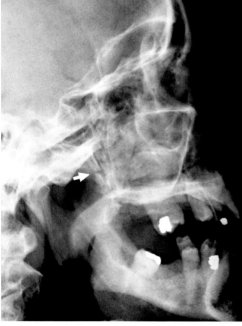

FIGURE 9   Postoperative radiograph.
Fixation with mini-plates and screws.

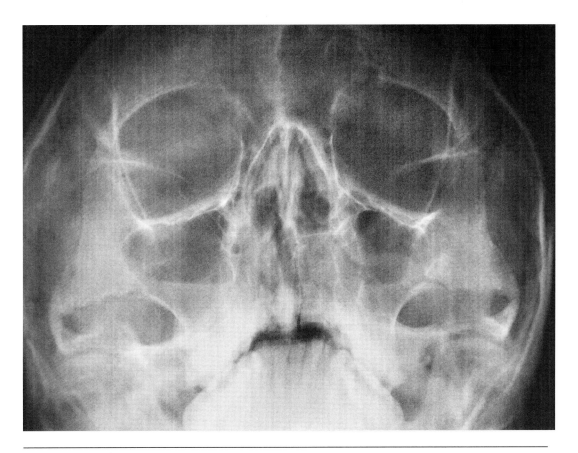

FIGURE 10 Patient 2B

Patient 2B A 39-year-old taxi driver ran into another car that had stopped short in front of him. His face hit the steering wheel. There was a bruise in the region of his upper lip and slight mobility of his maxilla.

• What injuries are present on the Waters view? (Figure 10)

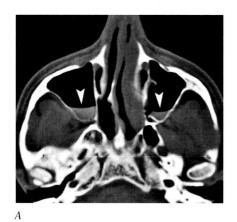
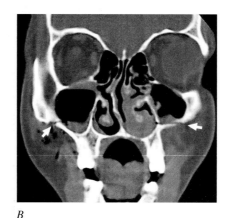
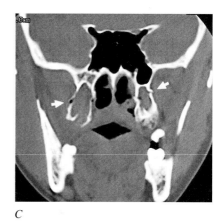

A　　　　　　*B*　　　　　　*C*

FIGURE 12　Patient 2B　CT – Le Fort 1.

(*A*) Axial CT showing bilateral maxillary sinus air/fluid levels (*arrowheads*).

(*B*) Coronal CT showing bilateral maxillary sinus air/fluid levels and fractures of the lateral walls of the maxillary sinuses (*arrows*). The fracture involves the medial wall of the maxillary sinus (lateral wall of the nasal fossa), a feature unique to Le Fort 1 fractures.

(*C*) On a posterior coronal image, bilateral pterygoid plate fractures are seen (*arrows*).

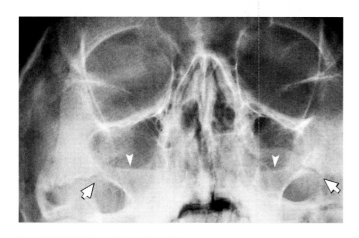

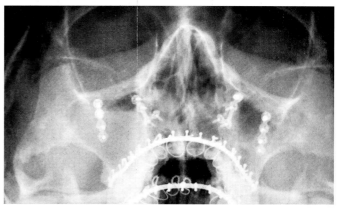

FIGURE 11　Patient 2B　Waters view – Le Fort 1.

Bilateral maxillary sinus air/fluid levels (*arrowheads*) and fractures of the lateral walls of the maxillary sinuses (*arrows*) (see Figure 5C).

FIGURE 13　Postoperative Waters view.

Fixation with mini-plates and screws. Additional stabilization is provided by maxillary and mandibular arch bars.

SUGGESTED READING

Rhea JT, Novelline RA: How to simplify the CT diagnosis of Le Fort fractures. *AJR* 2005;184:1700–1705.

INDEX

INDEX

Page numbers followed by *f* indicate figures; page numbers followed by *t* indicate tables.
Main chapter topics are boldface